Gastrointestinal Imaging Handbook

Gastrointestinal Imaging Handbook

Edited by Hudson Powell

hayle medical
New York

Hayle Medical,
750 Third Avenue, 9th Floor,
New York, NY 10017, USA

Visit us on the World Wide Web at:
www.haylemedical.com

ISBN: 978-1-63241-846-3

Cataloging-in-Publication Data

Gastrointestinal imaging handbook / edited by Hudson Powell.
p. cm.
Includes bibliographical references and index.
ISBN 978-1-63241-846-3
1. Gastrointestinal system--Radiography. 2. Diagnostic imaging.
3. Gastrointestinal system--Diseases--Diagnosis. I. Powell, Hudson.
RC804.R6 G37 2020
616.330 757 2--dc21

Table of Contents

Preface

Gastrointestinal imaging comprises of the techniques used for the imaging of the appendix and small bowel, liver and pancreas in the upper abdomen, and the colon and rectum. There has been immense progress in gastrointestinal imaging over the past decades, especially with advances in cross-sectional imaging such as magnetic resonance imaging and computed tomography. This has played an increasingly important role in the evaluation of gastrointestinal disorders. Further, advances in endoscopic techniques, especially the development of capsule endoscopy have enabled the direct mucosal visualization of the gastrointestinal tract. Cross-sectional imaging techniques allow the thickness of the gastric and bowel wall to be displayed, the deep pelvis ileal loops to be visualized without superimposition, and the mesentery and perienteric fat to be evaluated. This book is compiled in such a manner, that it will provide in-depth knowledge about the theory and practice of the use of gastrointestinal imaging in medical science. The aim of this book is to present researches that have transformed this discipline and aided its advancement. With state-of-the-art inputs by acclaimed experts of this field, this book targets students and professionals.

Significant researches are present in this book. Intensive efforts have been employed by authors to make this book an outstanding discourse. This book contains the enlightening chapters which have been written on the basis of significant researches done by the experts.

Finally, I would also like to thank all the members involved in this book for being a team and meeting all the deadlines for the submission of their respective works. I would also like to thank my friends and family for being supportive in my efforts.

Editor

Preface

1

Non-Enhanced T1-Weighted Liver Vessel Imaging at 7 Tesla

Anja Fischer[1,2*], Oliver Kraff[2], Stefan Maderwald[2], Karsten Beiderwellen[1,2], Mark E. Ladd[1,2,3], Michael Forsting[1], Thomas C. Lauenstein[1], Lale Umutlu[1,2]

1 Department of Diagnostic and Interventional Radiology and Neuroradiology, University Hospital Essen, Essen, Germany, **2** Erwin L. Hahn Institute for Magnetic Resonance Imaging, University Duisburg-Essen, Essen, Germany, **3** German Cancer Research Center (DKFZ), Heidelberg, Germany

Abstract

Objectives: Aim of the study was to assess the feasibility and to compare three non-enhanced T1-weighted (w) sequences for liver vessel imaging at 7 Tesla (T).

Material and Methods: 12 healthy volunteers were examined on a 7 T whole-body MR-system. The following non-enhanced sequences were acquired: T1w 2D FLASH, T1w 3D FLASH and Time of flight (TOF)-MRA. Qualitative image analysis was performed by two radiologists including over all image quality as well as vessel delineation of the liver arteries, liver veins and portal vein and the presence of artifacts using a five-point scale (5 = excellent vessel delineation to 1 = non-diagnostic). Contrast ratios (CR), SNR und CNR of the above named vessels in correlation to adjacent liver tissue were calculated for quantitative assessment. For statistical analysis, a Wilcoxon Rank Test was applied.

Results: All three sequences provided a homogenous hyperintense delineation of the assessed liver vessels. Qualitative image analysis demonstrated the superiority of TOF-MRA, providing best overall image quality (TOF 4.17, 2D FLASH 3.42, 3D FLASH 3.46; $p<0.01$) as well as highest image quality values for all analyzed liver vessel segments. TOF-MRA was least impaired by B_1 inhomogeneity (4.13) and susceptibility artifacts (4.63) out of all three sequences ($p<0.01$). Quantitative image analysis confirmed the superiority of TOF MRA showing significant higher CR values for all liver vessels (e.g. right hepatic artery TOF 0.47, 2D FLASH 0.09, 3D FLASH 0.11 with $p=0.02$ and 0.01, respectively). Providing the lowest standard deviation in noise, TOF showed highest values for SNR and CNR.

Conclusions: Non-enhanced T1w imaging in general and TOF MRA in particular, appear to be promising techniques for high quality non-enhanced liver vessel assessment at 7 T.

Editor: Jeroen Hendrikse, University Medical Center (UMC) Utrecht, Netherlands

Funding: The authors have no support or funding to report.

Competing Interests: The authors have declared that no competing interests exist.

* E-mail: anja.fischer@uk-essen.de

Introduction

Over the last decades, contrast-enhanced (ce) CT angiography and MR angiography (MRA) have been established as the imaging techniques of choice to assess liver vessel anatomy prior to hepatectomy or liver transplantation [1,2]. As CT angiography deploys ionizing radiation and the application of contrast agent in general bears the potential of side effects and is restricted in case of renal insufficiency [3], the focus of scientific research has shifted towards non-enhanced MRA techniques within the last few years. Several studies at lower field strength (1.5 Tesla) have demonstrated the diagnostic potential of non-contrast-enhanced liver vessel imaging, utilizing true steady-state free-precession sequences and time-spatial labeling inversion pulses. Shimada et al. reported initial results of 3D true SSFP imaging utilizing a spatial labeling inversion pulse to visualize hepatic arterial and venous vasculature, selectively achieving high arterial and venous vessel contrast and good suppression of the portal veins and surrounding static tissue [4–6].

In clinical routine, the standard magnetic field strength for imaging of hepatic vessels lies in 1.5 T MRI. The increase of the magnetic field strength to 3 T has been proven beneficial in terms of achieving higher spatiotemporal resolution, as well as enabling comparable or improved delineation of vessel structures [7]. With recent development in multi-channel transmit/receive RF (radiofrequency) body coil technology, the feasibility of ultra-high field imaging (7 T) of abdominal organs and vessel structures could be demonstrated [8–10]. A successful transformation of the increased signal-to-noise ratio into imaging at high spatiotemporal resolution could be observed, displaying highly defined anatomical details of parenchymatous organs and arterial vasculature [11,12]. Nevertheless, MR imaging at higher field strength also entails challenges, dealing with limitations based on increasing signal heterogeneities due to RF wavelength effects and restrictions due to increasing SAR (specific absorption rate) [13–15]. With SSFP and T2 TSE imaging being restricted at ultra-high-field strength, most studies on 7 Tesla non-enhanced MRA have focused on T1-weighted imaging, utilizing the inherently hyperintense vessel signal at 7 T.

Thus, non-enhanced MRA at 7 T has been successfully demonstrated for imaging of the intracranial and renal vasculature as well as vessels of the lower extremities [16–19].

The aim of this study was to investigate the feasibility of non-enhanced MR imaging of the arterial, venous and portal liver vessels comparing three T1w sequences at 7 Tesla.

Materials and Methods

Study Population

12 healthy volunteers were enrolled in this trial, including seven female and five male subjects. The average age was 31.2 years with a range of 23 to 44 years. The study was conducted in conformance with the Declaration of Helsinki and approved by the Ethics Commission of the Medical Faculty of the University Duisburg-Essen (study number 11-4898-BO). Written informed consent was obtained from each volunteer before the examination. After leaving the examination room all subjects were consulted about possible side effects.

Scanner and Coil System

Examinations were performed on a 7 Tesla whole-body MR system (Magnetom 7T, Siemens Healthcare Sector, Erlangen, Germany) in supine position. For image acquisition a custom-built eight channel body transmit/receive RF coil was utilized [20]. The body coil consisted of two arrays with four elements each placed ventral and dorsal on the upper abdomen. The field of view (FOV) was centered on the liver. In this region, manual adjustments, in particular B_0 shimming was performed utilizing a shim volume adapted to the region of interest. As MRI at higher field strength is known to be susceptible to transmit B_1 field inhomogeneities due to the reduced Larmor wavelength [21], static shimming of the eight individual transmit phases of the RF coil was performed to mitigate potential limitations and to achieve a more homogeneous excitation of the upper abdomen [22]. A phase increment of 90 degrees and equal amplitudes between neighboring elements (circularly polarized mode CP^{2+}) was found to be most compatible for this study in terms of image quality as it constrained the signal voids to a periaortal focus as shown in Figure 1. Here, flip angle maps obtained in transversal orientation with the Bloch-Siegert-Shift B1 mapping technique [23,24] demonstrate advantages of the CP^{2+} mode for the study objective in comparison to the CP^{+} mode. Furthermore, predefined phase settings allow an improved workflow as input power limits can be calculated prior to the study for the SAR supervision. For compliance with the International Electrotechnical Commission (IEC) guidelines [25], SAR calculations were performed in human adult male and female body models of the Virtual Family (CST Microwave Studio, Darmstadt, Germany) [26] prior to the study, resulting in a maximum permitted input power level of 24 W for which the localized 10 g-averaged SAR complies with the limit of 10 W/kg for both human body models used in the simulations. Given is the total RF power at the coil plug, which was equally split to all eight coil elements.

Sequence Protocol

With the increase of the magnetic field strength, sequence parameters need adjustments and modifications to provide best possible image quality while providing a good workflow for the whole imaging protocol and obeying RF power constraints. Therefore imaging parameters (e.g. repetition time (TR), echo time (TE), flip angle (α) and bandwidth) were adapted and modified to 7 Tesla in an exclusive group of three healthy volunteers prior to the start of the study. The examination protocol consisted of the following sequences:

1. T1w spoiled gradient-echo sequence (2D FLASH) in transversal orientation.
2. T1w spoiled gradient-echo sequence (3D FLASH) in transversal orientation.
3. T1w 2D FLASH Time-of-Flight (TOF) MRA in transversal orientation.

Aim of the optimization process was to achieve high contrast between vasculature and parenchyma at a high spatial resolution for the delineation of the vessels. However, nominal flip angles and transmit reference voltages in the sequences were set to allow continuous scanning without waiting times between individual scans to allow the subjects to cool down in case SAR limits would have been reached within the 6-minute averaging time-window requested by the safety guidelines. Achieving an acquisition time within breath-hold conditions for the rather high flip angle TOF sequence was found difficult. Best results regarding image quality and workflow were obtained by using a lower spatial resolution compared to FLASH acquisitions. However, to compensate for the reduced matrix the FOV of the TOF sequence was reduced to a minimum for whole-liver coverage. The above mentioned SAR limitations in the TOF sequence were also the rationale for including the other two gradient echo sequences in this study. Prior publications have demonstrated the feasibility of non-contrast enhanced MRA of those standard gradient echo sequences for intracranial or renal vessel imaging at 7 T [12,27]. Furthermore, it has to be mentioned, that 2D and 3D FLASH imaging were acquired at a higher spatial and temporal resolution which might be beneficial for a high quality vessel delineation and for clinical applicability providing a faster image acquisition. Imaging parameters of the above named sequences are summarized in Table 1. The total examination time was registered using a stop watch.

Data Analysis

All images were analyzed separately and blinded by two radiologists with 8 and 3 years experience in abdominal MRI on a standard Picture Archiving and Communication System (PACS) workstation (Centricity RIS 4.0i, GE Healthcare, USA). Qualitative image analysis was performed in the transversal source images for following vessel segments:

(1) *arterial*

a. proper hepatic artery (PHA)
b. 2nd order branch of the right hepatic artery in liver segment 5 (RHA)

(2) *portal venous*

a. main portal vein (PV)
b. 1st order branch of the right portal vein (RPV)

(3) *venous*

a. inferior vena cava (IVC)
b. middle hepatic vein (MHV).

Visual qualitative image analysis was carried out with regard to vessel delineation using a five-point scale (5 = excellent image quality with sharply defined vessels, 4 = good vessel delineation, 3 = moderate vessel delineation, 2 = poor vessel delineation, 1 = not visible or non-diagnostic) as well as overall image quality for each sequence. Additionally presence of artefacts was assessed

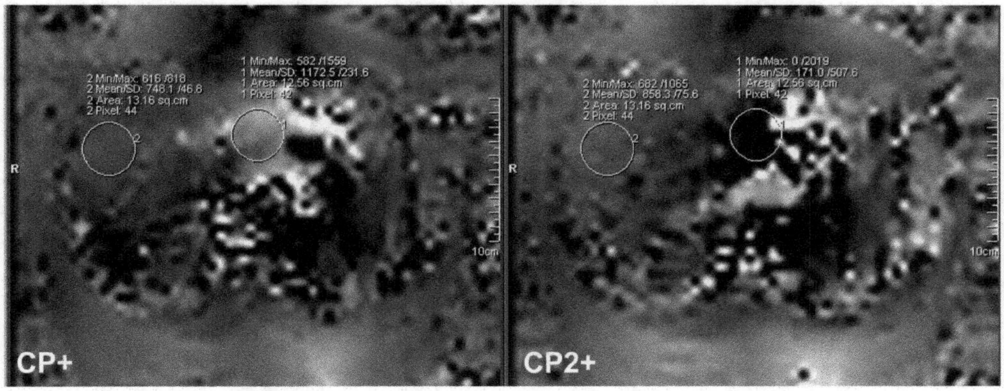

Figure 1. Flip angle maps obtained in two standard excitation modes in transversal orientation of the upper abdomen. Improved excitation of the liver is given with the CP^{2+} mode compared to the CP^{+} mode both in terms of general coverage, particularly of the right liver lobe as well as regarding mean reached flip angle. In the images, ROIs are displayed ventral of the aorta (ROI1) and within liver tissue of the right liver lobe (ROI2) yielding flip angle values encoded by a factor of 10.

for each sequence using five categories: 1 = massive impairment, non-diagnostic, 2 = strong impairment, 3 = moderate impairment, 4 = slight impairment or insignificant, 5 = no artifact present. The following artefacts were evaluated: (1) B_1 inhomogeneity, (2) inflow effects, (3) motion artefacts, (4) susceptibility artefact and (5) overall image impairment.

For quantitative image evaluation, contrast ratios ($CR = [S_{vessel} - S_{liver}] / [S_{vessel} + S_{liver}]$) of the above named vessel segments were assessed by placing ROIs (regions of interest) of identical size in the according vessel lumen and neighboring liver tissue.

Measurements of signal-to-noise and contrast-to-noise ratio (SNR, CNR) were performed for all vessel segments: $[SNR_{vessel} = Signal_{vessel}/noise]$, $[SNR_{liver} = Signal_{liver}/noise]$, $[CNR = SNR_{vessel} - SNR_{liver}]$. To accommodate for inhomogeneous noise due to the use of parallel imaging[28], it was measured by placing two maximum size ROIs out of the body and to use the mean value of the standard deviation of each noise value.

For statistical analysis, a Wilcoxon Rank Test was applied (Software: IBM SPSS Statistics 21). Score values for image quality and presence of artifacts were compared for each sequence. A p-value<0.05 was considered to establish statistically significant differences. In addition, interobserver reliability was calculated using the method of Landis et al. [29].

Results

All MR examinations at 7 T were successfully performed and well tolerated by the subjects without any side effects. The examination time amounted to 16 min (+/−2 min) including positioning, manual adjustments and data acquisition of the non-enhanced sequences.

Qualitative image analysis showed the superiority of TOF MRA, which provided best overall image quality (4.17 ± 0.38) as well as highest image quality values for all analyzed liver vessel segments and was least impaired by artifacts (overall artifacts 4.08 ± 0.28) (Fig. 2). 2D FLASH and 3D FLASH images revealed similar values, in terms of moderate to good overall image quality ratings (2D FLASH 3.42 ± 0.58, 3D FLASH 3.46 ± 0.51) and a low to moderate presence of artifacts (overall 2D FLASH 3.50 ± 0.51, 3D FLASH 3.46 ± 0.51). Nevertheless among the two sequences, 2D FLASH MRI yielded superior conspicuity of all assessed liver

Table 1. Sequence parameters.

	2D FLASH	3D FLASH	TOF
Repetition time TR [ms]	193	3.2	17
Echo time TE [ms]	3.57	1.36	4.7
Nominal Flip angle FA [°]	70	10	60
Bandwidth [Hz/pixel]	410	930	230
Slice orientation	transversal	transversal	transversal
Slices	42	104	20
Slice thickness [mm]	5	2	2.5
Field-of-view FOV [mm^2]	350	350	230
Acquisition matrix [pixel]	448×448	448×448	256×128
Parallel imaging with GRAPPA	Yes (R = 2)	Yes (R = 2)	Yes (R = 2)
Reference lines	48	48	48
Acquisition time TA [min:s]	0:52 (breathhold with 2 concatenations)	0:24	0:33 (breathhold with 5 concatenations)

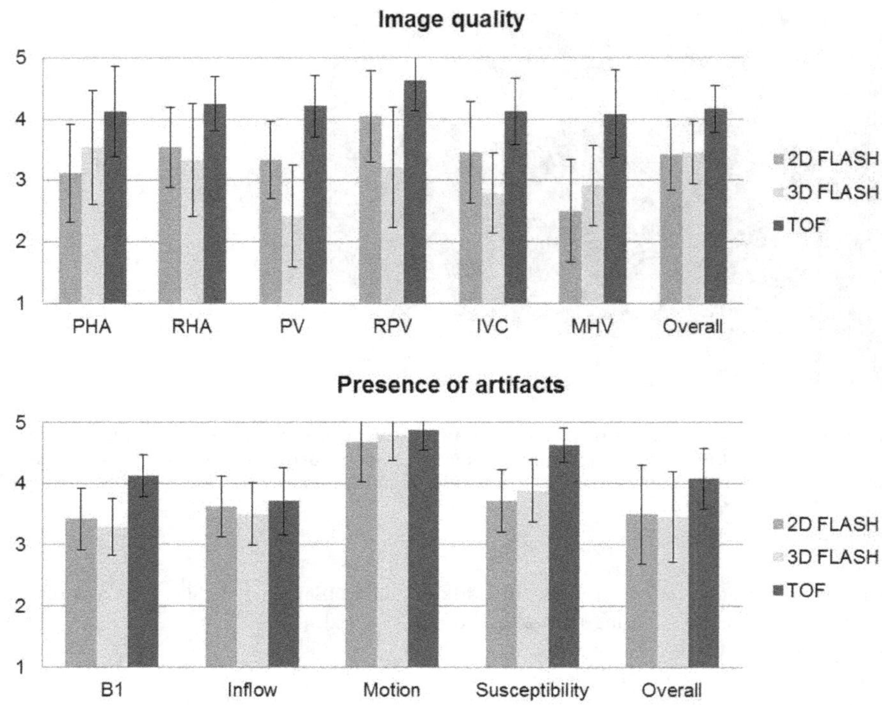

Figure 2. Qualitative analysis of image quality and presence of artifacts (5-point scales) for all analyzed liver vessel segments in all three sequences. (PHA = proper hepatic artery, RHA = 2nd order branch of right hepatic artery, PV = main portal vein, RPV = 1st order branch of right portal vein, IVC = inferior vena cava, MHV = middle hepatic vein).

vessels despite the common hepatic artery and the middle hepatic vein.

Quantitative image analysis confirmed the results of the qualitative image evaluation, in terms of superiority of the TOF sequence. TOF MRA showed highest CR values for the right portal vein (0.59±0.08), closely followed by the inferior vena cava and the middle hepatic vein (0.53±0.09, 0.50±0.08, respectively). In contrast, 2D and 3D FLASH imaging, achieved a considerably lower vessel contrast for all analyzed segments with values ranging from 0.07±0.05 (IVC at 3D FLASH) to 0.23±0.07 (RPV at 2D FLASH). TOF MRA provided comparable superiority for SNR and CNR measurements, yielding highest scores for SNR and CNR in all vessel segments (highest SNR and CNR for RPV: TOF SNR 129.73±33.98 and CNR 96.94±28.74, 2D FLASH SNR 97.75±23.33 and CNR 36.39±12.22, 3D FLASH SNR 60.44±16.88 and CNR 14.28±9.33). Mean scores for the qualitative analysis and the presence of artifacts are displayed in Figure 2. Figure 3 shows the mean CR, SNR and CNR values for all sequences. Detailed results for each sequence are described below.

T1w Spoiled Gradient-echo Sequence (2D FLASH)

Qualitative analysis of 2D FLASH imaging demonstrated a moderate delineation of the hepatic arteries (PHA 3.13±0.80, RHA 3.54±0.66) and veins (IVC 3.46±0.83, MHV 2.50±0.83). The sequence was moderately impaired by B_1 (3.42±0.50) and inflow (3.63±0.49) artifacts, mainly located in the periaortal region (Fig. 4). Signal loss due to susceptibility and motion artifacts caused only a slight disturbance of vessel delineation (mean values 3.71±0.81, 4.67±0.64, respectively).

Regarding quantitative evaluation, 2D FLASH imaging provided CR values ranging from 0.09 (RHA±0.07) to 0.23 (RPV±0.07), which were significantly lower compared to TOF imaging (RHA $p = 0.02$, RPV $p = 0.02$), yet marginally higher than for 3D FLASH MRI.

Assessment of interobserver reliability revealed a moderate agreement with a mean kappa value of 0.51 for qualitative analysis of all liver vessels. Regarding the presence of artifacts, a slightly higher strength of agreement was detected (mean 0.58).

T1w Spoiled Gradient-echo Sequence (3D FLASH)

Out of all three sequences, 3D FLASH MRI was the sequence to provide poorest vessel delineation, particularly for assessment of the main portal vein (2.42±0.83), inferior vena cava (2.79±0.66) and the middle hepatic vein (2.92±0.65) with statistically significant difference to TOF MRA (p-values ranging from to 0.00 to 0.012). Similar to 2D FLASH imaging, there was a moderate impairment caused by B_1 (3.29±0.46) and inflow artifacts (3.50±0.51) as well as a minor presence of susceptibility artifacts (3.88±0.74).

Quantitative analysis confirmed the predominantly moderate to poor vessel delineation at 3D FLASH imaging: CR values ranged from 0.07 (IVC±0.05) to 0.20 (MHV±0.10), being significantly lower compared to TOF imaging (IVC $p = 0.02$, MHV $p = 0.02$).

The interobserver agreement was rated moderate (mean 0.44) for vessel delineation and substantial (mean 0.63) for the presence of artifacts.

T1w Time-Of-Flight Sequence (TOF-MRA)

Analysis of all liver vessel segments demonstrated a significant superiority for TOF imaging, providing a homogeneous hyperintense delineation of all liver vessels (Fig. 5). Mean values of all assessed vessel segments were similar, ranging from 4.13±0.74 for assessment of the common hepatic artery to 4.13±0.54 for the inferior vena cava and 4.21±0.51 for the main portal vein. The right portal vein was the vessel segment to be best delineated with

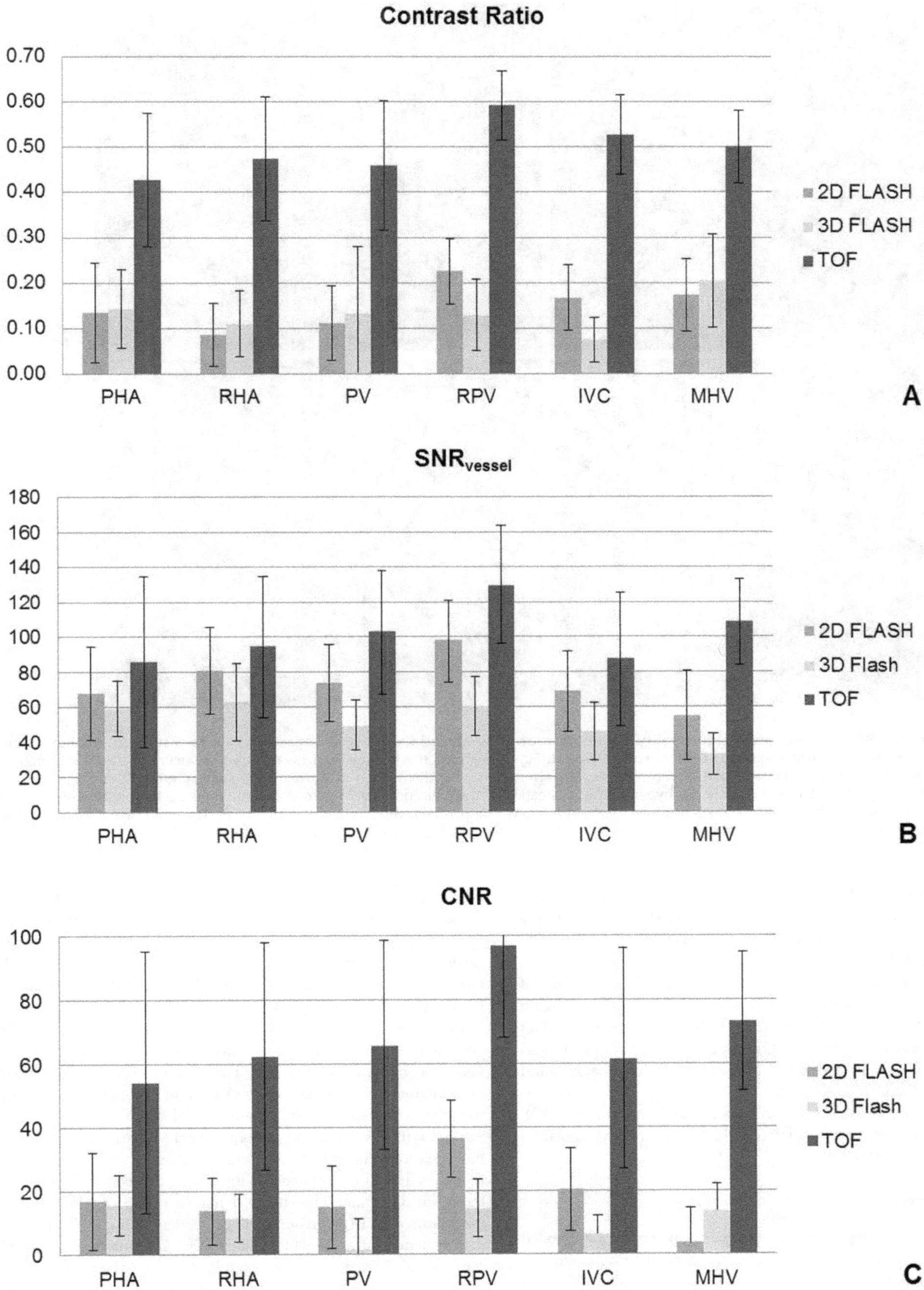

Figure 3. Quantitative analysis (A: Contrast ratios, B: SNR_{vessel}, C: CNR) for all analyzed liver vessel segments in all three sequences.

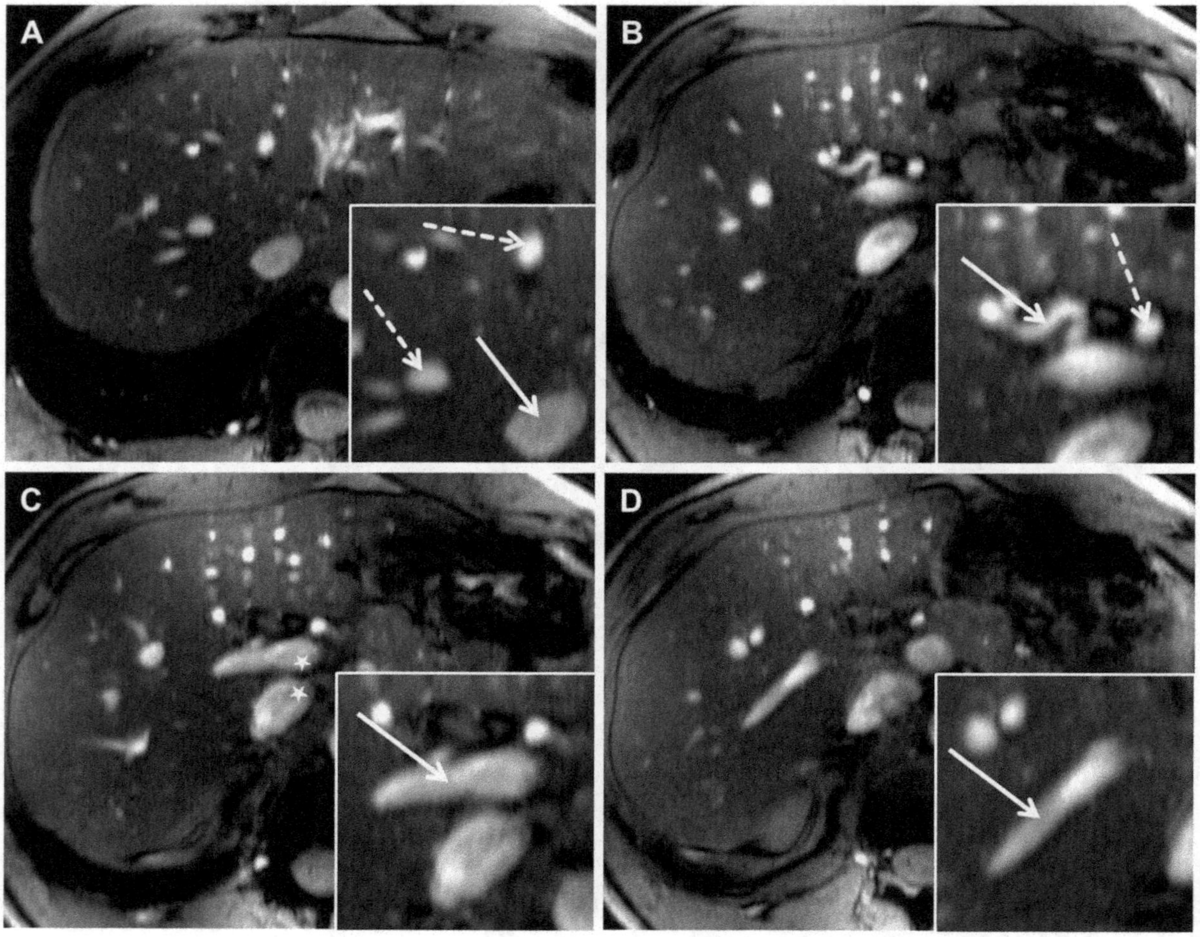

Figure 4. TOF MRA demonstrated high quality delineation of all analyzed liver vessel segments due to a hyperintensive vessel signal and an effective suppression of background signal. Figure A shows the inferior vena cava (arrow) as well as the right and middle hepatic veins (dashed arrow). A major part of the right hepatic artery (arrow) and a section of the common hepatic artery (dashed arrow) are visualized in Figure B. Figure C and D show the hyperintense delineation of the main portal vein (arrow) and the right portal vein (arrow). A slight intraluminal signal inhomogeneity could be depicted in the main portal vein and inferior vena cava (Figure C, star). Furthermore, signal drop outs due to susceptibility are visible in the stomach in the left ventral abdomen, but do not hamper vessel visualization (Figure B–D).

mean score values of 4.63±0.49. Furthermore, this sequence was least impaired by B_1 inhomogeneity (4.13±0.34) and susceptibility artifacts (4.63±0.49) out of all three sequences (p-value<0.01, respectively) (Fig. 6).

Quantitative analysis confirmed the high quality assessment of the arterial and venous liver vasculature with CR values ranging from 0.43±0.15 (PHA) to 0.59±0.08 (RPV). These CR values were considerably higher in TOF imaging compared to 2D and 3D FLASH imaging (p = 0.02) due to an effective background saturation of liver tissue signal.

Interobserver reliability was calculated moderate for the TOF sequence yielding mean values of 0.45 (image quality) and 0.40 (presence of artifacts).

Discussion

Noninvasive imaging techniques such as contrast-enhanced computed tomographic and magnetic resonance angiography have emerged to become excellent non-invasive alternatives to conventional catheter angiography for the evaluation of hepatic vasculature [30–35]. Gadolinium-based contrast agents for MRA were considered to be safe until first studies characterized Nephrogenic Systemic Fibrosis as a severe systemic side effect associated to the administration of gadolinium-based contrast agents in patients with acute or chronic renal insufficiency [36,37]. Owing to the onset of this severe side effect, the focus of research has shifted to non-contrast-enhanced MR angiographic techniques for the assessment of hepatic vasculature.

Recent studies at 1.5 Tesla have demonstrated the diagnostic potential of several strategies for liver vessel imaging without the need of contrast media [4,6,38]. The most common technique for non-enhanced MR angiography is based on the application of true steady-state free-precession sequences (SSFP).

Within the last few years ultra-high-field MR imaging at 7 Tesla has been introduced to in vivo human imaging. First approaches in neuro imaging revealed an interesting incidental finding, in terms of an inherently high signal intensity of the arterial vasculature in T1w imaging. This incidental finding has been shown beneficial and of high diagnostic value for non-enhanced intracranial MR angiographic applications [16,17,27,39]. With etiology remaining to be incompletely understood, a combination of steady-state and inflow effects as well as the utilization of local transmit/receive coils within a small excitation volume seem to be

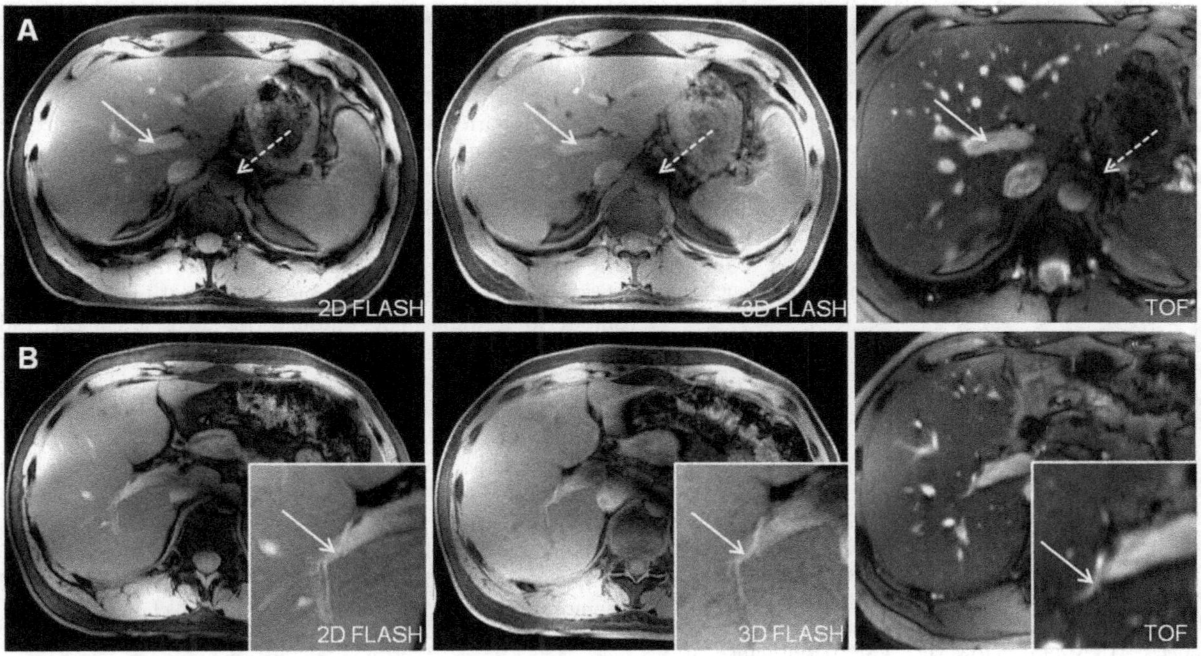

Figure 5. Depiction of the main portal vein (Figure A, arrows) and the right hepatic artery (Figure B, arrows) in all three sequences in one subject. 2D and 3D FLASH provided moderate to good image quality for both vessel segments with a slight advantage for 2D FLASH imaging due to a marginally higher contrast. TOF MRA was superior in the delineation of the liver arteries and veins from proximal to peripheral segments. Signal voids due to remaining B_1-inhomogeneity were shifted out of the liver to a periaortal focus, causing minor impairment of vessel delineation (dashed arrow in Fig. A).

accountable [40]. Thus, flowing spins are not pre-saturated by RF pulses when entering the imaging region [40].

Based on continuous development of multi-channel body coils and RF shimming technology at 7 T, the focus of research has expanded to whole-body applications, including abdominal imaging. Furthermore, the afore-mentioned hyperintense signal of the arterial vasculature could be confirmed for abdominal vessels [9,12,41,42]. Metzger et al. investigated the feasibility of non-enhanced renal MRA at 7 Tesla utilizing a respiratory triggered turbo-flash sequence [9,41]. In further 7 T studies, Umutlu et al. demonstrated the feasibility of non-enhanced as well as contrast-enhanced renal MRA. Their results showed promising results of non-enhanced renal arterial vessel imaging, utilizing T1w FLASH and TOF sequences with TOF MRA yielding best ratings in qualitative and quantitative analysis [12].

Our results go in line with previous publications on 7 T renal MRA in demonstrating the feasibility of high-quality T1w non contrast-enhanced imaging of abdominal vasculature at 7 Tesla. In accordance to a previous publication on non-enhanced renal MRA at 7 T by Umutlu et al. [12], our results also confirmed the considerable superiority of TOF MRA, regarding qualitative and quantitative evaluation due to sharply defined and homogeneously hyperintense vessel signal as well as an effective suppression of background signal. 2D and 3D FLASH imaging achieved a similar image quality and clearly lower contrast values with a slight advantage for the 2D FLASH sequence. Nevertheless, out of the three sequences, 3D FLASH imaging provided fastest acquisition (24 seconds) covering the entire liver during one breath-hold and offering high spatial resolution vessel imaging. Yet, in contrast to selective arterial vessel imaging, our results demonstrate the potential of T1w 7 T MRI not only for arterial vessels but for assessment of all three vessel types. TOF MRA revealed best delineation of the right portal vein and equivalently high quality delineation of the main portal vein as well as arterial and venous

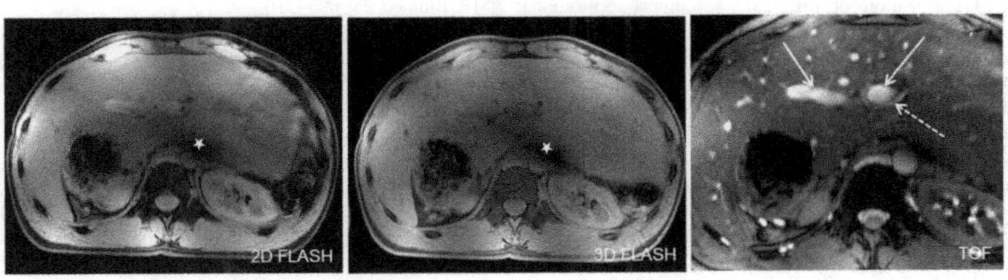

Figure 6. Figure 5 shows an anatomic variability of the upper abdomen in one healthy subject with a tall, centrally arranged liver and partially inverted situs, by means of mirrored location of spleen and stomach in the right upper abdomen. In this subject residual B_1-artifacts strongly impaired the conspicuity of central liver vessels in 2D and 3D FLASH imaging (stars in Figure A). Yet, being the sequence to be least impaired, TOF imaging allowed for a high-quality assessment of portal vein (arrow) and the left hepatic artery (dashed arrow). Figure B shows high quality delineation of the splenic artery and several small branches at the splenic hilus in all three sequences (arrows).

liver vasculature. Nevertheless, the comparatively long examination time for TOF-MRA has to be mentioned, as five imaging steps of 33 seconds each were necessary to cover the entire liver. Achieving an acquisition time within breath-hold conditions for the rather high flip angle TOF sequence was not possible. Best results regarding image quality and workflow were obtained by using a lower spatial resolution compared to FLASH acquisitions. However, to compensate for the reduced matrix the FOV of the TOF sequence was reduced to a minimum for whole-liver coverage. As an alternative, respiratory-gated imaging using a navigator is still restricted at 7 T due to an inhomogeneous excitation. At last, the breath-hold sequences acquired in the current study are advantageous regarding acquisition time compared to non-enhanced liver MRA studies at lower field strength based on SSFP imaging with acquisition times from 6–10 minutes [4,5].

Moreover, SSFP imaging is known to suffer from signal heterogeneity of the static magnetic field B_0 with increasing magnetic field strength, resulting in signal loss or dark banding artifacts [13]. An additional impairment of SSFP sequences can also be caused by SAR limitation, as SAR increases approximately with the square of the magnetic field and with the square of the flip angle. T2w Fast Spin Echo (FSE) imaging has also been proposed for non-enhanced MRA [43]. However, TSE performance at ultra-high field strength is strongly constrained by B_1 field signal alterations and by a lack of available RF power for generation of accurate refocusing pulses and high flip angles [13]. Hence, as described in previous trials on 7 T abdominal MRI, SSFP and T2w TSE imaging are strictly limited [10], leaving the exploitation of the inherently hyperintense vessel signal in T1 MRI to be a more promising method for non-contrast-enhanced liver vessel imaging at 7 Tesla.

Clearly, our initial study is not without some limitations. With increasing field strength, the Larmor wavelength is reduced to approximately 15 cm at 7 T, provoking significant B_1-field signal alterations and signal drop outs in large cross-sectional imaging [13]. These artifacts could be reduced in this trial with static RF shimming, pooling the majority of signal voids to a periaortal focus. Nevertheless, these residual B_1 artifacts caused a predominantly moderate impairment in 2D and 3D FLASH imaging, impeding the delineation of surrounding vessel structures as the main portal vein, the inferior vena cava and the common hepatic artery. Another limitation may be caused by the concomitant delineation of arterial, venous and portal venous vessels. Selective vessel delineation by dedicated vessel signal saturation would have been desirable. Yet, as stated in previous publications on 7 Tesla renal MRA [12], sufficient saturation of the inherently high vessel signal was not applicable, mainly based on B_1 inhomogeneities, SAR and peak RF power limitations associated with increasing field strength and limited coverage of the local transmit coil in contrast to a whole-body transmit coil used at clinical field strength. For body imaging at 7 T, hardware solutions in addition to improved pulse sequences are necessary. For example, Wu et al. have recently shown improved excitation homogeneity in liver MRI at 7 T with multi-spoke slice-selective parallel transmit RF pulse [44]. Additionally, further improvement of selective vessel signal suppression should be addressed in upcoming trials to improve dedicated vessel diagnostics. Finally, inflow effects depending on differences in slice thickness and TR between the three sequences, and in combination with aforementioned B1 inhomogeneities may have introduced a bias which might partially explain differences in the performance of the three sequences.

In conclusion, the initial results of our study demonstrate the feasibility of non-contrast-enhanced 7 Tesla liver vessel imaging and the challenges of this emerging technique. Non-enhanced T1w imaging in general and TOF MRA in particular, appear to be promising techniques for good quality liver vessel assessment at 7 T. Comparison trials to contrast-enhanced MRA in healthy subjects and patients with liver vessel pathologies should be addressed in future studies to assess the diagnostic competence of non-enhanced liver vessel MRI at 7 T.

Author Contributions

Conceived and designed the experiments: AF LU TCL OK. Performed the experiments: AF OK SM. Analyzed the data: AF KB. Contributed reagents/materials/analysis tools: MEL TCL MF. Wrote the paper: AF LU OK.

References

1. Saba L, Mallarini G (2008) Multidetector row CT angiography in the evaluation of the hepatic artery and its anatomical variants. Clin Radiol 63: 312–321.
2. Streitparth F, Pech M, Figolska S, Denecke T, Grieser C, et al. (2007) Living related liver transplantation: Preoperative magnetic resonance imaging for assessment of hepatic vasculature of donor candidates. Acta Radiol 48: 20–26.
3. Grobner T (2006) Gadolinium–a specific trigger for the development of nephrogenic fibrosing dermopathy and nephrogenic systemic fibrosis? Nephrol Dial Transplant 21: 1104–1108.
4. Shimada K, Isoda H, Okada T, Maetani Y, Arizono S, et al. (2009) Non-contrast-enhanced hepatic MR angiography with true steady-state free-precession and time spatial labeling inversion pulse: Optimization of the technique and preliminary results. Eur J Radiol 70: 111–117.
5. Shimada K, Isoda H, Okada T, Kamae T, Maetani Y, et al. (2009) Non-contrast-enhanced MR angiography for selective visualization of the hepatic vein and inferior vena cava with true steady-state free-precession sequence and time-spatial labeling inversion pulses: Preliminary results. J Magn Reson Imaging 29: 474–479.
6. Shimada K, Isoda H, Okada T, Kamae T, Arizono S, et al. (2009) Non-contrast-enhanced MR portography with time-spatial labeling inversion pulses: Comparison of imaging with three-dimensional half-fourier fast spin-echo and true steady-state free-precession sequences. J Magn Reson Imaging 29: 1140–1146.
7. Ramalho M, Altun E, Heredia V, Zapparoli M, Semelka R (2007) Liver MR imaging: 1.5T versus 3T. Magn Reson Imaging Clin N Am 15: 321–47, vi.
8. Vaughan JT, Snyder CJ, DelaBarre LJ, Bolan PJ, Tian J, et al. (2009) Whole-body imaging at 7T: Preliminary results. Magn Reson Med 61: 244–248.
9. Metzger GJ, Simonson J, Bi X, Weale P, Zuehlsdorff S, et al. (2010) Initial experience with non-contrast enhanced renal angiography at 7.0 tesla. ISMRM 403.
10. Umutlu L, Bitz AK, Maderwald S, Orzada S, Kinner S, et al. (2011) Contrast-enhanced ultra-high-field liver MRI: A feasibility trial. Eur J Radiol 82: 760–767.
11. Metzger GJ, Auerbach EJ, Akgun C, Simonson J, Bi X, et al. (2012) Dynamically applied B(1) (+) shimming solutions for non-contrast enhanced renal angiography at 7.0 tesla. Magn Reson Med 69: 114–126.
12. Umutlu L, Maderwald S, Kraff O, Kinner S, Schaefer LC, et al. (2012) A new look at renal vasculature: 7 tesla non-enhanced T1-weighted FLASH imaging. Investigative Radiology 36: 714–721.
13. Moser E, Stahlberg F, Ladd ME, Trattnig S (2012) 7-T MR-from research to clinical applications? NMR Biomed 25: 695–716.
14. Bernstein MA, Huston J 3rd, Ward HA (2006) Imaging artifacts at 3.0T. J Magn Reson Imaging 24: 735–746.
15. Ladd ME (2007) High-field-strength magnetic resonance: Potential and limits. Top Magn Reson Imaging 18: 139–152.
16. Umutlu L, Theysohn N, Maderwald S, Johst S, Lauenstein TC, et al. (2013) 7 tesla MPRAGE imaging of the intracranial arterial vasculature: Nonenhanced versus contrast-enhanced. Acad Radiol 20: 628–634.
17. Wrede KH, Dammann P, Monninghoff C, Johst S, Maderwald S, et al. (2014) Non-enhanced MR imaging of cerebral aneurysms: 7 tesla versus 1.5 tesla. PLoS One 9: e84562.
18. Fischer A, Maderwald S, Orzada S, Johst S, Schafer LC, et al. (2013) Nonenhanced magnetic resonance angiography of the lower extremity vessels at 7 tesla: Initial experience. Invest Radiol 48: 525–534.
19. Johst S, Orzada S, Fischer A, Schäfer L, Nassenstein K, et al. (2014) Sequence comparison for non-enhanced MRA of the lower extremity arteries at 7 tesla. PloS One 9: e86274.
20. Orzada S, Quick HH, Ladd ME (2009) A flexible 8-channel transmit/receive body coil for 7 T human imaging. ISMRM 2999.

21. Hoult DI, Phil D (2000) Sensitivity and power deposition in a high-field imaging experiment. J Magn Reson Imaging 12: 46–67.
22. Bitz AK, Brote I, Orzada S, Kraff O, Maderwald S, et al. (2009) An 8-channel add-on RF shimming system for whole-body 7 tesla MRI including real-time SAR monitoring. ISMRM 4767.
23. Sacolick LI, Wiesinger F, Hancu I, Vogel MW (2010) B1 mapping by bloch-siegert shift. Magn Reson Med 63: 1315–1322.
24. Duan Q, van Gelderen P, Duyn J (2013) Improved bloch-siegert based B1 mapping by reducing off-resonance shift. NMR Biomed 26: 1070–1078.
25. International Electrotechnical Commission (2002) Medical electrical equipment-part 2–33: Particular requirements for the safety of magnetic resonance diagnostic devices. IEC 60601-2-33.
26. Christ A, Kainz W, Hahn EG, Honegger K, Zefferer M, et al. (2010) The virtual family–development of surface-based anatomical models of two adults and two children for dosimetric simulations. Phys Med Biol 55: N23–38.
27. Maderwald S, Ladd SC, Gizewski ER, Kraff O, Theysohn JM, et al. (2008) To TOF or not to TOF: Strategies for non-contrast-enhanced intracranial MRA at 7 T. MAGMA 21: 159–167.
28. Dietrich O, Raya JG, Reeder SB, Ingrisch M, Reiser MF, et al. (2008) Influence of multichannel combination, parallel imaging and other reconstruction techniques on MRI noise characteristics. Magn Reson Imaging 26: 754–762.
29. Landis JR, Koch GG (1977) The measurement of observer agreement for categorical data. Biometrics 33: 159–174.
30. Carr JC, Nemcek AA Jr, Abecassis M, Blei A, Clarke L, et al. (2003) Preoperative evaluation of the entire hepatic vasculature in living liver donors with use of contrast-enhanced MR angiography and true fast imaging with steady-state precession. J Vasc Interv Radiol 14: 441–449.
31. Aslam R, Yeh BM, Yee J (2010) MR imaging evaluation of the hepatic vasculature. Magn Reson Imaging Clin N Am 18: 515–23, xi.
32. Lee MW, Lee JM, Lee JY, Kim SH, Park EA, et al. (2007) Preoperative evaluation of hepatic arterial and portal venous anatomy using the time resolved echo-shared MR angiographic technique in living liver donors. Eur Radiol 17: 1074–1080.
33. Lee MW, Lee JM, Lee JY, Kim SH, Park EA, et al. (2006) Preoperative evaluation of the hepatic vascular anatomy in living liver donors: Comparison of CT angiography and MR angiography. J Magn Reson Imaging 24: 1081–1087.
34. Sahani D, Mehta A, Blake M, Prasad S, Harris G, et al. (2004) Preoperative hepatic vascular evaluation with CT and MR angiography: Implications for surgery. Radiographics 24: 1367–1380.
35. Uchida K, Taniguchi M, Shimamura T, Suzuki T, Yamashita K, et al. (2010) Three-dimensional computed tomography scan analysis of hepatic vasculatures in the donor liver for living donor liver transplantation. Liver Transpl 16: 1062–1068.
36. Grobner T, Prischl FC (2007) Gadolinium and nephrogenic systemic fibrosis. Kidney Int 72: 260–264.
37. Lauenstein TC, Salman K, Morreira R, Tata S, Tudorascu D, et al. (2007) Nephrogenic systemic fibrosis: Center case review. J Magn Reson Imaging 26: 1198–1203.
38. Puippe GD, Alkadhi H, Hunziker R, Nanz D, Pfammatter T, et al. (2012) Performance of unenhanced respiratory-gated 3D SSFP MRA to depict hepatic and visceral artery anatomy and variants. Eur J Radiol 81: e823–9.
39. Monninghoff C, Maderwald S, Theysohn JM, Kraff O, Ladd SC, et al. (2009) Evaluation of intracranial aneurysms with 7 T versus 1.5 T time-of-flight MR angiography - initial experience. Rofo 181: 16–23.
40. Grinstead JW, Rooney W, Laub G (2010) The origins of bright blood MPRAGE at 7 tesla and a simultaneous method for T1 imaging and non-contrast MRA. ISMRM 1429.
41. Metzger GJ, Auerbach EJ, Akgun C, Simonson J, Bi X, et al. (2013) Dynamically applied B(1) (+) shimming solutions for non-contrast enhanced renal angiography at 7.0 tesla. Magn Reson Med 69: 114–26.
42. Umutlu L, Kraff O, Orzada S, Fischer A, Kinner S, et al. (2011) Dynamic contrast-enhanced renal MRI at 7 tesla: Preliminary results. Invest Radiol 46: 425–433.
43. Shimada K, Isoda H, Okada T, Kamae T, Arizono S, et al. (2009) Unenhanced MR portography with a half-fourier fast spin-echo sequence and time-space labeling inversion pulses: Preliminary results. AJR Am J Roentgenol 193: 106–112.
44. Wu X, Schmitter S, Auerbach EJ, Ugurbil K, Van de Moortele PF (2014) Mitigating transmit B 1 inhomogeneity in the liver at 7T using multi-spoke parallel transmit RF pulse design. Quant Imaging Med Surg 4: 4–10.

2

A New Conversation between Radiology and Pathology-Identifying Microvascular Architecture in Stages of Cirrhosis via Diffraction Enhanced Imaging *In Vitro*

Dou-dou Hu[1], Yu Chen[2], Ali Bihi[3], Xin-min Li[1], Tai-ling Wang[4], Bao-en Wang[1]*, Xin-yan Zhao[1]*

1 Liver Research Center, Beijing Friendship Hospital, Capital Medical University, Beijing, China, **2** Institute of High Energy Physics, Chinese Academy of Sciences, Beijing, China, **3** International School of Capital Medical University. Beijing, China, **4** Department of Pathology, China-Japan Friendship Hospital, Beijing, China

Abstract

Background/Aim: Diffraction enhanced imaging (DEI) is a synchrotron radiation X-ray phase-contrast imaging technique that can better reveal the microstructure of biological soft tissues than conventional X-rays. The aim of this study is to investigate the angio-architectural changes of the liver during fibrosis, cirrhosis and its subsequent regression by applying synchrotron radiation based DEI.

Methods: DEI experiments were performed at the 4W1A station of Beijing Synchrotron Radiation Facility. Twenty-four Sprague-Dawley rats were induced with liver fibrosis by carbon tetrachloride (CCl_4) for up to 10 weeks, after which spontaneous regression started and continued until week 30. Quantitative analysis of the DEI images yielded the mean vascular density and intercapillary distance, which was then re-confirmed by immunohistochemical analysis of CD34.

Results: Based on the DEI results, the mean vascular density was 1.4-fold higher in fibrotic rats (at week 6) and 2-fold higher in cirrhotic rats (at week 10) compared with the control ($p<0.05$). Accordingly, the intercapillary distance decreased to 563.89±243.35 μm in fibrotic rats and 392.90±92.68 μm in cirrhotic rats compared with 673.85±214.16μm in the control ($p<0.05$). During fibrosis regression at week 30, vascular density was 0.7-fold lower and intercapillary distance increased to 548.60±210.94 μm as compared with cirrhotic rats ($p<0.05$).In parallel to the DEI results, immunohistochemical analysis of CD34 showed similar changes.

Conclusion: Synchrotron-based DEI can conduct radiological as well as pathological analysis. Our results are consistent with previous reports indicating that angiogenesis is directly proportional to fibrosis progression. Furthermore, by clarifying the vascular characteristics of liver diseases, DEI reveals that cirrhosis cannot fully reverse during fibrosis regression.

Editor: Konradin Metze, University of Campinas, Brazil

Funding: The work was supported by a grant from the Beijing Nova program of China (Grant Number: 2009 B45, (http://210.76.125.50:8080/datainfo/public/kjxx.jsp) and a grant from National Natural Science Foundation of China (Grant Number: 81000178, http://159.226.244.22/portal/Proj_List.asp). The funders had no role in study design, data collection and analysis, decision to publish, or preparation of the manuscript.

Competing Interests: The authors have declared that no competing interests exist.

* E-mail: wangbbee@126.com (BW); Zhao_xinyan@ccmu.edu.cn (XZ)

These authors contributed equally to this work as first authors.

Introduction

Cirrhosis is currently ranked as the tenth leading cause of death in the Western World with a 10-year mortality of 34%–66% [1]. The golden sign pertaining to the pathology of cirrhosis includes fibrotic bands, regenerative nodules and vascular distortion that changes normal liver parenchyma [2]. In the past decades, researchers have mainly focused on collagen metabolism as well as antifibrotic therapies in order to inhibit the progression of disease and improve clinical outcomes. Besides collagen accumulation, cirrhosis also involves the formation of new vessels (angiogenesis) and the establishment of abnormal angio-architecture of the liver; this phenomenon has recently gained wider attention in the field of hepatology [3–5]. The vascular changes are chiefly attributed to microvascular changes within the intrahepatic circulation. These changes are regarded as one of the most important and newly discovered pathophysiological features of cirrhosis, and contribute to developing and maintaining portal hypertension as well as hindering the reversibility of cirrhosis [6,7].

Medical imaging techniques such as CT and MRI provide direct anatomical information of hepatic vessels, assisting doctors in decision making, yet the resolution of these techniques is too low to visualize small branches of the portal vein and/or the hepatic vein (< 200μm) [8]. Histopathology of liver tissues (mainly obtained by liver biopsy) is currently regarded as the gold standard for observing subtle vascular structures. However, traditional pathology can only show a given cross section of the microvascular architecture, often yielding discontinuous and incomplete information.

Therefore, it is imperative to develop tools that can detect the angio-architecture of the liver over a wider length scale, from "macro" down to "micro". We propose the use of synchrotron radiation-based DEI to better understand the changes in intrahepatic vessels during cirrhosis. The DEI set-up is an analyzer-based imaging technique that uses monochromatic and collimated synchrotron radiation beams together with an analyzer crystal placed between the sample and the detector, possessing high spatial resolution and high contrast resolution [9,10]. As a powerful tool, DEI provides not only the absorption contrast on which conventional imaging techniques rely, but also additional data on soft tissues that were previously accessible only by histopathology [11]. Although DEI has been used to study vascular changes in normal livers [12,13], it has not been used to study cirrhotic livers in a systemic manner. We believe that DEI has broader applicability in understanding pathological vascular changes during progression and regression of liver cirrhosis.

The aim of this study is to investigate changes in the microvasculature of liver tissues from CCl_4-induced rats during fibrosis, cirrhosis and regression stages using DEI to quantify the intrahepatic vascular remodeling in different periods of liver cirrhosis. Our study presents an illustrative view of microvasculature changes and an in-depth understanding of the pathogenesis of cirrhosis with regard to the angio-architecture. We postulate that DEI is a new radio-pathological method for assessing the severity of cirrhosis.

Materials and Methods

Animal Models

Twenty-four male adult Sprague-Dawley rats, weighing 180–220 g, were maintained in an environmentally controlled room (23±2°C, 55±10% humidity) with a 12-hour light/dark cycle and free accessed to food and water. Liver fibrosis was induced via administration of 2ml of CCl_4/olive oil (4:6, v/v) per kg body weight by intraperitoneal (i.p.) injection, twice per week for up to 10weeks. The twenty-four rats were euthanized in groups of six at different time intervals, i.e. at weeks 0 (control), 6, 10, and after spontaneous recovery at week 30. The livers from all animals were removed after euthanasia in accordance with the guiding principles for the care and use of laboratory animals approved by the Research Ethics Committee of the Beijing Friendship Hospital, Capital Medical University, China (Permit Number: 12-1004). Liver samples were fixed in neutral phosphate-buffered formalin (10%) and stored at room temperature (25±2°C) and relative humidity of 55±10% until histopathological and DEI analysis.

Experimental Setup

DEI experiments were performed at the 4W1A station of Beijing Synchrotron Radiation Facility (BSRF). A schematic of the experimental setup is shown in Fig. 1. The X-ray source is a wiggler that emits radiation over a wide energy range (5–20 keV), which is placed at a distance of 43 m from the sample. The size of the incident beam spot on the sample was approximately 20 mm (horizontal) ×11 mm (vertical). The electron energy in the storage ring was 2.5 GeV with a current of 150–250 mA. The white X-ray beam from the 4W1 wiggler was monochromatized by a perfect silicon [333] crystal. After passing through the sample, the X-rays were refracted by an analyzer crystal, identical to the monochromator crystal, and were detected by an X-ray CCD with a pixel size of 7.5 μm×7.5 μm. The spatial resolution of the images is about 30 microns. An aluminum absorber was used to attenuate X-rays of low energy. The DEI experiments were carried out by using the Si [333] diffraction plane of the two crystals to diffract 15 keV X-rays.

Principle of DEI

The white X-ray beam from the 4W1 wiggler was made monochromatic using a perfect silicon [333] crystal. After passing through the sample, the intensity of the monochromatic X-ray beam was reduced owing to absorption. Moreover, the incoming beam can be scattered and refracted by the sample through large angles, on the order of degrees, and through small angles, on the order of microradians. The analyzer crystal used in DEI was identical to the monochromator crystal. The silicon crystal has a very narrow angle acceptance range, on the order of microradians called Darwin width (W_D), which is related to the energy of the X-rays and the diffraction plane of the crystal. Only those photons deviating less than one W_D after passing through the sample can be reflected by the analyzer and detected by the detector (Fig. 2A-C).

The angular acceptance range of the analyzer is determined by the width of the rocking curve (RC), i.e. the intensity curve obtained by rocking the analyzer crystal around the Bragg angle with no sample in the beam (Fig. 2D). For the X-ray energy and crystal reflection used here, the width of this curve was a few microradians. Different kinds of images with enhanced contrast can be obtained at different positions on the RC.

Image Acquisition and Post-processing

Before DEI image acquisition, each liver sample was dehydrated for one to two hours by natural volatilization (23±2°C, 45±10% humidity) to obtain high quality images. Samples were set between two crystals, and a series of images were acquired when the analyzer crystal was set at different positions of the rocking curve of the system. The background images were obtained in the same way, with no sample present in the beam. Thus, two series of images were acquired, one with and one without sample. Each pixel yielded a sample RC and a reference RC. The center of the peak was calculated from both, resulting in a refraction angle image $\Delta\theta = \theta_{sample} - \theta_{reference}$. The width of the RC, which was related to the scattering image $W = (W^2_{sample} - W^2_{referencee})^{0.5}$, can also be obtained (Fig. 3). The integral of the RC will give the absorption image of the sample. Therefore, refraction, absorption and extinction images of the sample were simultaneously obtained by multiple-image radiography [14]. In general, refraction images have the best contrast; hence, we focus on this type of image in this paper.

Image Evaluation and Quantification

The mean vascular density was calculated in normal, fibrotic, cirrhotic and regressive livers from our animal models. First, in the direct method, the numbers of microvessels per mm^2 were independently counted in 10 randomly selected 1 mm^2 areas per liver sample by two researchers (X-y Zhao and D-d Hu), who were blinded to the stages of cirrhosis, and the mean numbers were calculated. Moreover, we calculated the intercapillary distance under surface edge of the liver in 10 non-overlapping areas to re-confirm the microvascular density, which was adopted from published method [15]. Results were expressed by mean ± SD.

Observation of Angiogenesis via Immunohistochemistry

Changes in microvasculature were evaluated by immunohistochemical analysis of CD34. Goat polyclonal antibodies against rat CD34 (LS-C150289, LifeSpan BioSciences, Seattle, WA, USA) was used according to the supplier's instructions. Slides were scanned at low magnification (100×) to identify areas with the greatest vascular density. Subsequently, the microvascular density (MVD) was determined by two pathologists, independently and in masked trials, on 10 non-overlapping areas at 200× magnification.

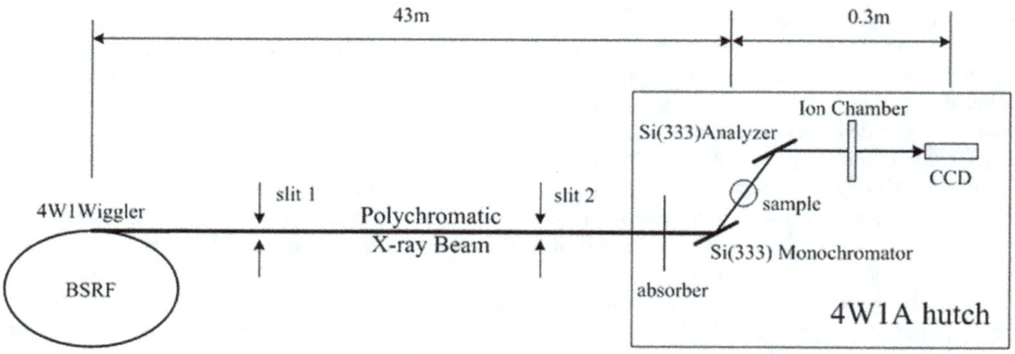

Figure 1. Experimental setup of Diffraction Enhanced Imaging (DEI). Schematic illustration of (DEI) experimental setup at the 4W1A Station in the Beijing Synchrotron Radiation Facility (BSRF).

Only immune-positive clusters of cells with a lumen were considered as individual vessels for the purposes of microvessel counting, consistent with the procedures described by Romanenko [16]. Vascular density was expressed as the mean number of CD34-positive microvessels per 0.785 mm^2.

Quantification of Fibrosis

Areas of fibrosis were stained by Sirius red and assessed in five non-overlapping areas at 100× magnification. The fibrosis area was analyzed using Image-Pro Plus 6.0 software (Media Cybernetics, Bethesda, Maryland, USA). The quantity of fibrosis was expressed as a relative percentage between the area of fibrosis and the total area.

Statistical Analysis

Error bars represented the mean ± SD and were analyzed by the nonparametric ANOVA test, using the software program SPSS ver. 17.0 (IBM, Chicago, IL, USA). All reported *p* values are

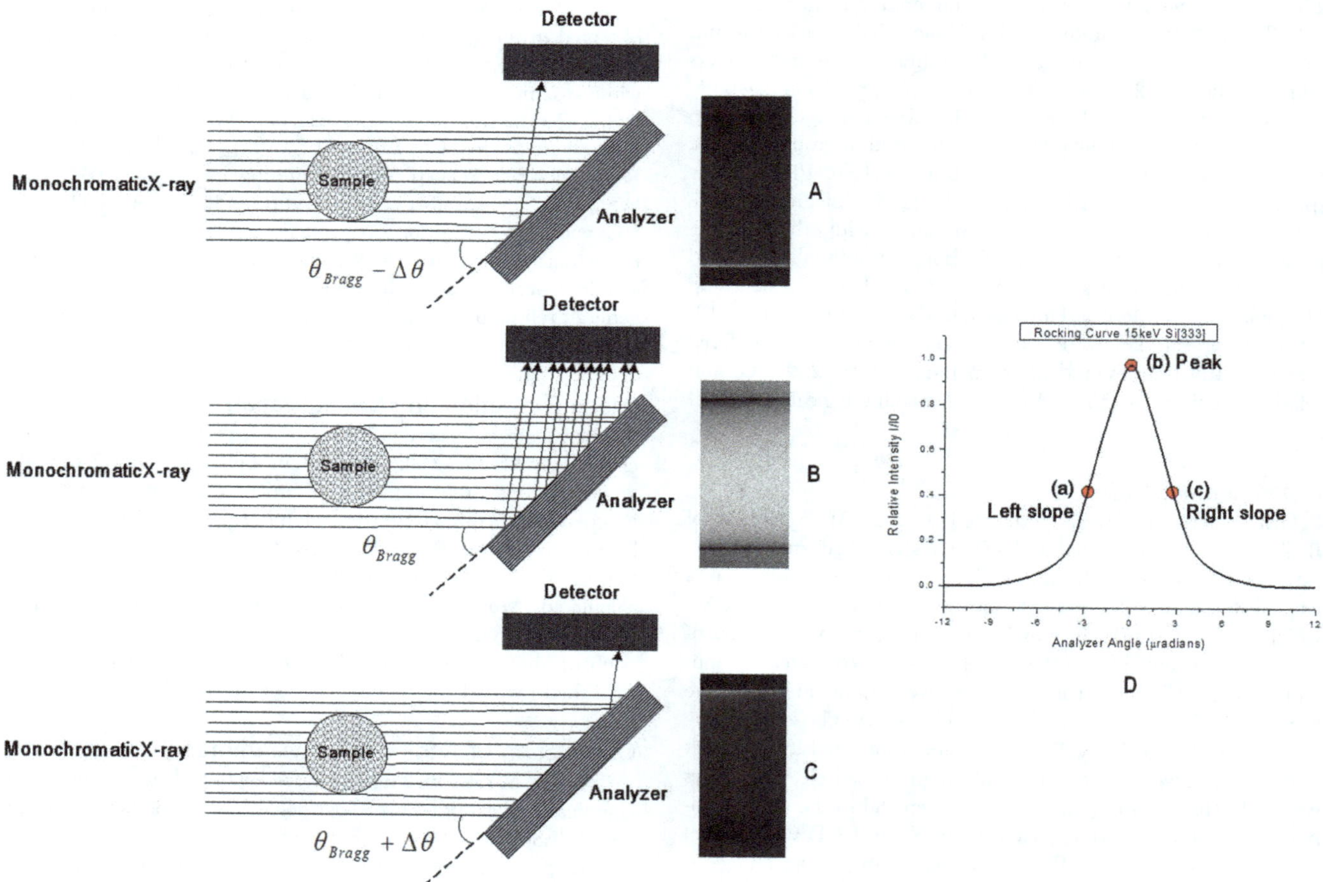

Figure 2. The analyzer crystal selects specifically X-rays which transmitted in a certain angle range incidence on the detector to produce high contrast images (A-C) relative to the position on the RC in (D). A schematic of RC with 15 keV X-rays and silicon [333] diffraction plane (D).

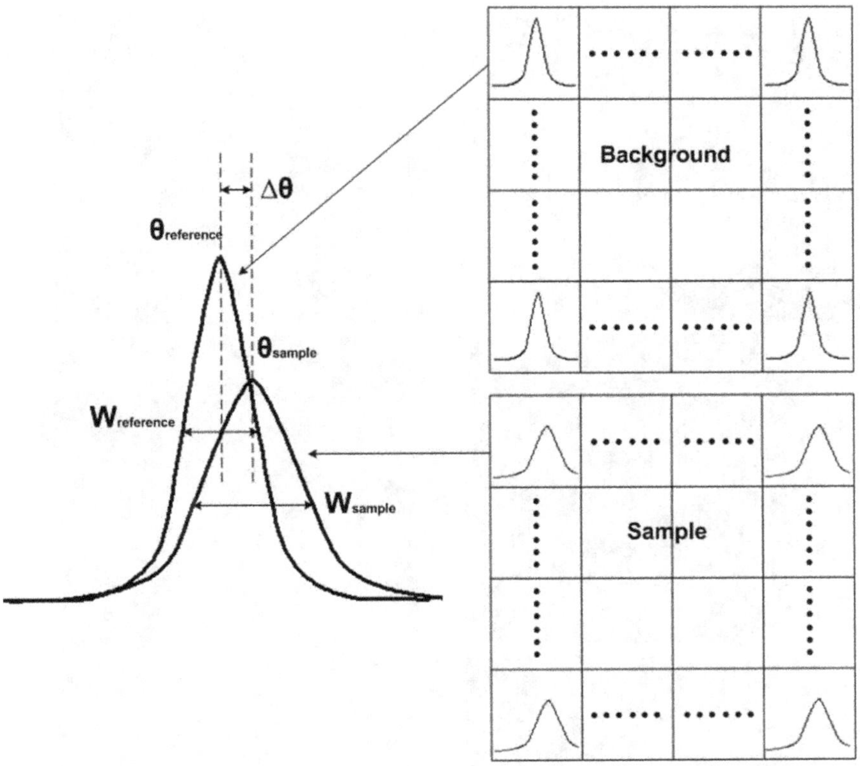

Figure 3. For every pixel, a sample RC and a reference RC can be obtained. The change of the peak, width, area interrelated to the refraction, scattering, absorption of the sample.

two-sided, and values with $p<0.05$ were considered statistically significant.

Results

Liver Fibrosis Progression and Regression in CCl_4-treated Rats

The progression of liver fibrosis in CCl_4-treated rats was revealed by Sirius red staining (Fig. $4C_{1\text{-}4}$). In normal livers, collagen was detected in low amounts around portal tracts and hepatic veins (Fig. $4C_1$). After CCl_4 induction for 6 weeks, collagen septa were detected (Fig. $4C_2$); cirrhosis was established at week 10, following which CCl_4 injection was stopped (Fig. $4C_3$). At week 30, the septa and collagen were reabsorbed and nodules became enlarged (Fig. $4C_4$). Figure 4F shows our quantitative analysis of fibrosis. Fibrotic and cirrhotic rats exhibited fibrosis areas of 1.92±0.44% and 9.30±1.50%, respectively, both of which were significantly higher than the fibrosis area in the control (0.16±0.5%, $p<0.05$). During cirrhosis regression, the fibrosis area decreased to 1.68±0.44% as compared with cirrhotic rats ($p<0.05$).

Imaging Vascular Changes via DEI

The morphology and branching of hepatic veins and portal veins in the liver lobe were visualized using DEI. In normal livers, the vascular structure resembled a tree, forming regular dichotomous branches (Fig. $4B_1$). Meanwhile, in CCl_4-treated rats, irregular and tortuous vasculature was observed after 6 weeks (Fig. $4B_2$). In week 10, the microvascular network presented numerous spikes, giving a "hairy" appearance (Fig. $4B_3$). During cirrhosis regression at week 30, the aberrant vascular density diminished considerably, exhibiting more delicate ramifications, though the final structure did not completely revert to that of the control (Fig. $4B_4$).

To complement the aforementioned qualitative study of morphological changes in general, quantitative analysis of the vascular density was performed. Compared with control rats, the mean vascular density was 1.4-fold higher in fibrotic rats and 2-fold higher in cirrhotic rats ($p<0.05$). The vascular density in cirrhotic rats decreased 0.7-fold ($p<0.05$) after 30 weeks regression (Fig. 4D). The changes in micro- vasculature were also quantified by intercapillary distance, which was inversely correlated with the vascular density [17]. The intercapillary width ranged from 563.89±243.35 μm in fibrotic rats to 392.90±92.68 μm in cirrhotic rats, compared with 673.85±214.16 μm in control rats, re-confirming that cirrhotic models had a higher vascular density. During regression, the intercapillary distance markedly increased (548.60±210.94 μm), but did not return to the normal condition (Fig. 4E).

In order to interpret increased vasculature, we compared the DEI images from CCl_4 model with bile duct ligation model (BDL, see Figure S1). Portal veins can be distinguished from hepatic veins based on the fact that portal veins are normally accompanied with bile ducts. By analysis of DEI images from these two different cirrhotic models (CCl_4 Vs BDL) along with their corresponding histopathological sections, we concluded that increased vasculature mainly belonged to portal vein systems as well as arterializations of hepatic sinusoids.

Identifying Vascular Changes by CD34 Immunolabeling

To affirm our DEI results regarding the vascular density and morphology, we stained liver tissue sections with an antibody

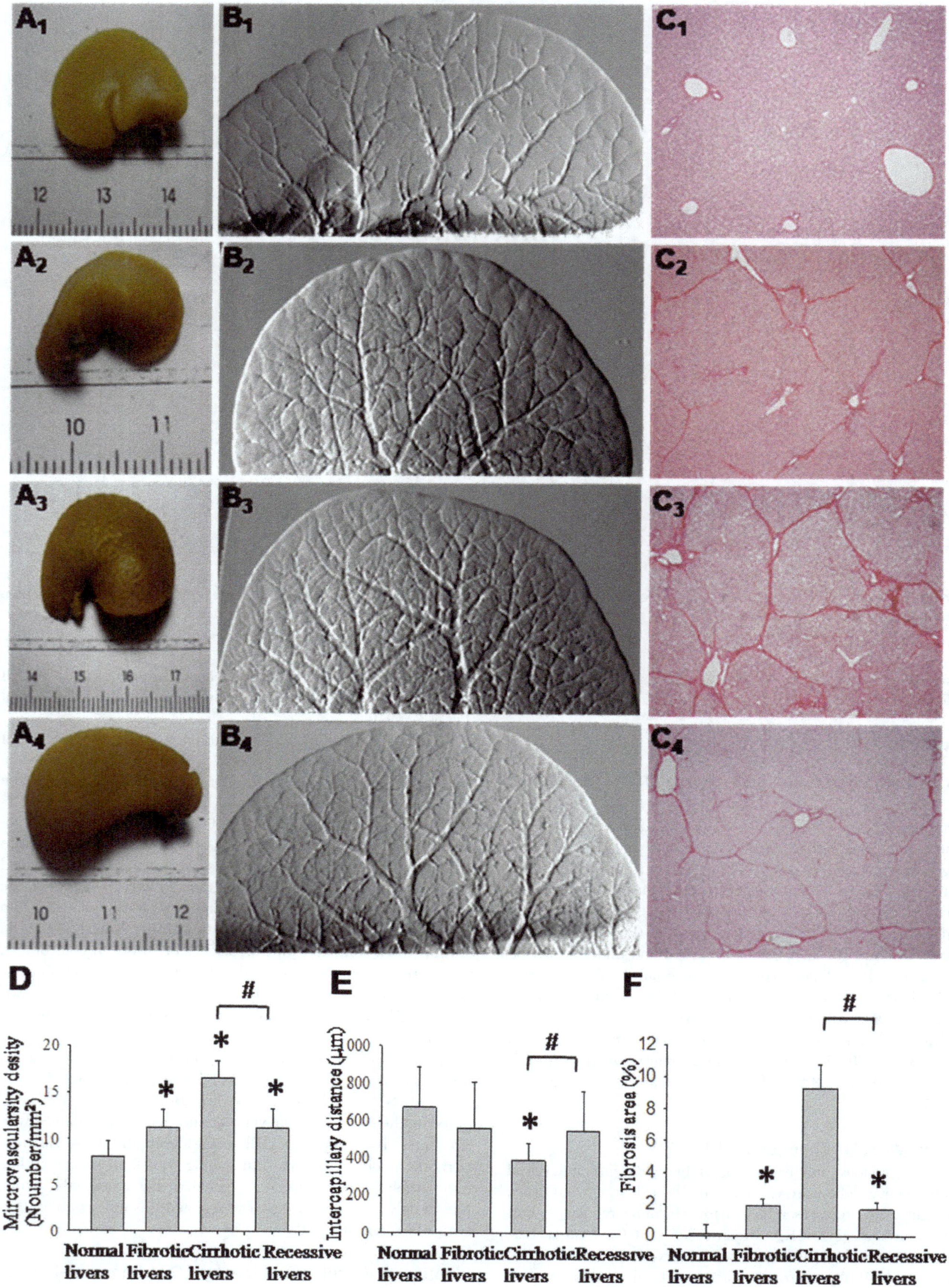
A1
B1
C1
12
13
14
A2
B2
C2
10
11
A3
B3
C3
14
15
16
17
A4
B4
C4
10
11
12
D
#
Mircrovascularsity desity (Noumber/mm²)
Normal livers
Fibrotic livers
Cirrhotic livers
Recessive livers
E
Intercapillary distance (μm)
F
Fibrosis area (%)

Figure 4. Illustration and quantification of microvasculature and fibrosis in corresponding stages of cirrhosis. Macroscopic observations of liver lobe (A_{1-4}) from representative control, fibrotic, cirrhotic and regressive rats, with corresponding DEI vasculature images (B_{1-4}) and fibrosis stained by Sirius-Red (C_{1-4}). The vasculature of control (B_1) became more dense at week 6 (B_2), further increasing in number at week 10 (B_3). After regression for 30 weeks, the number of micro-vessels decreased (B_4). The vascular density (D), intercapillary distance (E) and fibrosis area (F) were summarized and expressed as mean ± SD. *$p<0.05$ compared with control group. $^{\#}p<0.05$ compared with cirrhotic group.

against CD34, an endothelial antigen that is a direct marker for the degree of neoangiogenesis [18] and has been used to highlight vascular density. In normal livers, CD34 expression was restricted to the endothelium of portal veins and hepatic veins (Fig. 5A). In fibrotic livers (6 weeks), numerous CD34-positive vessels were detected in the fibrotic septa (Fig. 5B). In cirrhotic livers (10 weeks), the cirrhotic nodules became surrounded by a dense vascular plexus, and some scattered sinusoidal endothelial cells in these nodules also tested positive for CD34 (Fig. 5C). Conversely, at 30 weeks the number of CD34-labeled vessels decreased and only persisted within the thin fibrous septa (Fig. 5D).

Quantitative analysis of the CD34 staining of endothelial cells revealed an increase of the MVD, to 9.42±2.12 in fibrotic rats and 14.4±3.11 in cirrhotic rats, both of which were statistically significant compared with the MVD of the control group (7.1±2.30, $p<0.01$). After 30 weeks of cirrhosis regression, the MVD was 0.6-fold lower than that of cirrhotic rats ($p<0.05$), as shown in Fig. 5E.

Discussion

In this study, we explore the use of DEI as a radio-pathological diagnostic tool to study the vascular effects of liver cirrhosis. With the aid of DEI, we first re-confirm previous pathological findings such as the increase in angiogenesis over time during fibrogenesis [3,19]. Furthermore, during the regression phase of cirrhosis the quantity of blood vessels does in fact decrease but fails to completely return to normalcy [20,21]. This result corroborates with previous histopathological findings that cirrhosis is not fully reversible especially with regard to the changes in liver microvasculature [20]. The inability of the remodeled vasculature to returning to its original form is possibly due to the complexity of the angio-architecture, and the fundamental changes that it undergoes during the development of cirrhosis [20,21]. It is worth mentioning that our DEI image results are directly proportional to the results of immunohistochemistry staining of CD34.

More importantly, DEI can potentially be a new radio-pathological method to assess the severity of cirrhosis. Our results indicate that the vascular density of cirrhotic livers is related to the degree of fibrosis, where higher MVD corresponds to more severe cirrhosis. Current methods for determining the severity of cirrhosis and predicting prognosis include the Child-Pugh score and the Model for End-Stage Liver Disease score, both of which rely on functional markers such as albumin, INR, and creatinine [22], instead of evaluating the structural abnormalities corresponding to cirrhosis. Hence, the radio-pathological DEI technique is advantageous for evaluating the severity of cirrhosis by imaging the liver angio-architecture and anatomy; not only does it provide a view of soft tissues, but also a continuous and thorough view. This would complement existing diagnostic tools, allowing clinicians to determine the severity of cirrhosis with greater accuracy.

We selected DEI as a radio-pathological imaging technique because DEI can view the vascular tree in liver lobes, from visible macro-vessels down to small micro-vessels (30 μm) in a non-destructive, continuous and thorough fashion. Compared with traditional image profiles, DEI has the ability to differentiate soft tissues [23], thus achieving in-depth visualization of cirrhotic livers, in particular the microscopic blood vessels. Besides high phase contrast and high spatial resolution, other advantages of DEI include a wider view of the liver; instead of a small specimen as in liver biopsy (1/50,000th of the total liver tissue), it can display a total lobe (approximately 1/9th of the liver tissue) and consequently decrease the likelihood of sampling error. Finally, DEI is easy to perform, time-efficient, and exposes the tissue to a minimal radiation, lower than that of a traditional X-rays [24].

Compared with in vivo microangiography and optical angiography techniques, DEI has the disadvantage of assessing liver samples in vitro. Fresh liver samples are much closer to the in vivo condition than formalin fixed tissues. We initially attempted to perform DEI on fresh liver samples, but DEI was unable to visualize the microvasculature of these samples in the absence of contrast medium. Fresh livers contain fluid inside and outside the vessels, and the difference in electronic density is very small, exceeding the capacity of DEI. After dehydration, formalin volatilized over time, increasing the difference in electronic density

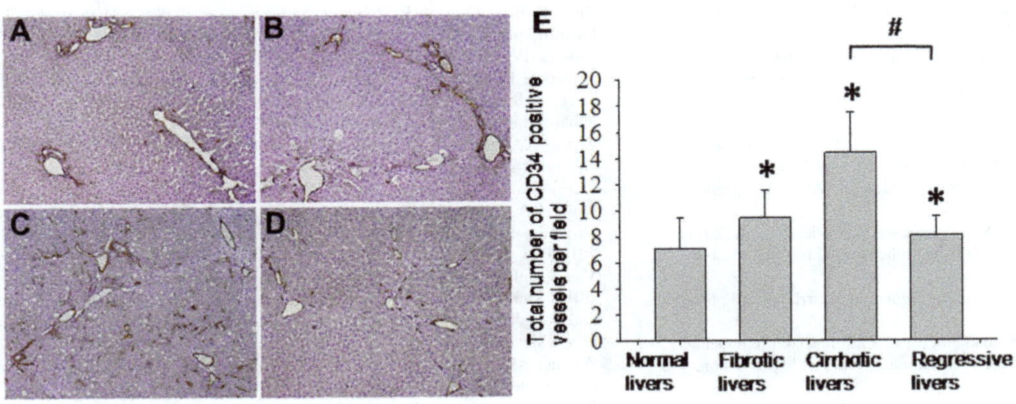

Figure 5. Angiogenesis or neo-vascularization was evaluated by immune- histochemical stain of CD34. CD34 positive microvasculature increases with time; control (A), fibrosis stage at week 6 (B), cirrhosis stage at week 10 (C) and regressive stage after cession of CCl_4 for 30 weeks (D). Results are expressed as mean ± SD. *$p<0.05$ compared with the control group. $^{\#}p<0.05$ compared with the cirrhotic group.

and enabling vessels to be detected by DEI. To our knowledge, microangiography is used to assess the hepatic artery systems (i.e. to detect microvascular lesions) rather than the portal or hepatic venous systems by injection of contrast medium into a peripheral artery. Optical microangiography was recently developed to visualize microcirculatory tissue beds in vivo. Since this new technique only can visualize superficial microvessels up to 2.00 mm beneath the tissue surface [25], and since the liver is located deep within the abdominal cavity, optical microangiography has not yet been used to study liver microcirculation. Therefore, unlike DEI, this method is unable to reveal the entire vascular tree of the liver lobe.

To explain the increased vascular density in cirrhotic livers, we carefully studied histopathological sections corresponding to the DEI images. We determined that the following factors caused the hypervascular changes during fibrosis progression. CCl_4 toxification induces necrosis of hepatocytes around central venules. Extinction of liver parenchyma leads to approximation of afferent (portal) and efferent (hepatic) venules [26]. Loss of hepatocytes and proliferation of fibrotic tissue change the original ratio between liver parenchyma and mesenchyma, increasing the density of vessels. Up-regulation of factors related to vascular development, i.e. vascular endothelial growth factor, angiopoietin-1 and platelet-derived growth factor (see Figure S2) drives vascularization or angiogenesis in diseased livers. We also confirmed that the newly developed vessels were portal venules and sinusoidal vascularizations (afferents) instead of hepatic venules (efferents).

One outstanding limitation of this two dimensional DEI technique adopted in the study is that surface vessels may obscure the internal vascular structure of the liver, which hindering differentiation afferent from efferent vessels within the entire liver lobe. To overcome this, we are currently evaluating three-dimensional DEI as a diagnostic tool. Three-dimensional DEI will be able to display all vascular structures; we presume that this method will provide more information. Besides three-dimensional DEI, in vivo DEI is the new direction of this image modality. To date, the DEI technique has been used to study joints, cartilage, brain and lungs in vivo [27–31]. DEI has higher sensitivity and specificity in the diagnosis of early breast cancer than traditional mammography [32]. However, most assessments of hepatic microvessels by DEI used ex vivo liver samples owing to the deep location, thickness and movement of the liver during respiration. These difficulties may be overcome by incremental changes in X-ray flux and more efficient CCD to increase the acquisition speed to video rates. In addition, large size beams compatible with the size of the animal are needed for in vivo applications. Despite these challenges, in vitro DEI may be able to visualize microvascular changes corresponding with cirrhosis, thus improving our understanding of the pathogenesis of cirrhosis. Moreover, it may aid in clinical decision-making by allowing real-time images that can clearly illustrate the stages of cirrhosis from a microvascular perspective.

In conclusion, synchrotron-based DEI is compatible with radiological and pathological analysis. Our results are consistent with previous reports that angiogenesis is directly proportional to fibrosis progression, and further reveal that the microvascular changes accompanying cirrhosis cannot fully reverse during fibrosis regression. DEI has the potential to be a new tool for assessing the prognosis of cirrhosis by the severity of microvascular abnormalities during various stages of the disease.

Supporting Information

Figure S1 Portal vein (red arrow), bile duct (red arrowhead) and central vein (yellow arrow) were illustrated by bile duct ligation rat models.

Figure S2 Quantitative analysis of angiogenic related factors. VEGF, Ang-1, PDGF mRNA (A) using real time polymerase chain reaction were showed**.** Enzyme-linked immunosorbent assay quantification of VEGF protein level (B). Change of angiogenic factors was parallel to the extent of vascular remodeling and severity of cirrhosis. Results are expressed the mean ±SEM. * $p<0.05$ compared with the control group. # $p<0.05$ compared with the cirrhotic group.

Acknowledgments

The authors gratefully acknowledge the assistance of the 4W1A station of Beijing Synchrotron Radiation Facility.

Author Contributions

Conceived and designed the experiments: TLW BEW XYZ. Performed the experiments: DDH YC XML. Analyzed the data: DDH YC TLW XYZ. Wrote the paper: DDH YC AB XYZ.

References

1. Sorensen HT, Thulstrup AM, Mellemkjar L, Jepsen P, Christensen E, et al. (2003) Long-term survival and cause-specific mortality in patients with cirrhosis of the liver: a nationwide cohort study in Denmark. J Clin Epidemiol 56: 88–93.
2. Zois CD, Baltayiannis GH, Karayiannis P, Tsianos EV. (2008) Systematic review: hepatic fibrosis - regression with therapy. Aliment Pharmacol Ther 28: 1175–1187.
3. Valfre dBL, Novo E, Cannito S, Busletta C, Paternostro C, et al. (2009) Angiogenesis and liver fibrogenesis. Histol Histopathol 24: 1323–1341.
4. Fernandez M, Semela D, Bruix J, Colle I, Pinzani M, et al. (2009) Angiogenesis in liver disease. J Hepatol 50: 604–620.
5. Coulon S, Heindryckx F, Geerts A, Van Steenkiste C, Colle I, et al. (2011) Angiogenesis in chronic liver disease and its complications. Liver Int 31: 146–162.
6. Iwakiri Y. (2012) Endothelial dysfunction in the regulation of cirrhosis and portal hypertension. Liver Int 32: 199–213.
7. Thabut D, Shah V. (2010) Intrahepatic angiogenesis and sinusoidal remodeling in chronic liver disease: new targets for the treatment of portal hypertension. J Hepatol 53: 976–980.
8. Zhang X, Liu XS, Yang XR, Chen SL, Zhu PP, et al. (2008) Mouse blood vessel imaging by in-line x-ray phase-contrast imaging. Phys Med Biol 53: 5735–5743.
9. Chapman D, Thomlinson W, Johnston RE, Washburn D, Pisano E, et al. (1997) Diffraction enhanced x-ray imaging. Phys Med Biol 42: 2015–2025.
10. Zhao Y, Brun E, Coan P, Huang Z, Sztrokay A, et al. (2012) High-resolution, low-dose phase contrast X-ray tomography for 3D diagnosis of human breast cancers. Proc Natl Acad Sci U S A 109: 18290–18294.
11. Faulconer LS, Parham CA, Connor DM, Kuzmiak C, Koomen M, et al. (2010) Effect of breast compression on lesion characteristic visibility with diffraction-enhanced imaging. Acad Radiol 17: 433–440.
12. Zhang X, Yang XR, Chen Y, Li HQ, Liu WY, et al. (2010) Diffraction - enhanced radiography of various mouse organs. AJR Am J Roentgenol 195: 545–549.
13. Lewis RA, Hall CJ, Hufton AP, Evans S, Menk RH, et al. (2003) X-ray refraction effects: application to the imaging of biological tissues. Br J Radiol 76: 301–308.
14. Van Steenkiste C, Trachet B, Casteleyn C, van Loo D, Van Hoorebeke L, et al. (2010) Vascular corrosion casting: analyzing wall shear stress in the portal vein and vascular abnormalities in portal hypertensive and cirrhotic rodents. Lab Invest 90: 1558–1572.
15. Wernick MN, Wirjadi O, Chapman D, Zhong Z, et al. (2003) Multiple-image radiography. Phys Med Biol 48: 3875–3895.
16. Romanenko AM, Ruiz-Sauri A, Morell-Quadreny L, Valencia G, Vozianov AF, et al. (2012) Microvessel density is high in clear-cell renal cell carcinomas of Ukrainian patients exposed to chronic persistent low-dose ionizing radiation after the Chernobyl accident. Virchows Arch 460: 611–619.
17. Van Steenkiste C, Trachet B, Casteleyn C, van Loo D, Van Hoorebeke L, et al. (2010) Vascular corrosion casting: analyzing wall shear stress in the portal vein

and vascular abnormalities in portal hypertensive and cirrhotic rodents. Lab Invest 90: 1558–1572.
18. Tanaka F, Otake Y, Yanagihara K, Kawano Y, Miyahara R, et al. (2001) Evaluation of angiogenesis in non-small cell lung cancer: comparison between anti-CD34 antibody and anti-CD105 antibody. Clin Cancer Res 7: 3410–3415.
19. Lemos QT, Andrade ZA. (2010) Angiogenesis and experimental hepatic fibrosis. Mem Inst Oswaldo Cruz 105: 611–614.
20. Desmet VJ, Roskams T. (2004) Cirrhosis reversal: a duel between dogma and myth. J Hepatol 40: 860–867.
21. Di VI, Baptista AP, Barbosa AA, Andrade ZA. (2005) Morphological signs of cirrhosis regression. Experimental observations on carbon tetrachloride-induced liver cirrhosis of rats. Pathol Res Pract 201: 449–456.
22. Gex L, Bernard C, Spahr L. (2010) [Child-Pugh, MELD and Maddrey scores]. Rev Med Suisse 6: 18031804, 1806–1808.
23. Keyrilainen J, Fernandez M, Fiedler S, Bravin A, Karjalainen-Lindsberg ML, et al. (2005) Visualisation of calcifications and thin collagen strands in human breast tumor specimens by the diffraction-enhanced imaging technique: a comparison with conventional mammography and histology. Eur J Radiol 53: 226–237.
24. Keyrilainen J, Fernandez M, Fiedler S, Bravin A, Karjalainen-Lindsberg ML, et al. (2005) Visualisation of calcifications and thin collagen strands in human breast tumour specimens by the diffraction-enhanced imaging technique: a comparison with conventional mammography and histology Eur J Radiol 53: 226–237.
25. Jia Y, Alkayed N, Wang RK. (2009) Potential of optical microangiography to monitor cerebral blood perfusion and vascular plasticity following traumatic brain injury in mice in vivo. J Biomed Opt 1: 040505.
26. Wanless IR, Nakashima E, Sherman M. (2000) Regression of human cirrhosis. Morphologic features and the genesis of incomplete septal cirrhosis. Arch Pathol Lab Med 124: 1599–1607.
27. Takeda T, Yoneyama A Wu J, Momose A, Hyodo K. (2012) In vivo physiological saline-infused hepatic vessel imaging using a two-crystal-interferometer-based phase-contrast X-ray technique. J Synchrotron Radiat 19: 252–256.
28. Yu Y, Xiong Z, Lv Y, Qian Y, Jiang S, et al. (2006) In vivo evaluation of early disease progression by X-ray phase-contrast imaging in the adjuvant-induced arthritic rat. Skeletal Radiol 35: 156–164.
29. Coan P, Wagner A, Bravin A, Diemoz PC, Keyrilainen J, et al. (2010) In vivo x-ray phase contrast analyzer-based imaging for longitudinal osteoarthritis studies in guinea pigs. Phys Med Biol 55: 7649–7662.
30. Donnelley M, Siu KK, Jamison RA, Parsons DW. (2012) Synchrotron phase-contrast X-ray imaging reveals fluid dosing dynamics for gene transfer into mouse airways. Gene Ther 19: 8–14.
31. Tanaka J, Nagashima M, Kido K, Hoshino Y, Kiyohara J, et al. (2013) Cadaveric and in vivo human joint imaging based on differential phase contrast by X-ray Talbot-Lau interferometry. Z Med Phys 23: 222–227.
32. Arfelli F, Bonvicini V, Bravin A, Cantatore G, Castelli E, et al. (2000) Mammography with synchrotron radiation: phase-detection techniques. Radiology 215: 286–293.

3

The Thermostable Direct Hemolysin from *Grimontia hollisae* Causes Acute Hepatotoxicity *In Vitro* and *In Vivo*

Yan-Ren Lin[1,2,7], Yao-Li Chen[3,7], Keh-Bin Wang[4], Yi-Fang Wu[1], Yu-Kuo Wang[1]*, Sheng-Cih Huang[1], Tzu-An Liu[5], Manoswini Nayak[1], Bak-Sau Yip[6]*, Tung-Kung Wu[1]*

1 Department of Biological Science and Technology, National Chiao Tung University, Hsin-Chu, Taiwan, Republic of China, **2** Department of Emergency Medicine, Changhua Christian Hospital, Changhua, Taiwan, Republic of China, **3** Transplant Medicine and Surgery Research Centre, Changhua Christian Hospital, Changhua, Taiwan, Republic of China, **4** Department of Nuclear Medicine, Kuang Tien General Hospital, Taichung, Taiwan, Republic of China, **5** Institute of Cellular and System Medicine, National Health Research Institutes, Zhunan, Miaoli County, Taiwan, Republic of China, **6** Department of Neurology, National Taiwan University Hospital Hsin Chu Branch, Hsin-Chu, Taiwan, Republic of China, **7** School of Medicine, Chung Shan Medical University, Taichung, Taiwan, Republic of China

Abstract

Background: G. hollisae thermostable direct hemolysin (Gh-TDH) is produced by most strains of *G. hollisae.* This toxin has been reported to be absorbed in the intestines in humans. Secondary liver injury might be caused by venous return of the toxin through the portal system. We aimed to firstly analyze the *in vitro* and *in vivo* hepatotoxicity of Gh-TDH.

Methods: Liver cells (primary human non-cancer cell and FL83B mouse cells) were treated and mice (BALB/c) were fed with this toxin to investigate its hepatotoxicity. Morphological examination and cytotoxicity assays using liver cells were also performed. Fluorescein isothiocyanate-conjugated toxin was used to analyze the localization of this protein in liver cells. Mice were subjected to liver function measurements and liver biopsies following toxin treatment and wild-type bacterial infection. PET (positron emission tomography)/CT (computed tomography) images were taken to assess liver metabolism during acute injury and recovery.

Results: The effect of hepatotoxicity was dose and time dependent. Cellular localization showed that the toxin was initially located around the cellular margins and subsequently entered the nucleus. Liver function measurements and liver biopsies of the mice following treatment with toxin or infection with wild-type *Grimontia hollisae* showed elevated levels of transaminases and damage to the periportal area, respectively. The PET/CT images revealed that the reconstruction of the liver continued for at least one week after exposure to a single dose of the toxin or bacterial infection.

Conclusions: The hepatotoxicity of Gh-TDH was firstly demonstrated. The damage was located in the periportal area of the liver, and the liver became functionally insufficient.

Editor: Cordula M. Stover, University of Leicester, United Kingdom

Funding: The authors thank National Chiao Tung University and the Ministry of Education, Aiming for Top University Plan (MOE ATU Program), and the National Science Council (NSC-99-2113-M-009 -004 -MY2) for financially supporting this research. The funders had no role in study design, data collection and analysis, decision to publish, or preparation of the manuscript.

Competing Interests: The authors have declared that no competing interests exist.

* E-mail: yu.kuo@yahoo.com.tw (Y-KW); neuron.nctu@gmail.com (B-SY); tkwmll@mail.nctu.edu.tw (T-KW)

Introduction

Diseases caused by different *Vibrio* species have been observed in large populations throughout the world, particularly in Asia, the United States, and Africa [1–3]. *V. cholera* and *V. parahaemolyticus* are the major etiological agents of vibriosis, which is associated with the ingestion of raw, undercooked, or contaminated seafood [1,2]. *Grimontia hollisae* (previously named *V. hollisae)* has been frequently reported to cause diseases in humans, including severe gastroenteritis, hypovolemia, and septicemia following the consumption of shellfish or oysters [4–6]. However, the mechanism of morbidity due to *G. hollisae* has not been thoroughly characterized. Although several specific laboratory examinations have detected *G. hollisae*, its incidence is likely highly underestimated because detection techniques are infrequently used throughout the world [7,8].

The toxin thermostable direct hemolysin (TDH) is composed of 165 amino acid residues and exhibits biological activities that include hemolytic activity, cytotoxicity, and enterotoxicity [9]. The toxic effects of TDH have been identified in a variety of *Vibrio* species, including *V. cholera* non-O1, *V. parahaemolyticus*, *V. mimicus*, *V. alginolyticus*, and *G. hollisae* [10–14]. In addition, TDH production has been observed in bacteria with similar *tdh* gene sequences and pathogenicities [15,16]. The *tdh* gene is present in all strains of *G. hollisae* but not in all *Vibrio* species [10]. The physical characteristics of *G. hollisae* TDH (Gh-TDH) are not well known. Some studies have reported that Gh-TDH is detoxified by aggregation into fibrils after heating at 60–70°C; the protein can be reversibly refolded into the toxic native form by rapid cooling after unfolding at higher temperatures [17]. The hemolytic activity of Gh-TDH is suppressed by the addition of Congo red [18]. In addition, the lipophilic effect of Gh-TDH has not been clearly characterized. The toxic effects of TDH have been localized mainly in the intestinal portion of the gastrointestinal tract [19–21]. However, a relationship between the TDH and the liver has not been reported or analyzed. In addition to being absorbed by the intestine, TDH may also cause secondary injury to the liver via effects on the venous return of the portal system. In this study, we analyzed the hepatotoxicity of TDH *in vivo* and *in vitro* to provide insights into the acute injury and recovery stages of THD-induced hepatotoxicity in living animals.

Materials and Methods

Bacterial Strains and Materials

G. hollisae strain ATCC 33564 was obtained from the Culture Collection and Research Center (Hsin-Chu, Taiwan). Phenyl Sepharose 6 Fast Flow and protein molecular weight standards were purchased from GE Healthcare (Piscataway, NJ). The protein assay kit was obtained from Bio-Rad (Hercules, CA). Protein purification chemicals were obtained from Calbiochem (La Jolla, CA).

Molecular Cloning, Protein Expression and Purification, and Characterization of *G. hollisae* Recombinant Thermostable Direct Hemolysin (Gh-rTDH)

Molecular cloning, protein expression, and purification of Gh-rTDH were performed according to previous publications [20,21]. The effect of endotoxin was excluded before the start of the experiment. For the purpose of this study, endotoxin contamination was excluded during protein preparation by anion-exchange chromatography using diethylaminoethane (DEAE) chromatographic matrices [22,23]. The protein identities of the SDS-PAGE bands corresponding to Gh-rTDH were confirmed by MALDI-TOF/TOF spectrometry.

Cytoviability and Morphological Examination of Gh-rTDH-treated Human Liver Cells and FL83B Cells

FL83B (BCRC 60325) and primary human non-cancer cells (which were kindly provided by the liver transplantation center of a medical center in central Taiwan; IRB number: 120305) were cultured for use in these studies. Following surface attachment, the cells were treated with Gh-rTDH at a concentration of 1 μg/ml for 24 hr at 37°C; the treatment dose was determined by using the initial results from the IC_{50} determination (1 μg/ml, as obtained from the MTT assay). Cellular morphology in the experimental group was observed microscopically at 4 time points (before and after exposure to Gh-rTDH for 8, 16, and 24 hr). Cells treated with PBS (mixed with culture medium) were used as the control group and were observed at the same time points as the experimental group. The cytoviability of human liver cells and FL83B cells was measured by MTT assay at 4 treatment durations (12, 16, 24, and 48 hr). In the MTT assay, cells were treated with PBS as a control and with Gh-rTDH at different concentrations (10 to 10^{-8} μg/ml mixed with culture medium and administered in a total volume of 250 μl). All experiments were independently performed five times.

Localization of the Gh-rTDH Protein in FL83B Cells

To investigate the localization of Gh-rTDH after its entry into FL83B cells, Gh-rTDH was conjugated with fluorescein isothiocyanate (FITC) to produce Gh-rTDH-FITC, and reactions were performed using the FluoReporter FITC Protein Labeling Kit (Molecular Probes) according to the manufacturer's protocol. Two batches of cells (plated at 1×10^4 cells/well) were independently treated with 10 μg/ml Gh-rTDH-FITC for 20 and 40 min, washed 3 times with PBS, and stained with propidium iodide (PI) for 5 min in the dark. Images were acquired by confocal microscopy (wavelength: $\lambda_{ex} = 488$ and $\lambda_{em} = 650$ nm).

In vivo Hepatotoxicity of Gh-rTDH in BALB/c Mice

A total of 114 six-week-old female mice were obtained from the National Laboratory Animal Center of Taiwan for the analysis of *in vivo* hepatotoxicity. All mice were fed normal diets. This study was carried out in strict accordance with the recommendations of the Guide for the Care and Use of Laboratory Animals of the National Institutes of Health. The protocol was approved by the Committee on the Ethics of Animal Experiments of National Chiao Tung University (Permit Number: 01001008). All surgery was performed under sodium pentobarbital anesthesia, and all efforts were made to minimize suffering.

Withdrawal of Blood for Liver Function Analysis (n = 25)

A total of 25 mice were assigned to one of 5 groups (n = 5 for each group). One group served as a control group and was administered PBS; the other 4 groups were administered different doses of Gh-rTDH (0.1, 1, 10, and 100 μg) in a single treatment. The dosage that might initiate organ injury in animals has not been reported (information on natural infection in humans is also lacking). Therefore, the treatment dosages were carefully determined and modified according to the initial results of the IC_{50} determination (1 μg/ml, as determined by the MTT assay described above). All mice were treated with the same volume (200 μl) and the same treatment time (10:00 a.m.) via gastric tubes without volume loss (i.e., vomiting). A total of 100 μl of whole blood was withdrawn from the orbital vascular plexus of each mouse through a capillary tube with no analgesics. Samples were taken at 8 time points: before treatment with PBS or Gh-rTDH and 4, 8, 16, 32, 64, 128, and 256 hr after treatment with PBS or Gh-rTDH. The blood samples were analyzed for the continuation of liver function as assessed by glutamic-oxaloacetic transaminase (GOT), glutamic-pyruvic transaminase (GPT), total/direct/indirect bilirubin, albumin, and globulin (Reagents Beckman Coulter). One-way ANOVA analysis was used to analyze the significance of differences between each treatment/time point. All analyses were performed with the SPSS statistical package for Windows (Version 15.0, SPSS Inc., Chicago, IL).

Withdrawal of Blood for Cardiotoxicity and Nephrotoxicity Analyses (n = 20)

A total of 20 mice were assigned to one of 4 groups (n = 5 in each group). One group served as the control group and was treated with PBS. The other 3 groups were treated with Gh-rTDH at doses of 1, 10, and 100 μg in a single administration via a gastric tube. A total of 100 μl of whole blood was withdrawn from each mouse at 5 time points: before treatment with PBS or Gh-rTDH and 4, 16, 64, and 256 hr after treatment with PBS or Gh-rTDH. Nephrotoxicity was assessed by determining the creatinine levels in the blood samples (Creatinine Reagent, Beckman Coulter), and cardiotoxicity was assessed by analyzing the levels of CK-MB (CK-MB Reagent Pack, Beckman Coulter) and troponin I (ADVIA Centaur TnI-Ultra Ready Pack).

Liver Biopsy (n = 9)

A total of 9 mice were assigned to one of 3 groups which were treated with PBS, 10 μg Gh-rTDH, or 100 μg Gh-rTDH (n = 3 in

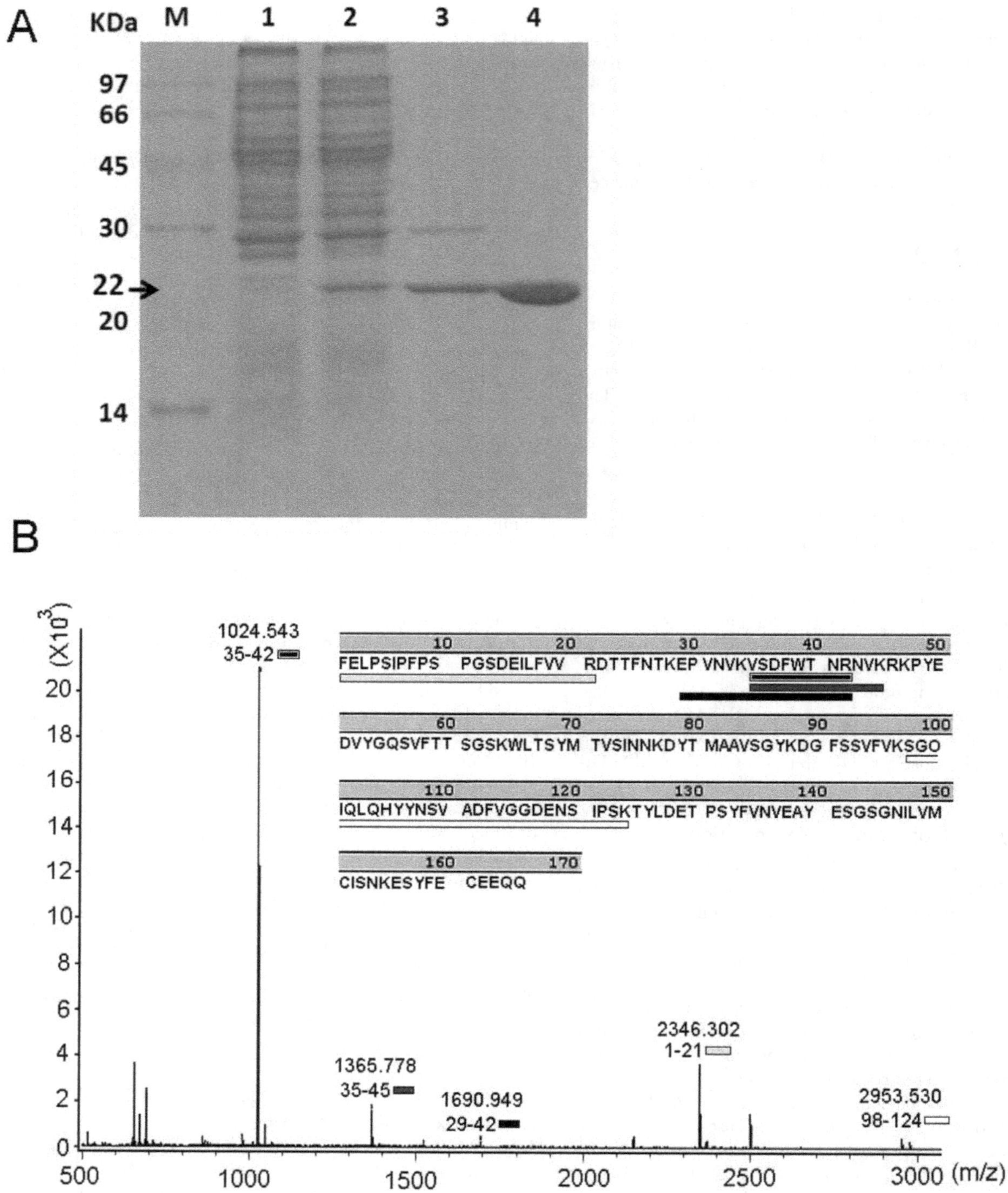

Figure 1. Identification of Gh-rTDH purified from G. hollisae. (A) SDS-PAGE analysis of Gh-rTDH. Marker proteins (M): phosphorylase b (97 kDa), albumin (66 kDa), ovalbumin (45 kDa), carbonic anhydrase (30 kDa), trypsin inhibitor (20 kDa), and α-lactoalbumin (14 kDa); lane 1: cell crude extract of BL21(DE3) pLysS containing the pCR2.1-TOPO plasmid alone; lane 2: crude protein expression in BL21(DE3) pLysS containing pCR2.1-TOPO-*Gh-tdh*; lanes 3 and 4: Phenyl Sepharose 6 Fast Flow purification yielded a homogenous protein with a molecular mass of ~22 kDa. (B) The tandem mass spectrum of the doubly charged tryptic peptide at *m/z* 1024.543 from the SDS-PAGE of Gh-rTDH revealed a unique hit matching ^{35}VSDFWTNR^{42} of the Gh-rTDH peptide sequence.

each group) in a single administration via a gastric tube. The livers of all mice were biopsied after 8 hr of treatment. Samples were prepared from tissue that was harvested at the time of sacrifice and subjected to H&E staining.

PET/CT Scan (n = 60)

A ^{18}F-FDG PET/CT scan was used to detect liver cell glucose metabolism in living animals after exposure to Gh-rTDH to monitor trends in glucose metabolism (GE Medical System). ^{18}F-FDG is an analog of glucose that can be used to measure glucose

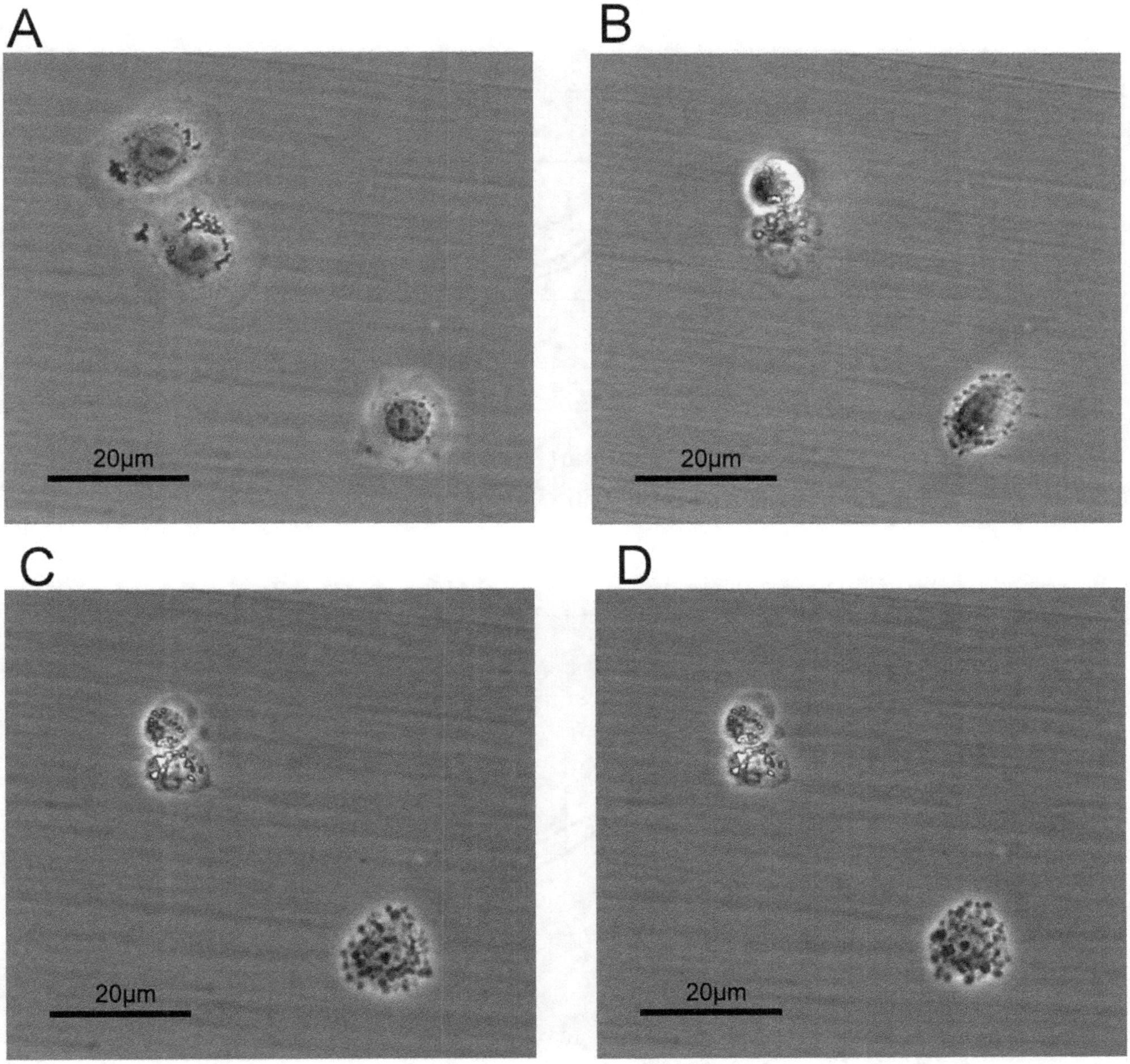

Figure 2. Liver cell morphology was affected by the administration of Gh-rTDH. The morphology of liver cells (FL83B) was clearly changed after the administration of 1 μg/ml Gh-rTDH for 24 hours at 37°C. The morphological changes included cell detachment and a loss of cell cytoplasm with cell shrinkage; they were the same cells that were recorded at different time points. Liver cells before (A) and after exposure to the Gh-rTDH protein for 8 hr (B), 16 hr (C), and 24 hr (D).

metabolism in organs and cells. A total of 60 mice were assigned to one of 4 dosage groups, and each group (n = 15) was treated with PBS or 1, 10, or 100 μg of Gh-rTDH in a single administration. Within each dosage group, mice were further sub-grouped to receive ^{18}F-FDG PET/CT scans over time; examinations were performed at 8, 72, and 168 hr (n = 5 for each time group) after treatment with Gh-rTDH. For this study, 0.07 mCi of ^{18}F-FDG was administered to each mouse by tail vein injection. Imaging was performed under appropriate general anesthesia (Isoflurane) one hour after ^{18}F-FDG injection. In this study, each mouse did not receive a ^{18}F-FDG PET/CT scan at each time point. The recurring general anesthesia might cause hepatotoxicity, which could influence the results of the study. For this analysis, the ^{18}F-FDG uptake value was calculated by using a region of interest approach (ROI). The ROIs of liver and muscle (left foot) were determined by a semi-quantitative method using the ratio of liver/muscle ^{18}F-FDG uptake.

Infection Models of *in vivo* Hepatotoxicity of *G. hollisae*, *Escherichia coli* Expressing Recombinant Gh-tdh (E. coli-TOPO-tdh), and the *E. coli*-TOPO Strain in BALB/c Mice (n = 126)

An animal infection model was established to evaluate the hepatotoxicity of bacterial infection. The *G. hollisae* (wild type), *E. coli*-TOPO-*tdh*, and *E. coli*-TOPO strains were cultured. A total of 75 mice were assigned to one of three major groups (n = 25 for each group) and infected with bacteria via oral administration. Two groups were infected with *G. hollisae* and *E. coli*-TOPO-*tdh* to

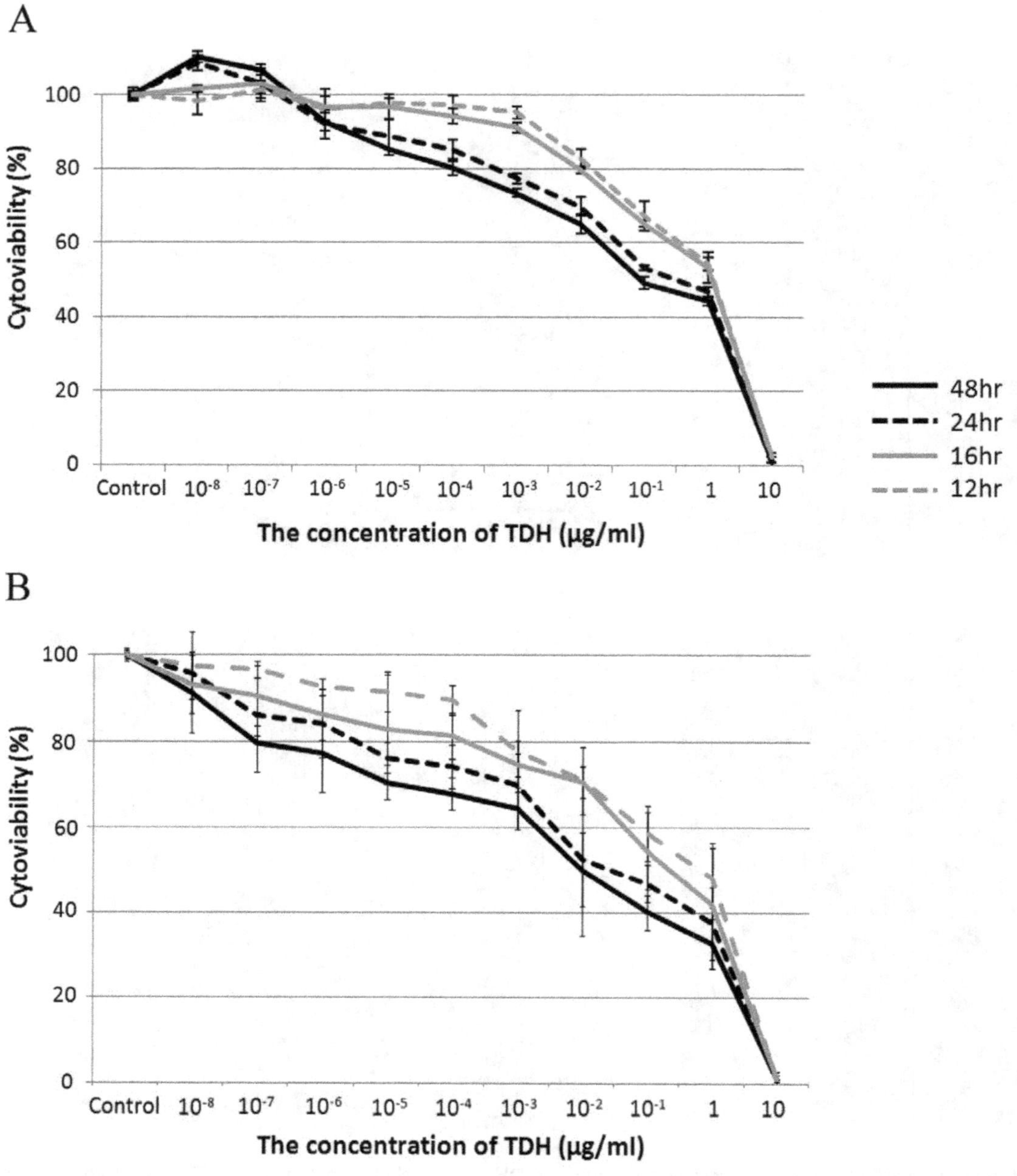

Figure 3. The MTT assay. The MTT assay revealed that the cytoviability of both (A) mouse and (B) human liver cells decreased in proportion to the concentration of Gh-rTDH over different treatment durations. Moreover, we noted that Gh-rTDH damaged liver cells *in vitro* when the concentration of Gh-rTDH exceeded 10^{-6} μg/ml.

demonstrate their hepatotoxicity; the third group was infected with *E. coli*-TOPO as a control. For each major group, five subgroups were established (n = 5 for each group) according to treatment dosage (10^7, 10^8, 10^9, 10^{10}, and 10^{11} organisms/ml, all with the same volumes). A total of 100 μl of whole blood was withdrawn at 8 different time points: before treatment with bacteria and 4, 8, 16, 32, 64, 128 and 256 hours after bacterial treatment. Blood samples were analyzed for continued liver function (GOT, GPT, total bilirubin, albumin, and globulin). In addition, 6 mice were treated with 10^{11} organisms/ml of *G. hollisae, E. coli*-TOPO-*tdh*, and *E. coli*-TOPO (n = 2 for each group). For these animals, liver biopsies and H&E staining (200X) were performed 8 hr after bacterial treatment. Finally, 54 mice were treated with *G. hollisae, E. coli*-TOPO-*tdh*, and *E. coli*-TOPO (n = 18 for each group) with a single administration. Within each group, mice were sub-grouped for treatment with bacteria at concentrations of 10^7, 10^9, and 10^{11} organisms/ml (n = 6 for each group). In each concentration group, mice received a PET/CT scan at 8, 72, and 168 hr (n = 2 for each group) after bacterial treatment.

Results

1. Identification of Gh-rTDH Purified from *G. hollisae*

SDS-PAGE of the homogeneous protein indicated a molecular mass of ~22 kDa. Moreover, the tandem mass spectrum of the doubly charged tryptic peptide at m/z 1024.543 from an SDS-PAGE of Gh-rTDH revealed a unique hit matching

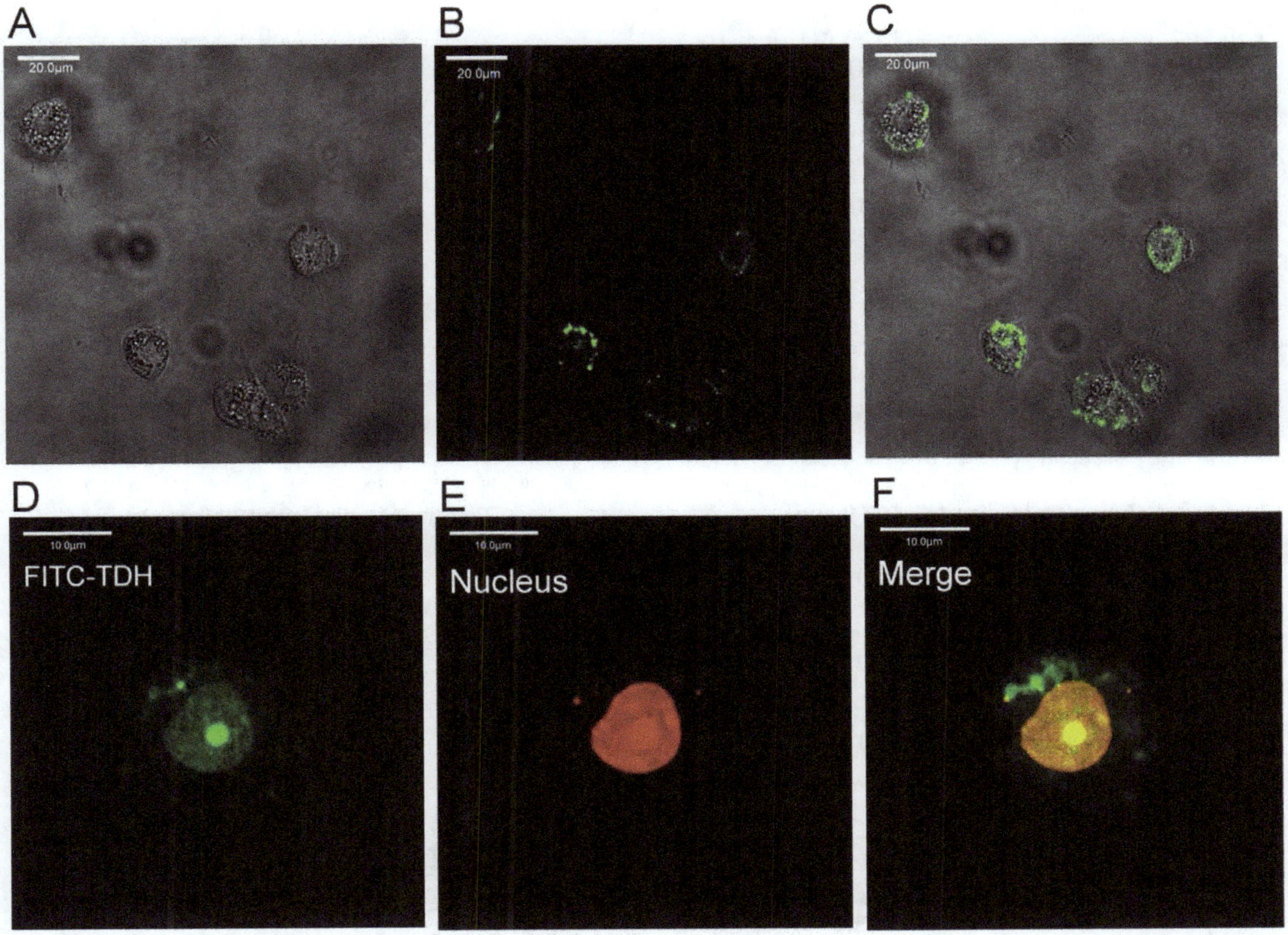

Figure 4. Subcellular localization of Gh-rTDH. Liver cells were treated with 10 μg/ml Gh-rTDH-FITC for 20 (A–C) or 40 (D–F) min at 26°C and were then observed by confocal microscopy. (A) The liver cells were observed without a FITC filter, (B) with a FITC filter, (C) and with A and B merged, confirming that Gh-rTDH-FITC (green) could bind around the liver cell margins. (D) Gh-rTDH-FITC (green) was taken up by the nuclei of liver cells. (E) Nuclei stained with PI (red). (F) The merge of D and E confirmed that Gh-rTDH-FITC was located in the nuclei of liver cells.

^{35}VSDFWTNR^{42} of the Gh-rTDH peptide sequence (by MALDI TOF/TOF spectrum) (Figure 1).

2. Hepatotoxicity was Demonstrated by *in vitro* Analyses

2.1 Gh-rTDH causes *in vitro* liver cell damage. Liver cell morphology was clearly affected by the administration of Gh-rTDH (Figure 2). In the control group (treated with PBS), we did not observe any morphological changes (or damage). The MTT assay revealed that the cytoviability of both mouse and human liver cells decreased in proportion to the concentrations of Gh-rTDH (Figures 3A and B). The hepatotoxicity caused by Gh-rTDH was both dose- and time-dependent. Very low concentrations of toxin ($>10^{-6}$ μg/ml) caused damage to the liver cells.

2.2 Gh-rTDH-FITC binds to the margins of liver cells and is taken up by their nuclei. Gh-rTDH-FITC was bound around the margin of liver cells after the administration of 10 μg/ml Gh-rTDH-FITC for 20 min (Figures 4A–C). Moreover, Gh-rTDH-FITC was translocated to the nuclei of liver cells after treatment with Gh-rTDH-FITC for 40 min; the locations of the nuclei were confirmed by PI staining (Figures 4D–F).

3. Acute Hepatotoxicity was Noted by *in vivo* Analyses

3.1 *In vivo* liver damage is quickly induced by Gh-rTDH. The levels of GOT and GPT were not elevated in the control group after the administration of a single dose of PBS. However, the mean GOT and GPT levels were clearly elevated in the group that was treated with 0.1 μg Gh-rTDH, and the highest levels were observed 8 hr after toxin administration. Similar findings were observed in other treatment groups. Higher doses of Gh-rTDH were clearly associated with more severe mouse liver injury (Figures 5A and B).

3.2 Gh-rTDH induces an acute hemolytic status *in vivo*. Total bilirubin levels were clearly elevated in the groups that were treated with Gh-rTDH, and an increased dosage of Gh-rTDH resulted in further increases in total bilirubin levels (Figure 5C). Moreover, the proportions of indirect bilirubin were much higher than the direct bilirubin within 8 hr after exposure to 1 μg or 100 μg Gh-rTDH (Figure 6). Thus, an acute hemolytic status could be induced *in vivo* by the administration of Gh-rTDH.

3.3 Gh-rTDH damages the albumin synthesis capacity of the liver and triggers the immune response. Albumin levels began to decrease at 32 hr after Gh-rTDH administration, and the decrease was proportional to the dosage. In the groups that were treated with Gh-rTDH, albumin levels progressively de-

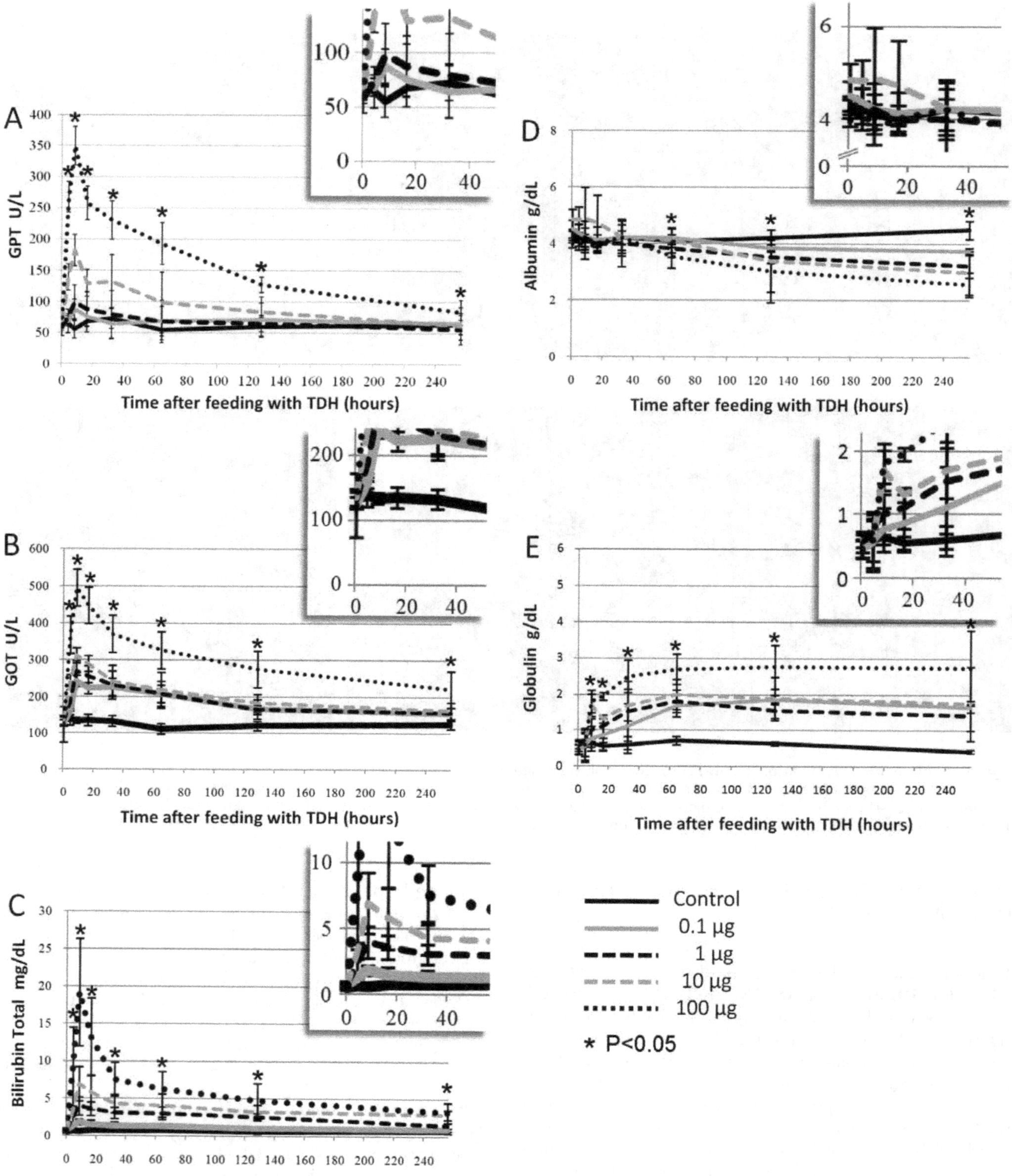

Figure 5. Liver function evaluation after a single administration of Gh-rTDH. The levels of liver function were abnormal after a single administration of Gh-rTDH. Six-week-old female BALB\c were treated with four different dosages of Gh-rTDH (0.1, 1, 10, and 100 µg), and the control group was treated with PBS (n = 5 for each group). Acute liver injury was demonstrated by elevated levels of (A) GPT and (B) GOT; the highest levels could be found at the 8th hr after feeding in both. (C) Hyperbilirubinemia and (D) hypoalbuminemia also occurred in the mice that were treated with Gh-rTDH. The hyperbilirubinemia was the most severe at the 8th hr, and hypoalbuminemia was noted after 32 hr of treatment with Gh-rTDH. (E) Globulin levels were gradually increased after exposure to Gh-rTDH. *A p-value <0.05 was considered statistically significant.

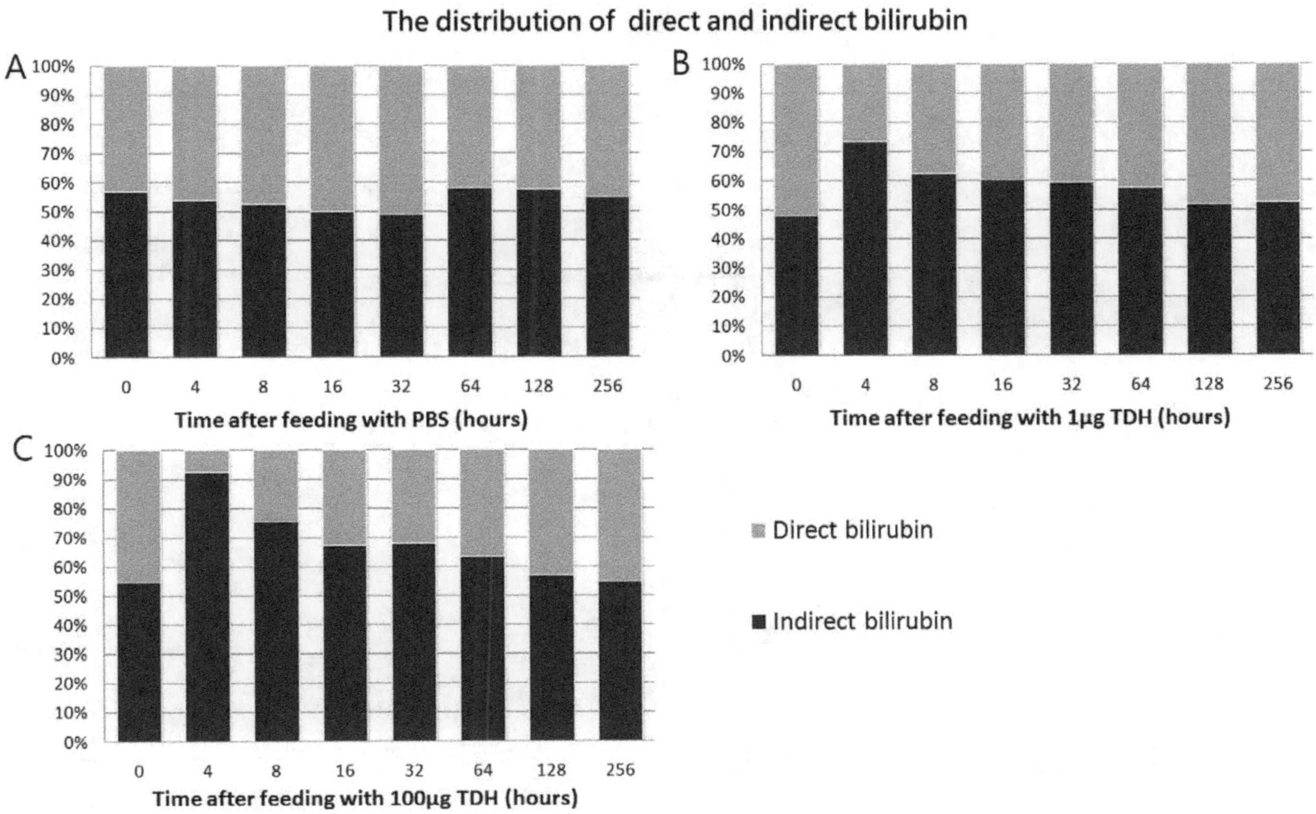

Figure 6. Gh-rTDH induces an acute hemolytic status. The distribution of direct and indirect bilirubin in mice that were fed with (A) PBS (control), (B) 1 μg of Gh-rTDH, or (C) 100 μg of Gh-rTDH.

creased and did not recover, even in the 256-hr treatment group (Figure 5D). These results indicate that albumin synthesis was damaged and did not recover during the initial 256 hr. By contrast, globulin levels were higher in the groups that received Gh-rTDH than in the control groups. This finding indicates that Gh-rTDH might trigger an immune system response in the circulation (Figure 5E).

3.4 Gh-rTDH might not cause *in vitro* cardiotoxicity and nephrotoxicity. Creatinine and CK-MB levels, which reflect kidney and heart injuries, were not elevated in Gh-rTDH-treated mice. The levels of creatinine and CK-MB did not change in proportion to the dosage of Gh-rTDH. The troponin I levels were also normal in all Gh-rTDH-treated mice (Figure 7).

3.5 Hepatic damage is located in the periportal area of the liver. No pathological changes were noted in the liver parenchyma of the control group (Figure 8A). In mice treated with 10 μg Gh-rTDH, biopsies revealed the preservation of liver parenchymal architecture with mild congestion over the periportal areas and spotty liver cell damage around the portal vein. The damage was clearly located in the periportal area of the liver (zone 1 of the liver acinus) (Figure 8B). Moreover, severe congestion with hemorrhage was noted in mice that were treated with 100 μg Gh-rTDH (Figure 8C). Similar findings were noted for each mouse group that was biopsied.

3.6 ^{18}F-FDG PET/CT scans reveal decreases in and recovery of metabolism in the livers of treated animals. A series of 3 images was acquired for each mouse, including CT, PET, and a merge of the CT and PET after the ^{18}F-FDG PET/CT scan. The red color in the merge images indicates ^{18}F-FDG uptake by cells (Figure 9A). We found that hepatic ^{18}F-FDG uptake in the livers of mice treated with Gh-rTDH was significantly lower than in mice that were given PBS; the decreased uptake was proportional to the dose of Gh-rTDH (Figure 9B). Moreover, we also noted that the ratios of liver/muscle ^{18}F-FDG uptake levels clearly decreased at the 8th hr after treatment with Gh-rTDH dose-dependently. In addition, the ratios of liver/muscle ^{18}F-FDG uptake levels recovered to a normal range and even crossed the normal range during the 72nd and 168th hr after treatment with Gh-rTDH. These results indicate that liver glucose metabolism initially decreased after exposure to Gh-rTDH but that recovery continued for at least one week after a single exposure to the toxin (Figure 9C).

3.7 *G. hollisae* and *E. coli*-TOPO-tdh but not *E. coli*-TOPO causes *in vivo* hepatotoxicity. GOT and GPT levels were not elevated after administration of *E. coli*-TOPO. However, the mean GOT and GPT levels were clearly elevated in the groups treated with *G. hollisae* or *E. coli*-TOPO-*tdh*, and the highest levels were observed 8 hr after bacterial treatment (data not shown). Higher concentrations of bacteria caused more severe liver injury. Acute hemolytic status, poor albumin synthesis, and more strongly induced immune system function were noted in mice that were fed *G. hollisae* and *E. coli*-TOPO-*tdh*. These patterns are similar to those observed in mice treated with Gh-rTDH. There was no pathological damage to the liver parenchyma in mice treated with *E. coli*-TOPO (Figure 8D). By contrast, spotty liver cell damage around the portal vein was noted in mice that were treated with *G. hollisae* (Figure 8E) or *E. coli*-TOPO-*tdh* (Figure 8F). The ^{18}F-FDG PET/CT images revealed that the mice treated with *G. hollisae* (Figure 9D) or *E. coli*-TOPO-*tdh* (Figure 9E) exhibited much less ^{18}F-FDG hepatic uptake than those treated with *E. coli*-TOPO

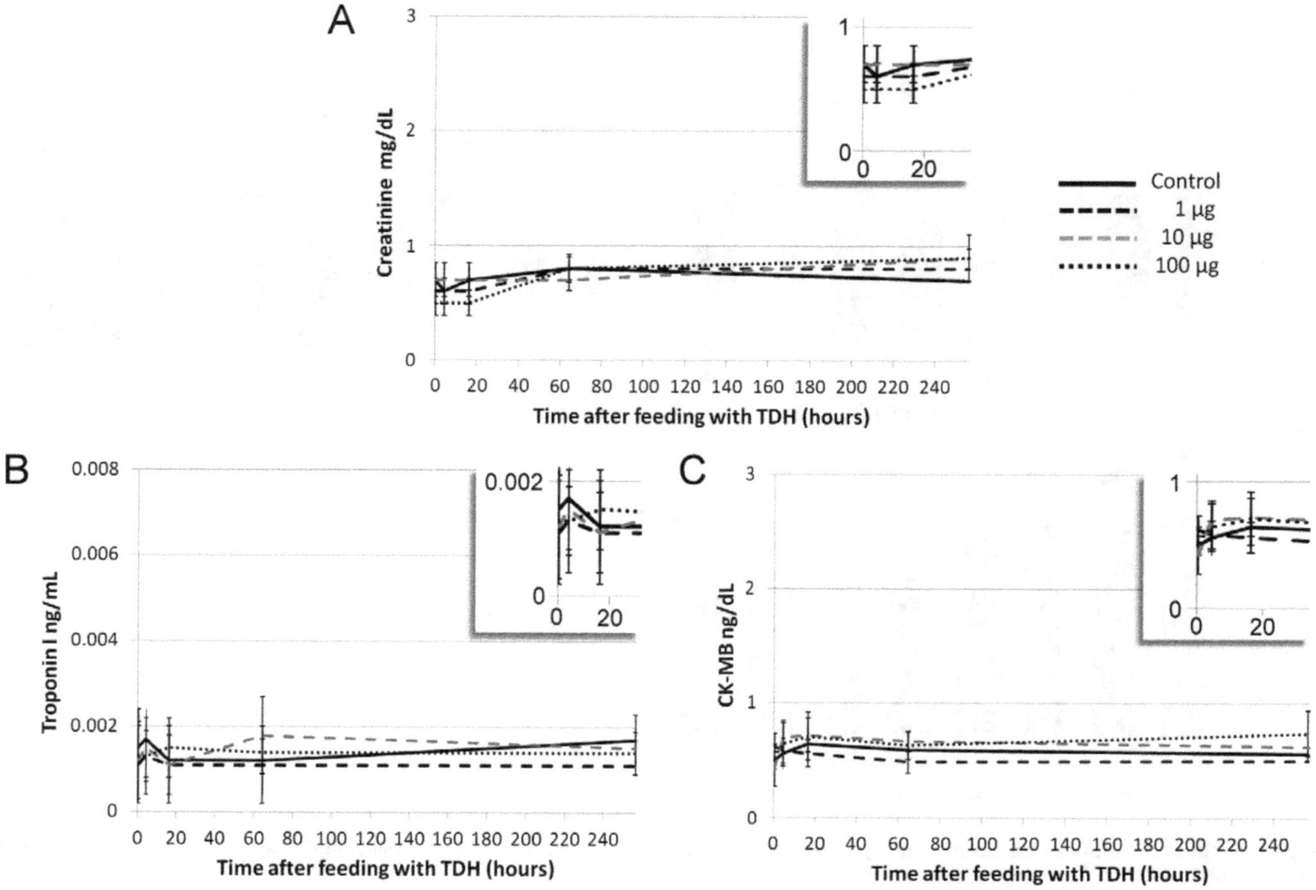

Figure 7. Gh-rTDH might not cause cardiotoxicity and nephrotoxicity. The levels of (A) creatinine, (B) CK-MB, and (C) troponin I did not significantly increase when mice were treated with different doses of Gh-rTDH.

(Figure 9F). Overall, the patterns of hepatotoxicity were notably similar between mice infected with *G. hollisae* or treated with Gh-rTDH. *E. coli*-TOPO did not cause significant liver injury.

Discussion

In this study, both human and mouse liver cells were treated with *G. hollisae* TDH, and the *in vitro* hepatotoxicity was demonstrated by direct observation and the MTT assay. The hepatotoxicity caused by Gh-rTDH was both dose- and time-dependent. Very low concentrations of TDH ($>10^{-6}$ μg/ml) damaged liver cells. We also noted that the MTT assays yielded a similar pattern over 12, 16, 24, and 48 hr under different toxin concentrations. One possible explanation is that when the concentration of toxin increased, cells were not only killed by this toxin but also probably suffered cell division suppression. Therefore, when we prolonged the treatment durations, the number of surviving cells did not clearly differ between the 4 time points. Naim et al. reported that *V. parahaemolyticus* TDH caused Rat-1 cell injury and that TDH might induce cytotoxicity by acting inside the cells [24]. In this study, we noted that the Gh-rTDH-FITC was taken up by liver cells via binding around the margin of the cell and was translocated to the nucleus within a short time period. Therefore, the destruction caused by *G. hollisae* TDH is notably quick and lethal to the liver cells.

Morros et al. firstly reported an account of a patient suffering a *G. hollisae* infection who presented with liver cirrhosis and hepatic encephalopathy in 1982 [25]. Previous studies demonstrated that *Vibrio* species infections could be more severe in patients with a history of impaired liver function [1,9]. However, evidence of hepatotoxicity caused by *G. hollisae* TDH has never been provided. In this study, we found that the GOT and GPT levels in mice treated with Gh-rTDH obviously increased, and acute liver injury was strongly suspected. Muscle injury was not favored as the major reason for the elevation of GOT/GPT, as a ^{18}F-FDG PET/CT scan did not show muscle injury. Moreover, liver biopsy revealed that the periportal areas of the livers were damaged and that the severity of the damage was associated with the dosage of Gh-rTDH. The periportal area in the liver is functionally well-known for its oxidative energy metabolism of fatty acids and amino acids, glucose release and glycogen formation, ammonia detoxification, protective metabolism, and the synthesis of albumin [26–28]. Therefore, mice with periportal area injury caused by Gh-rTDH might also suffer complications, which include malnutrition, protective system destruction, hepatic encephalopathy and hypoalbumenia. Clinically, the hypoalbumenia could be induced by decreased (hepatic) production or increased loss (gut tract loss). The result of hypoalbumenia in this study might be influenced by both mechanisms. The globulin levels also increased as the protective systems of the livers were damaged and the toxin triggered their immune systems in the circulation.

TDH is well-known for having strong hemolytic activity *in vitro* [9,16,24,29]. We further noted that the acute hemolytic status *in vivo* arose within 4 hours after treatment with Gh-rTDH and

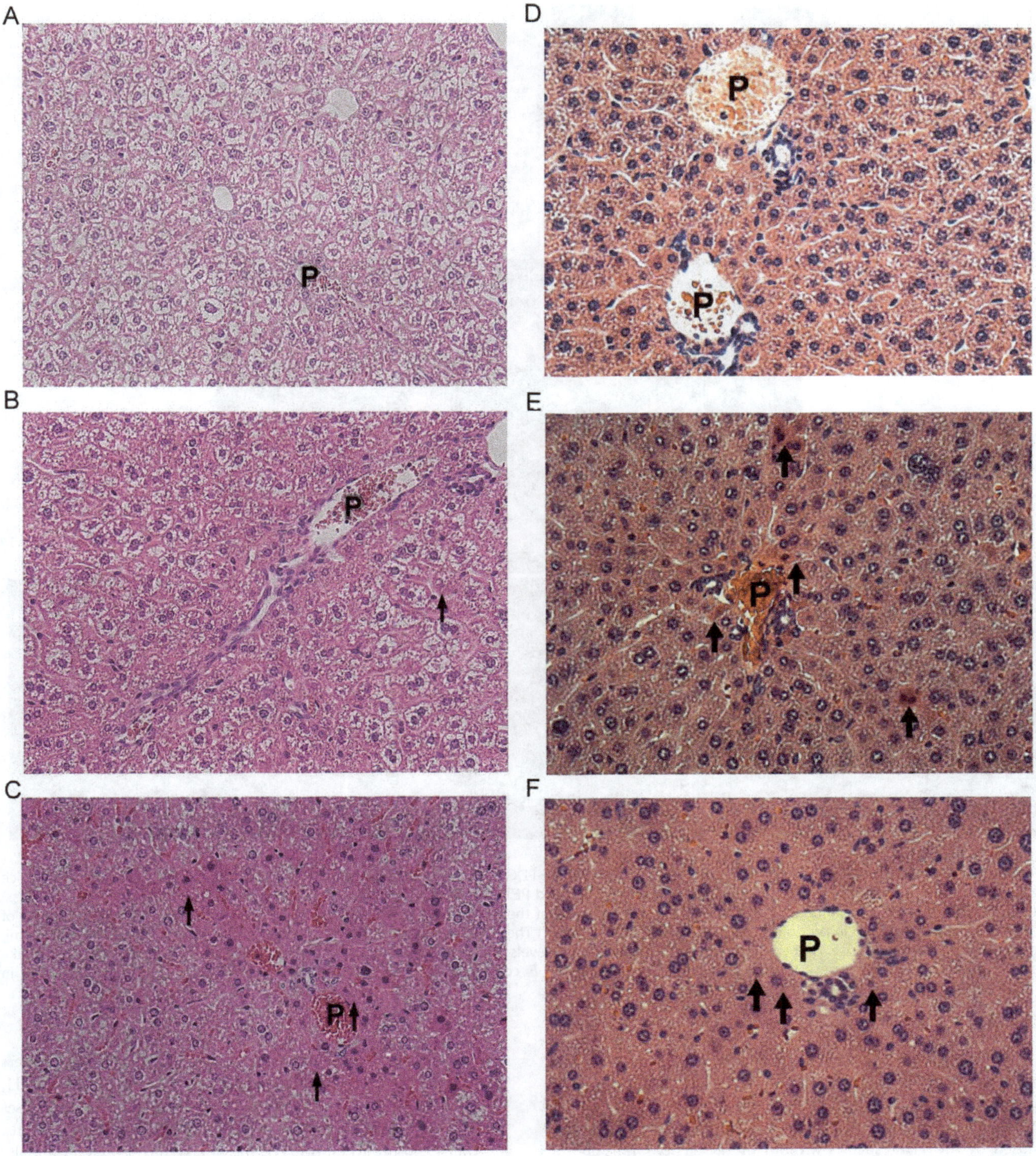

Figure 8. Liver biopsy (tissue harvested at the time of animal sacrifice) following Gh-rTDH ingestion and bacterial infection. Each image was acquired after 8 hr of toxin or bacterial exposure). The pathological images of liver parenchyma that were obtained from liver biopsies in mice were observed by microscopy at −400X (A, B, C) and −200X (D, E, F). (A) The parenchyma was homogeneous in mice treated with PBS (control group), and the liver cells around the portal vein were not damaged. (B) In mice treated with 10 μg Gh-rTDH, the parenchyma was mildly congestive over the periportal areas, and spotty damage (Councilman bodies) could be noted in the liver cells around the portal vein. (C) In mice fed 100 μg Gh-rTDH, the parenchyma was severely congestive with hemorrhage around the periportal areas, and most of the liver cells around the portal vein were damaged. These cells revealed confluent liver cell injury with intracytoplasmic acidophilic and ballooning change as well as nuclear pyknosis. Above all, these images demonstrated that Gh-rTDH was absorbed by the intestine and caused secondary injury to the liver via the venous return of the portal system. In mice fed *E. coli*-TOPO (D), the parenchyma was homogeneous and healthy. However, in mice fed *G. hollisae* (E) or *E. coli*-TOPO-*tdh* (F), cell damages were notable around the portal veins. P: portal vein, Arrows: damaged liver cells.

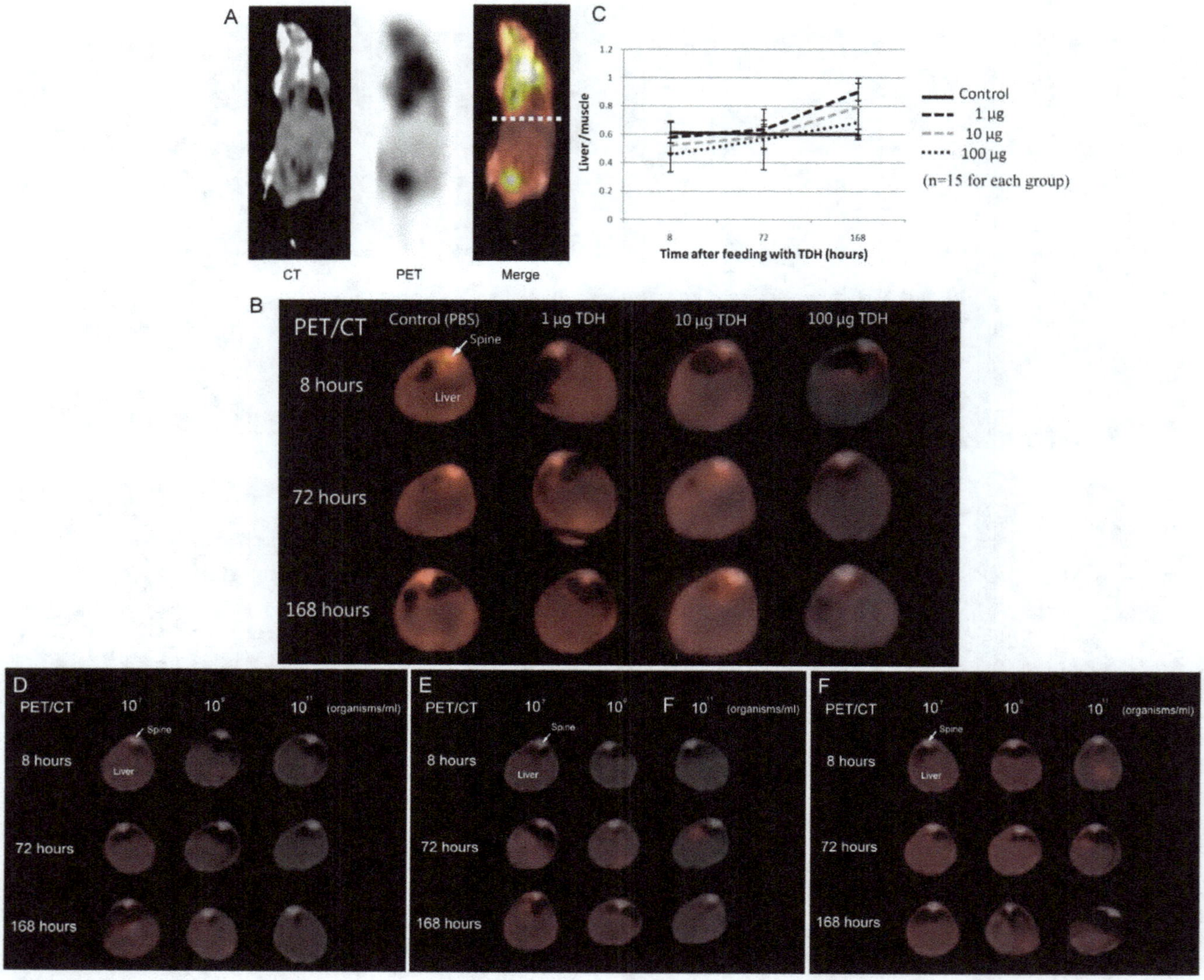

Figure 9. ^{18}F-FDG PET/CT scan. Mice were treated with 0.07 mCi ^{18}F-FDG by tail vein injection, and imaging was performed 1 hr later. (A) All mice received 3 series of images, including CT, PET, and a merge of CT and PET. The location of the liver is labeled by a dotted line where the cross-sectioned images were obtained. (B) These images are cross-sections of the livers. At 8, 72 and 168 hr after treatment with Gh-rTDH, the uptake of ^{18}F-FDG in livers decreased in proportion to the dosage of Gh-rTDH. (C) The ^{18}F-FDG uptake value was calculated using the ROI (liver/muscle, semi-quantification) in each mouse. Higher doses of toxin indicated lower levels of ^{18}F-FDG uptake. In the animal infection models, the ^{18}F-FDG uptake levels were clearly lower in mice that were fed (D) *G. hollisae* or (E) *E. coli*-TOPO-*tdh* than those fed (F) *E. coli*-TOPO. These decreases were in proportion to the levels of bacteria in the treatment.

increased in a dose-dependent manner. The acute hemolytic status *in vivo* results in acute anemia, which would exacerbate tissue hypoxia and organ hypoperfusion. Therefore, septicemia caused by *Vibrio* species with the *tdh* gene might be more critical than that caused by the *Vibrio* species without the *tdh* gene. Clinically, the hepatotoxicity might be caused via hemolysis. However, the pathological findings revealed that the hepatic injury was mainly located at the periportal areas, and the injury was not diffused. It is suspected that the major etiology is toxin absorption and injury to the liver via the venous return of the portal system.

Clinical ^{18}F-FDG PET/CT scans have been reported as excellent tools to survey organ metabolism in small animals [30]. Damage in the liver caused by Gh-rTDH can be demonstrated by blood withdrawal and liver biopsy. However, the conditions of recovery and organ metabolism in living animals were difficult to analyze. Therefore, ^{18}F-FDG PET/CT scans were performed for our assessment. We noted that the uptake of ^{18}F-FDG in the livers decreased in proportion to the administered dosages of Gh-rTDH, which indicate that the hepatic damage in the animals was dose-dependent. In other non-hepatic organs, damage was not obvious.

After exposure to Gh-rTDH, the uptake of ^{18}F-FDG gradually increased in trend. We suggest that the livers could finally reconstruct from the destruction of Gh-rTDH exposure, and these liver cells had undergone repair and proliferation via increasing their uptake of glucose, which is well-known as an unavoidable material in metabolism. The metabolism of glucose in the livers damaged by Gh-rTDH almost recovered to a normal range in the 72nd hour after exposure to TDH. Furthermore, the metabolism of glucose crossed the normal range in the 168th hour after exposure to Gh-rTDH, and the recovery was more predominant in mice treated with low dosages than in those treated with a high dosage of Gh-rTDH. The level of glucose uptake crossing the normal range noted that the metabolism of glucose was notably robust in these damaged livers in addition to ongoing strong recovery. According to our findings from the liver biopsies, the construction might be mainly located in the periportal area, which has been labeled as a major location of glucose and amino acid metabolism [26–28]. Therefore, the construction in the periportal area might contribute to the high level of ^{18}F-FDG intake in the liver during the recovery stage. Overall, this finding might provide strong evidence indicating that the reconstruction of liver continues for at least one week after a single Gh-rTDH exposure and that the damaged liver has the ability to recover from the Gh-rTDH related injury, even when exposed to a massive dosage of Gh-rTDH. Consistent with this observation is the finding that differential hepatotoxicity could be detected when mice were treated with different amounts of *G. hollisae and E. coli*-TOPO-*tdh* but were free from hepatotoxicity with *E. coli*-TOPO. The ^{18}F-FDG PET/CT results of the animal infection models showed that the severity of the liver injury was notably similar in mice treated with 100 μg of Gh-TDH and in mice treated with 10^{10} organisms of *G. hollisae*. Therefore, we suspected that 10^8 organisms of *G. hollisae* might produce 1 μg of TDH and cause liver injury *in vivo*. The results clearly demonstrate the *in vivo* hepatotoxicity of the *Gh-tdh* gene product.

In conclusion, *G. hollisae* TDH is reported as having *in vitro* and *in vivo* hepatotoxicity in our study. *G. hollisae* TDH damaged the liver in living animals and mainly attacked the periportal area, which is associated with the synthesis of albumin and the metabolism of glucose. Most importantly, the ^{18}F-FDG PET/CT scan revealed evidence that the reconstruction of the liver continued at least for one week after a single exposure of *G. hollisae* TDH. Furthermore, the damaged liver was shown to have an adequate ability to recover.

Author Contributions

Conceived and designed the experiments: YRL TKW. Performed the experiments: YKW YRL. Analyzed the data: YFW YRL. Contributed reagents/materials/analysis tools: YLC KBW SCH TAL MN BSY. Wrote the paper: YRL.

References

1. Morris JG Jr (2003) Cholera and other types of vibriosis: A story of human pandemics and oysters on the half shell. Clinical Infectious Diseases : An Official Publication of the Infectious Diseases Society of America 37: 272–280.
2. Yeung PS, Boor KJ (2004) Epidemiology, pathogenesis, and prevention of foodborne vibrio parahaemolyticus infections. Foodborne Pathogens and Disease 1: 74–88.
3. Lesmana M, Subekti DS, Tjaniadi P, Simanjuntak CH, Punjabi NH, et al. (2002) Spectrum of vibrio species associated with acute diarrhea in north jakarta, indonesia. Diagnostic Microbiology and Infectious Disease 43: 91–97.
4. Abbott SL, Janda JM (1994) Severe gastroenteritis associated with vibrio hollisae infection: Report of two cases and review. Clinical Infectious Diseases : An Official Publication of the Infectious Diseases Society of America 18: 310–312.
5. Gras-Rouzet S, Donnio PY, Juguet F, Plessis P, Minet J, et al. (1996) First european case of gastroenteritis and bacteremia due to vibrio hollisae. European Journal of Clinical Microbiology & Infectious Diseases : Official Publication of the European Society of Clinical Microbiology 15: 864–866.
6. Carnahan AM, Harding J, Watsky D, Hansman S (1994) Identification of vibrio hollisae associated with severe gastroenteritis after consumption of raw oysters. Journal of Clinical Microbiology 32: 1805–1806.
7. Rank EL, Smith IB, Langer M (1988) Bacteremia caused by vibrio hollisae. Journal of Clinical Microbiology 26: 375–376.
8. Hickman FW, Farmer JJ 3rd, Hollis DG, Fanning GR, Steigerwalt AG, et al. (1982) Identification of vibrio hollisae sp. nov. from patients with diarrhea. Journal of Clinical Microbiology 15: 395–401.
9. Raimondi F, Kao JP, Fiorentini C, Fabbri A, Donelli G, et al. (2000) Enterotoxicity and cytotoxicity of vibrio parahaemolyticus thermostable direct hemolysin in in vitro systems. Infection and Immunity 68: 3180–3185.
10. Nishibuchi M, Janda JM, Ezaki T (1996) The thermostable direct hemolysin gene (tdh) of vibrio hollisae is dissimilar in prevalence to and phylogenetically distant from the tdh genes of other vibrios: Implications in the horizontal transfer of the tdh gene. Microbiology and Immunology 40: 59–65.
11. Shinoda S, Nakagawa T, Shi L, Bi K, Kanoh Y, et al. (2004) Distribution of virulence-associated genes in vibrio mimicus isolates from clinical and environmental origins. Microbiology and Immunology 48: 547–551.
12. Cai SH, Wu ZH, Jian JC, Lu YS (2007) Cloning and expression of gene encoding the thermostable direct hemolysin from vibrio alginolyticus strain HY9901, the causative agent of vibriosis of crimson snapper (lutjanus erythopterus). Journal of Applied Microbiology 103: 289–296.
13. Yoh M, Honda T, Miwatani T (1986) Purification and partial characterization of a vibrio hollisae hemolysin that relates to the thermostable direct hemolysin of vibrio parahaemolyticus. Canadian Journal of Microbiology 32: 632–636.
14. Shinoda S (1999) Protein toxins produced by pathogenic vibrios. Journal of Natural Toxins 8: 259–269.
15. Yoh M, Honda T, Miwatani T, Tsunasawa S, Sakiyama F (1989) Comparative amino acid sequence analysis of hemolysins produced by vibrio hollisae and vibrio parahaemolyticus. Journal of Bacteriology 171: 6859–6861.
16. Nishibuchi M, Doke S, Toizumi S, Umeda T, Yoh M, et al. (1988) Isolation from a coastal fish of vibrio hollisae capable of producing a hemolysin similar to the thermostable direct hemolysin of vibrio parahaemolyticus. Applied and Environmental Microbiology 54: 2144–2146.
17. Fukui T, Shiraki K, Hamada D, Hara K, Miyata T, et al. (2005) Thermostable direct hemolysin of vibrio parahaemolyticus is a bacterial reversible amyloid toxin. Biochemistry 44: 9825–9832.
18. Wang YK, Huang SC, Wu YF, Chen YC, Lin YL, et al. (2011) Site-directed mutations of thermostable direct hemolysin from grimontia hollisae alter its arrhenius effect and biophysical properties. International Journal of Biological Sciences 7: 333–346.
19. Park KS, Ono T, Rokuda M, Jang MH, Iida T, et al. (2004) Cytotoxicity and enterotoxicity of the thermostable direct hemolysin-deletion mutants of vibrio parahaemolyticus. Microbiology and Immunology 48: 313–318.
20. Wang YK, Huang SC, Wu YF, Chen YC, Chen WH, et al. (2011) Purification, crystallization and preliminary X-ray analysis of a thermostable direct haemolysin from grimontia hollisae. Acta Crystallographica.Section F, Structural Biology and Crystallization Communications 67: 224–227.
21. Wang YK, Huang SC, Wu YF, Chen YC, Lin YL, et al. (2011) Site-directed mutations of thermostable direct hemolysin from grimontia hollisae alter its arrhenius effect and biophysical properties. International Journal of Biological Sciences 7: 333–346.
22. Anspach FB (2001) Endotoxin removal by affinity sorbents. Journal of Biochemical and Biophysical Methods 49: 665–681.
23. Petsch D, Anspach FB (2000) Endotoxin removal from protein solutions. Journal of Biotechnology 76: 97–119.
24. Naim R, Yanagihara I, Iida T, Honda T (2001) Vibrio parahaemolyticus thermostable direct hemolysin can induce an apoptotic cell death in rat-1 cells from inside and outside of the cells. FEMS Microbiology Letters 195: 237–244.
25. Morris JG Jr, Miller HG, Wilson R, Tacket CO, Hollis DG, et al. (1982) Illness caused by vibrio damsela and vibrio hollisae. Lancet 1: 1294–1297.
26. Jungermann K (1988) Metabolic zonation of liver parenchyma. Seminars in Liver Disease 8: 329–341.
27. Jungermann K (1986) Functional heterogeneity of periportal and perivenous hepatocytes. Enzyme 35: 161–180.
28. Jungermann K, Kietzmann T (1996) Zonation of parenchymal and nonparenchymal metabolism in liver. Annual Review of Nutrition 16: 179–203.
29. Wu TK, Wang YK, Chen YC, Feng JM, Liu YH, et al. (2007) Identification of a vibrio furnissii oligopeptide permease and characterization of its in vitro hemolytic activity. Journal of Bacteriology 189: 8215–8223.
30. Tatsumi M, Nakamoto Y, Traughber B, Marshall LT, Geschwind JF, et al. (2003) Initial experience in small animal tumor imaging with a clinical positron emission tomography/computed tomography scanner using 2-[F-18]fluoro-2-deoxy-D-glucose. Cancer Research 63: 6252–6257.

4

Novel Bioimaging Techniques of Metals by Laser Ablation Inductively Coupled Plasma Mass Spectrometry for Diagnosis of Fibrotic and Cirrhotic Liver Disorders

Pornwilard M-M[1,2,3], **Ralf Weiskirchen[1*]**, **Nikolaus Gassler[4]**, **Anja K. Bosserhoff[5]**, **J. Sabine Becker[2]**

1 Institute of Clinical Chemistry and Pathobiochemistry, RWTH University Hospital Aachen, Aachen, Germany, **2** Central Division of Analytical Chemistry, Forschungszentrum Jülich, Jülich, Germany, **3** Department of Chemistry and Center for Innovation in Chemistry, Mahidol University, Bangkok, Thailand, **4** Institute of Pathology, RWTH University Hospital Aachen, Aachen, Germany, **5** Institute of Pathology, University Hospital of Regensburg, Regensburg, Germany

Abstract

Background and Aims: Hereditary disorders associated with metal overload or unwanted toxic accumulation of heavy metals can lead to morbidity and mortality. Patients with hereditary hemochromatosis or Wilson disease for example may develop severe hepatic pathology including fibrosis, cirrhosis or hepatocellular carcinoma. While relevant disease genes are identified and genetic testing is applicable, liver biopsy in combination with metal detecting techniques such as energy-dispersive X-ray spectroscopy (EDX) is still applied for accurate diagnosis of metals. *Vice versa*, several metals are needed in trace amounts for carrying out vital functions and their deficiency due to rapid growth, pregnancy, excessive blood loss, and insufficient nutritional or digestive uptake results in organic and systemic shortcomings. Established *in situ* techniques, such as EDX-ray spectroscopy, are not sensitive enough to analyze trace metal distribution and the quantification of metal images is difficult.

Methods: In this study, we developed a quantitative biometal imaging technique of human liver tissue by laser ablation inductively coupled plasma mass spectrometry (LA-ICP-MS) in order to compare the distribution of selected metals in cryo-sections of healthy and fibrotic/cirrhotic livers.

Results: Most of the metals are homogeneous distributed within the normal tissue, while they are redirected within fibrotic livers resulting in significant metal deposits. Moreover, total iron and copper concentrations in diseased liver were found about 3-5 times higher than in normal liver samples.

Conclusions: Biometal imaging *via* LA-ICP-MS is a sensitive innovative diagnostic tool that will impact clinical practice in identification and evaluation of hepatic metal disorders and to detect subtle metal variations during ongoing hepatic fibrogenesis.

Editor: Matias A. Avila, University of Navarra School of Medicine and Center for Applied Medical Research (CIMA), Spain

Funding: The authors are grateful to the Deutsche Forschungsgemeinschaft (DFG grant number BE 2649/5-1) for instrumental support of the BrainMet laboratory. RW is sponsored by the SFB/TRR 57 and the IZKF Aachen. The funders had no role in study design, data collection and analysis, decision to publish, or preparation of the manuscript.

Competing Interests: The authors have declared that no competing interests exist.

* E-mail: rweiskirchen@ukaachen.de

These authors contributed equally to this work.

Introduction

Hepatic fibrosis, cirrhosis and hepatocellular carcinoma are characterized by a drastic increase of extracellular matrix proteins comprising collagens, glycoproteins, proteoglycans and hyaluronan [1,2]. The pathogenesis is triggered by various noxious agents (e.g. alcohol, drugs, viruses, and parasites), cholestasis, autoimmune reactions, metabolic diseases, or other exogenous or endogenous stimuli [1,2]. In addition, the overload with metals or trace elements that originates from hereditary disorders, nutritional oversupply, or occupational exposure is potentially causative for the pathogenesis of liver diseases. Hereditary hemochromatosis for example is the most common inherited disease of iron metabolism that results in toxic accumulation of iron in parenchymal cells of the liver [3]. This disease is most often associated with a polymorphism within the *HFE* gene that is quite common among white people resulting in an amino acid exchange (i.e. C282Y). Homozygous carriers usually have increased serum transferrin saturation levels and increased serum ferritin levels. In addition, non-*HFE* hepatic iron overload diseases originate from mutation in other genes such as transferrin receptor 2, hepcidin, hemojuvelin, and ferroportin [4]. Since these genes influence net iron concentration by affecting the synthesis and activity of the peptide hormone hepcidin that represents the master regulator of iron homeostasis, respective mutational alterations most often give rise to elevated concentrations of circulating iron and thus overload occurs. Conversely, iron deficiency resulting from decreased iron uptake, low absorption, rapid growth, pregnancy, and blood loss provoked by frequent blood donation or heavy menstrual periods, leads to anemia impairing proper body function.

Copper is a unique essential trace element playing an important function as a cofactor for a number of cellular processes [5]. Copper homeostasis is regulated by copper uptake in the gastrointestinal tract, distribution through the body, and excretion mainly into the bile. At the cellular level two copper transporters namely CTR1 and CTR2 regulate the intake, while copper efflux occurs *via* the ATP-dependent pumps ATP7B and ATP7A [6]. Hepatic copper accumulation can result from increased copper intake, inherited metabolic defects or from a reduced biliary excretion of copper. Wilson disease (WD) is an autosomal recessive disease caused by mutations of the WD gene *ATP7B* resulting in copper accumulation in different tissues. In liver, ATP7B is mainly expressed in hepatocytes and its loss is the basis for reduced hepatic biliary copper excretion and reduced incorporation of copper into ceruloplasmin [7]. Affected patients display hepatic and neurological disease with yet poorly understood pathomechanisms. In line, $Atp7b^{-/-}$ mutant mice display a gradual accumulation of hepatic copper inducing gross anatomic liver abnormalities in older mice with an irregular liver surface with protruding regenerative nodules of different sizes indicative for cirrhosis [8].

These examples underline that body metal homeostasis is crucial and metal deficiencies or dramatic build-ups should be prevented to avoid hepatic or other organic impairments. Therefore, indicative, non-invasive serum parameters (e.g. serum transferrin concentration and saturation, ferritin, haemoglobin, hematocrit, serum ceruloplasmin) and genetic testing of causative genes is widely propagated in diagnosis to identify metal disorders or predisposition for respective diseases. Moreover, the performance of liver biopsy to measure or stain *in situ* metal content in combination with scanning electron microscopy with energy-dispersive X-ray analysis (SEM-EDX) is traditionally the confirmatory test in cases in which the non-invasive markers suggest elevated metal concentrations. Unfortunately SEM-EDX is often not sensitive enough for trace element imaging. However, liver heterogeneity can result in wrong analytical data). Therefore, novel imaging techniques that provide information about the regional distribution of individual metals or groups of metals combined with a diagnostic score system further providing information about the extent of hepatic insult are urgent required.

Although potentially not causative, the outcome of hepatic fibrosis is also significantly modulated by variations in hepatic metal distribution and concentrations. Hepatic iron overload for example has been described in chronic hepatitis C as a cofactor affecting fibrosis progression and hepatic iron deposits were found in well-compensated chronic hepatitis B infection, especially in patients that were co-infected with hepatitis D virus [9]. Likewise, severe copper deficiency exacerbates liver injury and liver fibrosis in rats that underwent experimental bile duct ligation surgery [10], again demonstrating that variations in individual metal concentrations might not only be the result of ongoing hepatic fibrogenesis but are further important modulators in disease progression. Therefore, there is no doubt that accurate method allowing to measure hepatic metal concentrations or to detect metals deposits are of important diagnostic relevance not only in determination liver insult but further to predict overall disease outcome.

Magnetic resonance imaging (MRI) allows the mapping only of selected single metals (such as iron) in organs [11], but the quantification is often difficult [12]. Novadays, laser ablation inductively coupled plasma mass spectrometry (LA-ICP-MS) techniques with multi-element capability and high spatial resolution are herein discussed has been established to a new generation of sensitive analytical tools for imaging of metals in biological tissue.

Recently, LA-ICP-MS imaging technique has been applied as a reference standard method to validate the results from quantitative gadolinium enhanced MRI technique [12]. Although LA-ICP-MS imaging has been introduced in diagnosis of metal disorders in brain [13–16], this innovative technique has not been used in quantitative bioimaging of metals in human liver. A first report from Feldmann's working group from 2003 demonstrated for copper and zinc in sheep liver sections the capability of LA-ICP-MS for elemental mapping [17]. In another previous study, LA-ICP-MS imaging revealed that *staphylococcal aureus* liver abscesses from normal mice are enriched in Ca^{2+}, while these abscesses are devoid of detectable Zn^{2+} and Mn^{2+} [18]. These studies are encouraging and show that LA-ICP-MS is indeed a methodology that might be suitable to detect delicate metal alterations in liver that are the cause or a consequence of organ alteration or dysfunction.

The aim of the present study is to develop a novel quantitative imaging technique for trace metals and to characterize the distribution of various metals in cryo-sections of normal, fibrotic and cirrhotic human liver tissues. We demonstrate that most of the metals analyzed are regularly distributed within normal liver tissue, while they are redirected within fibrotic and cirrhotic livers resulting in defined deposits suggesting that this method is not only valuable in diagnosis of common metal disorders but also adequate to determine subtle changes during ongoing liver fibrogenesis.

Materials and Methods

Patients and informed consent

Liver samples were taken from internal tissue banks of the RWTH University Hospital Aachen or the University Hospital Regensburg in which liver tissue was used for experimental purposes that was acquired either from biopsies for routine clinical purposes or explants of cirrhotic livers that were obtained during liver transplantation. Each patient from which material is stored provided written informed consent and the study was approved by the local ethics committee at the RWTH Aachen University and the University of Regensburg. Liver fibrosis/cirrhosis was diagnosed mainly on the grounds of liver routine histology. Fibrotic/cirrhotic tissue samples used in this study were obtained from five independent patients (D1 – D5). Secluded tissue from tumour-free margins of resected hepatic metastasis within normal liver parenchyma (N1 – N5) served as controls.

Immunohistochemical characterisation of liver specimens

After being fixed in 4% buffered formalin for 24 h, the liver tissue was embedded into paraffin wax. A histological semi-quantitative examination of the liver was performed on sections after standard Sirius Red and H & E stains. Liver sections were stained with an anti-human α-SMA antibody using standard procedures. To assess the degree of fibrosis, a standard Ladewig staining was performed and the severity of liver biopsy lesions and overall immunological activity were graded and staged according to routine scoring guidelines of Desmet and Scheurer [19]. Patients with cirrhosis were stratified according to the Child-Pugh score. The characteristics of the biopsies used in this study are given in Table 1.

Table 1. Characteristics of biopsy samples used in this study.

No.	Internal Number / Origin	Remarks / Desmet-Scheuer Score	Etiology of disease
N1	NG237 / Aachen	no fibrosis/ 0	liver metastasis from colon adenocarcinoma
N2	NG238 / Aachen	no fibrosis/ 0	liver metastasis from breast adenocarcinoma
N3	NG265 / Aachen	no fibrosis/ 0	hepatocellular carcinoma
N4	27 (normal) / Regensburg	no fibrosis/ 0	no known disease history
N5	29 (normal) / Regensburg	no fibrosis/ 0	slight signs of steatosis due to alcohol abuse
D1	NG205 / Aachen	mild fibrosis, portal extracellular matrix deposits/ 1	liver metastasis from colon adenocarcinoma; fibrosis of unknown origin
D2	NG241 / Aachen	cirrhosis/ 4	hepatocellular carcinoma; cirrhosis in chronic HCV infection
D3	NG264 / Aachen	cirrhosis/4	hepatocellular carcinoma; cirrhosis of unknown origin
D4	8 (cirrhosis) / Regensburg	cirrhosis/ 4	cryptogenic cirrhosis, burned-out NASH
D5	23 (cirrhosis) / Regenburg	cirrhosis/ 4	cryptogenic cirrhosis, burned-out NASH

Scanning Electron Microscopy with EDX analysis (SEM-EDX)

Slices of 20 to 50 µm thickness were obtained from paraffin-embedded liver tissue, sputtered with a conductive silver paint to make contact on the surface, carbon-coated in a rotary evaporator, and then maintained in desiccators to prevent air-contact before analysis. Analysis of element content by EDX was rapidly performed within two days of preparation using an environmental scanning electron microscope (ESEM XL 30 FEG, FEI, PHILIPS, Eindhoven, The Netherlands) in a high vacuum environment operating at 15 to 20 kV. The slices were imaged by back-scattered electrons and analysed for the elemental composition of the element present. For quantitative analysis of the element concretions, the contributions of the C-coating and the embedding resin containing C, O and trace of Cl were computer-based subtracted from the quantitative data of each spectrum.

Metal imaging of liver tissue section by laser ablation inductively coupled plasma mass spectrometry (LA-ICP-MS)

A quadrupole-based inductively coupled plasma mass spectrometer (ICP-MS, XSeries 2, Thermo Scientific, Bremen, Germany) coupled to a laser ablation system (NWR 213, New Wave Research, Fremont, CA, USA) was used to study elemental distributions in tissue sections of human livers (30 µm thickness). Laser ablation of biological tissue was performed using a focused Nd:YAG laser beam in the scanning mode (wavelength 213 nm, repetition frequency 20 Hz, laser spot diameter 60 µm, scanning speed 60 µm s^{-1}, laser fluency 0.24 J cm^{-2}). The ablated material was transported by argon gas (as carrier gas) into the inductively coupled plasma (ICP). The ions formed in the atmospheric pressure ICP were extracted in the ultrahigh vacuum mass spectrometer via a differential pumped interface, separated in the quadrupole mass analyzer according to their mass-to-charge ratios and detected by an ion detector. No reference standard materials for quantification of metals in human liver were available. Therefore, SRM NIST 1577b (bovine liver) was used as standard reference material. The trace metal concentrations in the samples were determined by single point calibration using this SRM. Moreover, the selection of internal standard element is the important part for LA-ICP-MS analyzing. The appropriate internal standard element was chosen to correct for plasma instabilities and sample-to-sample variations in the ion signal intensity. In this work, sulphur was used as an internal standard element for all the analyses because sulphur in human livers present rather a homogeneous distribution and provide constant concentration (see below). The human liver tissue and the NIST standard reference material deposited on glass slide were mounted in the laser ablation chamber to perform LA-ICP-MS imaging of sample and standard reference material under identical experimental conditions. Mass spectrometric measurements by LA-ICP-MS for imaging of liver tissue were performed by line scanning ablation (line by line) with a focused laser beam under the optimized experimental parameters given in Table 2. The experimental parameters of LA-ICP-MS were optimized with respect to the maximum ion intensity of $^{63}Cu^{+}$ using a SRM 1577b

Table 2. Optimized experimental parameters used for LA-ICP-MS imaging of human liver samples.

ICP mass spectrometer	ICP-QMS, Thermo XSeries II
Rf power	1450 W
Cooling gas flow rate	16.0 L min^{-1}
Auxiliary gas flow rate	0.7 L min^{-1}
Carrier gas flow rate	1.0 L min^{-1}
Dwell time	20 ms
Extraction lens potential	3400 V
Mass resolution (m/Δm)	300
Scanning mode	peak hopping
Analysis time per liver sample (10 mm×10 mm)	4 hours
Laser ablation system	New Wave (NRW213)
Wavelength of Nd:YAG laser	213 nm
Laser fluence	0.24 J cm^{-2}
Repetition frequency	20 Hz
Laser spot size	60 µm
Scan speed	60 µm s^{-1}
Ablation mode	line scan

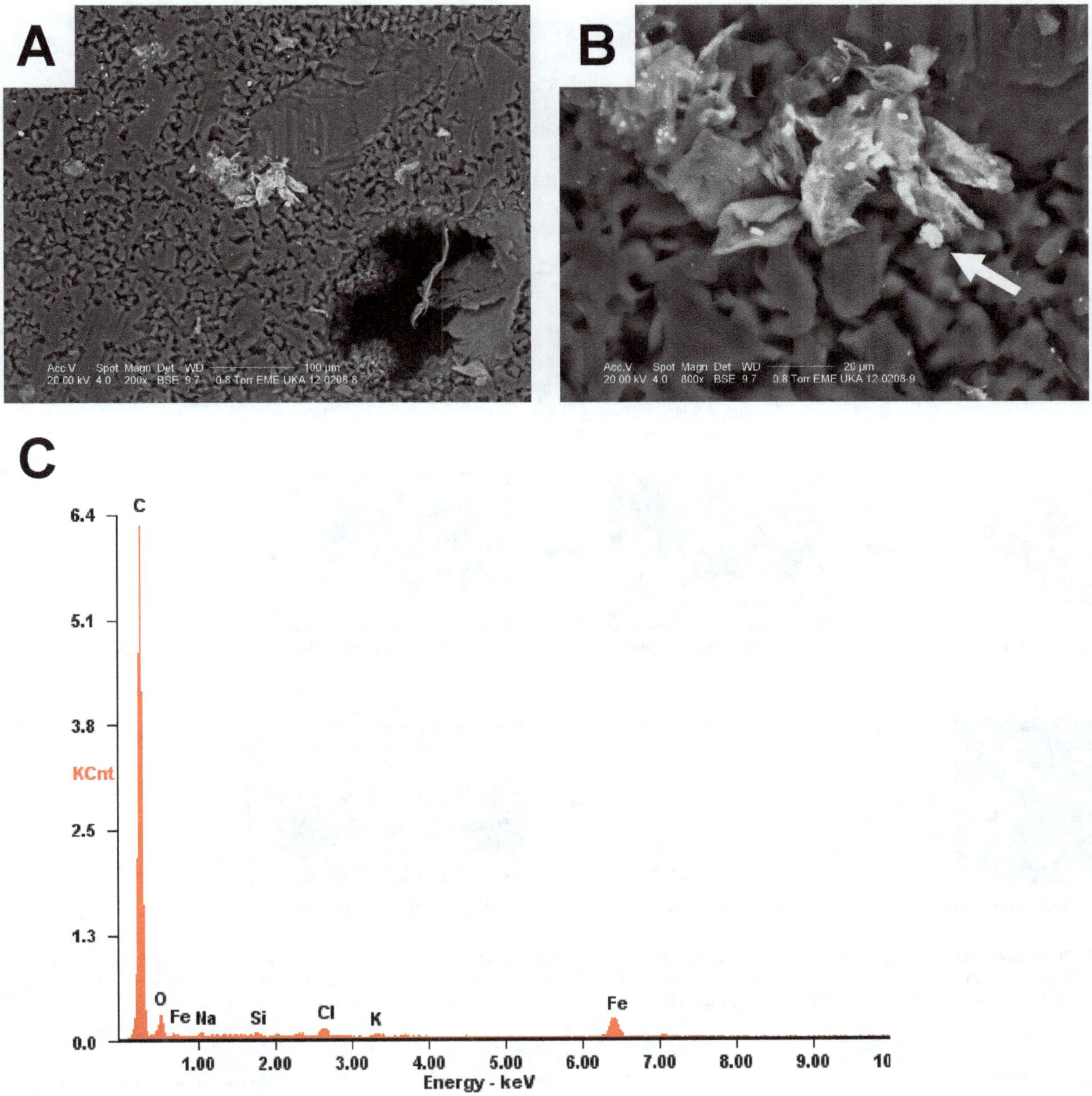

Figure 1. Representative SEM/EDX microanalysis in liver. (A) SEM overview of a paraffin embedded liver specimen from a patient (N1) suffering from fibrosis. **(B)** The metal deposit that was subsequently analysed by EDX is marked by a white arrow. **(C)** Resulting elemental EDX microanalyses of the marked mineral crust in **(B)**. The peaks in the spectrum are labelled with the EDX line of the corresponding element.

bovine liver standard. To validate the metal ion images, two isotopes of the same element were analyzed, whenever possible. From the continuous list of raw pixel values elemental images were reconstructed using the IMAGENA LA-ICP-MS Image Generation software created at Forschungszentrum Juelich [20]. Trace metal concentrations were calculated from ion intensities averaged throughout freely drawn regions of interest (ROIs) within ion intensity images using PMOD version 3.0 (details see www.pmod.com).

Results

Analysis of liver specimen by SEM-EDX

SEM-EDX is used for chemical analysis and determination of the elemental composition of microscopic particles or regions within a sample by *in situ* measuring the energy and intensity distribution of X-ray signals generated by a focused electron beam on the specimen (i.e. biopsy). It relies on the investigation of an interaction of some source of X-ray excitation and the sample resulting in a unique set of peaks on the X-ray spectrum that is characteristic for each element. In brief, the necessary equipment for this technique is based on an excitation source that transmits an electron beam, an X-ray detector that converts X-ray energy into voltage signals, a pulse processor and an analyzer that processed the signals and matches them to individual atoms. Based on the fact that this technique allows discriminating of metals, this technique is used to corroborate or even score metal disorder in organ tissue.

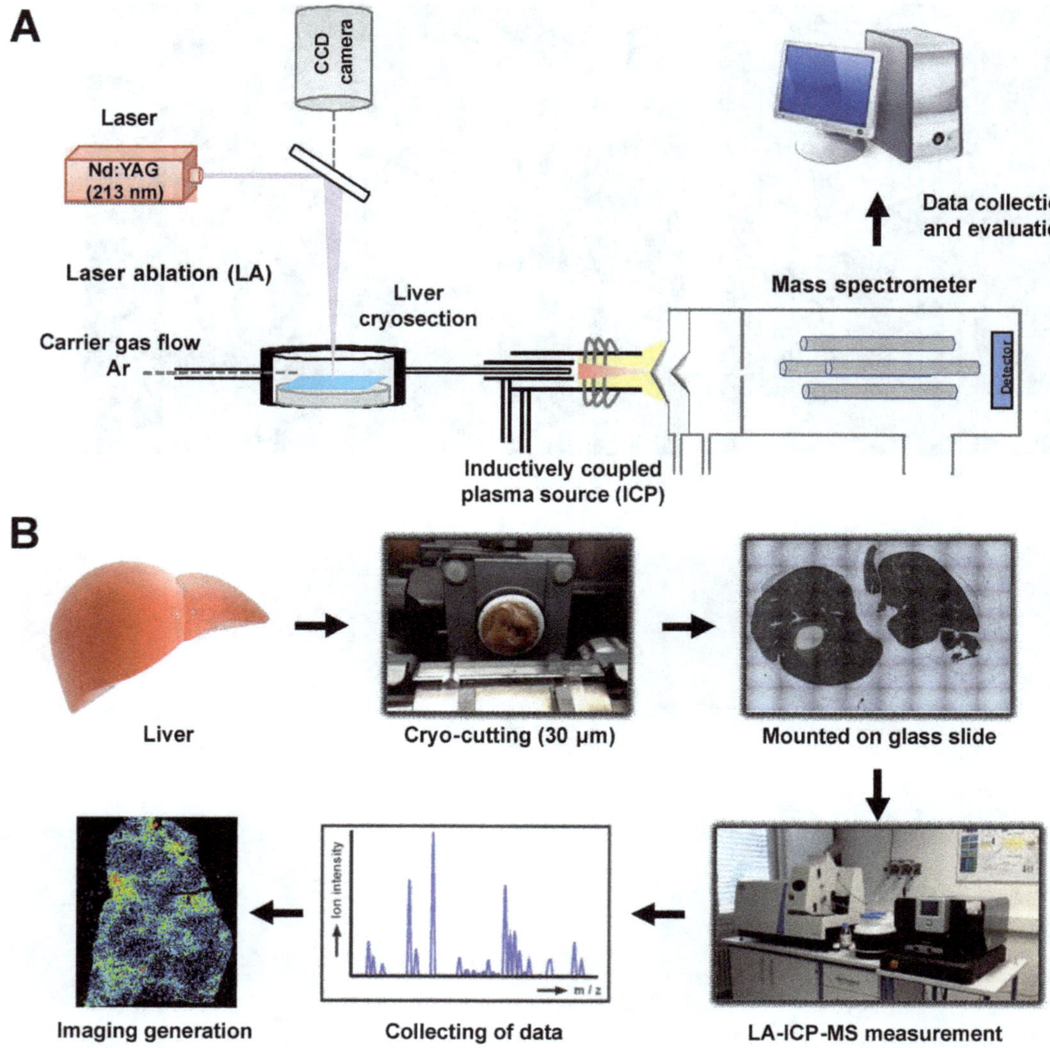

Figure 2. Principle and workflow of LA-ICP-MS for hepatic metal imaging. (A) Principle and **(B)** Workflow of imaging mass spectrometry from sample preparation of thin section by cryo-cutting, *via* the LA-ICP-MS measurement procedure by scanning of thin tissue section (line by line), acquisition and evaluation of analytical data including quantification using single point calibration (NIST SRM 1577b bovine liver).

When we applied this method to non-WD patients suffering from liver fibrosis or cirrhosis, we noticed that although it allows the identification of individual metal deposits (Figure 1), it was unsuitable to discriminate between normal, fibrotic or cirrhotic liver tissue. Moreover, the identification of metals by SEM-EDX is somewhat critical because several elements have overlapping peaks and data interpretation is somewhat enigmatic and only possibly by highly experienced investigators.

LA-ICP-MS analysis of liver tissues

The introduction of LA-ICP-MS technology has recently been successfully applied as a powerful imaging (mapping) technique to produce quantitative images of detailed regionally specific element distributions in thin tissue sections of human or rodent brain [21].

In an attempt to use this methodology for analysis of liver tissue, we established a protocol that allows quantitative metal imaging of liver tissue. In the final workflow, liver tissue is cryo-sected into specimen of 30 μM thickness and mounted on glass slides (Figure 2B). Mass spectrometric measurements is then performed in the LA-ICP-MS by line scanning ablation (line by line) with a focused laser beam under the optimized experimental parameters given in Table 1.

To evaluate the LA-ICP-MS imaging technique in liver specimen and to further analyse if the concentration or distribution of individual metals is altered in fibrotic or cirrhotic liver tissue, we thought to apply this imaging technique in a small set of histological well-characterized samples from normal, fibrotic and cirrhotic liver tissue (Figure 3).

Trace metal imaging and quantification in selected liver sections

The reproducibility of the LA-ICP-MS imaging technique for the analysis of 20 μm thin cross section of human brain tissues is already well studied [22]. 3% reproducibility had been observed for homogeneous tissues (thin cross sections of matrix-matched laboratory standards) and 5%–7% reproducibility for inhomogeneous tissue. Moreover, the applicability of LA-ICP-MS technique was demonstrated in Parkinson mouse brain 14 μm sections [23,24]. The reproducibility of 5% for Fe and Cu, 12% for Zn, and 11% for Mn was presented. In our study, the replicate

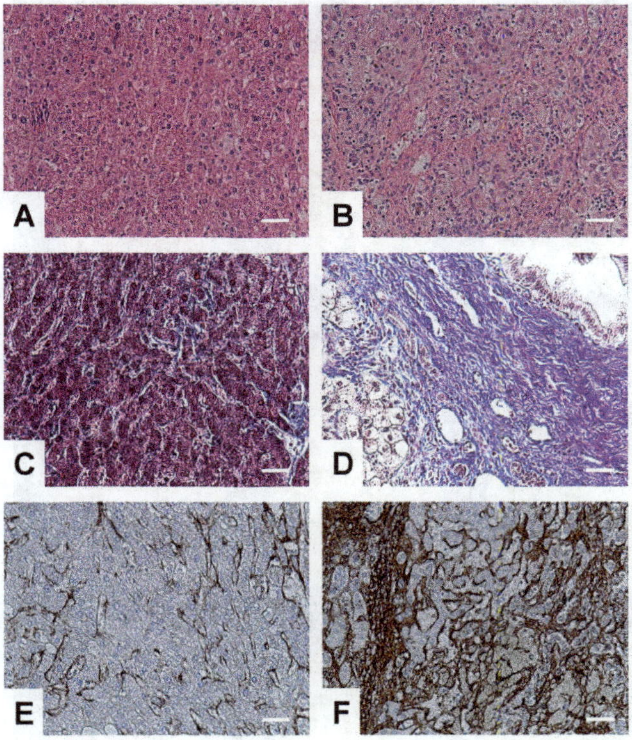

Figure 3. Representative immunohistochemical analysis of liver sections of patients enrolled in this study. (A, C, E) Normal (N1) and (B, D, F) cirrhotic liver tissues (D2) were stained with (A, B) hematoxylin and eosin, (C, D) Ladewig, or (E, F) probed with an antibody specific for α-SMA. The space bar in each figure represents 100 μM each.

measurement of 4 adjacent sections of the same human liver tissue (N3) were scanned using optimum condition of LA-ICP-MS in order to determine the reproducibility (see Figure 4). The reproducibility values calculated were 9% for S, 10% for Mn, 14% for Fe, 6% for Cu, 4% for Zn and Cd. Since sulphur is an abundant element showing an overall homogenous distribution in liver (see Figure 4, left panel), we used this non-metal as an internal standard.

Figure 5 shows LA-ICP-MS images of the detected elements (C, Na, Mg, P, K, Ca, Cr, Mn, Fe, Co, Cu, Zn, Mo, Ag, Cd, Sn, Hg, and Pb) in a fibrotic liver sample (N3). Ca, Mn, Fe, Cu, Zn, Mo, Cd, were detected with a higher abundance in fibrotic zones compared to normal zones, whereas the ion intensity measured of C, Na, Mg, P, K, Cr, Co, Ag, Sn, Hg, and Pb were not different between fibrotic and normal zones. This picture presents the potential of LA-ICP-MS to investigate the distribution of various essential and toxic elements. However, no quantification of some elements (C, P, Mo, Sn, and Hg) was possible due to the lack of certified concentrations in the bovine liver standard reference material used in this study.

Quantitative bioimages of Mn, Fe, Cu, Zn, and Cd of control and diseased (fibrotic and cirrhotic) human liver samples are illustrated in Figure 6 and Figure 7, respectively. In the case of control liver samples, Mn, Cu, Zn, and Cd images are homogeneous distributed. For Fe images, the hexagonal structure was found clearly in N1 and N3 control liver sections. These hexagonal shapes are corresponding to the structure of human liver lobule and reflect the typical histological pattern of iron deposition in the normal liver. As shown in the Fe image, Fe was distributed predominantly around the rim of lobule structure. Fe distribution presented a decreasing gradient from the rim area to the central area. However, these hexagonal structures cannot be investigated in disease liver tissue section (Figure 7).

The bioimaging approach of metals in fibrotic/cirrhotic liver tissue sections by LA-ICP-MS revealed inhomogeneous distribution of Mn, Fe, Cu, Zn, and Cd. Very low concentrations of metals were observed in fibrous septa areas when compared to nodules areas. Moreover, the concentrations of Fe and Cu in all disease liver (Figure 7) were significant higher than all control liver section (Figure 6). In contrast, Zn concentrations in control liver samples were higher than in disease liver. In comparison with the high Fe content region (mark within circle area), it's was found low concentration of Cu (Figure 7).

Figure 8 compares the average of trace metal concentrations measured in the control liver tissue (N1–N5) and disease liver tissue (D1–D5). The average concentrations of Mn, Fe, Cu, Zn, and Cd were 5.8, 493, 23, 140, and 1 $\mu g\ g^{-1}$ in control; were 4.9, 576, 35, 80, and 0.5 in disease (fibrotic/cirrhotic) liver samples. In the case of Mn and Cd, the different concentrations between control and disease are not significant. On the other hand, the concentration of Fe, Cu, and Zn are quite different between the control and disease liver. Fe and Cu concentrations in diseased liver are higher than in normal liver samples, while Zn concentrations are decreased in diseased samples suggesting that these changes can be used to predict the changing of liver state from healthy to diseased liver.

Discussion

Hereditary liver diseases resulting in metal intoxication are reasons for morbidity and mortality worldwide [25,26]. In addition, various liver diseases including both alcoholic and non-alcoholic steatohepatitis are associated with increased iron deposits [27,28]. Furthermore several trace elements are known to influence the outcome of hepatitis virus infections [29]. Although there have been great advancements in the establishment of novel genetic test systems and measurements of serum parameters that are indicative and suitable for identification of respective diseases or intoxications, metal stains in liver sections and other techniques like SEM-EDX measurements are traditionally the confirmatory diagnostic tests for hepatic metal poisoning and is one the first sight attractive because (i) the detectors have high sensitivity due to a wide solid angle collecting the X-rays emitted from the sample, (ii) the entire chemical composition of the analyzed specimen can be observed without wavelength scans, and (iii) analysis time are rather small [30]. However, the accuracy of techniques that are based on electron-microscopic analysis of liver sections such as SEM-EDX is limited by several factors. First the analysts performing the SEM have a bias and restrict their analysis to material deposits that are visible. Second several elements in EDX have overlapping peaks that under certain constellations does prevent precise assignment of signals to element. Third quantification of individual element concentration is impossible or only hardly to achieve. Finally, the accuracy of the spectrum can also be affected by the nature of the sample *per se* in that way that inhomogeneous samples result in inadequate or dissimilar excitations.

X-rays can be generated by any atom in the sample that is sufficiently excited by the incoming beam. These X-rays are emitted in any direction, and so they may not all escape the sample. The likelihood of an X-ray escaping the specimen, and thus being available to detect and measure depends on the energy of the X-ray and the amount and density of material it has to pass

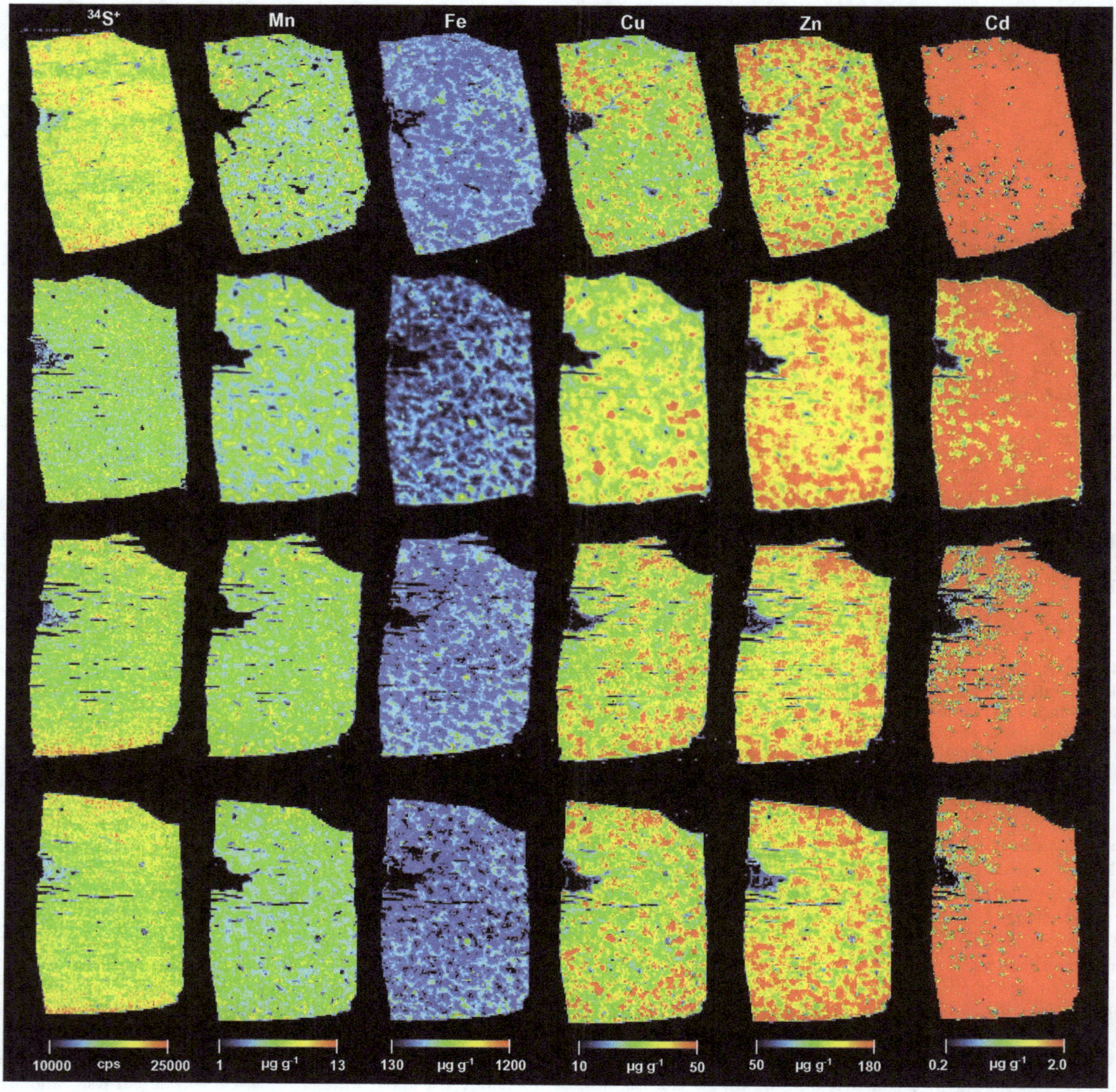

Figure 4. Reproducibility of imaging of elements in liver tissue sample. Representative spatial distribution of elements of interest (S, Mn, Fe, Cu, Zn, and Cd) in four adjacent sections from the same human liver tissue is depicted.

through. This can result in reduced accuracy in inhomogeneous and rough samples.

All these limitations of SEM-EDX measurements become evident in our experiment that is depicted in Figure 1 demonstrating that this method is not sensitive enough to illustrate trace metal distribution or even quantify individual metals in the analyzed liver specimens.

LA-ICP-MS on the other side is one of the most powerful and sensitive techniques for the analysis of a variety of solid samples because it provides good sensitivity for major, minor, trace, and ultra-trace elements with high sample throughput and without sample preparation which generates a large amount of waste as occurring in solution-based techniques [14]. Several years ago, the imaging analysis for biometal concentrations in human tissues obtained either by biopsy or postmortem was becoming an increasingly important function of the clinical laboratory.

The use of matrix matched reference material for quantification of analytical data is important because the ablation yield varies with the sample matrix. However, an appropriate matrix-matched standard reference material that for metal in human liver is not available. The most common quantification method for tissue in LA-ICP-MS is external calibration utilizing matrix-matched standards [24]. In the ongoing project, suitable matrix-matched tissue standards with well-defined concentrations of the biometals of interest were created and used for the calibration of the LA-ICP-MS technique. Several independent other studies have shown

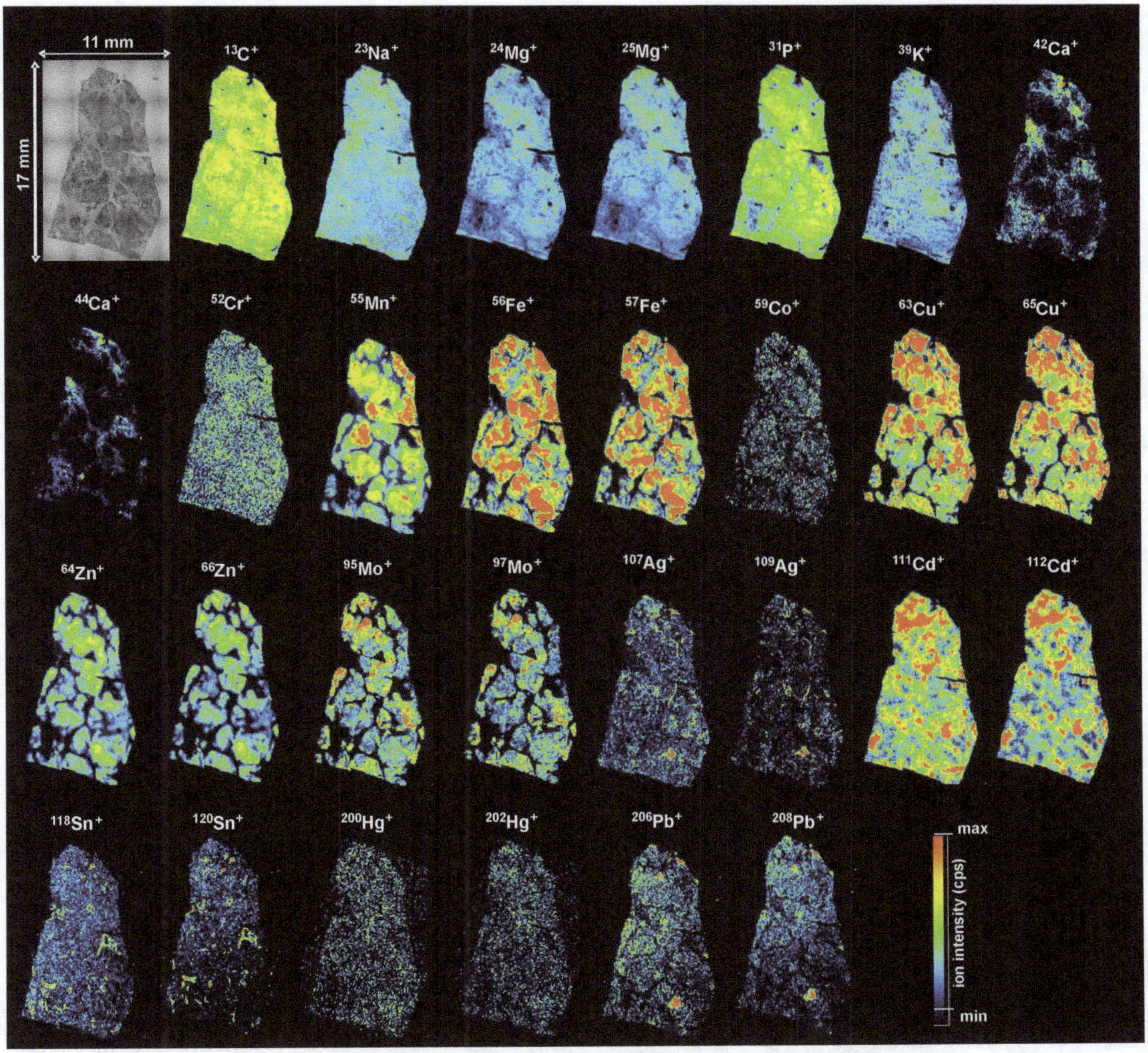

Figure 5. LA-ICP-MS imaging of essential and toxic metals and carbon in hepatic cirrhosis. Representative LA-ICP-MS maps of C, Na, Mg, P, K, Ca, Cr, Mn, Fe, Co, Cu, Zn, Mo, Ag, Cd, Sn, Hg, and Pb isotope as detected in cirrhotic human liver sample (D3).

that this one point calibration method also known as offset-only calibration gives a reasonable accuracy in quantification of various metals in LA-ICP-MS [12,17,31,32].

Human liver consists of two main lobes, left and right, which overlap slightly. Each lobe contains lobules that are the building blocks of the liver that are six-sided structures or hexagonal shapes. As shown in Figure 6, Fe-rich regions are found around the rim of hexagonal shape. In contrast, the concentrations of Fe become lower at the central of structure. Our results also support the previous finding, which investigated the distribution of Fe in liver tissue. Kinoshita and coworkers have been reported distribution in the lobule of human liver by synchrotron radiation X-ray fluorescence (SRXRF) microscopy [33]. In their report, Fe was distributed predominantly in periportal hepatocytes in the normal liver in a decreasing gradient from the periportal area (rim of hepatocyte) to the perivenous area (central of hepatocyte).

Mn is one of the important trace biometal, which can be detected in human liver. Mn is secreted in bile and concentration increase in cholestatic liver disease. The manganese content of the liver is very high as compared to its concentration in serum [34]. It has also been demonstrated that the liver has an important role in the excretion of manganese. Previous findings reported the increasing of whole blood Mn concentrations in patients with liver cirrhosis [35,36]. Moreover, they suggested that in cirrhosis of the liver failure of biliary excretion of Mn leads to overload and subsequent cerebral accumulation of this metal. Mn accumulates in mitochondria, a major source of superoxide, which can oxidize Mn^{2+} to the powerful oxidizing agent Mn^{3+} [37]. Oxidation of important cell components by Mn^{3+} has been suggested as a cause of the toxic effects of it. For our results, in fibrotic/cirrhotic tissue samples (Figure 7), Mn was increased to higher concentration in fibrotic and cirrhotic zones compared to non-tumor zones.

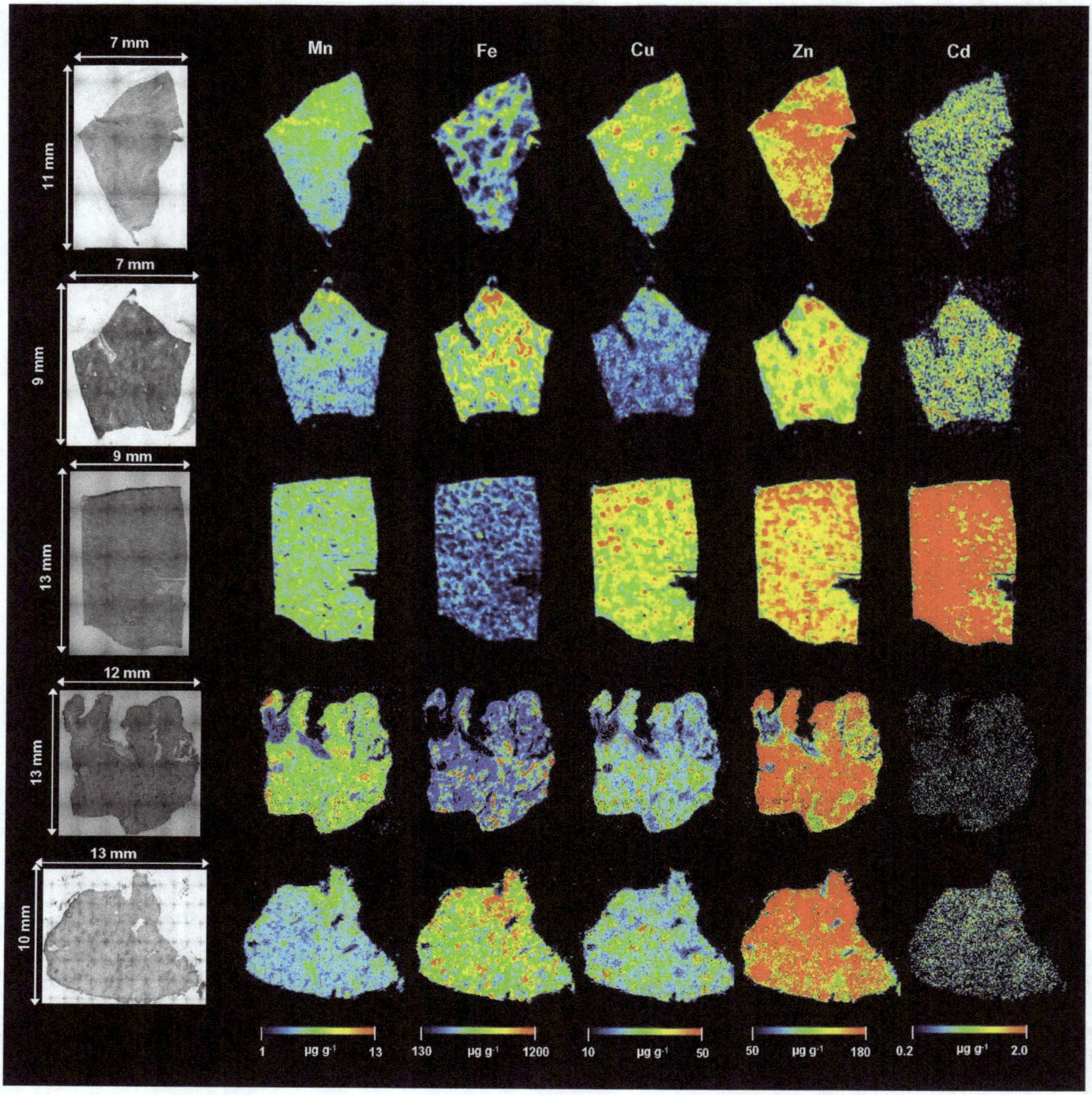

Figure 6. Selected LA-ICP-MS images in control liver samples. Images of Mn, Fe, Cu, Zn and Cd of control human liver samples (N1-N5) measured by LA-ICP-MS.

However, the average concentrations of Mn in control liver and disease samples (Figure 8) are not significant different.

In the animal model of liver fibrogenesis, iron acts as a "co-factor" of fibrogenesis [38]. Within the liver, iron related oxidative stress can lead to fibrosis and ultimately to cirrhosis [39]. When present in excess within the cell (hemochromatosis), iron can be toxic due to its ability to catalyze the formation of damaging radicals *via* a chemical reaction known as the Fenton reaction, which promote cellular injury and cell death. The results shown in this study could be in agreement with results from previous studies. In the control livers, the distributions of Fe are quite homogeneous. In contrast to disease livers, higher concentration of Fe was found in fibrotic or cirrhotic area when compared to normal area. For fibrotic liver, Fe concentration is higher than control tissue (Figure 8). However, the different between these values are not significant. In contrast to fibrotic tissue, the average concentrations of Fe in cirrhotic liver samples are higher than control liver about three times.

Not only Fe overload, the accumulation of too much Cu in WD is able to catalyze the development of liver disease. The major physiologic aberration is excessive absorption of copper from the small intestine and decreased excretion of copper by the liver. WD is an inherited metabolic disorder characterized by accumulation of copper in the tissue leading to progressive hepatic damage in the

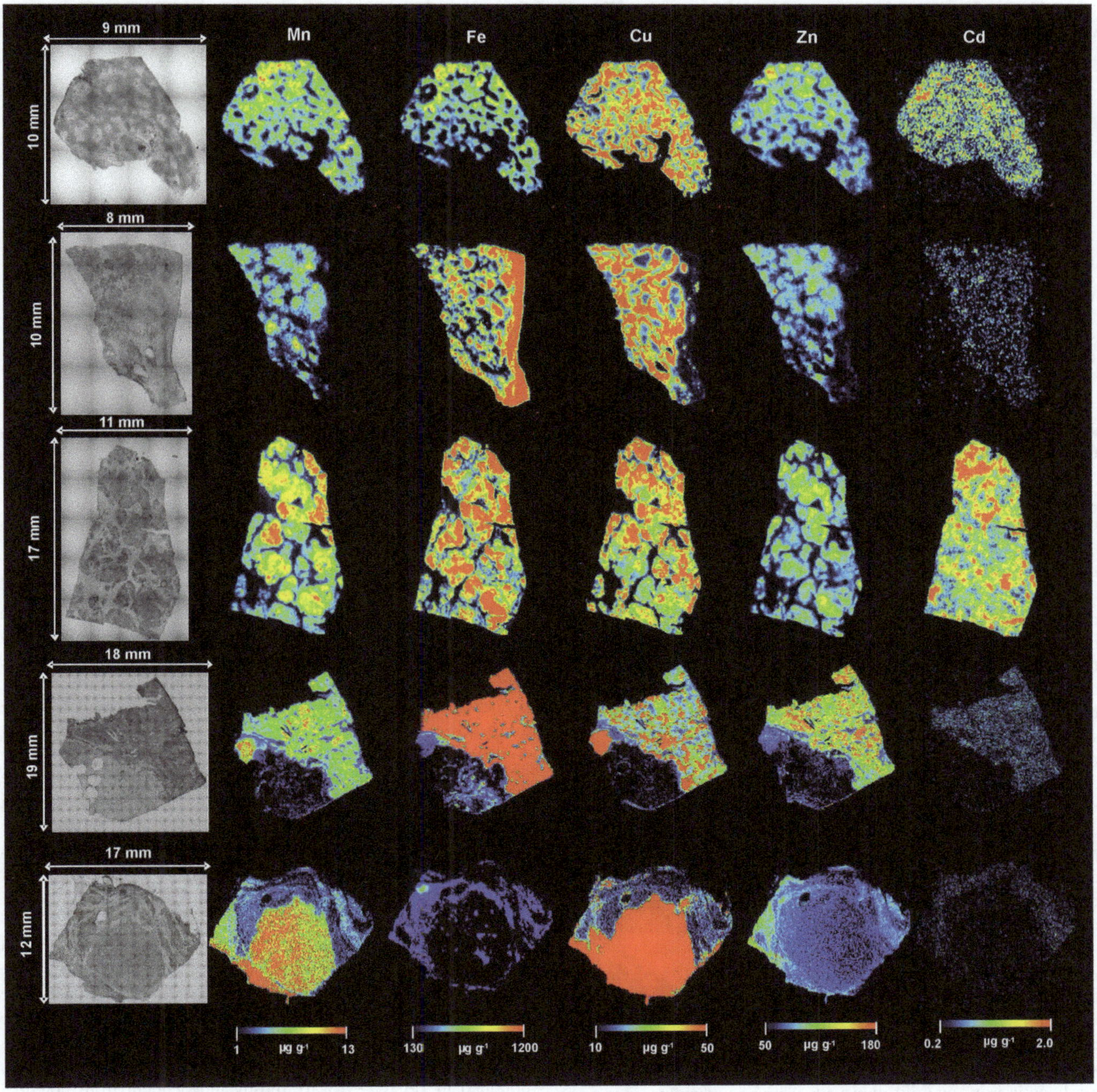

Figure 7. Selected LA-ICP-MS images in diseased liver. Images of Mn, Fe, Cu, Zn and Cd of fibrotic (D1) and cirrhotic human liver samples (D2-D5) measured by LA-ICP-MS.

liver and the other organs [40,41]. With progressive parenchymal damage, fibrosis and subsequently cirrhosis can be developed. In early stages of the disease, copper is mainly in the cytoplasm bound to metallothionein and is not histochemically detectable; in later stages, copper is found predominantly in lysosomes [41]. The amount of copper varies from nodule to nodule in cirrhotic liver and may vary from cell to cell in pre-cirrhotic stages. The absence of histochemically identifiable copper does not exclude WD, and this test has a poor predictive value for screening for WD. By use of LA-ICP-MS, we found inhomogeneous distributions in all fibrotic/cirrhotic liver sections analyzed. The average concentrations of fibrotic and cirrhotic are 204, and 210 µg g^{-1}, and 39.4 µg g^{-1} for control tissue samples. With these data, Cu is the important element that relates to the stage of liver failure and therefore used as an indicator for liver damage.

Zn is necessary for normal liver function and, the liver plays a central role in Zn homeostasis [42,43]. The liver is important for the regulation of zinc homeostasis, while zinc is necessary for proper liver function. It has long been speculated that Zn has a protective effect against liver fibrosis [42,44]. In our study, Zn concentrations in liver tissue were decreased from control (319 µg g^{-1}), fibrosis (223 µg g^{-1}), and cirrhosis (192 µg g^{-1}), respectively. Data obtained from our and previous studies suggest that ongoing liver disease correlates with reduced Zn levels. These findings fit

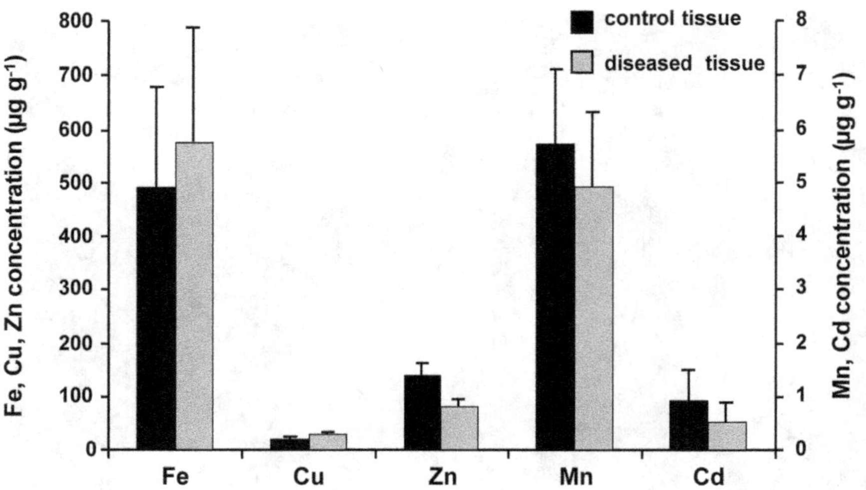

Figure 8. Quantitative metal distribution in liver samples. Comparative measurement of Mn, Fe, Cu, Zn, and Cd concentration in sections through the control (n = 5) and diseased (fibrotic/cirrhotic) (n = 5) liver tissue.

quite well with recent experimental observations showing that Fe and Cu act in an antagonistic fashion and iron is an important factor triggering copper deficiency in liver [45].

Cadmium is a highly toxic element present in food and water. It can deposit in the liver and kidney and strongly binds to macromolecules in the intracellular compartment and influences the metabolism of Fe, Ca, Zn, Mn and Cu [46,47]. Therefore, the overloading of Cd in liver may be disturbed the protective function of Zn to liver disease. However, Cd concentrations of control samples in our study are slightly higher than in fibrotic and cirrhotic samples. This result may be due to the fact that Cd concentration in liver tissue varies depending on many factors. The major route for cadmium intake for non-smoker is ingestion of cadmium in foodstuffs of natural origin or from the use of phosphate fertilizers and sludge on agricultural soils. Smokers have elevated blood and tissue concentrations of cadmium from cigarette smoke. As shown in Figure 8, the average concentration of the toxic trace metal Cd is not higher than 1 $\mu g\ g^{-1}$ in all tissue samples.

Considering all known hepatic diseases that are caused, promoted or modulated by accumulation of metals, there is a mandatory need for the establishment and evaluation of precise non-invasive metal imaging methods for diagnostics. In recent years, many studies have demonstrated the possibility of performing hepatic iron quantification with magnetic resonance imaging technology. However, a consensus has not been reached yet regarding the technique or the possibility to reproduce the same method of calculus in different equipments and intensive discussion for the establishment of consensus guidelines for clinical practice of hepatic iron quantification by magnetic resonance imaging techniques are conducted [48]. Since recent experimental and clinical studies have further demonstrated that different metals act as strong modifiers that influence the outcome of hepatic fibrogenesis [10,49], it is obvious that the quantitative trace metal determination in the diagnosis of disease progression will potentially become more important in future. The demonstration that LA-ICP-MS imaging representing one direct solid sampling technique for major, minor and trace element analysis is suitable for biometal analysis in normal and disease liver will therefore enrich the spectrum of diagnostic options. It allows to parallel measure the metal content in cryo-sections that become available in routine biopsy that still represent the gold standard for accurate assessment of the degree of fibrosis or presence of cirrhosis.

It would be an absolute goal to further analyze the sub-lobular and sub-cellular distribution of signals regarding different metals in both normal and disease conditions. In our study we noticed that the signals of several metals are more punctuated than others. However, the precise mapping of individual metals to cellular subpopulation of the liver is a complex venture and must be addressed in future studies. There are however already pioneering studies available that have already precisely co-localized aggregates and mercury deposits within cellular subpopulations of the liver [50]. Such studies would be fundamental for understanding the pathophysiological relevance of individual hepatic cells including Kupffer cells, hepatocytes, sinusoidal endothelial cells, hepatic stellate cells, and Pit cells (or even hepatic stem cells) in any kind of metal-induced liver disorders.

In summary, all these findings indicate that LA-ICP-MS is a novel powerful and innovative analytical technique that will have tremendous impact on diagnostics of metal disorders in liver. The fact that the obtained metal concentrations in liver tissue were the same in specimen that were obtained from two different hospitals (Aachen and Regensburg) further demonstrates that the results obtained in LA-ICP-MS are mostly independent from potential pre-analytical differences that may arise from sample collection. Although we presently do not know how individual hepatic disorders impact the distribution and location of individual metals or groups, it is known that metal overload or lack of individual metals may induce or contribute to the pathogenesis of liver disease. Therefore, LA-ICP-MS allowing quasi-simultaneous measurement of all metals and selected non-metals will provide an important add-on to routine diagnosis of liver sections or biopsies.

Acknowledgments

The authors are grateful to Dr. Manfred Bovi who has done the SEM-EDX microanalysis. We further would like to acknowledge the scientific input of Dr. Andreas Matusch (Institute of Neurosciences and Medicine, Juelich Research Centre, Germany) in this study. The paper is dedicated to Dr. M. Bovi (who died unexpectedly on June 12, 2012).

Author Contributions

Conceived and designed the experiments: RW JSB. Performed the experiments: PMM RW NG AKB. Analyzed the data: RW JSB. Wrote the paper: RW JSB.

References

1. Gressner AM, Weiskirchen R (2006) Modern pathogenetic concepts of liver fibrosis suggest stellate cells and TGF-β as major players and therapeutic targets. J Cell Mol Med 10: 76–99.
2. Lee UE, Friedman SL (2011) Mechanisms of hepatic fibrogenesis. Best Pract Res Clin Gastroenterol 25: 195–206.
3. Pietrangelo A (2010) Hereditary hemochromatosis: pathogenesis, diagnosis, and treatment. Gastroenterology 139: 393–408, 408.e1–2.
4. Pietrangelo A, Caleffi A, Corradini E (2011) Non-HFE hepatic iron overload. Semin Liver Dis 31: 302–318.
5. van den Berghe PV, Klomp LW (2009) New developments in the regulation of intestinal copper absorption. Nutr Rev 67: 658–672.
6. Wang Y, Hodgkinson V, Zhu S, Weisman GA, Petris MJ (2011) Advances in the understanding of mammalian copper transporters. Adv Nutr 2: 129–137.
7. Rosencrantz R, Schilsky M (2011) Wilson disease: pathogenesis and clinical considerations in diagnosis and treatment. Semin Liver Dis 31: 245–259.
8. Buiakova OI, Xu J, Lutsenko S, Zeitlin S, Das K, et al. (1999) Null mutation of the murine ATP7B (Wilson disease) gene results in intracellular copper accumulation and late-onset hepatic nodular transformation. Hum Mol Genet 8: 1665–1671.
9. Sebastiani G, Tempesta D, Alberti A (2012) Hepatic iron overload is common in chronic hepatitis B and is more severe in patients coinfected with hepatitis D virus. J Viral Hepat 19(2): e170–6.
10. Song M, Zhou Z, Chen T, Zhang J, McClain CJ (2011) Copper deficiency exacerbates bile duct ligation-induced liver injury and fibrosis in rats. J Pharmacol Exp Ther 339: 298–306.
11. Sirlin CB, Reeder SB (2010) Magnetic resonance imaging quantification of liver iron. Magn Reson Imaging Clin N Am 18: 359–381, ix.
12. Sussulini A, Wiener E, Marnitz T, Wu B, Müller B, et al. (2013) Quantitative imaging of the tissue contrast agent concentration of $[Gd\text{-}(DTPA)]^{2-}$ in articular cartilage by laser ablation inductively coupled plasma mass spectrometry. Contrast Media Mol Imaging 8: 204–209.
13. Becker JS (2010) Bioimaging of metals in brain tissue from micrometre to nanometre scale by laser ablation inductively coupled plasma mass spectrometry: State of the art and perspectives. Int J Mass Spectrom 289: 65–75.
14. Becker JS, Matusch A, Becker JS, Wu B, Becker AJ, et al. (2011) Mass Spectrometric Imaging (MSI) of metals using advanced BrainMet techniques for biomedical research. Int J Mass Spectrom 307: 3–15.
15. Qin Z, Caruso JA, Lai B, Matusch A, Becker JS (2011) Trace metal imaging with high spatial resolution: applications in biomedicine. Metallomics 3: 28–37.
16. Matusch A, Fenn LS, Depboylu C, Klietz M, Strohmer S, et al. (2012) Combined elemental and biomolecular mass spectrometry imaging for probing the inventory of tissue at a micrometer scale. Anal Chem 84: 3170–3178.
17. Kindness A, Sekaran NC, Feldmann J (2003) Two-dimensional mapping of copper and zinc in liver sections by laser ablation-inductively coupled plasma mass spectrometry. Clin Chem 49: 1916–1923.
18. Corbin BD, Seeley EH, Raab A, Feldmann J, Miller MR, et al. (2008) Metal chelation and inhibition of bacterial growth in tissue abscesses. Science 319: 962–965.
19. Desmet VJ (2003) Milestones in liver disease. Scoring chronic hepatitis. J Hepatol 38: 382–386.
20. Osterholt T, Salber D, Matusch A, Becker JS, Palm C (2011) IMAGENA: Image Generation and Analysis - an interactive software tool handling LA-ICP-MS data. Int J Mass Spectrom 307: 232–239.
21. Becker JS, Zoriy M, Matusch A, Wu B, Salber D, et al. (2010) Bioimaging of metals by laser ablation inductively coupled plasma mass spectrometry (LA-ICP-MS). Mass Spectrom Rev 29: 156–175.
22. Zoriy M, Becker JS (2007) Imaging of elements in thin cross sections of human brain samples by LA-ICP-MS: A study on reproducibility. Int J Mass Spectrom 264: 175–180.
23. Matusch A, Depboylu C, Palm C, Wu B, Höglinger GU, et al. (2010) Cerebral bioimaging of Cu, Fe, Zn, and Mn in the MPTP mouse model of Parkinson's disease using laser ablation inductively coupled plasma mass spectrometry (LA-ICP-MS). J Am Soc Mass Spectrom 21: 161–171.
24. Becker JS (2007) Inorganic mass spectrometry. Principles and applications. Springer, Berlin/Heidelberg
25. Brissot P, Bardou-Jacquet E, Jouanolle AM, Loréal O (2011) Iron disorders of genetic origin: a changing world. Trends Mol Med 17: 707–713.
26. Maxwell KL, Kowdley KV (2012) Metals and the liver. Curr Opin Gastroenterol 28: 217–222.
27. Corradini E, Pietrangelo A (2012) Iron and steatohepatitis. J Gastroenterol Hepatol 27(S2): 42–46.
28. Nelson JE, Klintworth H, Kowdley KV (2012) Iron metabolism in Nonalcoholic Fatty Liver Disease. Curr Gastroenterol Rep 14: 8–16.
29. Rashed MN (2011) The role of trace elements on hepatitis virus infections: a review. J Trace Elem Med Biol 25: 181–187.
30. Lechene CP, Warner RR (1977) Ultramicroanalysis: x-ray spectrometry by electron probe excitation. Annu Rev Biophys Bioeng 6: 57–85.
31. Feldmann J, Kindness A, Ek P (2002) Laser ablation of soft tissue using a cryogenically cooled ablation cell. J Anal At Spectrom 17: 813–818.
32. Guerra MB, Amarasiriwardena D, Schaefer CE, Pereira CD, Spielmann AA, et al. (2011) Biomonitoring of lead in Antarctic lichens using laser ablation inductively coupled plasma mass spectrometry. J Anal At Spectrom 26: 2238–2246.
33. Kinoshita H, Hori Y, Fukumoto T, Ohigashi T, Shinohara K, et al. (2010) Novel assessment of hepatic iron distribution by synchrotron radiation X-ray fluorescence microscopy. Med Mol Morphol 43: 19–25.
34. Versieck J, Barbier F, Speecke A, Hoste J (1974) Manganese, copper, and zinc concentrations in serum and packed blood cells during acute hepatitis, chronic hepatitis, and posthepatitic cirrhosis. Clin Chem 20: 1141–1145.
35. Hauser RA, Zesiewicz TA, Rosemurgy AS, Martinez C, Olanow C (1994) Manganese intoxication and chronic liver failure. Ann Neurol 36: 871–875.
36. Krieger D, Krieger S, Theilmann L, Jansen O, Gass P, et al. (1995) Manganese and chronic hepatic encephalopathy. Lancet 346: 270–274.
37. Gunter TE, Miller LM, Gavin CE, Eliseev R, Salter J, et al. (2004) Determination of the oxidation states of manganese in brain, liver, and heart mitochondria. J Neurochem 88: 266–280.
38. Pietrangelo A, Montosi G, Garuti C, Contri M, Giovannini F, et al. (2002) Iron-induced oxidant stress in nonparenchymal liver cells: mitochondrial derangement and fibrosis in acutely iron-dosed gerbils and its prevention by silybin. J Bioenerg Biomembr 34: 67–79.
39. Philippe MA, Ruddell RG, Ramm GA (2007) Role of iron in hepatic fibrosis: one piece in the puzzle. World J Gastroenterol 13: 4746–4754.
40. Schilsky ML, Scheinberg IH, Sternlieb I (1994) Liver transplantation for Wilson's disease: indications and outcome. Hepatology 19: 583–587.
41. Roberts EA, Schilsky ML (2008) Diagnosis and treatment of Wilson disease: an update. Hepatology 47: 2089–2111.
42. Stamoulis I, Kouraklis G, Theocharis S (2007) Zinc and the liver: an active interaction. Dig Dis Sci 52: 1595–1612.
43. Capocaccia L, Merli M, Piat C, Servi R, Zullo A, et al. (1991) Zinc and other trace elements in liver cirrhosis. Ital J Gastroenterol 23: 386–391.
44. de Sousa IK, Hamad Minervino AH, Sousa Rdos S, Chaves DF, Soares HS, et al. (2012) Copper deficiency in sheep with high liver iron accumulation. Vet Med Int 2012: 207950.
45. Ishikawa T (2012) Can zinc enhance response interferon therapy for patients with HCV-related liver disease? World J Gastroenterol 18: 3196–3200.
46. Spickett J, Lazner J (1979) Cadmium concentrations in human kidney and liver tissues from Western Australia. Bull Environ Contam Toxicol 23: 627–630.
47. Seth T, Agarwal L, Satija N, Hasan M (1976) The effect of lead and cadmium on liver, kidney, and brain levels of cadmium, copper, lead, manganese, and zinc, and on erythrocyte ALA-D activity in mice. Bull Environ Contam Toxicol 16: 190–196.
48. Alústiza JM, Castiella A, De Juan MD, Emparanza JI, Artetxe J, et al. (2007) Iron overload in the liver diagnostic and quantification. Eur J Radiol 61: 499–506.
49. Nobili V, Siotto M, Bedogni G, Ravà L, Pietrobattista A, et al. (2012) Levels of serum ceruloplasmin associate with pediatric nonalcoholic fatty liver disease. J Pediatr Gastroenterol Nutr 2012 Nov 14. [Epub ahead of print]. doi: 10.1097/MPG.0b013e31827aced4
50. Barst BD, Gevertz AK, Chumchal MM, Smith JD, Rainwater TR, et al. (2011) Laser ablation ICP-MS co-localization of mercury and immune response in fish. Environ Sci Technol 45: 8982–8988.

TWEAK/Fn14 Signaling is Required for Liver Regeneration after Partial Hepatectomy in Mice

Gamze Karaca[1], Marzena Swiderska-Syn[1], Guanhua Xie[1], Wing-Kin Syn[2,3], Leandi Krüger[1], Mariana Verdelho Machado[1], Katherine Garman[1], Steve S. Choi[1], Gregory A. Michelotti[1], Linda C. Burkly[4], Begoña Ochoa[5], Anna Mae Diehl[1]*

1 Division of Gastroenterology, Department of Medicine, Duke University Medical Center, Durham, North Carolina, United States of America, **2** Regeneration and Repair Group, The Institute of Hepatology, Foundation for Liver Research, London, United Kingdom, **3** Department of Hepatology, Barts Health NHS Trust, London, United Kingdom, **4** Departments of Exploratory Science, Discovery Biology, and Validation Biology, Biogen Idec Inc., Cambridge, Massachusetts, United States of America, **5** Department of Physiology, Faculty of Medicine, University of the Basque Country, Bilbao, Spain

Abstract

Background & Aims: Pro-inflammatory cytokines are important for liver regeneration after partial hepatectomy (PH). Expression of Fibroblast growth factor-inducible 14 (Fn14), the receptor for TNF-like weak inducer of apoptosis (TWEAK), is induced rapidly after PH and remains elevated throughout the period of peak hepatocyte replication. The role of Fn14 in post-PH liver regeneration is uncertain because Fn14 is expressed by liver progenitors and TWEAK-Fn14 interactions stimulate progenitor growth, but replication of mature hepatocytes is thought to drive liver regeneration after PH.

Methods: To clarify the role of TWEAK-Fn14 after PH, we compared post-PH regenerative responses in wild type (WT) mice, Fn14 knockout (KO) mice, TWEAK KO mice, and WT mice treated with anti-TWEAK antibodies.

Results: In WT mice, rare Fn14(+) cells localized with other progenitor markers in peri-portal areas before PH. PH rapidly increased proliferation of Fn14(+) cells; hepatocytic cells that expressed Fn14 and other progenitor markers, such as Lgr5, progressively accumulated from 12–8 h post-PH and then declined to baseline by 96 h. When TWEAK/Fn14 signaling was disrupted, progenitor accumulation, induction of pro-regenerative cytokines, hepatocyte and cholangiocyte proliferation, and over-all survival were inhibited, while post-PH liver damage and bilirubin levels were increased. TWEAK stimulated proliferation and increased Lgr5 expression in cultured liver progenitors, but had no effect on either parameter in cultured primary hepatocytes.

Conclusions: TWEAK-FN14 signaling is necessary for the healthy adult liver to regenerate normally after acute partial hepatectomy.

Editor: Patricia Aspichueta, University of Basque Country, Spain

Funding: This work was supported by R37 AA010154 and R01 DK077794 (to AMD). The funders had no role in study design, data collection and analysis, decision to publish, or preparation of the manuscript.

* E-mail: diehl004@mc.duke.edu

Introduction

Healthy adult livers regenerate efficiently after partial hepatectomy (PH). To reconstruct functional hepatic tissue, regeneration requires replacement of all cell types that were lost with the resected liver lobes. Replacement of mature hepatocytes and cholangiocytes is believed to be accomplished by replication of those cell types in the remaining liver. Mechanisms that replenish other cell populations, including progenitors, are unclear.[1]

Progenitors in healthy adult livers localize along canals of Herring (COH), vestiges of the fetal ductal plate that persist around adult liver portal tracts.[2] The COH-associated progenitor population of adult livers includes bipotent progenitors that are capable of differentiating along either the hepatocytic or biliary lineages depending on the demand for replacing the respective mature cell types.[3] This progenitor population expands during chronic liver injury, presumably to keep pace with chronically increased turnover rates of mature liver epithelial cells.[3] 70% of the portal tracts and associated COH are abruptly lost during PH. Thus, PH provides an enormous stimulus to regenerate the hepatic stem/progenitor compartment. Little is known about this process.

Bipotent liver epithelial progenitors express Fn14, a TNF-superfamily receptor for TWEAK (TNF-like weak inducer of apoptosis).[4,5] TWEAK is a cytokine that is produced by tissue macrophages and other cells during many types of injury.[4,6] TWEAK-Fn14 interactions promote the growth of Fn14(+) progenitors because knocking down Fn14 or neutralizing TWEAK in mice blocks the expansion of progenitor populations during chronic liver injuries that typically mobilize such cells, while TWEAK treatment promotes the expansion of progenitor populations.[4,7,8] The importance of TWEAK/Fn14 signaling in regulating liver progenitor populations was further substantiated by a recent report that bone marrow transplantation generated TWEAK-producing macrophages which stimulated outgrowth of liver progenitors.[6]

Hepatic expression of Fn14 mRNAs increases more than 50 fold within a few hours after PH.[9,10] The significance of this dramatic induction of Fn14 after PH is uncertain. Herein we evaluate the hypothesis that TWEAK-Fn14 signaling helps to replenish liver progenitor populations in regenerating livers after PH. Various approaches were used to quantify and localize changes in Fn14 expression following PH in healthy adult WT mice, and to map the timing of the Fn14 response to changes in other progenitor markers, proliferative activity in mature liver epithelial cells, recovery of liver mass, and overall survival. Results in WT mice were then compared to these same outcome measures in mice with targeted deletion of Fn14 or TWEAK, and WT mice that were treated with neutralizing anti-TWEAK antibodies. The findings confirm the hypothesis about TWEAK/Fn14 and reconstitution of hepatic progenitor pools, but also reveal that TWEAK/Fn14 signaling is required for otherwise healthy adults to regenerate mature liver epithelial cells, recover healthy liver mass, and survive following acute PH.

Materials and Methods

Reagents

Chemicals were obtained from Sigma-Aldrich Corporation (St. Louis, MO) unless stated otherwise.

Animal Experiments

In total, more than 200 mice were used in these studies. C57BL/6 wild type mice (WT, n = 80), Fn14 knockout (Fn14 KO) mice (n = 60), TWEAK knockout (TWEAK KO) mice (n = 10), and their respective littermate controls (n = 16), were maintained in animal facilities at Duke University. Both KO mice strains were generously provided by Biogen Idec Inc. (Cambridge, MA).[4,11] Animal surgery and care were approved by the Institutional Animal Care and Use Committee as governed by the National Institute of Health's "Guide for the Care and Use of Laboratory Animals", Duke University Animal Welfare Assurance Number A3195-01. Animals were sacrificed under general anesthesia and all efforts were made to minimize suffering during surgery.

8 to 10 week old male mice were subjected to 70% partial hepatectomy (PH) according to the method Higgins and Anderson as previously reported.[9] A minimum of 4 mice/group/time point were sacrificed at 12 hours (Fn14 KO mice and controls only), and 24 and 48 hours (all groups) after PH. Depending on availability of knockout mice, studies were repeated to increase sample size. Hence, at least 10 mice/group were sacrificed at the 12, 24 and 48 hour time points. More detailed list of experimental group division was provided in **Table S1**. In some studies, C57BL6 WT mice were injected i.p. with anti-TWEAK antibodies (200 μg/mouse, clone P2D10, Biogen Idec) or a comparable volume of control IgG immediately before PH and daily thereafter. To evaluate treatment effects on proliferative activity, all mice were routinely administered bromo-deoxyuridine (BrdU) intraperitoneally (50 μg/g body weight) 2 hours before sacrifice. Animals were weighed before PH and before sacrifice. Collected liver samples removed at the time of initial PH (0 hour time point) and regenerating liver samples that were harvested at 12, 24, or 48 hours post-PH were weighed and snap frozen in liquid nitrogen or formalin fixed for further analysis.

Immunohistochemistry and BrdU Labelling

Immunohistochemistry was performed as previously described.[12] Formalin-fixed paraffin-embedded liver tissues were cut into 5 μm thick sections and placed on glass slides. Sections were de-parafinized with xylene and dehydrated with ethanol, then incubated for 10 min in 3% hydrogen peroxide to block endogenous peroxidase. Antigen retrieval was performed by

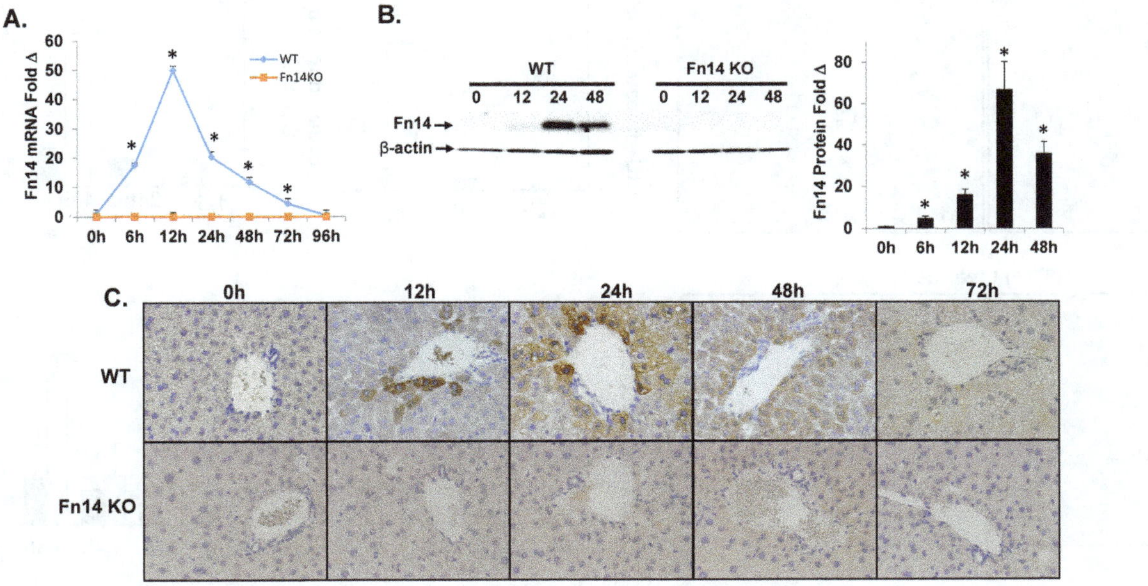

Figure 1. Partial hepatectomy triggers hepatic accumulation of Fn14(+) cells in WT mice. Healthy adult wild type (WT) mice (n = 80) underwent PH. Expression of Fn14 was evaluated at various time points by (A) qRT-PCR analysis, (B) Representative western blot, quantification of protein levels for Fn14 normalized to β-actin and (C) Immunohistochemistry (magnification 20×). To assure reagent specificity, similar analysis was done in mice that were genetically-deficient in Fn14(Fn14 KO). Mean +/− SEM results from all mice (n = 4–5/time point) are graphed relative to baseline, pre-PH (time 0), * $p<0.05$.

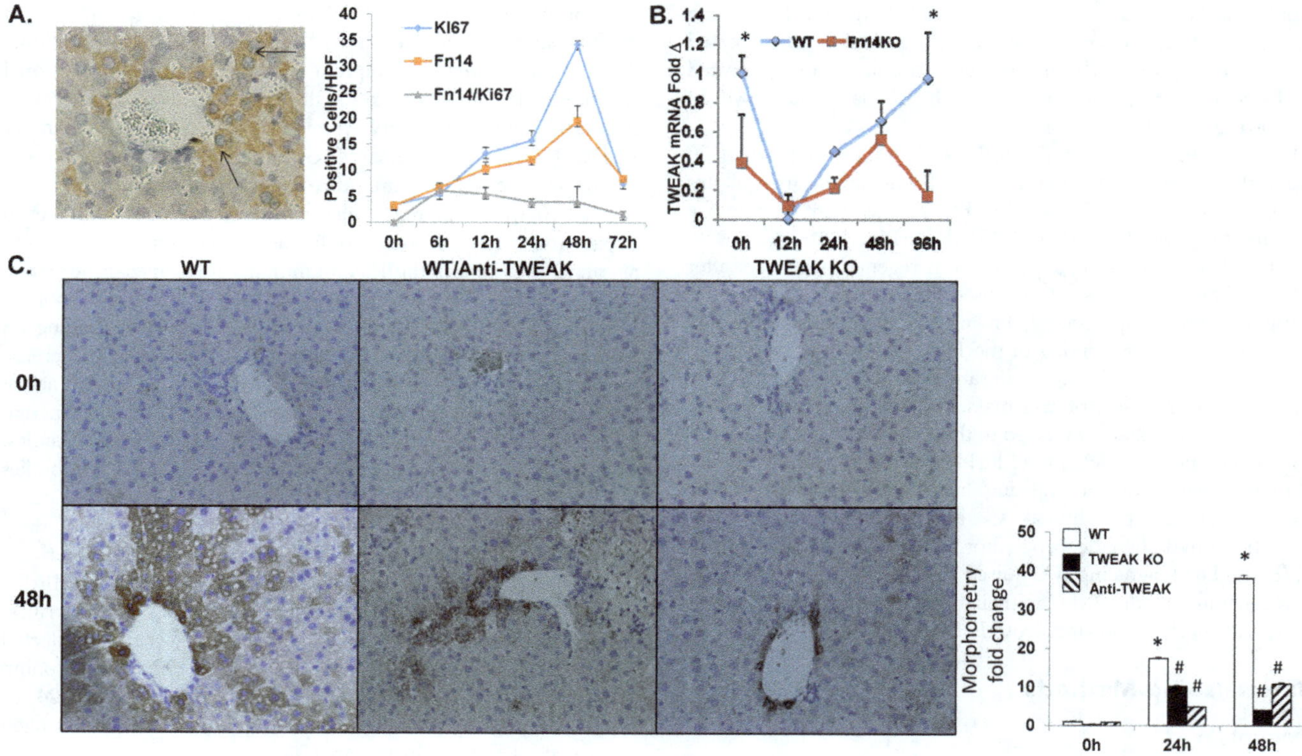

Figure 2. Post- PH growth of Fn14(+) cells is Fn14-dependent and requires TWEAK. (A) Liver sections from WT mice were double-stained for Fn14 (brown) and Ki67 (green), a proliferation marker. Representative image of liver from 6 h after PH is displayed. Arrow indicates double positive cells. Mean +/− SEM numbers of positive cells in 10 random 40× fields/section in 5 mice/group/time point. (B) qRT-PCR analysis of TWEAK mRNA expression in whole liver RNA from WT and Fn14 KO mice at various time points after PH; * $p<0.05$ vs WT. (C) Fn14 immunohistochemistry and morphometry analysis in WT mice, WT mice treated with Anti-TWEAK antibodies, TWEAK KO mice, and Fn14 KO mice at baseline (0 h) and 48 h after PH. * $p<0.05$ vs time 0, # p 0.05 vs WT. Representative images are displayed (magnification 20×).

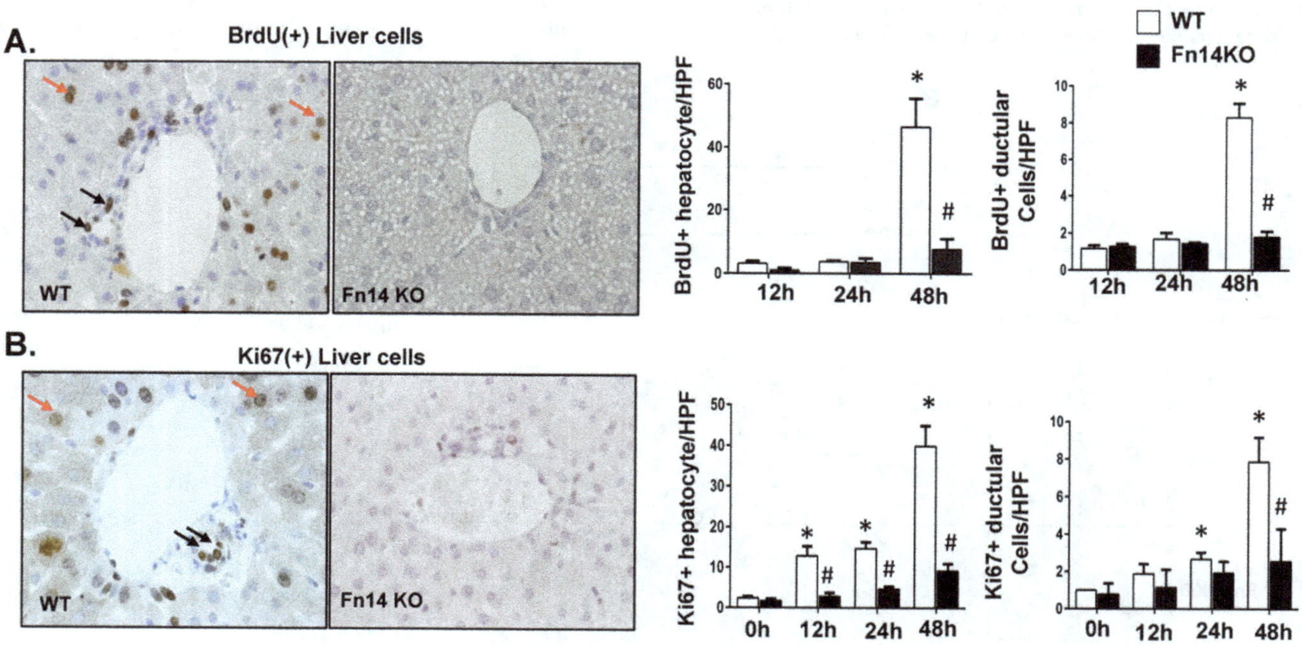

Figure 3. Deletion of Fn14 inhibits post- PH proliferation of hepatocytes and cholangiocytes. Fn14 KO mice and wild type (WT) mice underwent PH. Proliferative activity was evaluated by (A) BrdU incorporation and (B) Ki67 immunostaining. Representative images are displayed (magnification 20×). Arrows indicate Brdu(+) or Ki67(+) cells (red-hepatocyte, black-ductular cells). Labeled hepatocytes/ductular cells were counted in 10 randomly-selected 20× magnification fields/section. Mean +/− SEM results from all mice (n = 3–4/group/time point) are graphed relative to baseline, pre-PH (time 0) in WT group. * $p<0.05$ vs time 0, # $p<0.05$ vs WT. Representative images of 48 hours post-PH liver are displayed (magnification 20×).

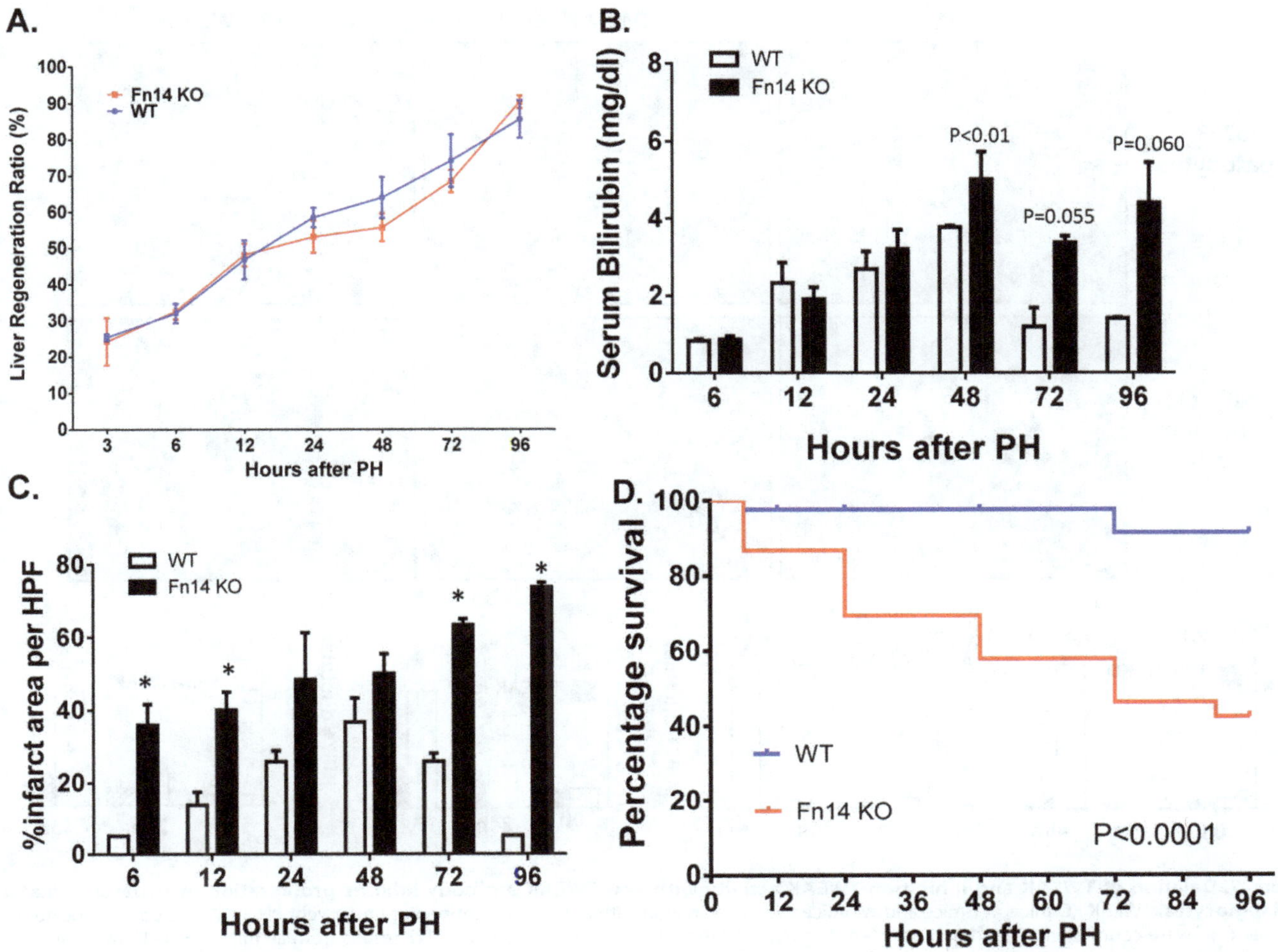

Figure 4. Deletion of Fn14 impairs liver regeneration and survival after PH. Healthy adult wild type (WT) and Fn14 KO mice underwent PH. (A) Liver regeneration ratios (assessed by dividing liver weight at sacrifice by the estimated original liver weight) were compared between WT and Fn14 KO mice at various time points post-PH. (B) Serum bilirubin levels were measured using a Total Bilirubin Test Kit (BIOTRON Diagnostics). (C) Percentage of infarct areas per high-powered field (HPF) were also quantified at in 50 randomly-chosen fields/section. Mean +/− SEM results from 3–4 mice/group/time point are shown. * p<0.01 vs WT. (D) Survival rates were compared between WT and Fn14 KO mice at various time points post-PH. The P values for survival curve are calculated using the log rank test.

heating in 10 mM sodium citrate buffer (pH 6.0) for 10 min or incubation with pepsin (00-3009; Invitrogen) for 5 min. Sections were blocked in Dako protein block (X9090; Dako) for 15 min and incubated with primary antibodies at 4°C overnight. Primary antibodies used were: keratin19 (Troma III, 1:400; Hydroma Bank), AFP (A0008, 1:400; Dako), Fn14 (314102, Biolegend), LGR5 (TA301323, Origene) HRP-conjugated anti-rabbit (K4003; Dako) secondary antibodies were used to visualize target proteins. DAB reagent (K3466; Dako) was applied in the detection procedure. Ki67 and BrdU staining were quantified by counting the numbers of hepatocytes and ductular cells with stained nuclei in ten randomly chosen 20X fields/section/mouse.

mRNA Quantification by Real Time RT-PCR

Total RNA was isolated using commercial reagents (TRIzol Reagents, Invitrogen). RNA concentration and purity was determined with NanoDrop ND-1000 Spectrophotometer (NanoDrop Technologies, Palo Alto, CA) and samples with a 260/280 nm absorbance ratio of >1.8 were used in subsequent analyses. mRNAs were quantified by QRT-PCR using 25 ng of cDNA, as described.[13] All samples were analyzed in duplicate. Gene expression levels were normalized to the reference gene S9, and fold change was calculated by the $2^{-\Delta\Delta Ct}$ method. Sequences of primers are listed in the **Table S2**.

Western Blot Analysis

Protein extracts were prepared by homogenization of liver tissue in RIPA buffer (R0278; Sigma) and quantified by Pierce BCA kit. Proteins were visualized by western analysis using the following primary antibodies; keratin 7 (sc-70936, Santa Cruz Biotechnology), alpha-fetoprotein (AFP, A0008, Dako), Fn14 (314102, Biolegend), LGR5 (TA301323, Origene) and β-actin (sc-47778, Santa Cruz Biotechnology).

Statistical Analysis

Results are expressed as mean ± SEM. Significance was established using the student *t*-test. P<0.05 was considered significant.

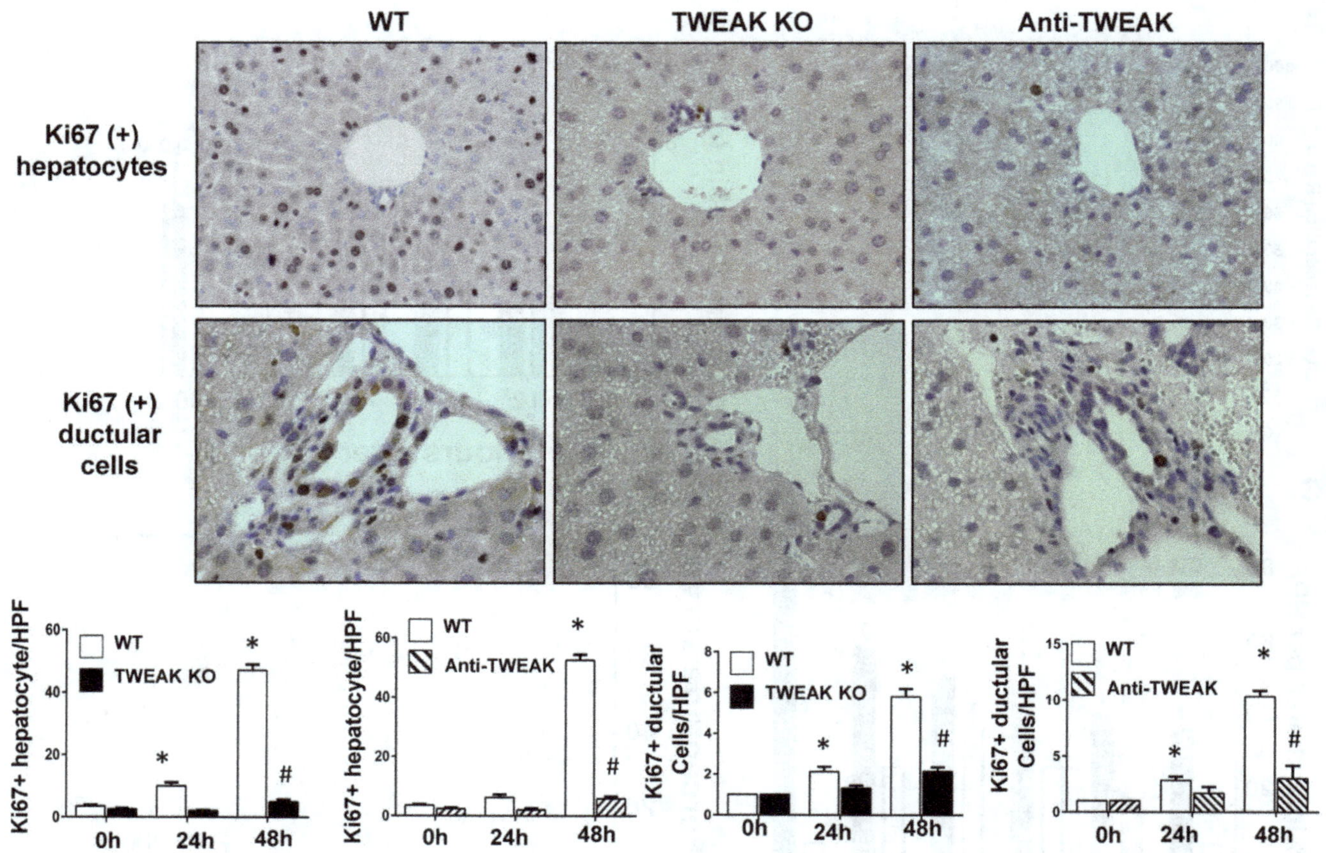

Figure 5. Deletion of TWEAK and inhibition TWEAK activity with anti-TWEAK antibody inhibits proliferation of hepatocytes and cholangiocytes. TWEAK KO mice, WT mice and WT mice that were treated with anti-TWEAK antibodies underwent PH. Ki67 labeled hepatocytes or ductular cells were counted in 10 randomly-selected 20× magnification fields/section. Mean +/− SEM results from all mice (n = 3–4/time point) are graphed relative to baseline, pre-PH (time 0) in WT group. * $p<0.05$ vs time 0, # p 0.05 vs WT. Representative images of 48 hours post-PH liver are displayed (magnification 20×).

Results

Partial Hepatectomy Triggers Hepatic Accumulation of Fn14(+) Cells in WT Mice

Healthy adult wild type (WT) mice (n = 80) underwent PH. Expression of Fn14 was evaluated at various time points by qRT-PCR analysis, Western blot, and immunohistochemistry. Similar analysis was done in mice that were genetically-deficient in Fn14 (Fn14KO) (n = 60). Consistent with earlier reports,[9,10] we found that Fn14 mRNA levels were barely detectable at baseline but increased around 50 fold following PH (**Figure 1A**). Transcript induction was maximal at 12 hours post-PH. Western blot analysis demonstrated a comparable induction of Fn14 protein which peaked about 12 hours later and remained 30 fold above basal levels through 48 hours post-PH (**Figure 1B**). Changes in whole liver content of Fn14 protein reflected a dramatic increase in Fn14-expressing cells (**Figure 1C and Figure S1**). These cells emerged around portal tracts and then rapidly accumulated in other parts of the liver lobule. Interestingly, however, the morphology of these Fn14(+) cells was not typical of bipotent liver epithelial progenitors, which are generally small cells with an oval nucleus. Rather, the cells that express Fn14 following PH appear hepatocytic. Given the kinetics of the RNA and protein data (**Figure 1A–B**), plus the fact that neither transcripts (**Figure 1A**) nor immunoreactivity (**Figure 1B–C and Figure S1**) were demonstrated in Fn14 KO liver, immunohistochemistry evidence for Fn14 expression by hepatocytic cells appears to be valid, and consistent with another report which demonstrated Fn14 expressing hepatocytes in injured human and mouse liver.[5]

Post-PH growth of Fn14(+) Cells is TWEAK/Fn14-Dependent.

To determine the mechanism for accumulation of these Fn14(+) hepatocytic cells, liver sections from WT mice were double-stained for Fn14 and Ki67, a proliferation marker[14] (**Figure 2A**). Numbers of Fn14/Ki67-double positive cells increased rapidly after PH and were 5 fold greater than baseline by 6 hours post-PH. Proliferative activity in the Fn14(+) compartment gradually declined thereafter, reaching baseline levels by 72 hours after PH. The early peak in Fn14(+) cells preceded increased proliferative activity in Fn14-negative cells, which occurred around 48 hours after PH, the expected time frame for maximal post-PH DNA synthesis in hepatocytes.[1] Interestingly, outgrowth of Fn14(+) cells occurred despite reduced hepatic expression of TWEAK mRNA, which decreased sharply during the initial 12 hours after PH and only returned to basal levels by 96 hours post-PH. TWEAK expression in Fn14 KO mice followed a similar pattern, albeit at generally lower levels, demonstrating that Fn14-expressing cells were not required for TWEAK production after PH (**Figure 2B**). To determine if TWEAK was necessary for accumulation of Fn14(+) cells, immunostaining for Fn14 was done on liver sections from TWEAK KO mice and WT mice treated

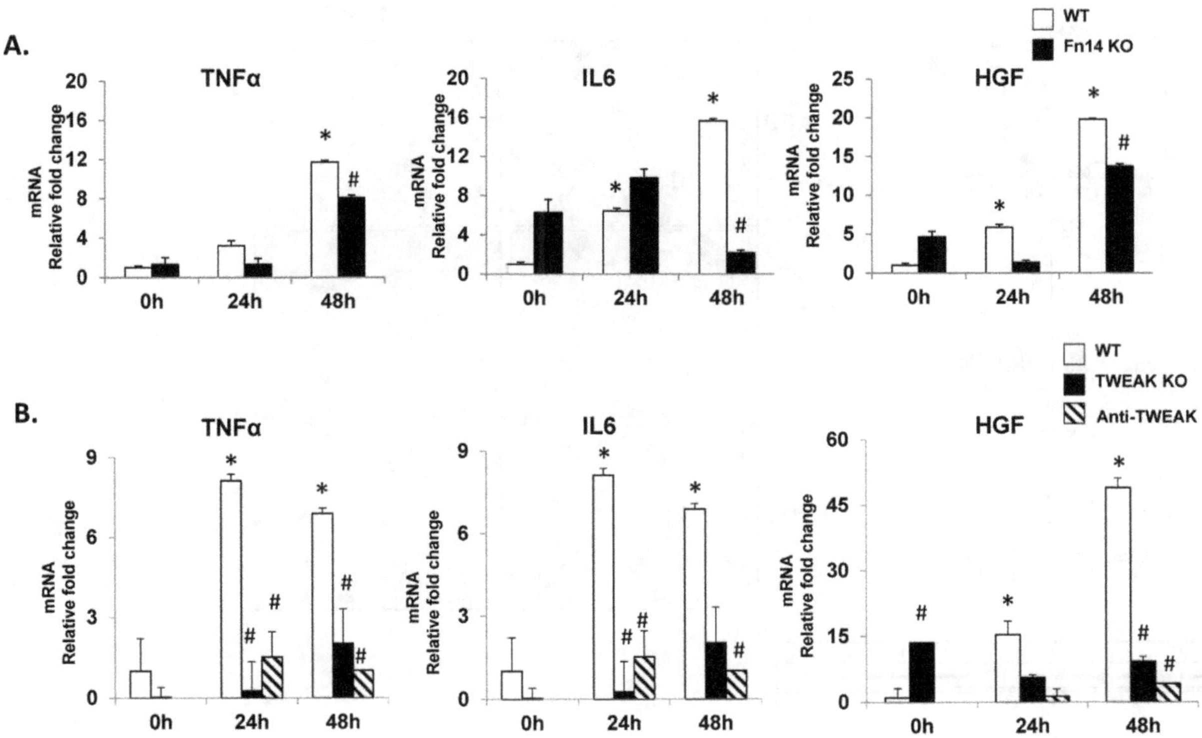

Figure 6. Inhibiting TWEAK/Fn14 signaling attenuates the induction of mitogens associated with liver regeneration. QRT-PCR analysis of whole liver expression of TNFα, IL6 and HGF mRNA in (A) WT and Fn14 KO mice (B) WT, TWEAK KO and WT mice treated with Anti-TWEAK antibodies after PH. Mean +/− SEM results from all mice (n = 3–4/time point) are graphed relative to baseline, pre-PH (time 0) in WT group. * p<0.05 vs time 0, # p<0.05 vs WT.

with either anti-TWEAK antibodies or an irrelevant IgG. Morphometry confirmed striking expansion of the Fn14(+) compartment during the initial 48 hours after PH in WT mice and demonstrated significant attenuation of this response in both TWEAK KO mice and WT mice treated with anti-TWEAK antibodies (**Figure 2C**). Thus, the outgrowth of Fn14(+) cells post-PH is TWEAK-dependent.

Deletion of Fn14 Inhibits Post-PH Proliferation of Hepatocytes and Cholangiocytes

Most of the proliferative cells at later time points (e.g., 24–72 hours) post-PH did not express Fn14 (**Figure 2A**). To resolve whether or not Fn14 activity was necessary for this late increase in liver cell proliferation, proliferative activity in hepatocytic and ductular cells was evaluated at various time points in WT and Fn14 KO mice by BrdU incorporation and Ki67 immunostaining. Both approaches demonstrated the expected increase in hepatocyte and ductular cell proliferation in WT mice. In contrast, deletion of Fn14 significantly inhibited the normal post-PH induction of proliferation in both compartments (**Figure 3**), demonstrating that Fn14 is required for optimal regeneration of mature hepatocytes and cholangiocytes following PH. Consistent with these data, net recovery of liver weight in the Fn14 KO group (assessed by regeneration ratio [15]) lagged somewhat behind that of WT mice from 24–72 hours post-PH (**Figure 4A**). Moreover, other outcome measures indicated that loss of Fn14 significantly subverted post-PH recovery of ***functional*** hepatic parenchyma. Rather, areas of infarcted liver increased steadily after PH in Fn14 KO mice (**Figure 4C, Figure S2**). This was accompanied by sustained hyperbilirubinemia and progressive mortality. (**Figure 4B,D**). Indeed, by 96 hours after PH, almost 60% of Fn14KO mice were dead compared to about 5% of WT mice, and serum bilirubin levels in surviving Fn14 KO mice were about three fold higher than in WT controls. Hence, loss of Fn14 signaling impairs proper liver regeneration and leads to liver failure after PH.

Deletion of TWEAK or Inhibition TWEAK Activity with Anti-TWEAK Antibody Inhibit Proliferation of Hepatocytes and Cholangiocytes

Post-PH outgrowth of Fn14(+) cells is TWEAK dependent (**Figure 2C**) and accumulation of Fn14(+) cells is necessary for optimal regeneration of Fn14-negative hepatocytes and cholangiocytes following PH (**Figure 3**). This suggests that TWEAK activity is also required for increased hepatocyte and ductular cell proliferative activity post-PH. To evaluate this possibility directly, TWEAK KO mice, WT mice treated with anti-TWEAK antibodies, and their respective controls underwent PH and numbers of Ki67-labeled hepatocytes/ductular cells were counted in representative sections of livers harvested at various time points post-PH. The results confirm that inhibiting TWEAK significantly inhibited post-PH proliferation of hepatocytes and cholangiocytes (**Figure 5**), demonstrating that TWEAK-Fn14 signaling is necessary for adult livers to regenerate successfully after PH.

TWEAK/Fn14 Signaling Stimulates Post-PH Replication of Mature Liver Epithelial Cells via Indirect Mechanisms

Although several earlier studies had demonstrated that TWEAK was unable to stimulate proliferation of healthy mature hepatocytes, evidence that deleting/neutralizing TWEAK or deleting its receptor blocked liver regeneration after PH prompted

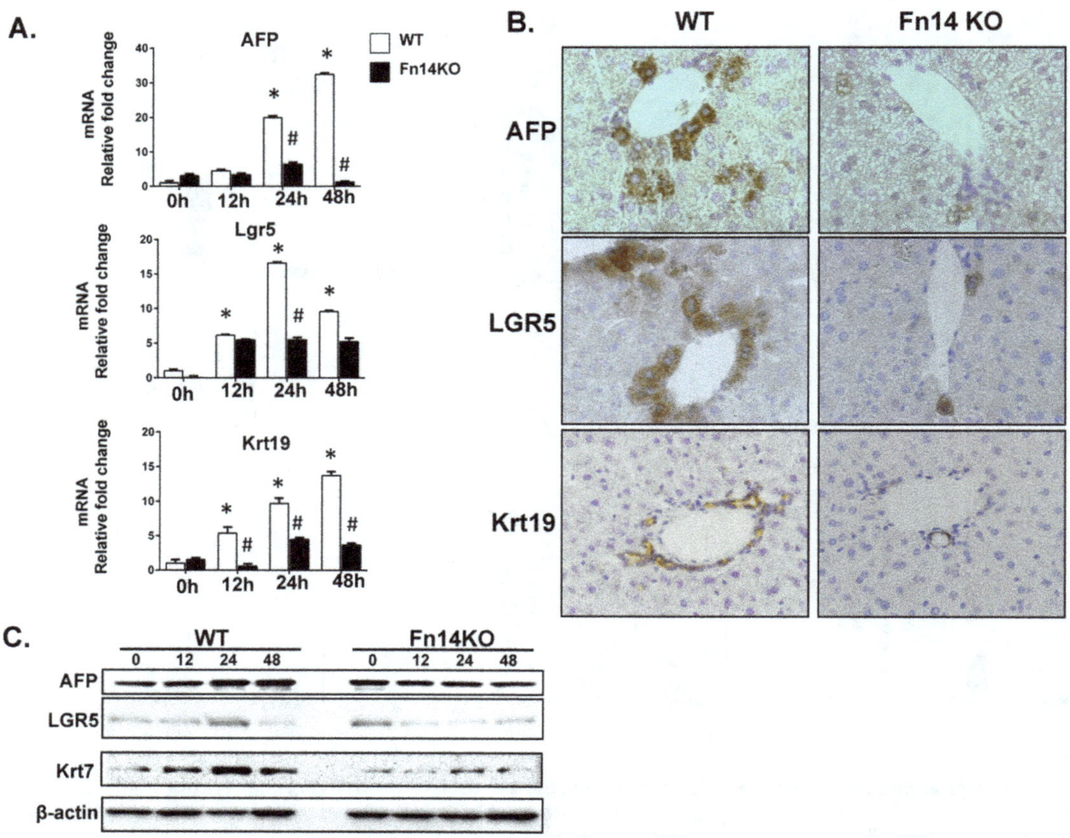

Figure 7. Deletion of Fn14 inhibits accumulation of progenitor cells after PH. Fn14 KO mice and wild type (WT) mice underwent PH. Expression of progenitor markers was evaluated at various time points by (A) qRT-PCR analysis, (B) Immunohistochemistry and (C) Western blot. Mean +/− SEM results from all mice (n = 5/time point) are graphed relative to baseline, pre-PH (time 0) in WT group, * $p<0.05$ vs time 0, # $p<0.05$ vs WT. Representative images of 48 hours post-PH liver are displayed (magnification 40×).

us to re-examine the direct effects of TWEAK on hepatocyte proliferation. To verify the biological activity of the recombinant TWEAK used for our studies, we tested its effect on a mouse liver progenitor cell line (603B cells) which we had previously characterized and found to exhibit features of liver progenitors.[16] FACS showed that, 603B cells uniformly expressed Fn14 protein (**Figure S3A**). Treating 603B cells with TWEAK increased their expression of AFP[17] and LGR5 [3], markers of hepatocytic progenitors (**Figure S3C**). Doses of TWEAK as low as 1 ng/ml also stimulated their growth (**Figure S3B**). However, as others reported,[4,7] we found that recombinant TWEAK was unable to stimulate proliferation of primary hepatocytes isolated from the livers of healthy adult mice even at doses as high as 10 ng/ml (**Figure S3B**), or when used in conjunction with IL6, a putative hepatotrophic cytokine (data not shown). Consistent with the inability of TWEAK to directly impact hepatocyte proliferative activity, neither qRT-PCR analysis (data not shown), nor flow cytometry (**Figure S3A**) were able to demonstrate expression of Fn14 by primary hepatocytes isolated from healthy adult mice livers. The aggregate data, therefore, demonstrate that after PH, TWEAK directly stimulates an early wave of replication in Fn14(+) progenitors, but promotes the subsequent proliferative surge of mature liver epithelial cells via indirect mechanisms.

One such mechanism might involve TWEAK/Fn14-related induction of other liver growth factors. Cytokines and growth factors that increase rapidly after PH function as co-mitogens to promote hepatocyte proliferation after PH. In this regard, tumor necrosis factor (TNF) alpha, interleukin (IL)-6 and hepatocyte growth factor (HGF) are particularly noteworthy because blocking the activities of any of these factors is sufficient to inhibit induction of hepatocyte DNA synthesis and liver regeneration following PH.[1] Quantitative RT-PCR analysis of whole liver RNA from Fn14 KO mice, TWEAK KO mice, WT mice treated with anti-TWEAK antibodies, and their respective wild-type controls demonstrated that inhibiting TWEAK-Fn14 signaling inhibited normal post-PH induction of each of these factors (**Figure 6**). Therefore, loss of TWEAK/Fn14-regulated growth factors likely contributed to the inhibited proliferation of mature-appearing hepatocytes and ductular cells that occurred after PH when TWEAK/Fn14 signaling was disrupted. Additional mechanisms might also be involved, however, including reduced availability of Fn14-positive progenitors to differentiate into more mature, Fn14-negative liver cells that proliferate in response to these other mitogens at later time points after PH. This possibility merits consideration because PH abruptly removes not only 70% of mature liver epithelial cells, but also 70% of the COH-associated progenitor cells.

Deletion of Fn14 Inhibits Accumulation of Progenitor Cells after PH

Consistent with the concept that PH provides a strong stimulus to regenerate the progenitor compartment, we observed increased expression of Fn14 in hepatocytic cells near COH within a few hours after PH (**Figure 1C, Figure S1**). To evaluate the effects of

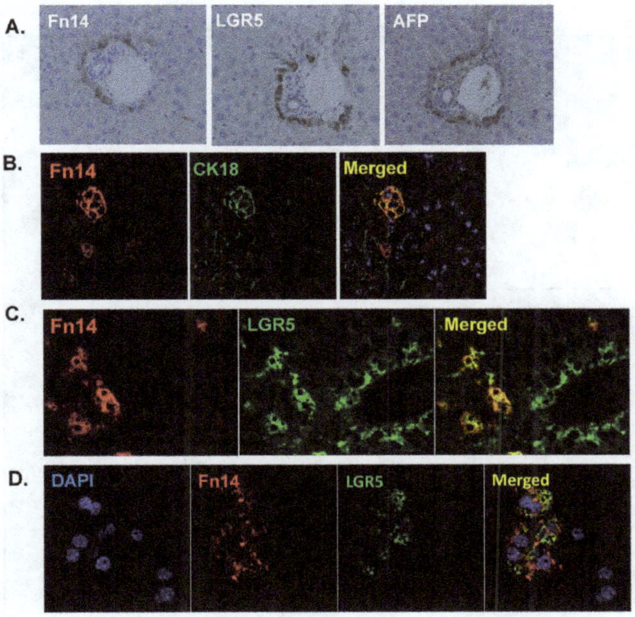

Figure 8. Liver Fn14(+) cells co-localize with progenitor cells. (A) Serial section staining for Fn14 and progenitor markers (AFP and LGR5) in WT mice 48 hours after PH (magnification 40×). (B) Confocal images of Fn14 and CK18 co-staining in WT mice liver 24 hours after PH (magnification 40×). Yellow indicates co-localization of these two markers. (C) Double immunofluorescence for Fn14 and LGR5 in WT mice liver 48 hours after PH (magnification 20×). Yellow indicates co-localization of these two markers. (C) Confocal images of Fn14 and LGR5 co-stained primary hepatocytes isolated from WT mice 24 hours after PH (magnification 63×).

PH on expression of other progenitor markers, and determine whether or not loss of Fn14 impacted this, expression of other progenitor markers was evaluated by immunohistochemistry, qRT-PCR analysis, and Western blot. At baseline, cells expressing AFP (a marker of hepatocytic progenitors) or LGR5 (an endodermal progenitor marker) were rarely observed, and expression of Krt19 (a marker for immature and mature ductular cells [18]) was restricted to intralobular bile ducts in both WT and Fn14KO mice (**Figure S4**). In WT mice following PH, hepatocytic cells expressing AFP and LGR5 emerged in periportal areas and gradually accumulated in other regions of the hepatic parenchyma, while Krt19 staining remained largely restricted to ductular structures around portal tracts. However, the post-PH accumulation of AFP, LGR5 and Krt19-expressing cells was severely attenuated in Fn14 KO mice (**Figure 7B and Figure S4**). These changes were substantiated by PCR and Western blot analysis, demonstrating significant post-PH increases in mRNA and protein expression of AFP, LGR5, Krt19, and Krt7 (another liver progenitor marker [18]) in WT mice, but consistent suppression of these responses in Fn14 KO mice (**Figure 7A,C**). Hence, Fn14 is required for progenitor cells to accumulate normally after PH. Moreover, careful inspection of serially-stained sections demonstrated that Fn14(+) cells were closely localized with LGR5(+) cells and AFP(+) cells at each time point, but distinct from cells that expressed Krt19 (**Figure 7, Figure 8A**), suggesting that Fn14 marks hepatocytic progenitors after PH. To confirm this finding, we performed double immunofluorescence staining of Fn14 and CK18 (an epithelial cytokeratin that is expressed by both mature hepatocytes and hepatocyte progenitors) on liver sections from WT mice after PH. In addition, double staining of Fn14 and LGR5 was assessed on both liver sections and isolated hepatocytes from WT mice after PH (**Figure 8B–D**). Fn14 co-localized with CK18 and LGR5 in a subpopulation of hepatocytes, providing strong evidence that Fn14 is expressed by hepatocytic progenitors and demonstrating that the hepatocyte compartment becomes enriched with such progenitors a day or so before Fn14-negative hepatocytes begin to proliferate.

TWEAK Is Required for Optimal Regeneration of Liver Progenitors after PH

Having shown that Fn14 is required for expansion of progenitor populations following PH (**Figure 7**), we wished to determine if TWEAK is also necessary for this aspect of post-PH regeneration. Therefore, we compared progenitor responses to PH in WT mice, TWEAK KO mice, and WT mice that were treated with anti-TWEAK antibodies. QRT-PCR and immunohistochemistry demonstrated that inhibiting TWEAK significantly inhibited post-PH induction of markers for hepatocytic progenitors (AFP and LGR5), and ductular cell precursors (Krt19) (**Figure 9**). Hence, TWEAK and its receptor, Fn14 are necessary for regeneration of both mature hepatocytes and cholangiocytes (**Figure 3 and 5**), and their respective precursors (**Figure 7 and 9**), following PH.

Discussion

Our results show, for the first time, that TWEAK/Fn14 signaling is required for optimal induction of various processes that are necessary for livers to regenerate after PH, including activation of hepatocyte/cholangiocyte proliferation, induction of key mitogenic factors, and accumulation of liver progenitors. These new observations extend earlier evidence that PH leads to rapid and strong up-regulation of hepatic Fn14 mRNA expression.[9,10]

Fn14 mRNAs are known to be expressed by liver cell lines that exhibit features of immature, relatively undifferentiated cells, and TWEAK promotes the proliferation of such cells in culture.[4,7] In addition, disrupting Fn14 or blocking TWEAK in animal models of liver regeneration that depend upon liver progenitors severely inhibits liver regeneration.[4,7,8] The present study provides novel evidence that TWEAK/Fn14 signaling is also necessary to expand liver progenitor populations and regenerate the liver following PH. Thus, it is reasonable to conclude that liver regeneration after PH also depends upon TWEAK-responsive Fn14(+) progenitors.

Evidence that progenitors mediate post-PH regeneration was unexpected because current dogma posits that the process is driven mainly by the replication of residual mature liver epithelial cells in the remnant liver.[19] Therefore, we used FACS analysis to determine if mature hepatocytes express Fn14 and tested whether or not TWEAK was able to increase their proliferative activity directly. We were unable to demonstrate Fn14 on the surface of primary hepatocytes isolated from healthy adult livers, and TWEAK was unable to induce these cells to proliferate. Our results are in accordance with earlier publications which also failed to demonstrate appreciable expression of Fn14 in mature hepatocytes in healthy adult livers.[4,7] Moreover, that earlier work demonstrated that hepatocyte proliferation was not increased in TWEAK-transgenic mice although such animals strongly expressed TWEAK in hepatocytes and maintained relatively high serum levels of TWEAK.[4] Thus, disruption of TWEAK/Fn14 signaling in mature hepatocytes does not explain why we observed inhibited proliferation of such cells in Fn14 KO and TWEAK KO mice.

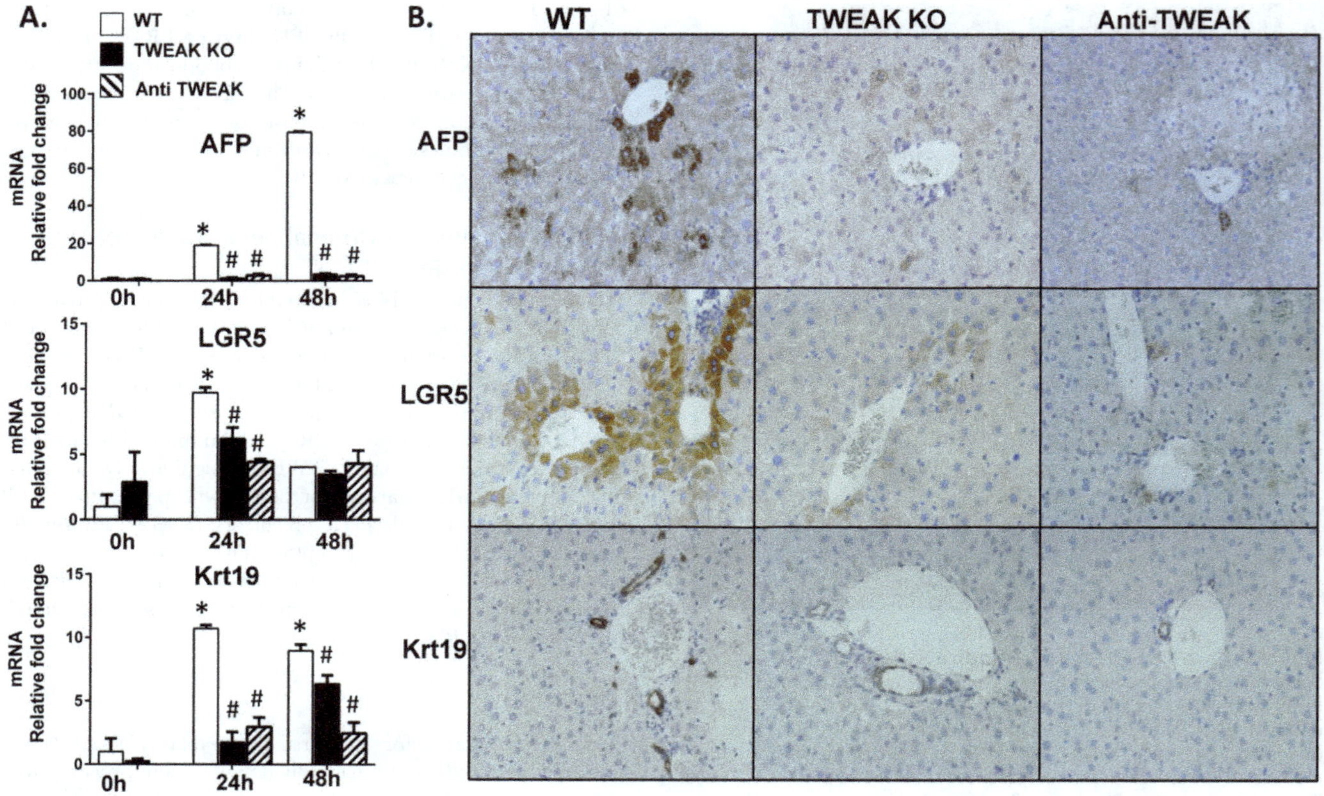

Figure 9. TWEAK is required for optimal liver regeneration after PH. TWEAK KO mice, WT mice and WT mice that were treated with anti-TWEAK antibodies underwent PH. Expression of progenitor markers was evaluated at various time points by (A) qRT-PCR analysis and (B) Immunohistochemistry. Mean +/− SEM results from all mice (n = 5/time point) are graphed relative to baseline, pre-PH (time 0) in WT group, * $p<0.05$ vs time 0, # $p<0.05$ vs WT. Representative images of 48 hours post-PH liver are displayed (magnification 20×).

Mice that were deficient in TWEAK or FN14 were noted to have defective induction of certain pro-regenerative cytokines (e.g., TNFα and IL6) and hepatocyte mitogens, such as HGF. Thus, it is conceivable that reduced availability of hepato-trophic factors contributed to the inhibited regenerative responses to PH that occurred when TWEAK/Fn14 signaling was disrupted. Another hypothesis that merits consideration is that some replicating hepatocytes in post-PH livers may be the recent progeny of Fn14(+) TWEAK-sensitive liver progenitors. These more mature liver cells no longer express Fn14 and hence, have lost the ability to replicate in response to TWEAK. Our data support this possibility. We found that TWEAK directly stimulated proliferation of Fn14(+) liver progenitors and increased their expression of AFP and LGR5 *in vitro*. We also demonstrated co-localization of Fn14 and these other progenitor markers in regenerating livers after PH, and confirmed co-expression of Fn14 and LGR5 in hepatocytic cells isolated from 24 hours post-PH livers. Recent lineage tracing studies that tracked the fate of LGR5(+) cells in regenerating livers after acute CCl_4-induced injury demonstrated that some of the repopulating hepatocytes were derived from LGR5(+) progenitors.[3] Our data suggest that the same process might occur after PH.

Moreover, our findings provide novel evidence that TWEAK/Fn14 signaling regulates accumulation of LGR5(+) cells during liver regeneration. In WT mice after PH, we showed that the increased proliferative activity and accumulation of Fn14(+)/LGR5(+) cells was TWEAK-dependent, and resulted in enrichment of the hepatocytic compartment with Fn14(+) progenitor cells before proliferative activity increased in hepatocytes that did not express progenitor markers. In livers that lacked Fn14 (or which had reduced TWEAK activity), LGR5(+) liver progenitors failed to accumulate normally after PH; proliferation of hepatocytes was severely inhibited; and the livers were unable to regenerate normally, resulting in progressive liver damage, liver dysfunction, and mortality rather than recovery. Based on the aggregate results, therefore, our working hypothesis is that many of the hepatocytes that normally repopulate adult livers after PH are the progeny of TWEAK-responsive progenitors that co-express Fn14 and LGR5. Testing this hypothesis requires lineage tracing approaches. Thus, future experiments that genetically label Fn14(+) cells and follow the fate of these cells after PH are needed to resolve this issue.

In summary, the current results prove that TWEAK/Fn14 signaling is required for the liver to regenerate normally following PH. The data demonstrate that key aspects of the regenerative response, including induction of hepatocyte/cholangiocyte proliferation, accumulation of hepato-trophic factors, and expansion of hepatic progenitor populations depend upon signaling that is activated when TWEAK engages its receptor, Fn14. These insights explain earlier observations that Fn14 expression is up-regulated dramatically after PH and improve understanding about mechanisms that control regeneration of adult livers after injury.

Supporting Information

Figure S1 Partial hepatectomy triggers hepatic accumulation of Fn14(+) cells in WT mice. Healthy adult wild type (WT) mice and

Fn14 KO mice underwent PH. Expression of Fn14 was evaluated at various time points by Immunohistochemistry (magnification 10×).

Figure S2 Deletion of Fn14 impairs liver regeneration after PH. Healthy adult wild type (WT) mice and Fn14 KO mice underwent PH. Representative H&E staining of liver sections from WT and Fn14 KO mice at different time points after PH were displayed (magnification 10×). Note Fn14 KO mice livers have more infarct areas than WT mice.

Figure S3 TWEAK promotes proliferation and differentiation of mouse bipotent epithelial liver progenitor cells (603B) but not primary mouse hepaotcyte. (A) FACS analysis of Fn14 protein expression by 603B and freshly isolated wild type primary mouse hepatocyte (mHep). (B) 603B cells and primary mouse hepatocyte (mHep) were cultured with 1 ng/ml recombinant TWEAK for 24 hours. 10 μM BrdU was added to the plates and cells were incubated for 2 hours. Cell proliferation were assessed by BrdU Cell Proliferation Assay Kit. * $p<0.05$. (C) 603B cells were treated with recombinant Tweak as described in (B) for 24 and 48 hours. mRNA was isolated and changes in α-Fetoprotein (AFP) and LGR5 gene expression were analyzed by qRT-PCR. Results are graphed relative to control at each time point.

Figure S4 Deletion of Fn14 inhibits progenitor response after PH. Wild type (WT) and Fn14 KO mice underwent PH. Expression of progenitor markers (AFP, LGR5 and Krt19) was evaluated at 0 and 48 hours after PH by Immunohistochemistry. Representative images are displayed (magnification 10×).

Table S1 Detailed usage of mice for PH.

Table S2 Sequence of mouse primers used in experiments.

Author Contributions

Conceived and designed the experiments: GK GX WKS SSC GAM AMD. Performed the experiments: GK MS GX LK MVM GAM BO. Analyzed the data: GK GX MVM KG SSC GAM AMD. Contributed reagents/materials/analysis tools: LB. Wrote the paper: GK GX GAM AMD.

References

1. Michalopoulos GK (2007) Liver regeneration. J Cell Physiol 213: 286–300.
2. Kuwahara R, Kofman AV, Landis CS, Swenson ES, Barendswaard E, et al. (2008) The hepatic stem cell niche: identification by label-retaining cell assay. Hepatology 47: 1994–2002.
3. Huch M, Dorrell C, Boj SF, van Es JH, Li VS, et al. (2013) In vitro expansion of single Lgr5+ liver stem cells induced by Wnt-driven regeneration. Nature 494: 247–250.
4. Jakubowski A, Ambrose C, Parr M, Lincecum JM, Wang MZ, et al. (2005) TWEAK induces liver progenitor cell proliferation. J Clin Invest 115: 2330–2340.
5. Affo S, Dominguez M, Lozano JJ, Sancho-Bru P, Rodrigo-Torres D, et al. (2013) Transcriptome analysis identifies TNF superfamily receptors as potential therapeutic targets in alcoholic hepatitis. Gut 62: 452–460.
6. Bird TG, Lu WY, Boulter L, Gordon-Keylock S, Ridgway RA, et al. (2013) Bone marrow injection stimulates hepatic ductular reactions in the absence of injury via macrophage-mediated TWEAK signaling. Proc Natl Acad Sci U S A 110: 6542–6547.
7. Tirnitz-Parker JE, Viebahn CS, Jakubowski A, Klopcic BR, Olynyk JK, et al. (2010) Tumor necrosis factor-like weak inducer of apoptosis is a mitogen for liver progenitor cells. Hepatology 52: 291–302.
8. Kuramitsu K, Sverdlov DY, Liu SB, Csizmadia E, Burkly L, et al. (2013) Failure of fibrotic liver regeneration in mice is linked to a severe fibrogenic response driven by hepatic progenitor cell activation. Am J Pathol 183: 182–194.
9. Ochoa B, Syn WK, Delgado I, Karaca GF, Jung Y, et al. (2010) Hedgehog signaling is critical for normal liver regeneration after partial hepatectomy in mice. Hepatology 51: 1712–1723.
10. Feng SL, Guo Y, Factor VM, Thorgeirsson SS, Bell DW, et al. (2000) The Fn14 immediate-early response gene is induced during liver regeneration and highly expressed in both human and murine hepatocellular carcinomas. Am J Pathol 156: 1253–1261.
11. Campbell S, Burkly LC, Gao HX, Berman JW, Su L, et al. (2006) Proinflammatory effects of TWEAK/Fn14 interactions in glomerular mesangial cells. J Immunol 176: 1889–1898.
12. Swiderska-Syn M, Syn WK, Xie G, Kruger L, Machado MV, et al. (2013) Myofibroblastic cells function as progenitors to regenerate murine livers after partial hepatectomy. Gut.
13. Michelotti GA, Xie G, Swiderska M, Choi SS, Karaca G, et al. (2013) Smoothened is a master regulator of adult liver repair. J Clin Invest.
14. Scholzen T, Gerdes J (2000) The Ki-67 protein: from the known and the unknown. J Cell Physiol 182: 311–322.
15. Kuramitsu K, Gallo D, Yoon M, Chin BY, Csizmadia E, et al. (2011) Carbon monoxide enhances early liver regeneration in mice after hepatectomy. Hepatology 53: 2016–2026.
16. Xie G, Karaca G, Swiderska-Syn M, Michelotti GA, Kruger L, et al. (2013) Cross-talk between notch and hedgehog regulates hepatic stellate cell fate. Hepatology.
17. Fausto N (2004) Liver regeneration and repair: hepatocytes, progenitor cells, and stem cells. Hepatology 39: 1477–1487.
18. Komuta M, Spee B, Vander Borght S, De Vos R, Verslype C, et al. (2008) Clinicopathological study on cholangiolocellular carcinoma suggesting hepatic progenitor cell origin. Hepatology 47: 1544–1556.
19. Michalopoulos GK (2011) Liver regeneration: alternative epithelial pathways. Int J Biochem Cell Biol 43: 173–179.

6

Semi-Supervised Segmentation of Ultrasound Images Based on Patch Representation and Continuous Min Cut

Anca Ciurte[1,2*], Xavier Bresson[3,4], Olivier Cuisenaire[3,4], Nawal Houhou[5], Sergiu Nedevschi[1], Jean-Philippe Thiran[2,3], Meritxell Bach Cuadra[2,3,4]

1 Department of Computer Science, Technical University of Cluj-Napoca, Cluj-Napoca, Romania, **2** Signal Processing Laboratory (LTS5), École Polytechnique Fédérale de Lausanne, Lausanne, Switzerland, **3** Department of Radiology, University Hospital Center and University of Lausanne, Lausanne, Switzerland, **4** Center for Biomedical Imaging, Signal Processing Core, Lausanne, Switzerland, **5** Swiss Institute of Bioinformatics (SIB), University Hospital Center and University of Lausanne, Lausanne, Switzerland

Abstract

Ultrasound segmentation is a challenging problem due to the inherent speckle and some artifacts like shadows, attenuation and signal dropout. Existing methods need to include strong priors like shape priors or analytical intensity models to succeed in the segmentation. However, such priors tend to limit these methods to a specific target or imaging settings, and they are not always applicable to pathological cases. This work introduces a semi-supervised segmentation framework for ultrasound imaging that alleviates the limitation of fully automatic segmentation, that is, it is applicable to any kind of target and imaging settings. Our methodology uses a *graph of image patches* to represent the ultrasound image and user-assisted initialization with labels, which acts as *soft priors*. The segmentation problem is formulated as a continuous minimum cut problem and solved with an efficient optimization algorithm. We validate our segmentation framework on clinical ultrasound imaging (prostate, fetus, and tumors of the liver and eye). We obtain high similarity agreement with the ground truth provided by medical expert delineations in all applications (94% DICE values in average) and the proposed algorithm performs favorably with the literature.

Editor: Arrate Muñoz-Barrutia, University of Navarra, Spain

Funding: This work is supported by PRODOC Project of Technical University of Cluj-Napoca and by the Center for Biomedical Imaging (CIBM) of the Geneva-Lausanne Universities and EPFL, and the foundations Leenaards and Louis-Jeantet, and by the FNS-205321-141283 and CTI-13741.1 funds. The funders had no role in study design, data collection and analysis, decision to publish, or preparation of the manuscript.

Competing Interests: The authors have declared that no competing interests exist.

* Email: Anca.Ciurte@cs.utcluj.ro

Introduction

Ultrasound (US) imaging provides a high image resolution and simplicity of use at much lower cost in comparison with other medical imaging modalities such as Magnetic Resonance imaging (MRI) or Computer Tomography (CT). These advantages make ultrasound a main image modality in medicine and its use becomes of particular interest in areas such echocardiography [1–3], obstetrics and gynecology [4], breast cancer [5] and intravascular diseases [6]. Indeed, US imaging is more and more used for image-guided therapy planning and navigation, and computer aided diagnosis. To this end, the development of efficient US image segmentation techniques of biological structures (e.g. different organs, heart chamber, fetus) or focal diseases (e.g. tumors, cysts) is needed.

US segmentation is very challenging due to the inherent speckle and some artifacts like shadows, attenuation and signal dropout. This often leads to weak (or missing) edges and also to the presence of fake edges, making standard unsupervised segmentation methods fail. Indeed, segmentation methods succeed on US imaging only when making use of application-specific constrains or priors. Several types of priors have been suggested in the literature [7]: those coming from *time* or *functional* data and those based on *shape* or *imaging physics*. In this work, we segment 2D B-mode US images without contrast enhancement. In consequence, we will not discuss the use of *time*-based constraints from different imaging frames or *functional*-based priors provided by contrast agent. However, such kind of priors could be included in our formulation if needed.

Anatomical shape priors are powerful for US image segmentation dealing very well with shadows and weak edges and they have been successfully used for different anatomical structures segmentation such as the heart [2,3], the prostate [8,9], the breast [10] or the kidney [11]. These priors can be encoded in the form of statistical shape models, usually derived from large data set segmentations, and they are often computationally expensive. Unfortunately, they are of limited use for pathological cases due to high variation in structure, shape, size and localization of lesions. Shape priors can be encoded in a simpler manner as for instance imposing a smooth boundary [2]. We will have such regularization in our approach.

Priors can also be related to the imaging physics, i.e. related to the observed intensities of the ultrasound image. For example, we consider intensity-based priors or learned texture as specific parametric intensity models to characterize the observed data. In this context, two different philosophical branches can be identified: those that consider speckle as information and those that consider it as noise. Since the gray level intensities in US images reflect the tissue density, some approaches use denoising filters in order to reduce the speckle structure and smooth the images (e.g. [12]). On the contrary, other approaches benefit of the texture information contained by speckle. As proved by Oosterveld et al. [13] by realistic simulations, the statistical and speckle characteristics of echographic texture change according to the density and spatial distribution of scatterers within the resolution cell.

A wide range of image features are used for modeling US observed data (see [7] for an extended review). Intensity features are often used by means of analytical models of the gray-level distribution (Rayleigh distribution being the most used model [4] but also Exponential, Gamma and Gaussian). Note that all these models are well-suited for the received signal while, in practice, clinical ultrasound devices log-compress the signal before visualization [14]. The main drawbacks of these gray-level distribution models are related to distribution parameter estimation and to its dependency on the imaging system settings such as dynamic range and gain. Intensity gradient features can also be used [1]. However, they strongly assume that there are homogeneous regions and thus, a very low level of speckle noise. Texture features have also proved to be successful in US segmentation, particularly statistical patterns of the intensity due to their advantage of being independent of the imaging system physics [5].

Contribution of this work

We consider in this work an alternative approach for characterizing the ultrasound data. Rather than using analytical distribution models or texture patterns to represent ultrasound images, we make use of *graph of intensity patches* as image representation. In contrast with most intensity or texture-based methods, the use of patches as image features allows us to be more independent of the imaging system and no assumption on the echogenicity of the object has to be done. Our choice of patch feature is also supported by previous works in the literature. Patch features were first introduced for texture synthesis [15] and image denoising [16] for natural images. In [17], Coupé et al. extended the non-local means filter [16] to reduce speckle noise in US images, by defining a particular similarity measure between patches. In [18,19], the patch-based approach was also successfully used for spatio-temporal registration and for motion or/and elasticity estimation in US image sequences of the heart. As far as we know, our preliminary work [20], published in 2011, was the first paper that introduces the use of intensity patches in US segmentation. Besides, we use the Pearson distance between patches as it proves to be a robust distance to speckle, as shown by [17].

Given the graph US image representation, we then address the segmentation problem with an efficient and *interactive* extraction algorithm of the foreground object, where the background cannot be trivially subtracted. Our segmentation method is thus fundamentally semi-supervised, that is, initial *labels* are defined on the image, acting as *soft priors*. Interactive soft priors were introduced in Computer Vision with user-assisted segmentation algorithms such as *Interactive Graph Cuts* [21], Lazy Snapping [22] and *GrabCut* [23]) and also in Medical Imaging (like CT [24] and US [12] segmentation. This quick and easy way to interact with images can provide the priors needed to make our segmentation accurate, robust and applicable to different kind of targets or imaging parameters. From the interaction point of view, our algorithm may be equivalent to a large variety of US segmentation methods proposed in the literature. Several state-of-the-art methods [7] require initial clicks or other types of interaction, like defining a region of interest or much tedious manual training. Moreover, depending on the application's specificities, the label initialization can be automatized, as in [20] for retinoblastoma segmentation.

Our segmentation method is based on the patch-based continuous graph cut approach for natural image segmentation introduced in [25]. Continuous graph cut methods have seen a rapid development over the recent years [26–32]. These methods find their theoretical roots in Strang [33] but the interest of applying them to real-world applications like medical imaging and computer vision has been triggered only recently. Nevertheless, continuous graph cut methods are quite attractive and offer new features that we will discuss in a further section.

A preliminary version of this work was presented in [20]. The main differences and improvements of the proposed work with respect to our previous work are as follows. Firstly, we introduce a new minimization algorithm that speeds up by at least an order of magnitude our previous optimization algorithm proposed in [20]. Secondly, we perform several tests of the proposed ultrasound segmentation methodology to identify clinical targets, namely, prostate, fetus, liver tumors and eye. Eventually, we carry out a thorough study of the robustness of our segmentation algorithm with respect to initialization.

As shown in [7], most US segmentation methods are usually limited to a specific target (as for instance the endocardial border [2,3,34,35], breast mass [5,36–38], prostate [8,12,39,40], and liver [41,42]). The major advantage of our segmentation framework, as regards the state-of-the-art, is its flexibility and easiness to use, while obtaining equivalent or better accuracy. However, this prevents us from selecting one approach in the literature for comparison that would not be equivalent in terms of flexibility. We will thus focus on one clinical context for method comparison, the segmentation of the prostate. This is one of the main areas of application of US in cancer treatment [40]. We have chosen the most recent, and methodologically close, semi-supervised approach presented in the literature [12], that makes use also of graph theory and soft priors using initial labels.

We now summarize the main methodological contributions of the proposed US segmentation method:

- An efficient representation of US images based on graph of intensity patches (naturally adapted to any echogenicity and imaging systems),
- A fast minimization algorithm for the minimum cut problem,
- An easy use of soft priors based on interactive user labels (unlike hard priors such as shape or temporal constrains),
- A study of accuracy and reproducibility of our algorithm with respect to different initial labels and users;

and the main application-oriented contributions are:

- A flexible framework, applicable to different US segmentation problems (eye, liver, prostate and fetus),
- A high accuracy of segmentation results as compared to manual delineations of expert raters, with mean Dice values around 94% in all data sets.

A related work on ultrasound image segmentation were recently introduced in [43,44] in the context of echocardiographic sequences. This work also promotes the use of intensity patches for ultrasound segmentation. More precisely, the authors of [43,44] define a sophisticated image representation model with multiscale signal analysis and sparse coding technology, which make the image representation rich but also time-consuming. We directly use image patches as image representation and show that this simple image representation is quite flexible and accurate to deal with multiple segmentation scenarios. Besides, [43,44] make use of the level set method (LSM) as segmentation method. The LSM is a PDE-based segmentation technique, which speed is limited by the Courant-Friedrichs-Lewy (CFL)'s condition. Discrete and continuous graph cut techniques (like the one introduced in this work) are more recent segmentation techniques and are not limited by the CFL condition, thus faster than the LSM (at least by an order of magnitude).

The proposed paper is organized as follows. In the first section, our mathematical framework and minimization scheme are presented. In the second section, the parameter setting and datasets are introduced. In the third section, we study the accuracy, repeatability and computational speed with respect to the initialization step. Then, quantitative results are presented for liver, eye tumors, fetal head estimation, and prostate. Eventually, a discussion is presented in the last section.

Methodology

The general block diagram of the proposed US segmentation method is shown in Figure 1. With a given US image as an input, the method first models the image with a graph representation of patches; next, the user provides markers inside (and outside, if needed) the object as initialization, serving as method initialization; finally, the novel numerical scheme for the minimization process is applied. Note that, in practice, if the segmentation result is not satisfying, our framework offer the possibility to re-initialize the labels and segment again, without re-computing the image modeling step. We will denote our new fast Patch-based Continuous Min-Cut segmentation by *fP-CMC* to distinguish it from our previous version *P-CMC* in [20].

Modeling of US images

Let an image I be defined as a vector in $\mathbb{R}^N$ where N is the number of pixels in the image. In this work, we represent US images as a graph of image patches. Therefore we introduce a graph $G=(V,E,W)$, where the set $V=\{x_1,...,x_N\}$ contains the nodes of the graph, the set E contains the edges (i.e. the connections between the nodes) and $W=\{w(x_i,x_j), \forall(x_i,x_j)\in E\}$ is the weight matrix that encodes the similarity between two points ($w(x_i,x_j)$ is small when x_i is different from x_j and $w(x_i,x_j)$ is large when x_i is similar to x_j). Each node x_i of the graph G represents a pixel in the image I. The following graph weight is considered:

$$w(x_i,x_j)=\begin{cases}\exp\left(-\dfrac{d(F(x_i),F(x_j))}{\sigma^2}\right) & \text{for } x_j\in\mathcal{N}_a(x_i)\\ 0 & \text{otherwise}\end{cases}, \quad (1)$$

where $d(F(x_i),F(x_j))$ expresses the proximity between the image descriptors located at x_i and x_j, $\mathcal{N}_a(x_i)$ is a neighborhood window centered at x_i of size $a\times a$, and the parameter σ is the scaling parameter of the weight matrix (using a standard Gaussian kernel with 0-mean and variance σ^2). In our case, the image descriptors $F(x_i)$ and $F(x_j)$ are $b\times b$ image patches centered at x_i and x_j, respectively. Note that the proposed segmentation framework is flexible enough to support any types of image descriptor. A standard distance d that measures the similarity between image patches is the ℓ^2 norm, a.k.a. the mean square difference, as used in [25] for natural image segmentation. Our patch feature is more adapted for US image segmentation than most texture descriptors used in the literature in several ways: it does not need multiple resolution characterization, it does not need any adjustment for ultrasound imaging (except from the patch size that can be easily set), it has no trouble in segmenting small areas (as some texture-based methods do) and, it is extremely easy to be computed.

Speckle model and Pearson distance

In the context of US imaging, patch distance is hard and critical to define. We need to consider the complex image formation of the US images such as local correlation due to periodic arrangements of scatterers and finite beam width, envelop detection and logarithm amplification of radio-frequency signals, and additive Gaussian noise of sensors. Consequently, we choose the following speckle model, that was proved in [45] to fit well the log-compressed US images:

$$I(x)=\tilde{I}(x)+\sqrt{\tilde{I}(x)}\eta(x), \quad (2)$$

where $\tilde{I}$ is the original image, I is the observed image and $\eta\sim N(0,\sigma^2)$ is a Gaussian noise. Thus, for each pixel x can be made the assumption that

$$I(x)|\tilde{I}(x)\sim N(\tilde{I}(x),\tilde{I}(x)\sigma^2). \quad (3)$$

An extensive study was performed by Coupé et al. [17] that proved the higher performance of the Pearson distance against the L2 norm to measure the similarities between patches in US images. Thus, we choose to use the Pearson distance between patches for segmentation since it is better adapted to the speckle:

$$d(F(x_i),F(x_j))=\frac{1}{2}\sum_{k=1}^{B}\frac{(F^k(x_i)-F^k(x_j))^2}{F^k(x_j)}, \quad (4)$$

where $F(x)=(F^1(x),\ldots,F^B(x))\in\mathbb{R}^B$, where $B=b\times b$ is the

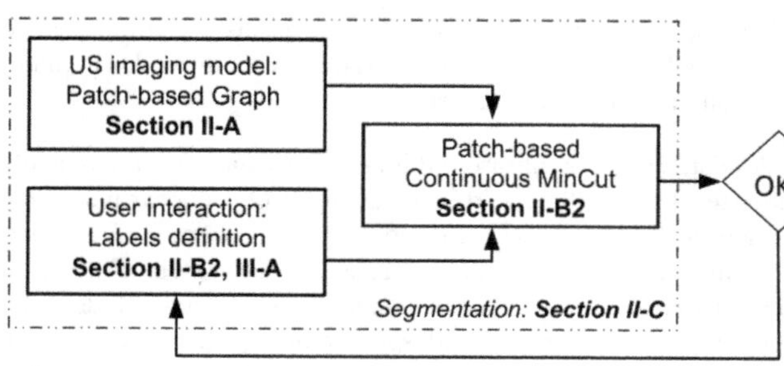

Figure 1. Our segmentation framework.

number of pixels in the patch F centered at x and $F^k(x)$ is the intensity of kth element of the patch.

Segmentation model

Continuous graph cut model. An efficient approach to solve the US segmentation problem is to cast the problem as a *continuous* graph partitioning problem such as [25,33]. In this work, we design a continuous graph cut model to carry out the US segmentation task with soft label priors.

Continuous graph cut methods, such as see [26–32], have seen a rapid development in the recent years based on new attractive properties. Different from discrete graph cut methods such as [21,23,46,47], which are generaly based on combinatorial optimization techniques, continuous graph cut techniques are fundamentally different: they are built on continuous tools like elliptic Partial Differential Equation (PDEs), variational methods and continuous convex optimization techniques like augmented Lagrangian, Uzawa-type primal-dual, iterative shrinkage techniques, etc. Mathematical fields like Functional Analysis offer strong tools to analyze the well-posedness of these continuous graph cut techniques. The main advantages of the continuous formulation of the graph cut methods are 1) sub-pixel accuracy, 2) easy to code (a few lines of Matlab) and 3) easy to parallelize with significant speedups.

Let us now introduce our continuous graph cut methodology, which benefits from these mentioned new features. Graph partition methods aim at segmenting a graph V into two subsets, A and A^c, such that $A \bigcup A^c = V$, $A \bigcap A^c = \emptyset$ and the inter-similarity between A and A^c being minimized. Partitioning a graph into two sets A and A^c can be achieved by minimizing the cut operator defined as:

$$cut(A,A^c) = \sum_{x_i \in A,\ x_j \in A^c} w(x_i,x_j), \tag{5}$$

which is equivalent to:

$$cut(A,A^c) = \sum_{x_i,\ x_j \in V} w(x_i,x_j) u_A(x_i) u_A(x_j), \tag{6}$$

when u_A is an indicator function of the set A. More specifically, we have $u_A = (u_A(x_1),...,u_A(x_N)) \in \mathbb{R}^N$ with $u_A(x_i)$ is the ith element of the vector u_A and N is the number of pixels in the image. Function u_A is an indicator function of the set A when $u_A(x) = 1$ for $x \in A$ and $u_A(x) = 0$ for $x \in A^c$. It is known that minimizing the cut operator (5) is equivalent to minimizing the graph-based H^1 norm as long as binary indicators, i.e. $u_A \in \{0,1\}$, are considered [48]. The graph-based H^1 norm is defined as:

$$\begin{aligned} H^1_w(u_A) &= \sum_{x_i \in V} |\nabla_w u_A(x_i)|^2 \\ &= \frac{1}{2} \sum_{x_i,\ x_j \in V} w(x_i,x_j)(u_A(x_i) - u_A(x_j))^2 = cut(A,A^c) \end{aligned}$$

$$\text{for } u_A(x) = \begin{cases} 1 & \forall x \in A \\ 0 & \forall x \in A^c \end{cases} \tag{7}$$

Observe that the weighted graph Laplacian naturally corresponds to a finite difference approximation of the continuous Laplacian operator and it also corresponds to the non-local operator of diffusion on graph.

Segmentation with labels. The proposed segmentation algorithm aims at minimizing the cut operator (or graph-based H^1 norm) given some labels to identify the objects of interest and the background. The object labels l_O are defined as $u(x) = 1$ for $x \in l_O$ and the background labels l_B are defined as $u(x) = 0$ for $x \in l_B$. We now formulate the segmentation method as a discrete minimization problem:

$$\min_{u \in \{0,\ 1\}} H^1_w(u) \quad \text{s.t.} \quad u(x) = \begin{cases} 1 & \forall x \in l_O \\ 0 & \forall x \in l_B \end{cases}, \tag{8}$$

where $H^1_w(u)$ is defined in (7) and l_O, l_B are provided by the user. As Shi and Malik observed in [48], minimizing the cut can favor small sets. An easy way to overcome this issue, while smoothing the irregularities along the cut boundary, is to use the total variation (TV) norm (i.e. the ℓ^1 norm of the gradient) as follows:

$$\min_{u \in \{0,\ 1\}} H^1_w(u) + \beta\, TV(u) \quad \text{s.t.} \quad u(x) = \begin{cases} 1 & \forall x \in l_O \\ 0 & \forall x \in l_B \end{cases}, \tag{9}$$

with $\beta > 0$, $TV(u) = \sum_{x_i \in V} |\nabla u(x_i)| = \sum_{x_i \in V} \sqrt{(\partial_x u)^2 + (\partial_y u)^2}$ where ∂_x, ∂_y are the discrete spatial derivative operators in the x,y-directions. The discrete minimization problem (9) is a combinatorial problem difficult to solve because the set of minimization is the binary function ($u \in \{0,1\}$) which is not convex. The natural approach is to relax the binary constraint to the closest convex set which is naturally $u \in [0,1]$. We thus consider the following continuous minimization problem:

$$\min_{u \in [0,\ 1]} H^1_w(u) + \beta\, TV(u) \quad \text{s.t.} \quad u(x) = \begin{cases} 1 & \forall x \in l_O \\ 0 & \forall x \in l_B \end{cases}, \quad \beta > 0, \tag{10}$$

which is convex, therefore providing a unique solution for any initial condition. Another nice consequence of (10) is the opportunity to develop efficient continuous minimization schemes, based on recent development for ℓ^1 optimization (for the compressed sensing field). The proposed segmentation model (9) was already introduced in [25] (based on [24]). However, we will present in the next section a novel and (much) faster minimization algorithm to solve (10).

Efficient minimization algorithm

This section introduces a fast minimization algorithm for (10) based on augmented Lagrangian method and splitting technique such as [49–53]. The minimization problem (10) is equivalent to (splitting step):

$$\min_{\substack{u:\ V \to [0,1] \\ v:\ V \to \mathbb{R} \\ q:\ V \to \mathbb{R}^2}} \sum_{x_i \in V} |\nabla_w u(x_i)|^2 + \beta \sum_{x_i \in V} |q(x_i)| \quad \text{s.t.} \quad \begin{cases} u = v \\ q = \nabla v \\ u(x_i) = 1 \quad \forall x_i \in l_O, \quad u(x_i) = 0 \quad \forall x_i \in l_B \end{cases}. \tag{11}$$

Adding new variables by a splitting step is a standard approach that can solve a difficult minimization problem by equivalently solving easier sub-minimization problems. Indeed, the constrained minimization problem (11) can be solved by the following iterative unconstrained minimization problems (augmented Lagrangian step):

$$\begin{cases} (u^{k+1},v^{k+1},q^{k+1}) = \underset{u\in[0,1],v,q}{\arg\min} & \sum_{x_i} |\nabla_w u|^2 + \beta \sum_{x_i} |q| \\ & + \langle \lambda_1^k, u-v \rangle + \frac{r_1}{2} \|u-v\|_2^2 \\ & + \langle \lambda_2^k, q-\nabla v \rangle + \frac{r_2}{2} \|q-\nabla v\|_2^2 \; s.t. \begin{cases} u(x_i)=1 & \forall x_i \in l_O \\ u(x_i)=0 & \forall x_i \in l_B \end{cases}, \\ \lambda_1^{k+1} = \lambda_1^k + r_1(u^{k+1}-v^{k+1}) & \\ \lambda_2^{k+1} = \lambda_2^k + r_2(q^{k+1}-\nabla v^{k+1}) & \end{cases} \tag{12}$$

where $||\cdot||_2^2$ and $\langle .,. \rangle$ are the standard l^2 norm and scalar product and $r_1, r_2 > 0$. Then, we consider the solution of the three sub-minimization problems in (12). The first sub-minimization problem is:

$$\begin{array}{l} \underset{u\in[0,1]}{\min} \quad \sum_{x_i} |\nabla_w u|^2 + \frac{r_1}{2} \sum_{x_i} \left(u - \left(v - \frac{\lambda_1}{r_1} \right) \right)^2, \\ u=(x_i)=1 \quad \forall x_i \in l_O \\ u=(x_i)=0 \quad \forall x_i \in l_B \end{array} \tag{13}$$

The Euler-Lagrange equation of (13) is:

$$-\Delta_w u + r_1 \left(u - \left(v - \frac{\lambda_1}{r_1} \right) \right) = 0,$$

$$(-\Delta_w + r_1) u = r_1 v - \lambda_1, \tag{14}$$

where $-\Delta_w$ is the graph Laplacian. The linear system of equations (14) can be solved efficiently with a conjugate gradient method (with e.g. Matlab). Then, the constraints $u\in[0,1]$ and $u(x_i)=1 \; \forall x_i \in l_O$, $u(x_i)=0 \; \forall x_i \in l_B$ are simply imposed to the solution of (14). The second sub-minimization problem to solve is:

$$\min_v \frac{r_1}{2} \sum_{x_i} \left(v - \left(u + \frac{\lambda_1}{r_1} \right) \right)^2 + \frac{r_2}{2} \sum_{x_i} |\nabla v - \left(q + \frac{\lambda_2}{r_2} \right)|^2. \tag{15}$$

Table 1. Algorithm 1.

Initialization: $u^{k=0}, v^{k=0}, q^{k=0} = 0$
While $\|u^{k+1} - u^k\|_2^2 \geq \epsilon)$ **do**
Compute: u^{k+1} with Eq. (14)
Constrain: $u^{k+1} \in [0,1]$ and $u^{k+1}(x_i) = 1 \; \forall x_i \in l_O$, $u^{k+1}(x_i) = 0 \; \forall x_i \in l_B$
Compute: v^{k+1} with Eq. (16)
Compute: q^{k+1} with Eq. (18)
Update:
$\lambda_1^{k+1} = \lambda_1^k + r_1(u^{k+1} - v^{k+1})$
$\lambda_2^{k+1} = \lambda_2^k + r_2(q^{k+1} - \nabla v^{k+1})$
end while

Fast optimization scheme for US image segmentation

The Euler-Lagrange equation of (15) is:

$$r_1 \left(v - \left(u + \frac{\lambda_1}{r_1} \right) \right) - r_2 \mathrm{div} \left(\nabla v - \left(q + \frac{\lambda_2}{r_2} \right) \right) = 0,$$

$$(-r_2 \Delta + r_1) v = -r_2 div \left(q + \frac{\lambda_2}{r_2} \right) + r_1 \left(u + \frac{\lambda_1}{r_1} \right), \tag{16}$$

which can be solved quickly with fast Fourier transform (FFT) or discrete cosine transform (DCT) depending on the boundary condition. The third and last sub-minimization problem is:

$$\min_q \beta \sum_{x_i} |q| + \frac{r_2}{2} \sum_{x_i} \left| q - \left(\nabla v - \frac{\lambda_2}{r_2} \right) \right|^2, \tag{17}$$

which solution is given by soft-thresholding [54]:

$$q = \max \left(|e| - \frac{\beta}{r_2}, 0 \right) \frac{e}{|e|}, \quad \text{with} \quad e = \nabla v - \frac{\lambda_2}{r_2}. \tag{18}$$

The pseudo-code is given in Table 1. to summarize the proposed algorithm. Finally, the stopping condition is chosen to be $\|u^{k+1} - u^k\|_2^2 < \epsilon$ and $\epsilon = 10^{-6}$ in all experiments.

Parameter setting

A detailed study of the parameters a, b and σ has previously been done in the context of image denoising for natural [55] and ultrasound images [17]. We briefly re-visit here after the parameter setting in the context of B-mode US segmentation.

Searching window size (a) - It has a great impact on the computational time. The size of searching window is also related to the "non-local character" of the method, since the similar patches are chosen inside this window and not only from the nearest neighbors.

Patch size (b) - The patch size is known to be related to the texture pattern size and to the target object scale [17], [55]. In ultrasound, texture pattern is provided by speckle. High values of b imply an increased computational time of weighted matrix w and the segmentation becomes coarser and a loss of details is noticed. Thus, we set $b=3$ to ensure the highest precision and a fast computation [56].

Scaling parameter (σ) - It stands for the typical distance between similar patches, which depends on the noise level [55]. For the proposed speckle model, according to Eq. (3), we have a level of noise equal to $\tilde{I}(x)\sigma^2$. Thus, the selection of σ parameter depends on the distribution of the gray levels inside the reference patch ($\tilde{I}(x)$). That implies that σ also depends on speckle characteristics such as speckle size and if it is fully developed or not. Based on the same assumption defined in Eq. (3), the level of noise $\tilde{I}(x)\sigma^2$ has a high variation because of the speckle appearance. This leads to a low power of discrimination between two different tissues with close density properties (meaning a low contrast in US image). A value of $\sigma = 4e-3 \pm 3e-3$ performs goods results in case of US images, with a higher sensitivity for the mentioned cases of tissues with close density properties.

Regularization weight (β) - It controls the smoothness of the contour and eliminates the misclassification of small subsets of pixels resulted by the min-cut algorithm. Optimal results in ultrasound segmentation are performed for β values between

Table 2. Data sets overview.

Target	US system	Frequency (MHz)	Estimated speckle size	Isotropic resolution ($mm^2/pixel$)	No images	Image size
Liver -depth: 8 cm -depth: 16 cm	Logiq 7	3 × 65.5	2 × 4	0.2×0.2 0.4×0.4	15 15	640 × 480
Fetus	Siemens Medical Systems	2.0–3.6	0.22 × 0.22-	0.33 × 0.33	22 -	800 × 600
Eye	OTI Ophthalmic Technologies Inc.	12.5	3 × 6	0.1 × 0.1	20	206 × 217
Prostate	-	-	2 × 4	-	6	356 × 468

$1e-4$ and $1e-1$. Larger β value, smoother the contour is. The sub-parameters r_1 and r_2 occurred in the augmented Lagrangian step (Eq. 12) are both fixed to 0.5.

For all the tests and clinical applications presented in this paper we used the following setting: $a=5$, $b=3$, $\sigma=0.004$ and $\beta=0.01$.

Data sets

Our data set contain a wide variety of ultrasound images in order to proof its flexibility and performance for different imaging systems, image resolution, speckle size and targets. It contains a total number of 78 images from which 20 ophthalmic, 30 liver, 22 fetal and 6 prostate images. Table 2 summarize the characteristics of each data set. Besides the US images, we dispose of manual delineation performed by medical experts for the ophthalmic, liver and prostate data sets and of manual biometric measurements for the fetal data set, which were used as ground truth in our tests.

Ethics Statement

The patient information from all data used in our study was anonymized and de-identied by physicians prior to our analysis. All studies presented are approved by the corresponding committee/ institutional review board: Switzerland (Cantonal Research Ethics Committee of Vaud), France (Comite de Protection des Personnes), Romania (local Ethical Committee of the University of Medicine and Pharmacy Cluj-Napoca) and Canada (Health Science Research Ethics Board at Western University).

Opthalmic imaging

Ultrasound is still in its early years as regards ophthalmology. However, its use is constantly increasing [57,58] for diagnosis, planning, therapy and follow up of treatments. We present the segmentation of B-scan US of the retinoblastoma. The clinical value of this work is related to a larger project that aims at improving the radiotherapy planning and treatment of retinoblastoma in childhood by fusion of CT, ultrasound and fundus of photograph [59]. Our clinical eye data set contains 20 ophthalmic US images which are 2D slices of the 3D volumes from 6 eyes with retinoblastoma (including both calcified and non calcified tumors). US eye images were acquired at *Jules Gonin Hospital*, Lausanne, Switzerland with Ophthalmic Technologies Inc. (OTI), having an isotropic resolution of 0.1×0.1 mm^2 and image size of 206×217 pixels.

Liver

Liver ultrasound aims at finding abnormalities, such as scarring (cirrhosis), masses (both cancer and non cancer) and blockage of the blood vessels. These findings help determine the diagnosis and therapy and also whether the patient is good or not as transplant candidate. In clinical practice, liver diagnosis requires additional examination with other invasive methods like biopsies, with the associated morbidity and mortality risk. Therefore, the automated segmentation of ultrasound images would provide a reliable non-invasive and quantitative approach in diagnosing liver diseases.

We will present the lesion segmentation of US liver imaging from 15 different patients diagnosed with hepatocarcinoma (HCC). These application does not aim at illustrating any clinical value but a quantitative validation thanks to the available manual delineations. The US liver images were acquired at 3rd *Medical Clinic*, Cluj-Napoca, Romania using Logiq7 system at a frequency of 5.5MHz, with isotropic resolution of 0.4×0.4 mm^2 ($depth=16$ cm) and 0.2×0.2 mm^2 ($depth=8$ cm) respectively and image size of 640×480 pixels. The data set contains two images per patient, one for each resolution, summing up a number of 30 images.

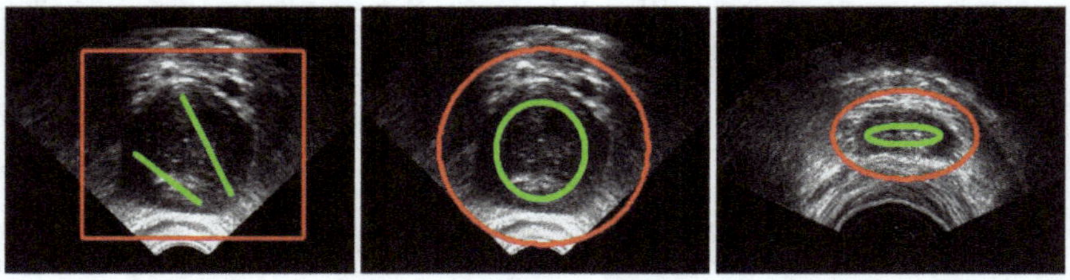

(a) Lines (b) Ellipses (c) Free hand

Figure 2. Different types of initialization using basic shapes like lines or ellipses, and free hand initialization. Yellow and light blue correspond to foreground and background labels respectively.

Fetal imaging

Ultrasound imaging is the gold standard modality for exploration, biometric measurements and diagnosis in fetal imaging. In this context, the development of efficient US image segmentation techniques of biological structures such as the head, femur or abdomen of the fetus are crucial towards a high quality perinatal follow up and diagnosis. Here we aim at segmenting the head of the fetus to estimate later on the head circumference (HC) as an indirect measure of fetal growth. Our data set contains 22 US images from 22 different fetuses ranging from 24 to 35 weeks of gestational age (GA). Images were acquired in clinical practice at *Hôpital Femme Mère Enfant*, Lyon, France with Siemens Medical Systems at $2.0-3.6M\ Hz$ with spatial resolution of isotropic pixels between 0.22 to $0.33mm$. Let us note that only four fetuses can be considered as healthy while the rest are suspected of developmental brain delay. Inner head circumference computed by expert radiologist will be used as gold standard. Our previous method *P-CMC* [20] was evaluated on a different dataset to estimate the outer HC in [60].

Prostate

Transrectal ultrasound (TRUS) is a key tool for prostate cancer diagnosis. Prostate volumes and boundaries are essential biomarkers in the diagnosis, treatment, and follow up of prostate cancer [7]. This has encourage many researches to develop segmentation tools for prostate boundary detection [40]. The testing data set contains 6 prostate US images, the ones introduced and used for tests in [12].

Let us note that the software and data set for testing presented in this paper will be made publicly available at http://www.unil.ch/mial/page86599.html website upon acceptance of the manuscript.

Results

Method evaluation

The overlap measures that we use to estimate the agreement between the segmentation result and the ground truth (GT) are: Dice coefficient metric (DCM) [61] and area overlap (AO, or accuracy overlap) [12]. They are defined as follows:

$$DCM = \frac{2|Seg \cap GT|}{|Seg| + |GT|},$$

where by Seg and GT we refer to the set of segmented, respectively ground truth points, and

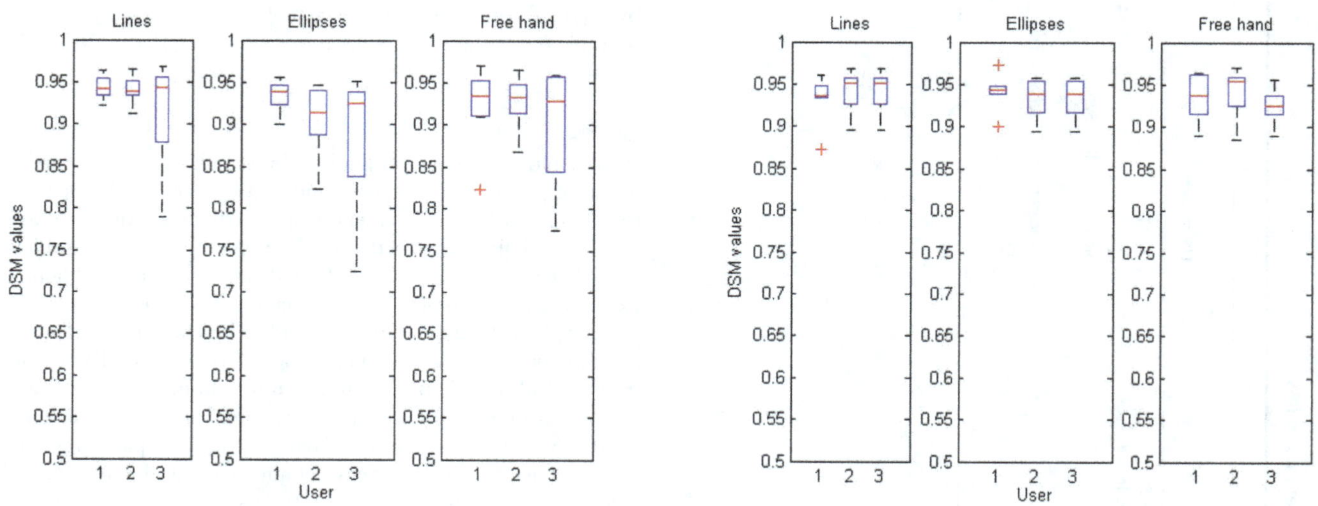

(a) Retinoblastoma (b) Prostate

Figure 3. Box-plot of inter-user initialization variability and of the robustness with respect to different labels: central red mark is the median, edges of the box are the 25th and 75th percentiles, whiskers extend to extreme values, and outliers are plotted by a red cross.

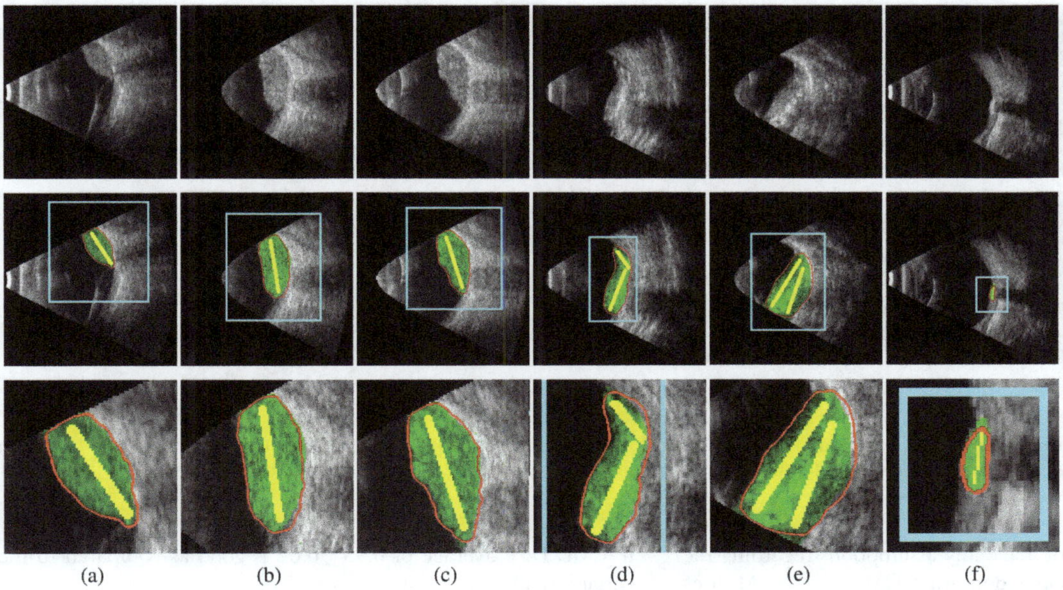

Figure 4. Eye tumor segmentation: ground truth is in transparent green, *fP-CMC* segmentation is in red, foreground and background labels are in yellow and light blue respectively.

$$AO = \frac{|TP|}{|TP| + |FN| + |FP|} \times 100,$$

By |.| we denote the set cardinal and TP, FN and FP are the *true positive*, *false negative* and *false positive* sets respectively. Added to overlap measures for segmentation agreement, speed in number of iterations and computational time are also shown. Our algorithm is implemented in Matlab and it was tested on an INTEL Core 2 Duo, 2.66 GHz, 2 GB of RAM.

Robustness to initialization

Our segmentation method is designed in an interactive framework which allows the user to easily and quickly initialize the algorithm for any target of interest. Let us remind that, depending on the specific application, the initialization process can be easily automatized [20]. However, we promote here some initial user interaction in favor of a great gain in flexibility: we will be able to segment many different targets. Having some initial interaction is not new in US segmentation. A large range of state-of-the-art methods must define initial clicks and even heavier interactions (please refer to Table II and III in [7] as regards interaction type for breast and prostate segmentation respectively). In this sense, our algorithm is not different from algorithms in the literature.

To this end, we present a robustness study with different type of initializations: simple straight lines, one click-drag and drop for generating predefined shapes like ellipses or circles, or freely drawing scribes (as they have prove to be largely used in interactive segmentation applications [47,62]. The initialization requires the selection of at least one *object*, and, optionally, of one or more *background* areas.

We test the robustness of our method for both eye and prostate imaging. Some examples of different types of initial labels (lines, ellipses and free hand) are shown in Figure 2. Moreover, three different users have drawn the initial labels to study also the inter-user variability. Results are shown in the boxplots of Figure 3. For a given user, DCM is in average 0.93 for both eye and prostate imaging with ± 0.2 and ± 0.3 of variance respectively. Therefore, this demonstrate a high robustness as regards different types of initializations. Moreover, inter-user variability for a given label is also highly robust (around 0.925 ± 0.3). We applied the Wilcoxon two-sided rank sum test, a non-parametric alternative to paired-

Table 3. Quantitatively evaluation of retinoblastoma segmentation against expert delineations used as ground truth.

Figure		4(a)	4(b)	4(c)	4(d)	4(e)	4(f)
DCM	*P-CMC*	0.95	0.93	0.94	0.89	0.95	0.72
	fP-CMC	0.96	0.95	0.95	0.93	0.95	0.90
Iterations	*P-CMC*	6217	4529	3031	3914	4287	1241
	fP-CMC	46	50	52	32	33	29
Convergence Time (s)	*P-CMC*	75	55	39	42	130	14
	fP-CMC	18	21	21	13	13	12

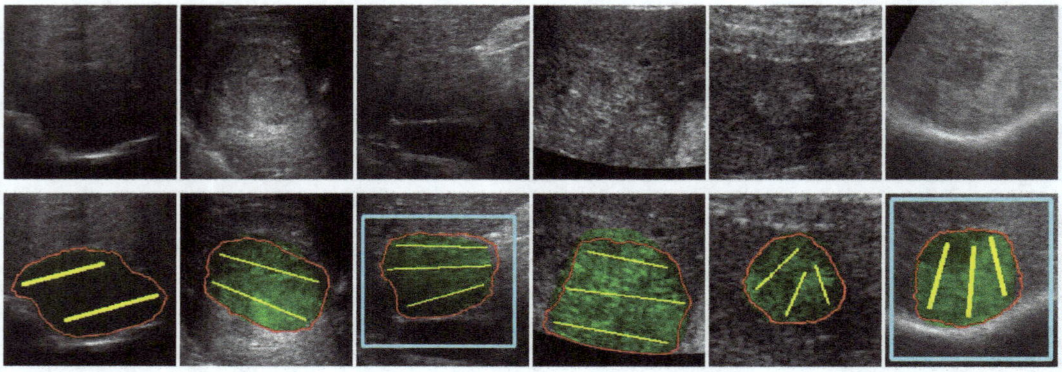

Figure 5. Liver tumor segmentation. Image resolution is $0.4 \times 0.4mm^2$ for (a), (b) and (c), and $0.2 \times 0.2mm^2$ for (d), (e) and (f). Ground truth is in transparent green, *fP-CMC* segmentation is in red, foreground and background labels are in yellow and light blue respectively.

student test since it does not make any assumptions regarding the distributions of the data population, on DCM statistics. All tests accepted the null hypothesis at 5% significance level, that is, differences between each boxplot are not statistically significant. Therefore we can conclude that all types of initialization are valid for segmentation and that results are repeatable by different users.

Additional study concerning the spatial filling of the initial labels can be found in File S1 attached to the manuscript.

Validation

Quantitative assessment is presented for the eye, the liver, the prostate, and the fetus. The color code used in figures 4, 5, 7 and 9 is as follows: foreground and background labels are in yellow and light blue respectively, fP-CMC segmentation is in solid red contour, and ground truth is in transparent green (except for figure 7 where ground truth segmentation is not available, only the fetal head circumference value).

Segmentation of eye tumors. Segmentation results of US image segmentation are shown in Figure 4 (input images in the first line, segmentation results in the second one and zoom on the results in the third one). The Dice coefficient metric and computational time, in comparison with the previous *P-CMC* method [20], are presented in Table 3. DCM is 0.94 with a standard deviation of 0.02 was obtained in average for the 8 images of the eye data set. The speed-up of the novel method is clear visible from the reduced time of convergence and number of iterations presented. We measure the intra- and inter-observer variability of two raters that manually delineated the ground truth retinoblastoma. The inter-observer Dice average and variance is of 0.88 ± 0.22 and the intra-observer variability is of 0.91 ± 0.06. The *fP-CMC* Dice average of 0.93 ± 0.02 is good as compared to the variability measurements.

Segmentation of liver tumors. A region of interest of 250×250 was defined from the original images (first row of Figure 5). Segmentation results are shown in second row of Figure 5 for different resolutions: (a) to (c) have a resolution of 0.4×0.4 mm^2 and (d) to (f) have a resolution of 0.2×0.2 mm^2. Similar results were obtained for all images in the US liver data set. Overlap measure and computational time are presented in Table 4. The average DCM of the 30 images of the liver data set is 0.9397 with standard deviation of 0.01. This performance proofs a good accuracy and high robustness for these challenging imaging. Moreover, as regards our previous method, the number of iterations till convergence and the computational time are reduced significantly, by a factor of 1000 and 15 respectively. A box-plot representation of the DCM is visualized in Figure 6, where the first box corresponds to the US liver data set of $depth = 16cm$ and the second one to the data set of $depth = 8cm$. The same accuracy is almost reached for both image resolutions but slightly higher variability is obtained for acquisitions at $8cm$ depth.

Fetal head segmentation. We proceed to define two elliptic labels inside and outside the fetus head (see yellow and cyan contours in Fig. 7) by a mouse click (press, drag and release). Then, the head is segmented with the *fP-CMC* (red contour in Fig. 7). From there, the axis of elongation of the obtained binary segmentation is computed with the following formulation [63]:

$$\tan(2\Phi_i) = 2\frac{\sum_r \sum_c (r-\bar{r}_i)(c-\bar{c}_i)I_i(r,c)}{\sum_r \sum_c (c-\bar{c}_i)^2 I_i(r,c) - \sum_r \sum_c (r-\bar{r}_i)^2 I_i(r,c)}, \quad (19)$$

Table 4. Quantitatively evaluation of the liver tumors against manual segmentation by an expert radiologist as ground truth.

Figure		5(a)	5(b)	5(c)	5(d)	5(e)	5(f)
DCM	*P-CMC*	0.94	0.95	0.94	0.93	0.91	0.92
	fP-CMC	0.96	0.95	0.95	0.95	0.93	0.95
Iterations	*P-CMC*	17566	11786	10103	19163	17732	19605
	fP-CMC	48	85	80	48	43	84
Convergence Time (s)	*P-CMC*	300	245	359	379	471	281
	fP-CMC	20	35	33	20	18	35

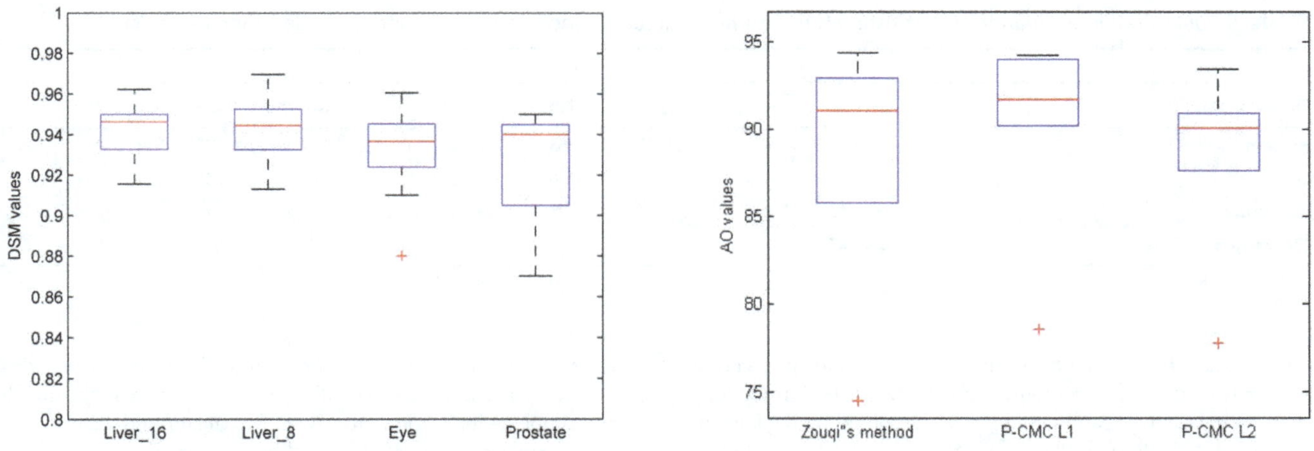

(a) Dice Coefficient Measure (b) Area Overlap

Figure 6. Box-plots of B-mode segmentations: (a) DCM values for liver tumors with a depth of 8 (Liver_8) and 16 (Liver_16), eye tumors and prostate; (b) Area overlap (AO) values in prostate segmentation of *fP-CMC* (using two different types of initial labels: *init 1* and *init2*) vs. GC-FIS [12].

where r, c corresponds to the rows and columns in the binary image I (1- for the object and 0 for the background) and $\overline{c}$, $\overline{r}$ are the coordinates for the centers of mass. The axis of elongation will correspond to Occipito-Frontal Diameter (OFD) measure, and then Biparietal Diameter (BPD) is computed for the angle ($\Phi+90°$), for the same center of mass. Finally, HC is computed from the BPD and OFD measurements using the expression [64]:

$$HC=\pi(BPD+OFD)/2. \tag{20}$$

Some visual segmentation results are shown in Figure 7 with their corresponding quantitative measures as in Table 5. Estimated HC metric as compared with radiologist computation for all images is plotted in Figure 8 in form of Bland-Altman plot [64] where the error in the HC estimation (difference in mm) is represented as a function of the estimated HC measure (in mm). Further, we compare our estimation errors with the inter-user variability of HC measurement reported in previous studies [65]. Sarris et al [65] recently presented, among other fetal ultrasound measurements, a variability study of HC measurements (in mm) between 3 different users over 175 images from 140 fetuses (ranging from 14 to 41 weeks of gestational age). They reported an average variability of $0.9mm$ and the 95% confidence intervals at $+13mm$ and $-11.1mm$. Our average error is smaller ($0.03mm$) and our error distribution fall within those confidence interval. In this sense, we can say that our estimated HC is equivalent to the one measured by hand by the radiologist.

Segmentation of prostate. In this application we compare our *fP-CMC* segmentation to previous published works [12] that are based on graph cut segmentation with a fuzzy interference system (*GC-FIS*). Both *fP-CMC* and *GC-FIS* methodologies are comparable in terms of interactivity and of semi-supervision with labels within a graph-cut based segmentation framework. However, contrary to our philosophy of considering speckle as image information, GC-FIS assumes a preprocessing step for image denoising in order to reduce the speckle noise by using 'stick filter' and smooths the image. The user interaction in GC-FIS differs a lot of ours indeed. In GC-FIS, few points lying on the object contour must be selected first. These points are further used to generate the contours for the inside and the outside labels, being

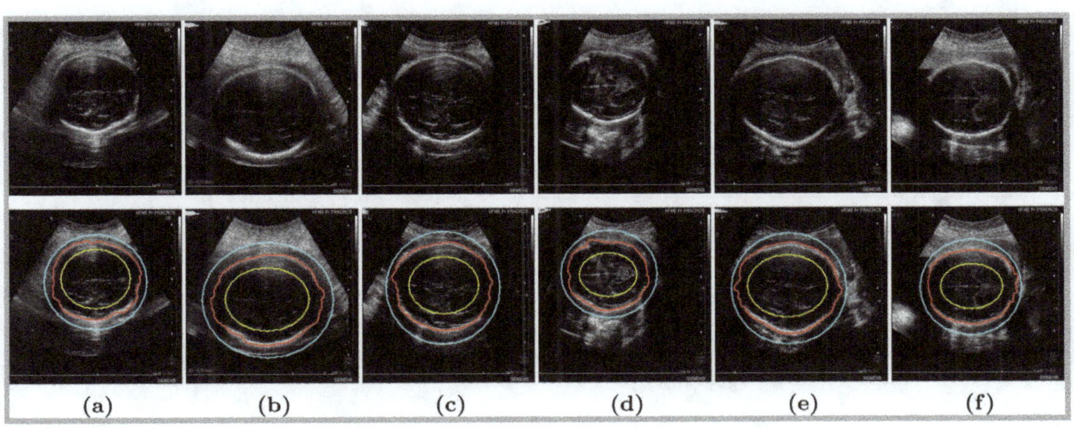

Figure 7. Fetal head segmentation: *fP-CMC* segmentation is in red, initial labels (ellipses) are in yellow and light blue for object and background, respectively.

Table 5. Quantitative evaluation of the estimated fetal head circumference versus biometry provided by radiologists.

Figure		7(a)	7(b)	7(c)	7(d)	7(e)	7(f)
HC (mm)	*fP-CMC*	253	265	257	250	255	251
	GT	260	256	267	262	257	254
Iterations	*fP-CMC*	2	2	3	2	3	2
Convergence Time (s)	*fP-CMC*	7	6	8	6	8	8

automatically defined in the normal direction and at a certain distance from the object contour. Segmentation is performed next, using the interactive graph-cut approach proposed by Boykov and Jolly in [21]. Please note that GC-FIS is thus based on a discrete optimization approach, while we have a continuous formulation. Finally, the contour is refined in a post processing step using a FIS, where each point is evaluated and marked as weak or strong boundary points. The misclassified (weak) points are used next to add more appropriate hard constraints and to further re-perform the segmentation.

For sake of comparison we force us to define labels as close as possible as defined by *GC-FIS*. Accordingly, in Fig. 9, for the initial labels shown in the 1st row we obtain the segmentation results as shown in the 2nd row. We will denote these results by *fP-CMC-L1*. Rather than using these *complex* labels, we will run our algorithm with much simple and intuitive initialization (as performed in all previous clinical applications), by straight lines for the foreground and without background labels. Results are denoted by *fP-CMC-L2* and shown in 3th row of Fig. 9.

In Table 6 we present the quantitative results for both methods in terms of area overlap (AO). Results with *fP-CMC-L1* are very close to *GC-FIS* or slightly better: an overall accuracy average of 90.06 of *fP-CMC-L1* against 88.28 obtained with *GC-FIS*. We have considerably reduced the variability of the results, proving again the robustness of the *fP-CMC* (see boxplots in Fig. 6). Results with *fP-CMC-L2*, (average accuracy of 88.3) are slightly worse than *fP-CMC-L1* and equivalent to *GC-FIS*. We believe though that this decrease in accuracy is acceptable when considering the much more simple initialization step without background labels. The DCM boxplot for *fP-CMC-L2* are shown in Fig. 6.

Conclusion

The most important methodological contributions of our work are the use of a graph of intensity patches for representing the ultrasound image and a fast minimization scheme for the continuous min cut problem. This new formulation has considerably reduced the computation time as regards our previous version [20]. Intuitively, our proposed graph cut method can be seen as a heat diffusion process on the graph of image patches. The heat diffusion propagates the information of the inside and outside labels selected by the user. Regions of interest that wish to be segmented entirely depend on the choice of the labels, i.e. which image patches are selected to be diffused. In other words, our segmentation method can segment both homogeneous and heterogeneous US regions, offering high-quality results with a large flexibility to work on different targets.

In practice, most parameters are easily set. Actually, we found that for many different B-mode sequence and scanners, the same parameter values provided high accurate results (all parameters are equally set for all clinical applications presented). The only parameter that may required an initial fine tuning according to B-

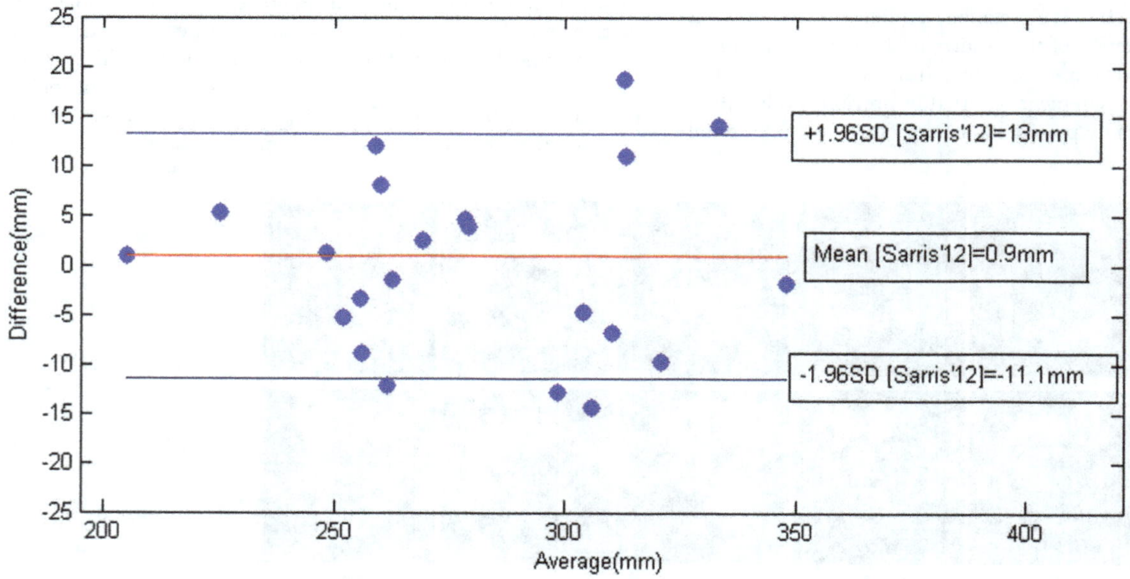

Figure 8. Inter-subject variability. Error measurements of our method w.r.t. the confidence interval at 95% and Bland-Altman plot of inter-subject variability from [65].

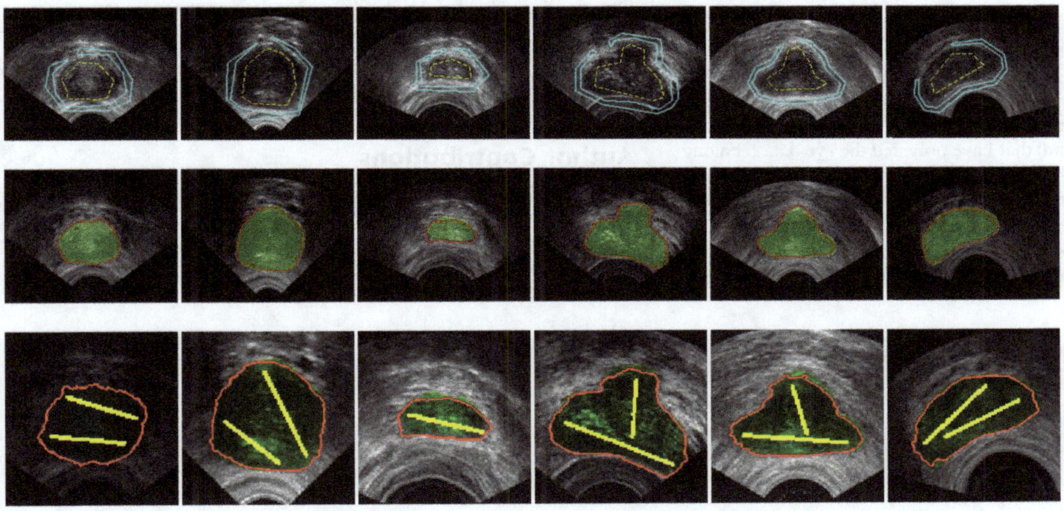

(a) (b) (c) (d) (e) (f)

Figure 9. Segmentation of US prostate data set. 1st and 2nd rows: initialization labels as in [12] (yellow for object and blue for background) and *fP-CMC-L1* segmentation in red. 3th row: initial labels in yellow and *fP-CMC-L2* segmentation in red contour. Ground truth is in transparent green area. We refer to [12] for visual comparison with GC-FIS results.

mode sequence is the scaling parameter σ which is more sensitive when the contrast between foreground and background is low, but which can be overcame with a proper label initialization. We showed that despite the semi-supervision, our segmentation framework provides highly accurate and quantitatively similar results for different types of labels and users. Indeed, setting the initial labels (by few clicks, lines, circles, etc.) is extremely easy and fast. The user interaction in the label definition might be seen as a limitation of our method but, in our opinion, ultrasound image analysis is particularly suited for an interactive segmentation framework since, in clinical practice, physicians are used to extract simple biometric measures from few click interactions. Moreover, in cases where ultrasound image quality is really challenging, our framework allows the expert to define labels close to the final object thus providing not only a faster convergence but also more reproducible segmentations. Nevertheless, in an application basis, the label definition process can easily be automatized if needed [20].

We have evaluated the segmentation results of the *fP-CMC* framework in several clinical contexts (some of them aimed at quantitative validation purposes more than real clinical applications). We have reported segmentation accuracy in average of 93% for all clinical applications (Fig. 6). This proofs a high practical value of our method in terms of flexibility and easy of use as compared to state of the art methods (limited and optimized for a specific organ and/or image sequence). Our interactive patch-based philosophy is rather different from most existing segmentation techniques for B-mode ultrasound imaging. Nevertheless, we have compared our method to the closest methodology in terms of interactive discrete graph cut segmentation [12] applied to the prostate.

We have presented a segmentation method for 2D US images since 2D US is widely accepted in clinical practice (except for the eye, all our images where in 2D). However, following the increasing number of 3D US imaging, the extension to 3D images is does not change the mathematics neither the algorithm introduced in this work. Plus, initialization could be easily extended to 3D, for instance considering a few group of 2D slices where the user clicks or to make use of 3D objects (sphere or ellipsoids) as initial labels. We assume that in 3D we would keep the same robustness as in the 2D case. However, this would require confirmation with new experiments, which is out of the scope of the paper.

Finally, we promote here the use of soft priors (semi-supervision with labels) for the ultrasound segmentation. Nevertheless, we agree that the use of strong shape, temporal and/or intensity, priors can be for a specific target more powerful that our soft priors. Note that strong priors can be easily included in our mathematical formulation. Future work goes into exploring other image features to be included in the patch representation (and the corresponding patch distance function) in order to better represent the echogenicity present in US imaging.

Table 6. Comparison with GC-FIS [12] using overall accuracy (AO).

Figure	9(a)	9(b)	9(c)	9(d)	9(e)	9(f)
AO-*fP-CMC-L1*	94.18	92.28	78.56	94.00	91.12	90.22
AO-*fP-CMC-L2*	87.65	93.43	77.79	90.92	90.02	90.15
AO [12]	94.35	92.92	74.54	91.40	85.81	90.71

Acknowledgments

The authors would like to thank Prof. Radu Badea and Monica Lupsor, MD-PhD (3rd Medical Clinic, University of Medicine and Pharmacy, Cluj-Napoca, Romania) for providing the liver data set and the manual segmentations too. More, we thank Prof. Francis Munier (Jules Gonin Hospital, Lausanne, Switzerland) that have provided the eye data set along the manual segmentations of the tumors. Our acknowledgment goes also to Prof. Laurent Guibaud and Dr. Benoit Morel (Department of pediatric and fetal imaging, Hôpital Femme Mère Enfant, Lyon, France) that provided the fetal images and biometric measures for the fetal head circumference study. We would like to thank also M. Zouqi (University of Western Ontario, Canada) for his kind cooperation in providing the prostate images. Our acknowledgment also goes to Marcel Arditi, PhD (Bracco Imaging Group SpA, Switzerland) for his thoughtful discussions on ultrasound physics.

Author Contributions

Conceived and designed the experiments: AC XB OC NH SN J-PT MBC. Performed the experiments: AC XB OC MBC. Analyzed the data: AC XB OC MBC. Contributed reagents/materials/analysis tools: AC XB OC NH MBC. Wrote the paper: AC XB MBC.

References

1. Corsi C, Saracino G, Sarti A, Lamberti C (2002) Left ventricular volume estimation for real-time three-dimensional echocardiography. IEEE Trans on Medical Imaging 21: 1202–1208.
2. Paragios N, Jolly MP, Taron M, Ramaraj R (2005) Active Shape Models and Segmentation of the Left Ventricle in Echocardiography, volume 3459 of *Lect. Notes in Computer Science*. 131–142 pp.
3. Chen Y, Huang F, Tagare HD, Rao M (2007) A coupled minimization problem for medical image segmentation with priors. Int J of Computer Vision 71: 259–272.
4. Anquez J, Angelini E, Bloch I (2008) Segmentation of fetal 3D ultrasound based on statistical prior and deformable model. In: IEEE International Symposium on Biomedical Imaging (ISBI). pp. 17–20.
5. Chen DR, Chang RF, Kuo WJ, Chen MC, Huang YL (2002) Diagnosis of breast tumors with sonographic texture analysis using wavelet transform and neural networks. Ultrasound Med Biol 28: 1301–1310.
6. Unal G, Bucher S, Carlier S, Slabaugh G, Fang T, et al. (2008) Shape-driven segmentation of the arterial wall in intravascular ultrasound images. IEEE Trans Inf Technol Biomed 12: 335–347.
7. Noble JA, Boukerroui D (2006) Ultrasound image segmentation: A survey. IEEE Trans on Medical Imaging 25: 987–1010.
8. Gong L, Pathak S, Haynor D, Cho P, Kim Y (2004) Parametric shape modeling using deformable superellipses for prostate segmentation. Medical Imaging, IEEE Transactions on 23: 340–349.
9. Pingkun Y, Sheng X, Turkbey B, Kruecker J (2011) Adaptively learning local shape statistics for prostate segmentation in ultrasound. Biomedical Engineering, IEEE Transactions on 58: 633–641.
10. Chang RF, Wu WJ, Moon WK, Chen WM, Lee W, et al. (2003) Segmentation of breast tumor in three-dimensional ultrasound images using three-dimensional discrete active contour model. Ultrasound in Medicine and Biology 29: 1571–1581.
11. Xie J, Jiang Y, tat Tsui H (2005) Segmentation of kidney from ultrasound images based on texture and shape priors. Medical Imaging, IEEE Transactions on 24: 45–57.
12. Zouqi M, Samarabandu J (2009) 2D ultrasound image segmentation using graph cuts and local image features. In: Computational Intelligence for Image Processing. pp. 33–40.
13. Oosterveld BJ, Thijssen JM, Verhoef WA (1985) Texture in B-mode echograms: 3-D simulations and experiments of the effects of diffraction and scatterer density. Ultrasonic Imag 7: 142–160.
14. Tao Z, Tagare HD, Beaty J (2006) Evaluation of four probability distribution models for speckle in clinical cardiac ultrasound images. IEEE Trans on Medical Imaging 11: 1483–1491.
15. Efros AA, Leung TK (1999) Texture synthesis by non-parametric sampling. In: ICCV. pp. 1033–1038.
16. Buades A, Coll B, Morel JM (2005) A review of image denoising algorithms, with a new one. Multiscale Modeling & Simulation 4: 490–530.
17. Coupé P, Hellier P, Kervrann C, Barillot C (2009) Nonlocal means-based speckle filtering for ultrasound images. IEEE Trans Image Process 18: 2221–2229.
18. Ledesma-Carbayo MJ, Kybic J, Desco M, Santos A, Suhling M, et al. (2005) Spatio-temporal nonrigid registration for ultrasound cardiac motion estimation. IEEE Trans Image Process 27: 1113–1126.
19. Revell J, Mirmehdi M, McNally D (2005) Computer vision elastography: speckle adaptive motion estimation for elastography using ultrasound sequences. IEEE Trans Image Process 24: 755–766.
20. Ciurte A, Houhou N, Nedevschi S, Pica A, Munier F, et al. (2011) An efficient segmentation method for ultrasound images based on a semi-supervised approach and patch-based features. In: IEEE International Symposium on Biomedical Imaging (ISBI). pp. 969–972.
21. Boykov Y, Jolly MP (2001) Interactive graph cuts for optimal boundary and region segmentation of objects in n-d images. In: ICCV. volume 1, pp. 105–112.
22. Li Y, Sun J, Tang CK, Shum HY (2004) Lazy snapping. In: ACM SIGGRAPH.
23. Rother C, Blake A, Kolmogorov V (2004) Grabcut - interactive foreground extraction using iterated graph cuts. In: ACM SIGGRAPH.
24. Unger M, Pock T, Cremers D, Bischof H (2008) Tvseg - interactive total variation based image segmentation. In: British Machine Vision Conference (BMVC).
25. Houhou N, Bresson X, Szlam A, Chan TF, Thiran JP (2009) Semi-supervised segmentation based on non-local continuous min-cut. In: Scale Space and Variational Methods in Computer Vision. volume 5567, pp. 112–123.
26. Chan T, Esedoglu S, Nikolova M (2006) Algorithms for Finding Global Minimizers 575 of Image Segmentation and Denoising Models. SIAM Journal on Applied Mathematics 66(5): 1632–1648.
27. Bresson X, Esedoglu S, Vandergheynst P, Thiran J, Osher S (2007) Fast Global Minimization of the Active Contour/Snake Models. Journal of Mathematical Imaging and Vision 28(2): 151–167.
28. Chambolle A, Cremers D, Pock T, Bischof H (2009) A Convex Approach for Computing Minimal Partitions. In: IEEE Conference on Computer Vision and Pattern Recognition. pp. 810–817.
29. Bae E, Yuan J, Tai XC (2009) Global Minimization for Continuous Multiphase Partitioning Problems Using a Dual Approach. International Journal of Computer Vision 92(1): 112–129.
30. Yuan J, Bae E, Tai XC, Boykov Y (2010) A Study on Continuous Max-Flow and Min-Cut Approaches Part I: Binary Labeling. UCLA CAM Report 10–61.
31. Lellmann J, Schnörr C (2011) Continuous Multiclass Labeling Approaches and Algorithms. SIAM Journal on Imaging Sciences 4(4): 1049–1096.
32. Nieuwenhuis C, Toppe E, Cremers D (2013) A Survey and Comparison of Discrete and Continuous Multi-label Optimization Approaches for the Potts Model. International Journal of Computer Vision.
33. Strang G (1983) Maximal flow through a domain. Mathematical Programming 26: 123–143.
34. Cheng J, Foo SW, Krishnan S (2006) Watershed-presegmented snake for boundary detection and tracking of left ventricle in echocardiographic images. Information Technology in Biomedicine, IEEE Transactions on 10: 414–416.
35. Mignotte M, Meunier J, Tardif JC (2001) Endocardial boundary etimation and tracking in echocardiographic images using deformable template and markov random fields. Pattern Analysis and Applications 4: 256–271.
36. Chiang HH, Cheng JZ, Hung PK, Liu CY, Chung CH, et al. (2010) Cell-based graph cut for segmentation of 2D/3D sonographic breast images. In: IEEE International Symposium on Biomedical Imaging. pp. 177–180.
37. Aleman-Flores M, Alvarez L, Caselles V (2008) Breast nodule ultrasound segmentation through texture-based active contours. In: Progress in Industrial Mathematics at ECMI 2006, Springer Berlin Heidelberg, volume 12 of *Mathematics in Industry*. pp. 858–862.
38. Xiao G, Brady M, Noble J, Yongyue Z (2002) Segmentation of ultrasound b-mode images with intensity inhomogeneity correction. Medical Imaging, IEEE Transactions on 21: 48–57.
39. Shen D, Zhan Y, Davatzikos C (2003) Segmentation of prostate boundaries from ultrasound images using statistical shape model. Medical Imaging, IEEE Transactions on 22: 539–551.
40. Shao F, Ling K, Ng W, Wu R (2003) Prostate boundary detection from ultrasonographic images. J Ultrasound Med 22: 605–623.
41. Cvancarova M, Albregtsen F, Brabrand K, Samset E (2005) Segmentation of ultrasound images of liver tumors applying snake algorithms and gvf. International Congress Series 1281: 218–223.
42. Lee WL, Chen YC, Chen YC, Hsieh KS (2005) Unsupervised segmentation of ultrasonic liver images by multiresolution fractal feature vector. Information Sciences 175: 177–199.
43. Huang X, Dione D, Compas C, Papademetris X, Lin B, et al. (2012) A dynamical appearance model based on multiscale sparse representation: Segmentation of the left ventricle from 4d echocardiography. In: Ayache N, Delingette H, Golland P, Mori K, editors, Medical Image Computing and Computer-Assisted Intervention MICCAI 2012, Springer Berlin Heidelberg, volume 7512 of *Lecture Notes in Computer Science*. pp 58–65.
44. Huang X, Dione DP, Compas CB, Papademetris X, Lin BA, et al. (2014) Contour tracking in echocardiographic sequences via sparse representation and dictionary learning. Medical Image Analysis 18: 253–271.

45. Loupas T, McDicken WN, Allan PL (1989) An adaptive weighted median filter for speckle suppression in medical ultrasonic images. IEEE Transactions on Circuits and Systems 36: 129–135.
46. Boykov Y, Kolmogorov V (2004) An experimental comparison of min-cut/max-ow algorithms for energy minimization in computer vision. EEE Transactions on Pattern Analysis and Machine Intelligence 26: 1124–1137.
47. Boykov Y, Funka-Lea G (2006) Graph Cuts and Efficient ND Image Segmentation. International Journal of Computer Vision 70(2): 109–131.
48. Shi J, Malik J (2000) Normalized cuts and image segmentation. Pattern Analysis and Machine Intelligence 22: 888–905.
49. Glowinski R, Marrocco A (1975) Sur l'Approximation, par Eléments Finis d'Ordre Un, et la Résolution, par Pénalisation-Dualité, d'une Classe de Problèmes de Dirichlet Non Linéaires. Laboria.
50. Glowinski R, Tallec PL (1989) Augmented Lagrangian and Operator-Splitting Methods in Nonlinear Mechanics. SIAM.
51. Bioucas-Dias J, Figueiredo M (2007) A new TwIST: Two-step iterative shrinkage/thresholding algorithms for image restoration. Image Processing, IEEE Transactions on 16: 2992–3004.
52. Goldstein T, Osher S (2009) The split bregman method for L1-regularized problems. SIAM J Img Sci 2: 323–343.
53. Setzer S (2011) Operator splittings, bregman methods and frame shrinkage in image processing. Int J Comput Vision 92: 265–280.
54. Donoho D (1995) De-noising by soft-thresholding. Information Theory, IEEE Transactions on 41: 613–627.
55. Duval V, Aujol JF, Gousseau Y (2010). On the parameter choice for the non-local means.
56. Lee A, Pedersen K, Mumford D (2003) The nonlinear statistics of high-contrast patches in natural images. International Journal of Computer Vision 54: 83–103.
57. Fledelius HC (1997) Ultrasound in ophthalmology. Ultrasound in Medicine and Biology 23: 365–375.
58. Fenster A, Downey D, Cardinal H (2001) Three-dimensional ultrasound imaging. Phys Med Biol 46: 67–99.
59. Cuadra MB, Gorthi S, Karahanoglu FI, Salvador F, Pica A, et al. (2009) Model-based segmentation and fusion of 3d computed tomography and 3d ultrasound of the eye for radiotherapy planning. In: Computational Vision and Medical Image Processing. pp. 53–58.
60. Rueda S, Fathima S, Knight C, Yaqub M, Papageorghiou A, et al. (2013) Evaluation and comparison of current fetal ultrasound image segmentation methods for biometric measurements: A grand challenge. Medical Imaging, IEEE Transactions on.
61. Dice LR (1945) Measures of the amount of ecologic association between species. Ecology 26: 297–302.
62. Grady L (2006) Random walks for image segmentation. Pattern Analysis and Machine Intelligence, IEEE Transactions on 28: 1768–1783.
63. Flusser J (2000) On the independence of rotation moment invariants. Pattern Recognition 33: 1405–1410.
64. Altman D, Chitty L (1997) New charts for ultrasound dating of pregnancy. Ultrasound Obstet Gynecol 10: 174–191.
65. Sarris I, Ioannou C, Chamberlain P, Ohuma E, Roseman F, et al. (2012) Intra- and interobserver variability in fetal ultrasound measurements. Ultrasound in Obstetrics and Gynecology 39: 266–273.

7

Stereotactic Body Radiotherapy-Induced Arterial Hypervascularity of Non-Tumorous Hepatic Parenchyma in Patients with Hepatocellular Carcinoma: Potential Pitfalls in Tumor Response Evaluation on Multiphase Computed Tomography

Mee Jin Park[1¤], So Yeon Kim[1*], Sang Min Yoon[2], Jong Hoon Kim[2], Seong Ho Park[1], Seung Soo Lee[1], Yedaun Lee[1], Moon-Gyu Lee[1]

1 Department of Radiology and Research Institute of Radiology, University of Ulsan College of Medicine, Asan Medical Center, Seoul, Korea, **2** Department of Radiation Oncology, University of Ulsan College of Medicine, Asan Medical Center, Seoul, Korea

Abstract

Purpose: To evaluate temporal changes in contrast enhancement patterns of non-tumorous hepatic parenchyma with a focus on arterial hypervascularity on multiphase computed tomography (CT) in patients with hepatocellular carcinoma (HCC) treated with stereotactic body radiotherapy (SBRT).

Methods: We retrospectively identified 61 patients who had undergone multiphase contrast-enhanced CT at one, three, and six months after SBRT. Irradiated versus non-irradiated liver parenchyma was delineated by cross-correlation with the dose-volume histogram of SBRT plan. Serial changes in the contrast enhancement patterns of the irradiated versus non-irradiated liver parenchyma were evaluated by two abdominal radiologists in consensus. We compared the frequency of the contrast enhancement patterns according to the follow-up period using the Fisher-Freeman-Halton exact test.

Results: The irradiated non-tumorous hepatic parenchyma showed that the prevalence of arterial hypervascularity increased during the follow-up period ($P<.01$): 11.5% (7/61) in one, 45.9% (28/61) in three, and 54.1% (33/61) in six months. Contrast wash-out on the delayed phase was uncommon: 1.6% (1/61) in one, 3.3% (2/61) in three, and 0% in six months.

Conclusion: The incidence of arterial hypervascularity of the irradiated hepatic parenchyma gradually increased until six months after SBRT, which could interfere with the accurate evaluation of treatment response. The lack of wash-out on the delayed phase in the hypervascular area would distinguish SBRT-related change from residual/recurred HCC.

Editor: Sang Hoon Ahn, Yonsei University College of Medicine, Korea, Republic of

Funding: This study was supported by Grant [2013-546] from the Asan Institute for Life Science, Seoul, Korea, and Grant [2012R1A1A1012731] by Basic Science Research Program through the National Research Foundation of Korea (NRF) funded by the Ministry of Education, Science and Technology, Korea. The funders had no role in study design, data collection and analysis, decision to publish, or preparation of the manuscript.

Competing Interests: The authors have declared that no competing interests exist.

* E-mail: sykimrad@amc.seoul.kr

¤ Current address: Department of Radiology, Ajou University School of Medicine, Suwon, Gyeonggi-do, Korea

Introduction

Hepatocellular carcinoma (HCC) is a major health problem worldwide, with more than half a million new cases yearly [1]. Traditional treatment modalities for HCC include surgical resection, percutaneous ablation, and transarterial chemoembolization [2]. Stereotactic body radiotherapy (SBRT) is an emerging treatment option for patients with inoperable HCC because it offers a high local tumor control probability and a high safety profile [3–5]. SBRT is a technique that uses precisely targeted three-dimensional conformal radiation delivered via multiple portals in various directions in a hypofractionated regimen under image guidance [6]. Although SBRT is designed to accurately deliver a high dose of radiation to a confined target while minimizing radiation to normal tissue [3,7,8], neighboring non-tumorous hepatic parenchyma are exposed to irradiation and may thus present with radiation-induced changes.

Many previous imaging studies on radiation-induced changes of the liver reported changes associated with conventional radiotherapy rather than SBRT [9–14]. Radiation-induced changes associated with SBRT are expected to differ from those associated with conventional radiotherapy because of the complex and distinct mode of radiation dose delivery of SBRT as well as delivered radiation dose [15]. With the increasing use of SBRT, it is important to be familiar with the radiation-induced changes of the liver after SBRT on multiphase computed tomography [16], as this information will help us to accurately assess treatment responses [17–21].

There have been a few published studies regarding the multiphase CT findings of non-tumorous hepatic parenchyma after SBRT [16,22–24]. Two of these studies briefly mentioned arterial hypervascularity as a form of focal liver reaction in the irradiated hepatic parenchyma, but without describing the incidence or temporal changes of arterial hypervascularity [16,22]. As arterial hypervascularity is also a key diagnostic feature of HCC [25], we need to determine the characteristics of

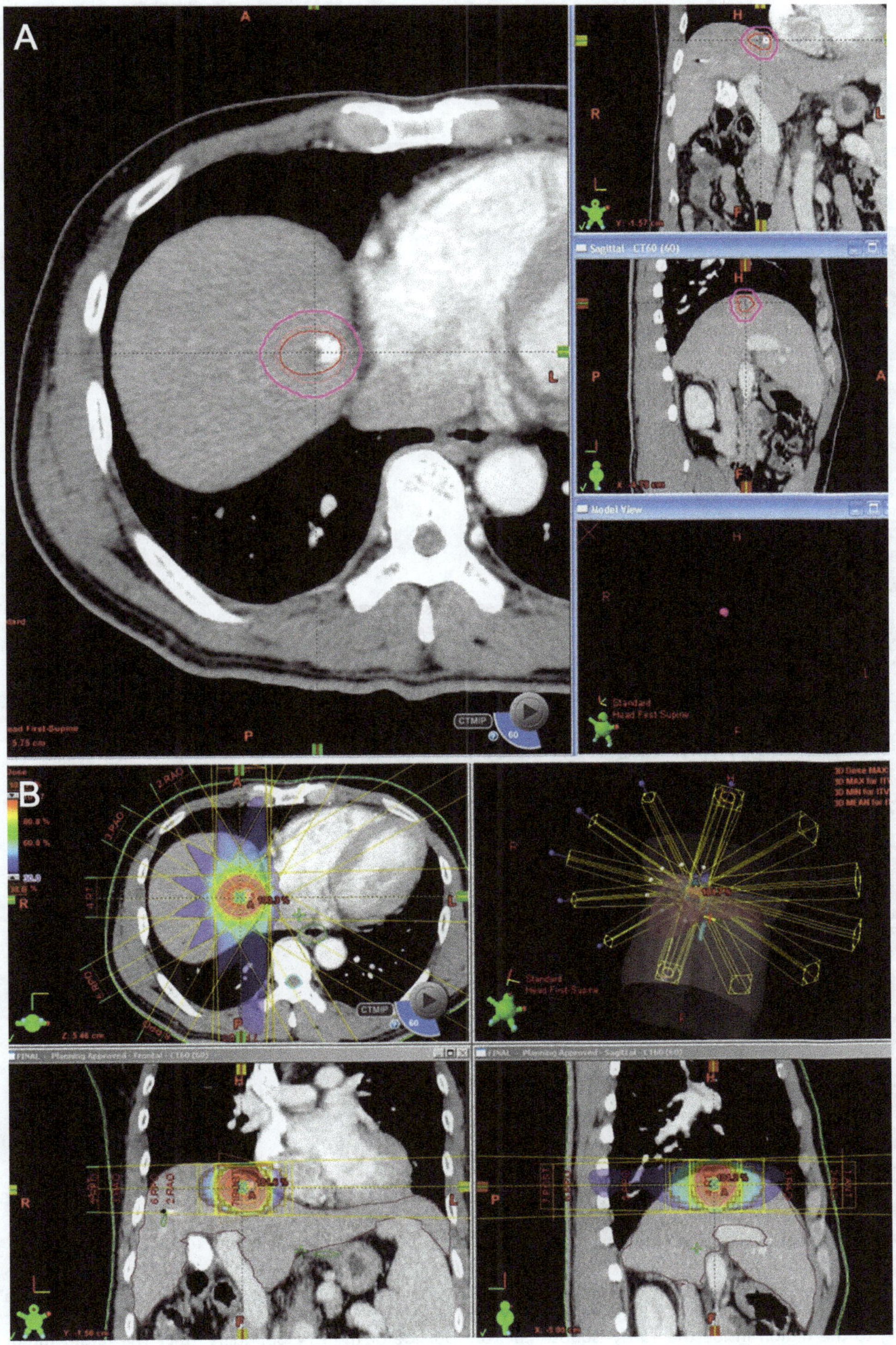

Figure 1. An example of delineation of the target volume and treatment planning: Planning for SBRT. (A) The planning target volume (purple circle) is expanded to cover the gross tumor volume (red circle). (B) Using six coplanar photon beams, a highly conformal isodose distribution is obtained three-dimensionally. The dose distribution is demonstrated on the color map as a percentage of the total radiation dose.

Table 1. CT scanning parameters.

Parameters	Sensation 16 (n = 60)	LightSpeed VCT (n = 52)	LightSpeed plus (n = 40)	LightSpeed 16 (n = 16)	LightSpeed QX/I (n = 12)	Definition AS+ (n = 3)
Number of detectors	16	64	4	16	16	4
Effective tube current-time production (mAs)†	200	200	200	200	250	200
Tube voltage (kVp)	120	120	120	120	120	120
Collimation (mm)	1.5	0.625	1.25	0.625	1.25	1.25
Rotation time (sec)	0.5	0.5	0.6	0.5	0.6	0.6
Pitch	1	1	0.75	1	0.75	0.75

†Automatic tube current modulation was used.

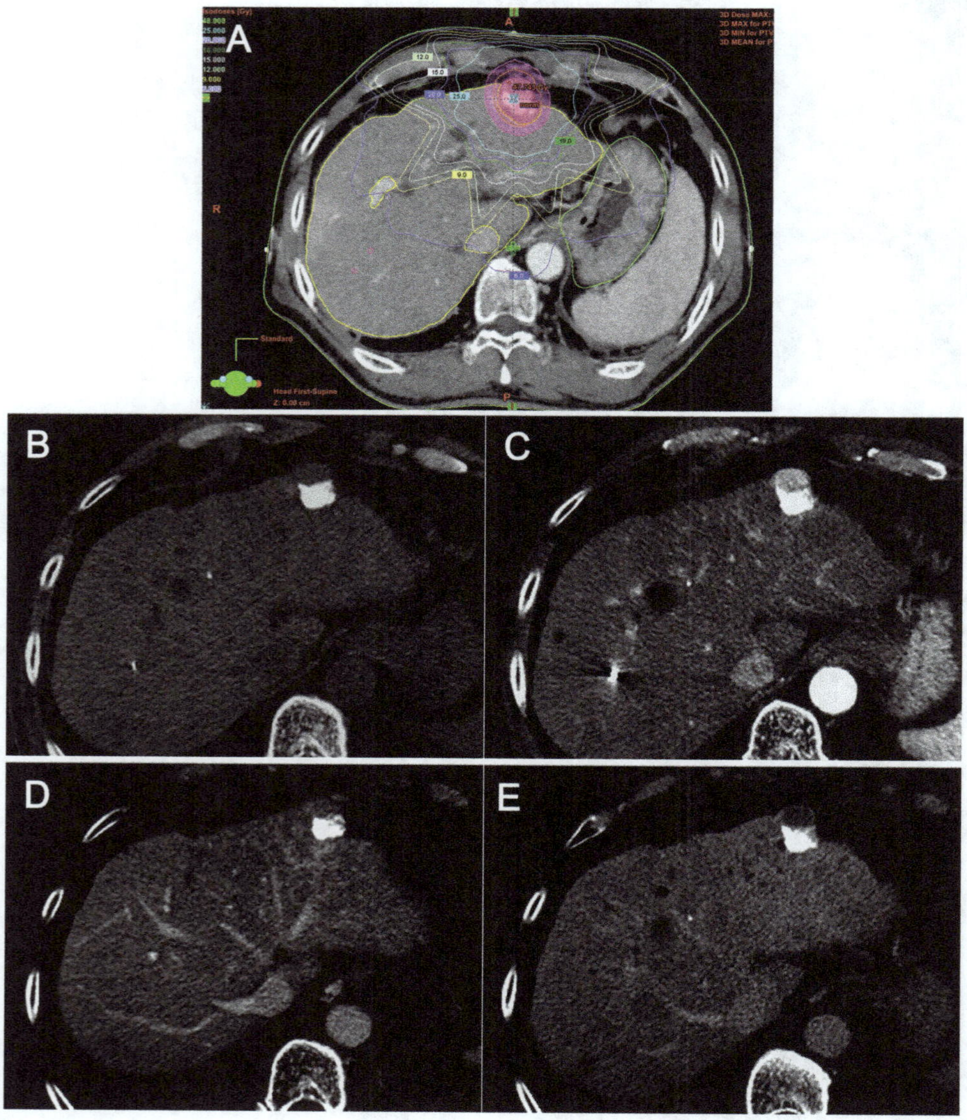

Figure 2. Typical hepatic parenchymal change seen on one month after SBRT. (A) As seen on the isodose curve for planning SBRT with a total dose of 45 Gy, the planning target volume (PTV, purple circle) is expanded to cover the gross tumor volume (red circle). The irradiated hepatic parenchyma is delineated corresponding to the region inside the 15-Gy isodose line, but outside of the PTV boundary. (B-E) The target tumor (arrowheads) in the left lateral segment of the liver, was treated with transarterial chemoembolization prior to SBRT. Residual tumor is noted (arrowheads) with arterial enhancement and washout on the portal and delayed phases adjacent to lipiodol. One-month f/u CT images after SBRT demonstrate that there is no significant change in the irradiated hepatic parenchyma or in the tumor (arrowheads) in any phase including noncontrast (B), arterial (C), portal (D), and delayed (E) phases. A fiducial marker (arrows) is also seen.

arterial hypervascularity of non-tumorous hepatic parenchyma after SBRT and differentiate them from recurred or residual HCC. Considering that multiple follow-up CT scans are generally available following the treatment of HCC, we suggest that temporal changes in the enhancement patterns of the irradiated hepatic parenchyma are also important to note.

Therefore, the purpose of our study is to evaluate temporal changes in contrast enhancement patterns of non-tumorous hepatic parenchyma on multiphase CT with a focus on arterial hypervascularity in patients with HCC treated with SBRT.

Materials and Methods

The institutional review board of Asan Medical Center approved this study, and informed consent was waived due to the retrospective nature of the study. All the data of patient records and information were anonymized and de-identified prior to analysis.

Study Patients

A computerized search of our institution's medical records revealed 93 patients (mean age ± SD, 60.8±7.3 years), including 75 men (60.3±7.0 years) and 18 women (62.9±8.4 years), with HCC treated using SBRT between March 2007 and December 2009. At our institution, indication of SBRT for the patients with HCC was as follows: (1) HCC not suitable for surgery or percutaneous ablative therapies; (2) HCC confined to the liver without extrahepatic metastases; HCC less than 6 cm in the longest diameter or up to 3 lesions; (4) HCC with no evidence of major vascular invasion; (5) a liver function of Child-Pugh class A or B; (6) adequate residual functional liver volume (more than 700 cc); and (7) a sufficient distance (more than 2 cm) from the adjacent organs at risk such as duodenum, stomach, colon, and spinal cord. The diagnosis of HCC was made non-pathologically according to the noninvasive diagnostic criteria proposed by the American Association for the Study of Liver Diseases in 93 patients [26].

Among these 93 patients, 65 had follow-up multiphase CT scans one, three, and six months after SBRT. Four of the 65 patients were excluded because of potentially confounding processes affecting contrast enhancement patterns of the irradiated hepatic parenchyma, i.e. (1) ethanol injection during the follow-up period (n = 2), (2) metal artifact from the gold fiducial markers detected in the liver and thus impairing the image quality in a very small target volume (n = 1), and (3) portal vein thrombus causing hepatic perfusion abnormality (n = 1). The remaining 61 patients (mean age ± SD, 61.7±8.3 years), including 52 men (61±8 years) and nine women (65.6±9.4 years), were finally included in the analyses.

In the study population, 50 of these had a single lesion and the remaining 11 patients had two or more lesions. For the 11 patients with multiple HCCs, only the largest lesion was included in further analysis to avoid clustering effects. The size of the 61 HCCs ranged from 0.3 to 3.7 cm (mean size ± SD, 1.8 cm±0.9 cm). Among the 61 HCCs, 19 HCCs were treated with transcatheter arterial chemoembolization (TACE) in combination with SBRT for the lesion of interest. Child-Pugh class of liver cirrhosis was also assessed one, three and six months after SBRT.

Treatment with SBRT

All patients underwent CT-based simulation (LightSpeed®RT 1, GE, Milwaukee, WI, USA) for SBRT. Prior to CT simulation, gold fiducial markers were inserted under US-guidance surrounding the target tumor. Implanted markers are typically separated by 3~5 cm in distance between markers and they indicate the location of tumors for SBRT. CT simulation was performed with free breathing using a four-dimensional (4D) CT respiratory gating system (Real-time position management™ system, Varian, Palo Alto, CA, USA) to evaluate the extent of tumor motion during entire respiratory cycles. The 'gross tumor volume (GTV)' was calculated as the sum of the tumor position within a gating phase. It was further expanded by a 5-mm margin and corresponded to the 'planning target volume (PTV)' (Fig. 1).

SBRT was planned using five to nine coplanar or non-coplanar beams with energies of 6 to 15 MV (Eclipse™, Varian, Palo Alto, CA, USA). A dose of 10–20 Gy (median, 15 Gy) per fraction was given over 3–4 consecutive days to a total dose of 30–60 Gy (median, 45 Gy) to the isodose line covering the PVT (generally 85–90% of the isodose line) (Fig. 1). The pretreatment tumor position was verified on the basis of fiducial markers detected by the on-board imaging system (On-Board Imager®, Varian, Palo Alto, CA, USA) which is part of a linear accelerator (CL21iX, Varian, Palo Alto, CA, USA) and includes a two-dimensional (2D) kilovoltage radiograph and cone-beam CT.

Table 2. Multiphase CT attenuation in the irradiated hepatic parenchyma in 61 patients.

Time interval	CT attenuation	Phase			
		Non-contrast	Arterial	Portal	Delayed
1 month	Low	16 (26.2%)	3 (4.9%)	9 (14.8%)	1 (1.6%)
	Iso	45 (73.8%)	51 (83.6%)	44 (72.1%)	52 (85.2%)
	High	0 (0%)	7 (11.5%)	13.1 (8%)	8 (13.1%)
3 months	Low	41 (67.2%)	7 (11.5%)	12 (19.7%)	2 (3.3%)
	Iso	20 (32.8%)	26 (42.6%)	20 (32.8%)	29 (47.5%)
	High	0 (0%)	28 (45.9%)	29 (47.5%)	30 (49.2%)
6 months	Low	48 (78.7%)	5 (8.2%)	8 (12.3%)	0 (0%)
	Iso	12 (19.7%)	23 (37.7%)	16 (24.7%)	30 (49.2%)
	High	1 (1.6%)	33 (54.1%)	37 (60.7%)	31 (50.8%)
P Values		<.01	<.01	<.01	<.01

Data are number of patients with percentages in parentheses. Sum of the percentages may not be 100% due to rounding of the numbers.

CT Imaging

CT scans were obtained with 4 to 64 multidetector CT scanners (Definition AS or Sensation 16 Siemens, Erlangen, Germany; LightSpeed, GE medical Systems, Milwaukee, WI, USAs) in the unenhanced, arterial, portal, and delayed venous contrast-enhanced phases (Table 1). The effective tube current time product was generally 200 mAs. The other parameters were described in detail in Table 1. Patients were given 2 mL/kg of iopromide (Ultravist 370; Schering, Berlin, Germany) or iopamidol (Isovue 370; Bracco, Milan, Italy) intravenously at a rate of 4 mL/sec via the antecubital vein. Arterial phase images were obtained using a bolus tracking technique with a trigger enhancement threshold at the upper abdominal aorta of 100 HU. After the threshold was reached, a diagnostic delay time of 25 seconds was used for the arterial phase. Portal and delayed phase images were obtained 72 and 180 seconds, respectively, following contrast injection.

Interpretation of CT Images

The images were evaluated in consensus by two abdominal radiologists (M.J.P and S.Y.K with 5 and 9 years, respectively, of clinical experience in abdomen CT). Irradiated versus non-irradiated

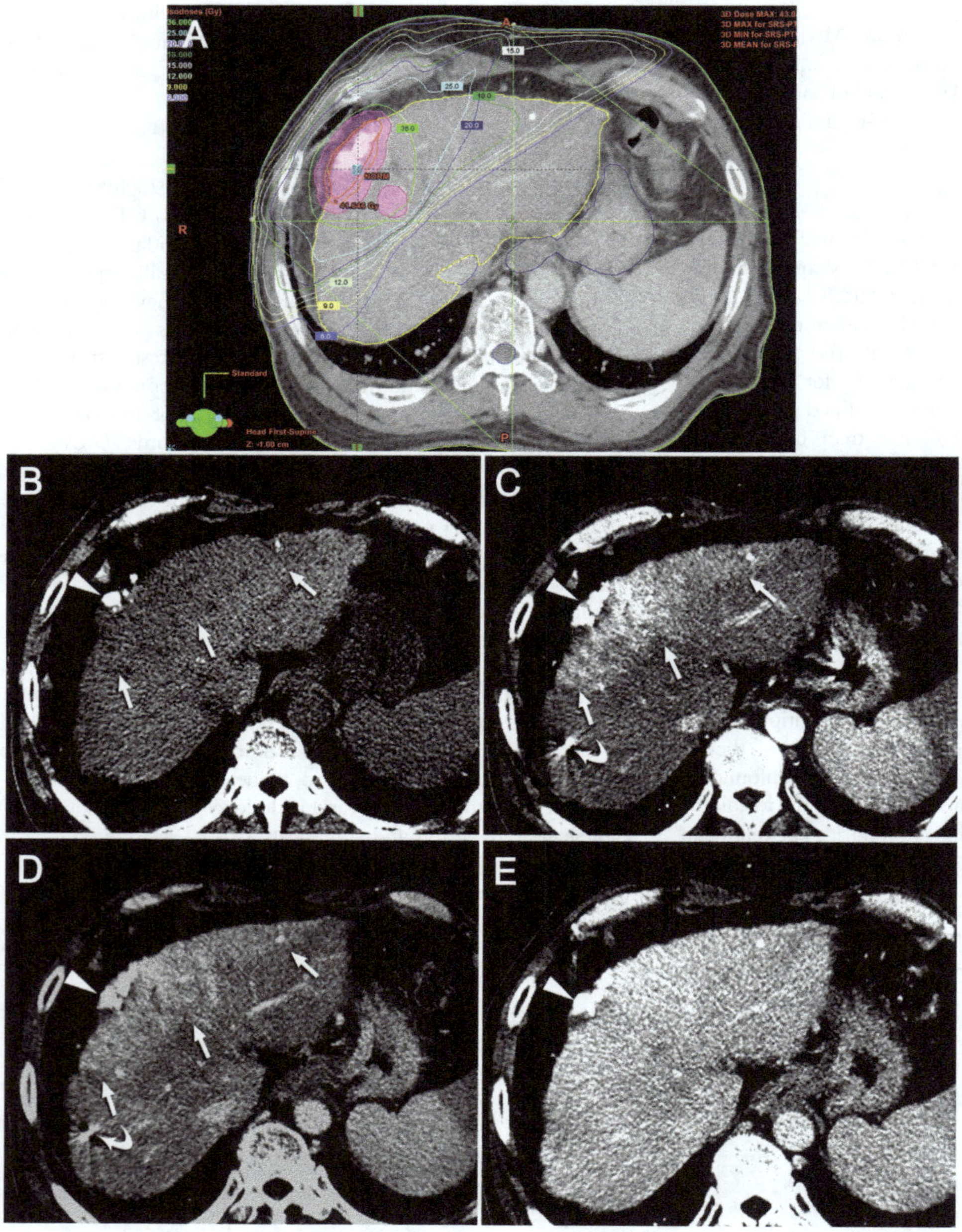

Figure 3. Typical hepatic attenuation difference seen on three months after SBRT. (A) Dose distribution is demonstrated on the isodose curve for SBRT. The planning target volume (PTV, purple circle) as well as the gross tumor volume (red circle) in the peripheral portion of the right lobe of the liver, was treated with 36 Gy of the total radiation dose. The irradiated hepatic parenchyma is delineated corresponding to the region inside the 15-Gy isodose line but outside the PTV boundary. (B-E) Multiphase CT images obtained three months after SBRT depict low attenuation (arrows) on noncontrast CT (B), high attenuation (arrows) on the arterial (C) and portal (D) phases, and isoattenuation on the delayed (E) phase, respectively. The target tumor (arrowheads) in the peripheral portion of the right lobe of the liver was treated using transarterial chemoembolization prior to SBRT. Fiducial markers are also seen (curved arrows).

liver parenchyma was delineated in each patient by cross-correlation with the dose-volume histogram of CT for the SBRT treatment plan (Fig. 2). As previous studies [5,22] suggested a threshold dose for hepatic attenuation differences in irradiated hepatic parenchyma from 13.7 Gy, a 15-Gy isodose curve on the dose-volume histogram was used as the outer boundary for the delineation of irradiated hepatic parenchyma. The calculated dose was verified on the follow-up CTs by visual comparison of the initial isodose lines and the margin of radiation reaction. The 15-Gy boundary also enclosed the tumor volume (PTV) irradiated on the dose-volume histogram. In order to exclude the possible tumor area with sufficient margin, we used PTV on the dose-volume histogram and one-year follow up CTs as a reference. In 55 patients with no recurrent tumor on one-year follow up CT in the irradiated area, we used PTV as a reference line for the possible tumor area. In 6 patients who had residual or recurrent HCCs on one-year follow-up CT in the irradiated area, we used the boundary of residual or recurrent tumors as a reference line for the possible tumor area. Therefore, we defined the irradiated non-tumorous hepatic parenchyma as corresponding to the region inside the 15-Gy isodose line but outside the PTV boundary or outside the boundary of the recurrent tumor on one-year follow up CTs (Fig. 1).

The hepatic attenuation difference (HAD) between the irradiated and non-irradiated hepatic parenchyma was determined on the non-contrast, arterial, portal, and delayed phase images at liver windows (window level, 70–100 HU; window width, 130–150 HU) on each follow-up CT scans [27]. If the presence of HAD was uncertain, the observers measured the CT attenuations

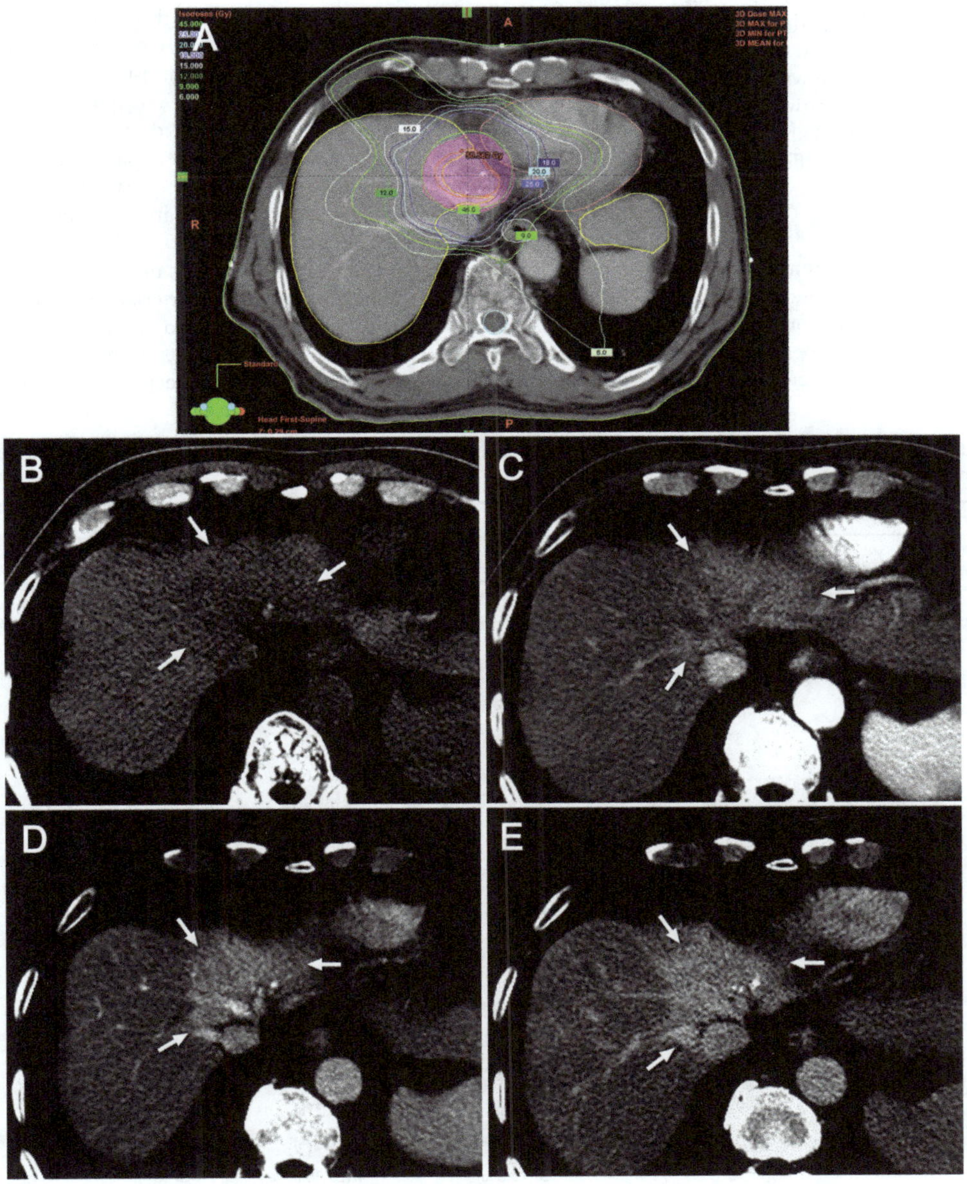

Figure 4. Typical hepatic attenuation difference seen on six months after SBRT. (A) The isodose curve for SBRT depicts the planning target volume (PTV, purple circle) as well as the gross tumor volume (red circle) for the treatment of hepatocellular carcinoma in left lobe of the liver. The total radiation dose for this patient was 45 Gy. The irradiated hepatic parenchyma is delineated corresponding to the region inside the 15-Gy isodose line but outside the PTV boundary. (B-E) Irradiated hepatic parenchyma appears as low attenuation (arrows) on noncontrast CT (B) and as high attenuation on the arterial (C), portal (D), and delayed (E) phase, respectively.

of the irradiated and non-irradiated hepatic parenchyma. A difference of at least 10 HU between the two regions was defined as a significant HAD [22,23].

Temporal changes of HAD within a study patient were evaluated according to the follow-up period. For patients who presented with HAD on the follow-up CTs, the time interval from the treatment to the first appearance of arterial hypervascularity and any form of HAD, was analyzed. For patients showing arterial hypervascularity, the HAD patterns seen on other phases were evaluated in order to identify the imaging features mimicking or differing from HCC.

Statistical Analyses

The Fisher-Freeman-Halton exact test was used to compare the frequency of HAD according to the follow-up period. In addition, comparisons were made using the same test between the following subgroups: (1) patients treated with SBRT only vs. those treated with TACE in combination with SBRT; (2); patients in Child-Pugh A vs. B and (3) patients with single disease vs. those with multiple lesions. Statistical analysis was performed using software (SPSS, version 19, SPSS, Chicago, IL, US). For all statistical analyses, a *P*-value <.05 was considered to indicate a significant difference.

Results

The CT findings of the irradiated hepatic parenchyma are summarized in Table 2. The areas and shapes of HAD corresponded well to the 15-Gy isodose line seen on the dose-volume histogram of the SBRT treatment plan. Hypervascularity on the arterial phase in the irradiated hepatic parenchyma was observed only in 11.5% (7/61) of our patients on the one-month follow-up CT examination. On subsequent follow-up CT scans, the incidence of arterial hypervascularity increased up to 54.1% (33/61) on the six-month follow-up CT. The temporal changes in arterial hypervascularity were, therefore, statistically significant (*P*<.01). On non-contrast CT, the irradiated hepatic parenchyma increasingly showed low attenuation compared to the nonirradiated hepatic parenchyma, which was seen in 26.2% (16/61) on the one-month follow-up CT and in 78.7% (48/61) on six-month follow-up CT. On the portal phase, the irradiated hepatic parenchyma was commonly seen as hyperattenuation after the three-month follow-up period; 47.5% (29/61) in three months and 60.7% (37/61) in six months after SBRT. Delayed phase images demonstrated isoattenuation or hyperattenuation in the majority of cases during any follow-up period. Hypoattenuation on the delayed phase was rarely seen on the follow-up CT scanning, i.e. 1.6% (1/61) on one month, 3.3% (2/61) on three-month, and none on the six-month follow-up CT scans. The temporal changes in the enhancement patterns on the non-contrast, portal, and delayed phases were also statistically significant. The typical image features on each follow-up period were presented in Fig. 2–4.

When the temporal changes in the enhancement patterns within a patient were analyzed, the time intervals between SBRT and the first appearance of arterial hypervascularity in the irradiated hepatic parenchyma were one month in 11.5 (7/61)% of the patients, three months in 34.4% (21/61), and six months in 14.8% (9/61). At the time of the first appearance of arterial hypervascularity, the same areas were seen as low attenuation in 57.1% (4/7), 57.1% (12/21), and 11.1% (1/9) of the patients on non-contrast CT. However, irradiated parenchyma was not seen in any of these

Table 3. Multiphase CT attenuation in the irradiated hepatic parenchyma in between patients treated with SBRT only vs. those treated with TACE in combination with SBRT.

Subgroups	Time interval	CT attenuation	Phase			
			Noncontrast	Arterial	Portal	Delayed
Patients	1 month	Low	10 (23.8%)	2 (4.8%)	5 (11.9%)	0 (0%)
with		Iso	32 (76.2%)	35 (83.3%)	33 (78.6%)	38 (90.5%)
SBRT		High	0 (0%)	5 (11.9%)	4 (9.5%)	4 (9.5%)
only	3 months	Low	31 (73.8%)	2 (4.8%)	6 (14.3%)	1 (2.4%)
(n = 42)		Iso	11 (26.2%)	20 (47.6%)	12 (28.6%)	21 (50.0%)
		High	0 (0%)	20 (47.6%)	24 (57.1%)	20 (47.6%)
	6 months	Low	33 (78.6%)	2 (4.8%)	4 (9.5%)	0 (0%)
		Iso	9 (21.4%)	16 (38.1%)	12 (28.6%)	25 (59.5%)
		High	0 (0%)	24 (57.1%)	26 (61.9%)	17 (40.5%)
	P Values		<.01	<.01	<.01	<.01
Patients	1 month	Low	6 (31.6%)	1 (5.3%)	4 (21.1%)	1 (5.3%)
with		Iso	13 (68.4%)	16 (84.2%)	11 (57.9%)	14 (73.7%)
combined		High	0 (0%)	2 (10.5%)	4 (21.1%)	4 (21.1%)
therapy	3 months	Low	10 (52.6%)	5 (26.3%)	6 (31.6%)	1 (5.3%)
(n = 19)		Iso	9 (47.4%)	6 (31.6%)	8 (42.1%)	8 (42.1%)
		High	0 (0%)	8 (42.1%)	5 (26.3%)	10 (52.6%)
	6 months	Low	15 (78.9%)	3 (15.8%)	4 (21.1%)	0 (0%)
		Iso	3 (15.8%)	7 (36.8%)	4 (21.1%)	5 (26.3%)
		High	1 (5.3%)	9 (47.4%)	11 (57.9%)	14 (73.7%)
	P Values		<.01	<.01	0.1	<.01

Data are number of patients with percentages in parentheses. Sum of the percentages may not be 100% due to rounding of the numbers.

patients as low attenuation on either the portal or the delayed phase. The time intervals between SBRT and the first appearance of any form of HAD in the irradiated hepatic parenchyma were one month in 39.3% (24/61), three months in 55.7% (34/61), and six months in 3.3% (2/61). In only one of 61 study patients (1.6%) did the irradiated hepatic parenchyma appear completely isoattenuated on any phase of CT during the follow-up period.

In the subgroup analysis, the group treated with SBRT only and the group with combined therapy of TACE and SBRT, were similar in their contrast enhancement patterns in the irradiated hepatic parenchyma: the incidence of arterial hypervascularity increased gradually until six months after SBRT up to 57.1% (24/42) in those with SBRT only, while up to 47.4% (9/19) in those with combination therapy of TACE and SBRT; on the portal and delayed phase images, the majority of the irradiated hepatic parenchyma appeared iso- or hyper-attenuation (Table 3). The temporal changes in the enhancement patterns on each phase were statistically significant for both groups ($P<.01$) except for the portal phase of the combined therapy subgroup ($P=0.1$). In the subgroup of Child-Pugh class A, the incidence of arterial hypervascularity in the irradiated hepatic parenchyma increased significantly during the follow up period from 10% (5/50) to 52.5% (21/40) ($P<.01$) (Table 4). Contrast washout on the delayed phases images was rarely seen in this group (only 1 patient on the 3-month follow-up CT). Similar phase-specific enhancement patterns were observed in the subgroup of Child-Pugh class B. However, temporal changes in the subgroup of Child-Pugh class B were not statistically significant, possibly because of the small number of the patients in each follow-up division (Table 4). Contrast enhancement patterns between the subgroups of a single HCC (n = 50) and multiple HCCs (n = 11) were also similar at each specific follow-up period (Table 5). The temporal changes were statistically significant in the patients with a single HCC, although the temporal changes in the arterial and delayed phase images in the patients with multiple HCCs did not show statistical significance, possibly due to the small number of the patients with multiple HCCs.

Discussion

Our study demonstrated that HAD in the irradiated non-tumorous hepatic parenchyma occurred in almost all of our patients after SBRT during the six-month follow-up period. Arterial hypervascularity in the irradiated non-tumorous hepatic parenchyma was observed in the considerable population of the patients and the incidence increased during the follow-up period, i.e. 11.5% of patients in one month, 45.9% in three months, and 54.1% in six months. According to the modified RECIST criteria recently suggested as a reliable method for assessing the tumor response in HCC clinical trials by American Association for the Study of Liver Diseases (AASLD)-Journal of the National Cancer Institute (JNCI), changes in the area of arterial enhancement is considered important in the evaluation of tumor response.[25] Therefore, arterial hypervascularity in the irradiated non-tumorous hepatic parenchyma is clinically important as it can create difficulties in evaluating the tumor response of HCC. In addition, the temporal changes of arterial hypervascularity in the irradiated hepatic parenchyma could also interfere with the accurate

Table 4. Multiphase CT attenuation in the irradiated hepatic parenchyma in subgroups according to Child-Pugh class A vs. B.

Subgroups	Time interval	CT attenuation	Phase			
			Noncontrast	Arterial	Portal	Delayed
Child-Pugh	1 month	Low	13 (26.0%)	3 (6.0%)	8 (16.0%)	1 (2.0%)
Class A	(n = 50)	Iso	37 (74.0%)	42 (84.0%)	36 (72.0%)	43 (86.0%)
		High	0 (0%)	5 (10.0%)	6 (12.0%)	6 (12.0%)
	3 months	Low	32 (69.6%)	6 (13.0%)	11 (23.9%)	2 (4.3%)
	(n = 46)*	Iso	14 (30.4%)	19 (41.3%)	15 (32.6%)	20 (43.5%)
		High	0 (0%)	21 (45.7%)	20 (43.5%)	24 (52.2%)
	6 months	Low	32 (80.0%)	5 (12.5%)	6 (15.0%)	0 (0%)
	(n = 40)†	Iso	8 (20.0%)	14 (35.0%)	10 (25.0%)	16 (40.0%)
		High	0 (0%)	21 (52.5%)	24 (60.0%)	24 (60.0%)
	P Values		<.01	<.01	<.01	<.01
Child-Pugh	1 month	Low	3 (27.3%)	0 (0%)	1 (9.1%)	0 (0%)
Class B	(n = 11)	Iso	8 (72.7%)	9 (81.8%)	8 (72.7%)	9 (81.8%)
		High	0 (0%)	2 (18.2%)	2 (18.2%)	2 (18.2%)
	3 months	Low	8 (57.1%)	1 (7.1%)	1 (7.1%)	0 (0%)
	(n = 14)*	Iso	6 (42.9%)	7 (50.0%)	5 (35.7%)	8 (57.1%)
		High	0 (0%)	6 (42.9%)	8 (57.1%)	6 (42.9%)
	6 months	Low	13 (72.2%)	0 (0%)	2 (11.1%)	0 (0%)
	(n = 18)†	Iso	4 (22.2%)	9 (50.0%)	6 (33.3%)	12 (66.7%)
		High	1 (5.6%)	9 (50.0%)	10 (55.6%)	6 (33.3%)
	P Values		.05	.22	.21	.47

Data are number of patients with percentages in parentheses. Sum of the percentages may not be 100% due to rounding of the numbers.
* One patient with Child-Pugh class C was excluded on 3 months follow up.
†Three patients with Child-Pugh class C was excluded on 6 months follow up.

Table 5. Multiphase CT attenuation in the irradiated hepatic parenchyma in subgroups according to single HCC vs. multiple HCCs.

Subgroups	Time interval	CT attenuation	Phase			
			Noncontrast	Arterial	Portal	Delayed
Single	1 month	Low	14 (28.0%)	3 (6.0%)	8 (16.0%)	1 (2.0%)
(n = 50)		Iso	36 (72.0%)	42 (84.0%)	36 (72.0%)	42 (84.0%)
		High	0 (0%)	5 (10.0%)	6 (12.0%)	7 (14.0%)
	3 months	Low	32 (64.0%)	7 (14.0%)	12 (24.0%)	2 (4.0%)
		Iso	18 (36.0%)	21 (42.0%)	16 (32.0%)	23 (46.0%)
		High	0 (0%)	22 (44.0%)	22 (44.0%)	25 (50.0%)
	6 months	Low	39 (78.0%)	5 (10.0%)	8 (16.0%)	0 (0%)
		Iso	10 (20.0%)	18 (36.0%)	13 (26.0%)	23 (46.0%)
		High	1 (2.0%)	27 (54.0%)	29 (58.0%)	27 (54.0%)
	P Values		<.01.	<.01	<.01	<.01
Multiple	1 month	Low	2 (18.2%)	0 (0%)	1 (9.1%)	0 (0%)
(n = 11)		Iso	9 (81.8%)	9 (81.8%)	8 (72.7%)	10 (90.9%)
		High	0 (0%)	2 (18.2%)	2 (18.2%)	1 (9.1%)
	3 months	Low	9 (81.8%)	0 (0%)	0 (0%)	0 (0%)
		Iso	2 (18.2%)	5 (45.5%)	4 (36.4%)	6 (54.5%)
		High	0 (0%)	6 (54.5%)	7 (63.6%)	5 (45.5%)
	6 months	Low	9 (81.8%)	0 (0%)	0 (0%)	0 (0%)
		Iso	2 (18.2%)	5 (45.5%)	3 (27.3%)	7 (63.6%)
		High	0 (0%)	6 (54.5%)	8 (72.7%)	4 (36.4%)
	P Values		<.01	.17	.04	.24

Data are number of patients with percentages in parentheses. Sum of the percentages may not be 100% due to rounding of the numbers.

evaluation of treatment response. In our study, the first appearance of arterial hypervascularity in the irradiated hepatic parenchyma reached its peak on the three-month follow up CTs. As the treatment response of HCC after SBRT also appeared after three months [5,22,23], the temporal changes of the treatment response seen in a tumor could coincide with that of the arterial hypervascularity seen in the irradiated hepatic parenchyma.

In this context, post-SBRT arterial hypervascularity of non-tumorous hepatic parenchyma could be misinterpreted as pseudoprogression, a term originally applied to high-grade glioma showing a temporal increase in contrast-enhancing lesion size after concurrent radiation therapy and temozolomide [28]. However, on multiphase contrast-enhanced CT, we found that some features of the contrast-enhancement patterns of the non-tumorous hepatic parenchyma related to SBRT, differed from the known typical findings of HCC [18-21], even though we did not perform tumor response evaluation itself and our study was limited in the evaluation of tumor recurrence due to lack of pathologic proof. Based on our observation in this study, and the lack of contrast wash-out seen on the delayed phase would be suggested as the helpful features for differentiating radiation-induced changes in the non-tumorous hepatic parenchyma and tumor progression, when we encounter arterial hypervascularity in the irradiated liver after SBRT. These findings are consistent with those of previous studies reporting imaging findings after SBRT [22,23].

The changes we found in the contrast enhancement patterns in the irradiated hepatic parenchyma after SBRT differed from those seen after conventional radiation therapy [9–14]. In particular, hepatic arterial hypervascularity has not yet been reported following conventional radiation therapy [9–14]. This difference could possibly be explained by the differences in radiation dose and distribution in SBRT and conventional radiation therapy. Nevertheless, the underlying histolopathologic mechanism of SBRT-related change in the irradiated non-tumorous hepatic parenchyma has not yet been clearly elucidated. To our knowledge, there has been no published report indicating the difference in the underlying histolopathologic mechanism between SBRT and conventional radiation therapy, although venoocclusive disease has been suggested as the mechanism of the parenchymal changes seen after SBRT [10,29]. However, the study regarding the pathologic change in the liver after SBRT analyzed only two specimens [29] as it was difficult to obtain surgical specimens after SBRT. To date, SBRT is generally recommended as a treatment option for patients with inoperable HCC [3–5,7]. However, a recent study recommends SBRT as a bridge to transplantation in transplantation-eligible patients [5]. When this application becomes increasingly used, further studies with extensive histopathologic correlation can be performed in order to determine the difference in the underlying mechanism which explains the different imaging findings obtained after SBRT and conventional radiation therapy.

As some patients of our study population were treated with combination of TACE and SBRT, we investigated and compared the effects of the combined therapy versus SBRT only on the contrast enhancement patterns and their temporal changes by performing the subgroup analysis. These two subgroups were similar in their contrast enhancement patterns and temporal changes. Two additional subgroup analyses (single vs. multinodular lesions and Child-Pugh A vs. B) also revealed contrast enhancement patterns similar between the paired subgroups across the follow-up periods.

Our study has several limitations. First, lack of pathologic proof for the areas of presumed irradiated nontumorous hepatic parenchyma in all patients. Considering that the current indication of SBRT is mainly confined to the patients with HCC as mentioned in the previous paragraph, it was difficult to obtain surgical specimens after SBRT [3–5,7]. Thus, we tried to exclude the possible tumor area using both planning CT for SBRT and one-year follow-up CTs. However, lack of pathologic correlation would decrease the reliability of our study regarding the differentiating post-radiotherapy arterial hypervascularity and residual tumor. Second, to delineate the irradiated hepatic parenchyma, we correlated the isodose line of the SBRT treatment planning CT with the follow-up CT images using visual comparison. For the exact and objective definition of the irradiation of hepatic parenchyma, a co-registration technique over multiple time points would be required.

In conclusion, after SBRT, arterial hypervascularity of non-tumorous hepatic parenchyma was increasingly seen on follow-up CT scans and it could potentially interfere with an accurate treatment response. The lack of wash-out on the delayed phase and the shape and area of the radiation field would, therefore, help to differentiate radiation-induced arterial hypervascularity from residual HCC.

Acknowledgments

The authors thank Bonnie Hami for editorial assistance in preparing the manuscript.

Author Contributions

Conceived and designed the experiments: SYK SMY JHK. Performed the experiments: MJP SYK SMY. Analyzed the data: MJP SYK. Contributed reagents/materials/analysis tools: YL SHP SSL M-GL. Wrote the paper: MJP SYK.

References

1. Parkin DM, Bray F, Ferlay J, Pisani P (2001) Estimating the world cancer burden: Globocan 2000. Int J Cancer 94: 153–156.
2. Llovet JM (2005) Updated treatment approach to hepatocellular carcinoma. J Gastroenterol 40: 225–235.
3. Herfarth KK, Debus J, Lohr F, Bahner ML, Rhein B, et al. (2001) Stereotactic single-dose radiation therapy of liver tumors: results of a phase I/II trial. J Clin Oncol 19: 164–170.
4. Tse RV, Hawkins M, Lockwood G, Kim JJ, Cummings B, et al. (2008) Phase I study of individualized stereotactic body radiotherapy for hepatocellular carcinoma and intrahepatic cholangiocarcinoma. J Clin Oncol 26: 657–664.
5. Cardenes HR, Price TR, Perkins SM, Maluccio M, Kwo P, et al. (2010) Phase I feasibility trial of stereotactic body radiation therapy for primary hepatocellular carcinoma. Clin Transl Oncol 12: 218–225.
6. Potters L, Steinberg M, Rose C, Timmerman R, Ryu S, et al. (2004) American Society for Therapeutic Radiology and Oncology and American College of Radiology practice guideline for the performance of stereotactic body radiation therapy. Int J Radiat Oncol Biol Phys 60: 1026–1032.
7. Wulf J, Hadinger U, Oppitz U, Thiele W, Ness-Dourdoumas R, et al. (2001) Stereotactic radiotherapy of targets in the lung and liver. Strahlenther Onkol 177: 645–655.
8. Lax I, Blomgren H, Naslund I, Svanstrom R (1994) Stereotactic radiotherapy of malignancies in the abdomen. Methodological aspects. Acta Oncol 33: 677–683.
9. Okumura T, Itai Y, Tsuji H, Matsueda K, Matsuzaki Y, et al. (1994) Focused radiation hepatitis after Bragg-peak proton therapy for hepatocellular carcinoma: CT findings. J Comput Assist Tomogr 18: 821–823.
10. Willemart S, Nicaise N, Struyven J, van Gansbeke D (2000) Acute radiation-induced hepatic injury: evaluation by triphasic contrast enhanced helical CT. Br J Radiol 73: 544–546.
11. Chiou SY, Lee RC, Chi KH, Chia-Hsien Cheng J, Chiang JH, et al. (2001) The triple-phase CT image appearance of post-irradiated livers. Acta Radiol 42: 526–531.
12. Ahmadi T, Itai Y, Onaya H, Yoshioka H, Okumura T, et al. (1999) CT evaluation of hepatic injury following proton beam irradiation: appearance, enhancement, and 3D size reduction pattern. J Comput Assist Tomogr 23: 655–663.
13. Unger EC, Lee JK, Weyman PJ (1987) CT and MR imaging of radiation hepatitis. J Comput Assist Tomogr 11: 264–268.
14. Reed GB, Jr., Cox AJ, Jr. (1966) The human liver after radiation injury. A form of veno-occlusive disease. Am J Pathol 48: 597–611.
15. Lo SS, Fakiris AJ, Chang EL, Mayr NA, Wang JZ, et al. (2010) Stereotactic body radiation therapy: a novel treatment modality. Nat Rev Clin Oncol 7: 44–54.
16. Price TR, Perkins SM, Sandrasegaran K, Henderson MA, Maluccio MA, et al. (2012) Evaluation of response after stereotactic body radiotherapy for hepatocellular carcinoma. Cancer 118: 3191–3198.
17. Bartolozzi C, Lencioni R, Caramella D, Falaschi F, Cioni R, et al. (1994) Hepatocellular carcinoma: CT and MR features after transcatheter arterial embolization and percutaneous ethanol injection. Radiology 191: 123–128.
18. El-Serag HB, Marrero JA, Rudolph L, Reddy KR (2008) Diagnosis and treatment of hepatocellular carcinoma. Gastroenterology 134: 1752–1763.
19. Kim T, Murakami T, Takahashi S, Tsuda K, Tomoda K, et al. (1999) Optimal phases of dynamic CT for detecting hepatocellular carcinoma: evaluation of unenhanced and triple-phase images. Abdom Imaging 24: 473–480.
20. Iannaccone R, Laghi A, Catalano C, Rossi P, Mangiapane F, et al. (2005) Hepatocellular carcinoma: role of unenhanced and delayed phase multi-detector row helical CT in patients with cirrhosis. Radiology 234: 460–467.
21. Zech CJ, Reiser MF, Herrmann KA (2009) Imaging of hepatocellular carcinoma by computed tomography and magnetic resonance imaging: state of the art. Dig Dis 27: 114–124.
22. Herfarth KK, Hof H, Bahner ML, Lohr F, Hoss A, et al. (2003) Assessment of focal liver reaction by multiphasic CT after stereotactic single-dose radiotherapy of liver tumors. Int J Radiat Oncol Biol Phys 57: 444–451.
23. Sanuki-Fujimoto N, Takeda A, Ohashi T, Kunieda E, Iwabuchi S, et al. (2010) CT evaluations of focal liver reactions following stereotactic body radiotherapy for small hepatocellular carcinoma with cirrhosis: relationship between imaging appearance and baseline liver function. Br J Radiol 83: 1063–1071.
24. Takeda A, Oku Y, Sanuki N, Kunieda E, Koike N, et al. (2012) Dose volume histogram analysis of focal liver reaction in follow-up multiphasic CT following stereotactic body radiotherapy for small hepatocellular carcinoma. Radiother Oncol 104: 374–378.
25. Lencioni R, Llovet JM (2010) Modified RECIST (mRECIST) assessment for hepatocellular carcinoma. Semin Liver Dis 30: 52–60.
26. Bruix J, Sherman M, Practice Guidelines Committee AAftSoLD (2005) Management of hepatocellular carcinoma. Hepatology 42: 1208–1236.
27. Mayo-Smith WW, Gupta H, Ridlen MS, Brody JM, Clements NC, et al. (1999) Detecting hepatic lesions: the added utility of CT liver window settings. Radiology 210: 601–604.
28. Hygino da Cruz LC, Jr., Rodriguez I, Domingues RC, Gasparetto EL, Sorensen AG (2011) Pseudoprogression and pseudoresponse: imaging challenges in the assessment of posttreatment glioma. AJNR Am J Neuroradiol 32: 1978–1985.
29. Olsen CC, Welsh J, Kavanagh BD, Franklin W, McCarter M, et al. (2009) Microscopic and macroscopic tumor and parenchymal effects of liver stereotactic body radiotherapy. Int J Radiat Oncol Biol Phys 73: 1414–1424.

8

Imaging Liver Lesions using Grating-Based Phase-Contrast Computed Tomography with Bi-Lateral Filter Post-Processing

Julia Herzen[1,2]*, Marian S. Willner[2], Alexander A. Fingerle[3], Peter B. Noël[3], Thomas Köhler[4], Enken Drecoll[5], Ernst J. Rummeny[3], Franz Pfeiffer[2]

1 Institute of Materials Science, Helmholtz-Zentrum Geesthacht, Geesthacht, Germany, **2** Physics Department & Institute of Medical Engineering, Technische Universität München, Garching, Germany, **3** Department of Radiology, Technische Universität München, Munich, Germany, **4** Philips Technologie GmbH, Innovative Technologies, Research Laboratories, Hamburg, Germany, **5** Institute of Pathology, Technische Universität München, Munich, Germany

Abstract

X-ray phase-contrast imaging shows improved soft-tissue contrast compared to standard absorption-based X-ray imaging. Especially the grating-based method seems to be one promising candidate for clinical implementation due to its extendibility to standard laboratory X-ray sources. Therefore the purpose of our study was to evaluate the potential of grating-based phase-contrast computed tomography in combination with a novel bi-lateral denoising method for imaging of focal liver lesions in an ex vivo feasibility study. Our study shows that grating-based phase-contrast CT (PCCT) significantly increases the soft-tissue contrast in the ex vivo liver specimens. Combining the information of both signals – absorption and phase-contrast – the bi-lateral filtering leads to an improvement of lesion detectability and higher contrast-to-noise ratios. The normal and the pathological tissue can be clearly delineated and even internal structures of the pathological tissue can be visualized, being invisible in the absorption-based CT alone. Histopathology confirmed the presence of the corresponding findings in the analyzed tissue. The results give strong evidence for a sufficiently high contrast for different liver lesions using non-contrast-enhanced PCCT. Thus, ex vivo imaging of liver lesions is possible with a polychromatic X-ray source and at a spatial resolution of ~100 μm. The post-processing with the novel bi-lateral denoising method improves the image quality by combining the information from the absorption and the phase-contrast images.

Editor: Ming-Lung Yu, Kaohsiung Medical University Hospital, Kaohsiung Medical University, Taiwan

Funding: The Authors JH, MSW and FP acknowledge financial support through the DFG Cluster of Excellence Munich-Centre for Advanced Photonics (MAP), the DFG Gottfried Wilhelm Leibniz program and the European Research Council (ERC, FP7, StG 240142). This work was carried out with the support of the Karlsruhe Nano Micro Facility (KNMF, www.kit.edu/knmf), a Helmholtz Research Infrastructure at Karlsruhe Institute of Technology (KIT). The funders had no role in study design, data collection and analysis, decision to publish, or preparation of the manuscript.

* E-mail: julia.herzen@hzg.de

Introduction

Focal liver lesions are a common finding in ultrasound and computed tomography (CT) examinations often presenting without clinical symptoms [1–3]. Whether a hepatic lesion requires treatment, follow-up imaging, or does not need further attention depends on the dignity (benign vs. malignant) and entity of the finding [4]. Furthermore, in oncology the liver is the most common site of metastasis from gastrointestinal tumors. Accurate assessment of tumor spread and treatment response are important for therapy planning [5].

Non-enhanced CT is very limited for the detection and characterization of focal hepatic lesions due to its low soft-tissue contrast. The use of iodine contrast agents greatly improves detectability of lesions; however, the characterization especially of subcentimetric findings remains challenging [6]. Also, in some patients iodine-based contrast media can cause anaphylactic reactions, acute renal failure, or hyperthyroidism [7–9]. Drug interactions with metformin, an oral antidiabetic agent, have been described [10]. The gold standard for the detection and characterization of focal hepatic lesions remains magnetic resonance imaging (MRI) with the application of diffusion weighted imaging (DWI) and liver-specific contrast agents [11,12]. Contraindications for MRI include cardiac pacemakers and patients suffering from claustrophobia. Additionally, long scanning times can be a limitation due to motion artifacts or limited patient tolerance, as well as the limited spatial resolution compared to CT.

Conventional multi-slice CT uses the attenuation of x-rays by photo-electric absorption and Compton scattering processes in the examined object as the sole source of contrast. Therefore, structures containing elements with high Z number, like calcium in bones, give high contrast whereas soft tissues such as muscle, parenchymatous organs and adipose tissue show rather low contrast. On the other hand, phase-contrast computed tomography (PCCT) exploits the physical effect of the phase shift x-rays experience when passing through an object.

Different phase-contrast methods have been developed over the last decades [13]. All these methods can be divided into three main groups: (1.) the direct methods measuring the phase shift (Bonse-

Hart interferometer) [14,15], (2.) the propagation based methods measuring the 2nd derivative of the phase shift [16], and (3.) the differential methods measuring the 1st derivative of the phase shift by using e.g. the analyzer-based [17,18] or the grating-based method [19,20]. Only the grating-based phase-contrast computed tomography (PCCT) has been successfully expanded to standard, polychromatic X-ray tubes [21]. This method provides a three-dimensional map of the attenuation coefficients and the electron density distribution of the specimen at the same time. Several recent articles have shown the potential of the grating-based PCCT for clinical applications demonstrating a remarkable improvement of soft-tissue contrast without the use of contrast media [22–25].

The purpose of our experimental proof-of-principle study was to evaluate the potential of grating-based PCCT for the detection and characterization of focal lesions in ex-vivo human liver specimens using a standard laboratory x-ray tube setup. Furthermore, we aimed to apply a novel post-processing denoising method on the tomographic data to demonstrate the possible quality improvement of the images.

Materials and Methods

Grating interferometry

The principle of grating-based PCCT and its projection acquisition is explained in detail in [19–21]. The x-rays are attenuated and refracted when they pass through the object. The refraction causes a change in the direction of the x-ray path, which only can be measured indirectly using for example an interferometer as shown in Figure 1. This method provides the phase-contrast and the absorption-contrast images simultaneously. The device used with coherent synchrotron sources consists of two x-ray optical gratings [26,27]: the phase grating produces an interference pattern in discrete distances downstream the x-ray beam, and the analyzer grating is used to detect the pattern of several micrometer periods with a standard x-ray imaging detector by scanning the analyzer grating with respect to the phase grating [21]. The method can be transferred to standard laboratory sources by adding an additional source grating, which increases the coherence of the X-ray source.

Experimental setup

For the experimental setup a three grating interferometer has been used in combination with an ENRAF Nonius rotating anode X-ray tube and a single photon counting detector (Pilatus II, Dectris, Baden, Switzerland) with a pixel size of 172×172 µm^2 and a silicon sensor thickness of 450 µm. Gratings with periods of 5.4 µm (Microworks, Karlsruhe, Germany) in a symmetric setup have been chosen: Both inter-grating distances have been set to 875 mm. The phase grating made of Nickel had a height of 8 µm and introduced a phase-shift of Π at the design energy of 22.8 keV. The golden source and analyzer grating structures were 50 µm high. The 6th Talbot order for the design energy of 23 keV was chosen and the mean visibility of the interferometer reached 13%. The X-ray filtration consisted of the following components:

- Beryllium window of the X-ray tube with a thickness of 0.25 mm
- Silicon wafers of source, phase and analyzer grating with a thickness 0.5 mm each
- Silicon disk with a thickness of 1 mm
- Approximately 2.25 m of air.

Beryllium window and silicon wafers of the gratings are not chosen based on advanced simulations but are parts of the individual components of the set-up. The silicon disk has been introduced to further reduce low energy photons without relevant reduction of photon flux.

The target material of the X-ray tube was Molybdenum and a tube voltage of 35 kVp has been applied in all tomography scans. The tube current has been set to 70 mA resulting in a total tube power of 2.45 kW. Altogether, without an object in the beam, an average count of 630 photons per second has been collected in each pixel of the detector. The actual size of the focal spot is 3×0.3 mm^2, the effective source size is only 0.3×0.3 mm^2 due to an inclination of the anode surface with respect to the optical axis of the beam.

The whole interferometer has been installed 60 cm away from the source, each sample was placed 70 mm in front of the phase grating and the detector 40 mm behind the analyzer grating, which gives a sample magnification of 1.72 and an effective pixel size of 0.1×0.1 mm^2.

Liver samples

All samples were acquired through the Institute of Pathology, Technische Universität München. They were initially resected for clinical reasons independently of this study. The patients provided their written consent to the use of tissue samples for educational and scientific purposes in general. The use of these specimens and the way how written consent was obtained has been fully approved by the ethics committee at the Faculty of Medicine of the Technische Universität München.

After excision a selected representative tissue sample was excised and put in a 50 ml plastic container in a 4% neutral-buffered formaldehyde solution. The following five different liver specimens with lesions have been chosen: 1.) a metastasis of a low-grade adenocarcinoma in a steatotic liver, 2.) a cholangiocellular carcinoma in a liver with macrosteatosis and pilosis, 3.) a hepatocellular carcinoma in a cirrhotic liver, 4.) a subcapsular hematoma and 5.) a metastasis of a mucinous adenocarcinoma of the colon. Histological sections of the specimens were prepared with a standard hematoxylin and eosion (H&E) staining. The slice thickness was 5 micrometers. Histology and PCCT slices were manually correlated using prominent features for the correct orientation.

Image acquisition

The liver samples were put into cylindrical plastic containers of 30 mm diameter that were scanned in air. 1200 projections over 360° were recorded per tomography scan. Every 20 projections 5 reference projections without the sample were recorded for background correction. Each projection was obtained by the phase stepping method [19] using eleven images with 5 seconds exposure time acquired over one period of the source grating. The total scan time was approximately 25 h.

Image reconstruction and post processing

The beam divergence is approximately 1.1° and allows to perform a standard parallel beam filtered back-projection using a Ram-Lak filter to reconstruct the absorption-contrast data and a Hilbert filter to reconstruct the phase-contrast data [21]. The reconstructed slice thickness of 100 µm is given by the effective pixel size of the detector, and the vertical number of detector pixels limits the number of slices to 195. Joined bilateral filtering as described in [28] was used as post processing in order to reduce the noise level. This method exploits the fact that the absorption and phase-contrast images are perfectly registered with respect to

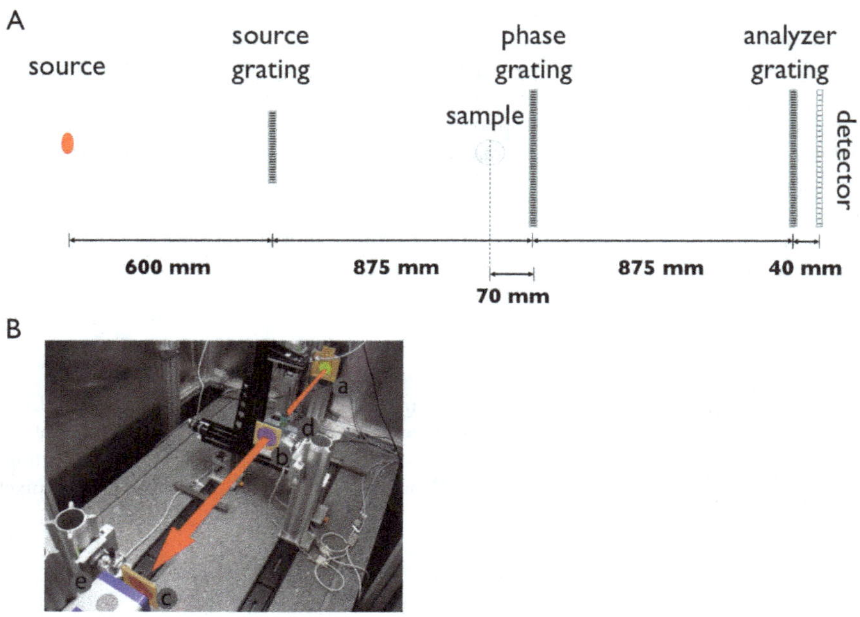

Figure 1. Schematic and a photograph of the grating-based imaging setup. A) Schematic top view of the grating-based imaging setup. The X-ray tube is a rotating anode with a Molybdenum target working with max. 60 kVp and 80 mA. The grating-interferometer consists of a source grating (to increase the coherence), a phase grating, an analyzer grating and a detector. The specimen is rotated in this setup. B) Photograph of the grating-based PCCT setup using conventional X-ray sources consisting of three gratings arranged in a symmetrical setup: (a) source grating marked yellow, (b) phase grating marked purple and (c) analyzer grating marked red, (d) the specimen mounted to a hanging rotation stage and (e) the detector. A red arrow marks the X-ray beam path.

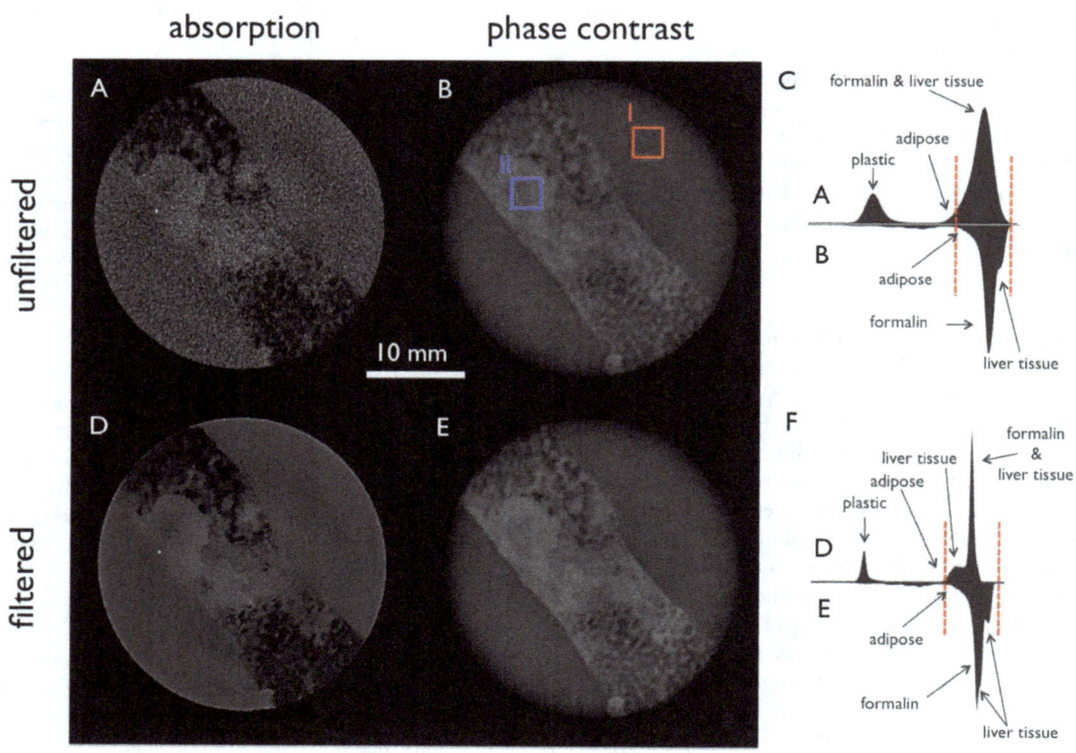

Figure 2. Comparison of unfiltered and filtered tomographic slices of a metastasis of a low-grade adenocarcinoma in a steatotic liver. Axial slices of the conventional absorption-based (A, D) and the phase-contrast (B, E) tomography windowed using the same window level and window width. The histograms of both unfiltered (C) and filtered (F) tomographic datasets demonstrate the filtering result and the red dashed markers show the window level. The areas I (red, surrounding formalin) and II (blue, high-contrast tumor in (B) mark the regions of 30×30 pixels, which were averaged for CNR calculation.

Table 1. Comparison of CNRs for unfiltered and filtered tomographic slices of a metastasis of a low-grade adenocarcinoma in a steatotic liver shown in Figure 2.

	absorption unfiltered	absorption filtered	phase-contrast unfiltered	phase-contrast filtered
CNR between ROI I and II	0.39	1.24	5.34	8.63

For the calculation of the CNRs the areas I (red, surrounding formalin) and II (blue, high-contrast tumor) marked in Figure 2B were used, which correspond to 30×30 pixels.

each other by performing edge-preserving filtering where edges are detected simultaneously in both images. This method overcomes at least partially the problem of standard edge-preserving filtering where edges with a contrast-to-noise-ratio (CNR) less than 1 are typically not detected as edges and are thus smoothed. Due to the simultaneous detection of edges in both images, edge detection becomes more reliable and thus, a mutual benefit is created. For the liver samples here, the noise levels, which are free parameters in the joined bilateral filter, were estimated as the local standard deviation of reconstructed image values in homogeneous regions. The filter was applied using a 13^3 neighborhood. The contrast-to-noise ratios (CNR) of two different regions (30×30 pixels each) of one sample relative to the surrounding formalin were calculated in absorption and phase-contrast tomogram before and after the denoising. The regions used for the CNR calculation are marked in Figure 2B The following equation was used to determine the CNRs:

$$CNR=\frac{|S_a-S_b|}{\sigma_S}, \tag{1}$$

where S_a and S_b represent the averaged measured signals in the region a and b, respectively, and σ_S is the error of the averaged signal. Here we set $\sigma_S=\sigma_a$, which is the standard deviation of the averaged signal S_a outside the specimen, to avoid higher noise values when averaging over inhomogeneous tissue. Please note that this implies the assumption that the noise is equally distributed over the whole image and the standard deviation σ_a of the homogenous region outside the specimen represents the noise level in the image.

Results

Figure 2 compares the unfiltered and the filtered tomographic slices of a metastasis of a low-grade adenocarcinoma in a steatotic

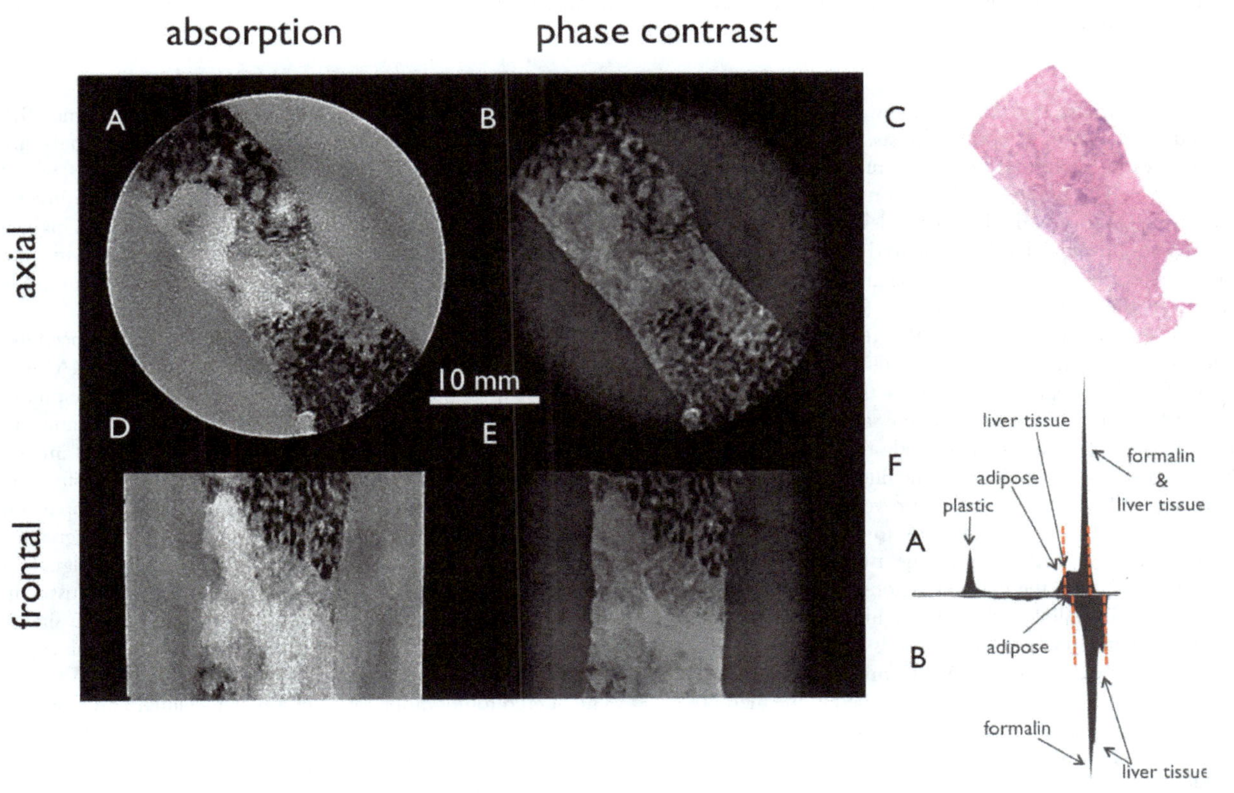

Figure 3. Filtered tomographic slices of a metastasis of a low-grade adenocarcinoma in a steatotic liver filtered with the 3D bilateral filter. Conventional absorption-based (A, D) and phase-contrast (B, E) CT images of the liver specimen in two different planes. H&E stain (C) corresponds to image A and B, respectively. (F) shows the histogram of the filtered absorption image (top) and the filtered phase-contrast image (bottom) with red dashed lines marking the window level in the shown slices.

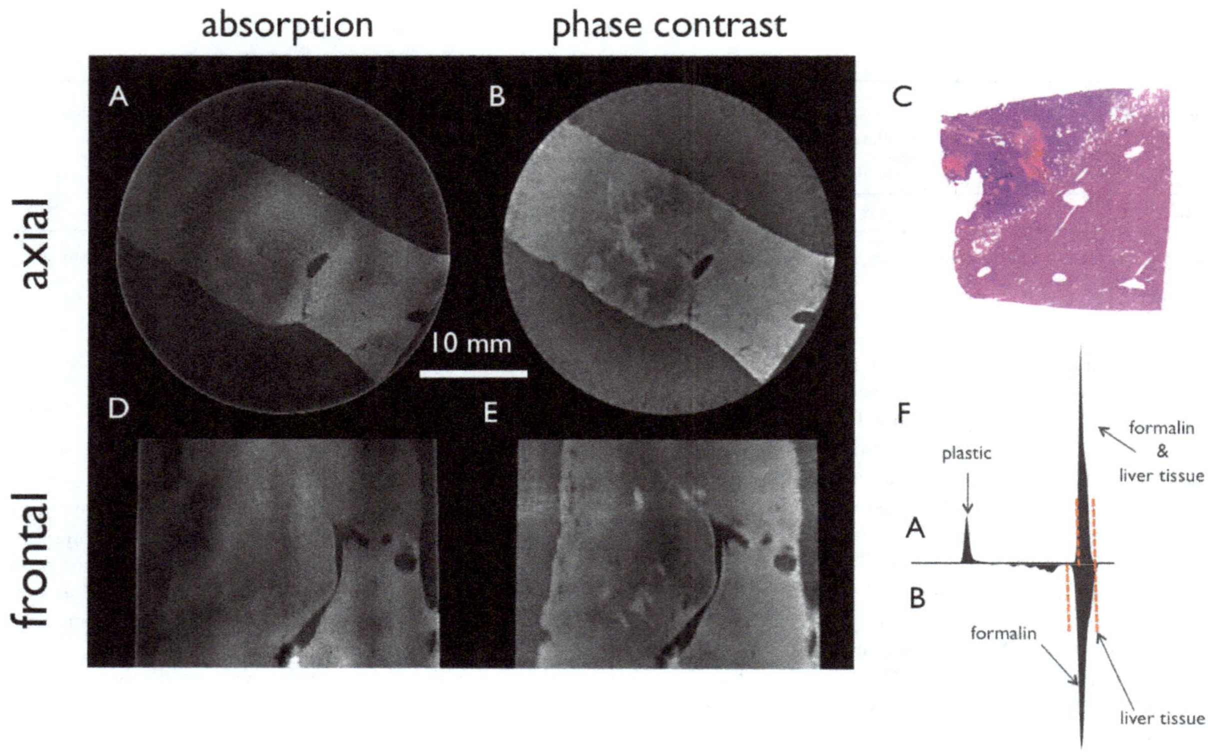

Figure 4. Tomographic slices of a cholangiocellular carcinoma in a liver with macrosteatosis and pilosis filtered with the 3D bilateral filter. Conventional absorption-based (A, D) and phase-contrast (B, E) CT images of the liver specimen in two different planes. H&E stain (C) corresponds to image A and B, respectively. (F) shows the histogram of the filtered absorption image (top) and the filtered phase-contrast image (bottom) with red dashed lines marking the window level in the shown slices. The absorption images (A, D) profit strongly from the filtering, but the information is still complementary.

liver. For this comparison the same window level and window width was used for the slices of both contrasts, which is indicated by red dashed lines in the histograms of the unfiltered (C) and of the filtered slices (F). The unfiltered absorption images (A) show a very low soft-tissue contrast and a high noise level. The areas with steatotic liver tissue show low density compared to the surrounding formalin, while the infiltrating tumor tissue in the center has a higher density. In the phase-contrast images (B, E) the steatotic liver tissue has also a low signal, but the tumor tissue shows intermediate to high signal with more details compared to the absorption images. Both signals profit from the post processing with the bilateral filter, but especially the absorption-contrast image contains many structural details inside the tumor after the filtering. For the remaining samples only the filtered images will be shown. To quantify the image-quality improvement the CNR of one region inside the tumour compared to the formalin was calculated for both signals. Note, that the two tomograms are intrinsically registered, thus, the marked regions-of-interest (ROIs) I (red, surrounding formalin) and II (blue, high-contrast tumor tissue) in Figure 2B correspond to 30×30 pixels and are exactly the same for the slices shown in Figures 2A, 2D, and 2E. These ROIs were averaged to determine the CNRs as described in the methods and materials section, where the signal S_a was chosen from the ROI I and the signal S_b from the ROI II. The resulting CNRs are given in Table 1.

In Figure 3 only the filtered tomographic slices of the same metastasis as shown in Figure 2 are depicted. The conventional absorption based (3A, 3D) and phase-contrast (3B, 3E) CT images of the liver specimen are shown in two different planes axial and frontal. The H&E stained histopathology image (3C) shows a corresponding region of the specimen like in 3A and 3B, respectively. The histograms (3F) of both filtered signals are presented to indicate the different windowing of the images, which is set to a visual optimum for each signal. The absorption images (3A, 3D) profit mostly from the post-processing in the higher-density area of the infiltrating tumor tissue in the center, while the areas with steatotic liver tissue with low density lead to an CNR improvement of this region in the phase-contrast image.

Figure 4 shows filtered tomographic slices of a cholangiocellular carcinoma in a liver with macrosteatosis and pilosis. (4A, 4D) present the conventional absorption-based and (4B, 4E) the phase-contrast CT slices of the liver specimen in two different planes. In (4C) the H&E stained slice corresponding to the regions of images 4A and 4B is shown. Even after the bilateral filtering the soft-tissue contrast in absorption images (4A and 4D) is low in comparison with the phase-contrast images (4B, 4E), which show low signal for the tumor tissue in the center of the slice with high signal in necrotic/hemorrhagic areas compared to the normal liver tissue in the upper left and lower right parts (4B) with intermediate signal. Here, the windowing is chosen to a visual optimum of each signal and is indicated in the histograms (4F).

The filtered tomographic slices of a hepatocellular carcinoma in a cirrhotic liver are shown in Figure 5. The patient had received a transcatheter arterial chemoembolisation (TACE) prior to excision. In the absorption images (5A, 5D) the HCC nodules (marked with red arrows in 5A) in the right center are visible due to the high density of the retained Lipiodol. Lipiodol is a composition of iodine with poppyseed oil, nowadays mainly used for chemoembolization procedures where a chemotherapeutic agent is mixed with the oily liquid. Chemoembolization interrupts the tumors

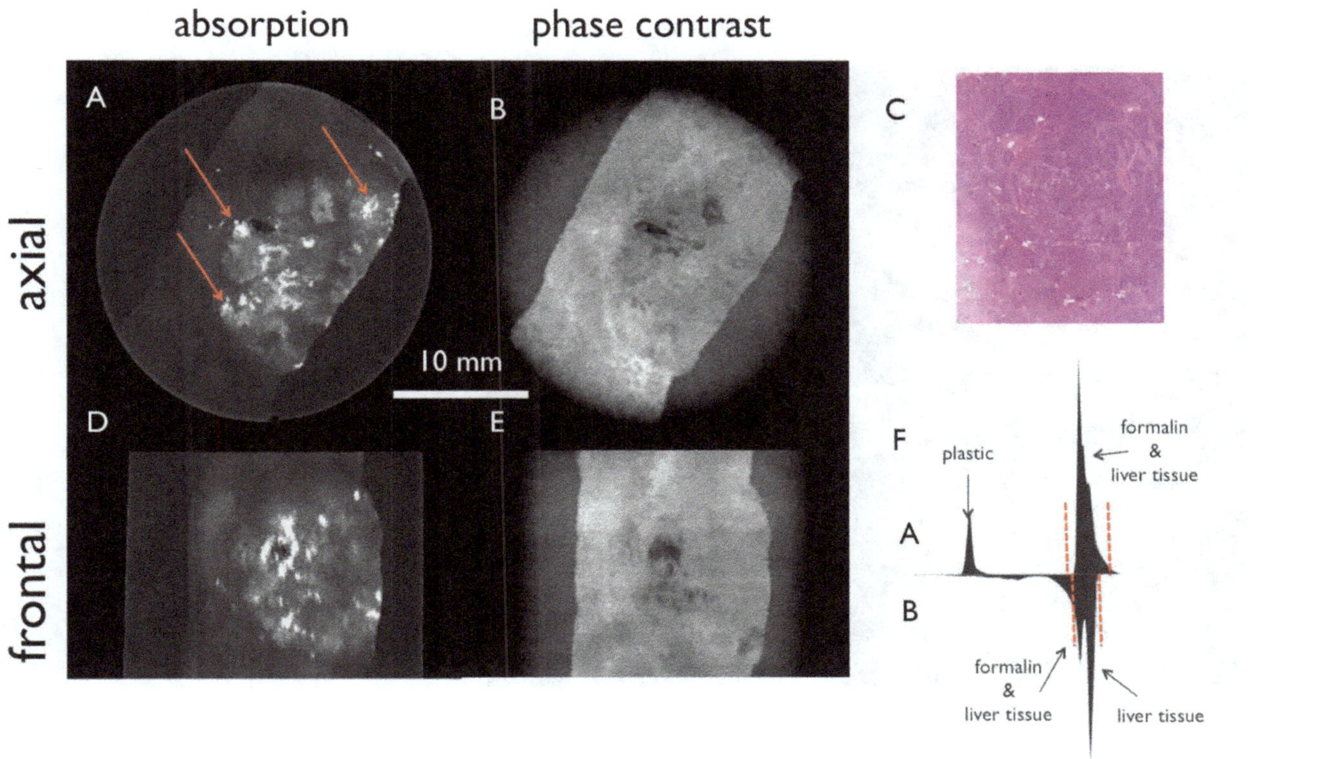

Figure 5. Filtered tomographic slices of a hepatocellular carcinoma in a cirrhotic liver. The patient had received transcatheter arterial chemoembolisation (TACE). Conventional absorption-based (A, D) and phase-contrast (B, E) CT images of the liver specimen in two different planes. H&E stain (C) corresponds to image A and B, respectively, and (F) shows the histogram of the absorption (top) and the phase-contrast image (bottom) with red dashed lines marking the window level. In the absorption images (A, D) the HCC nodules in the right center (marked with red arrows in A) are visible due to the high density of the retained Lipiodol. In the phase-contrast images (B, D) the fibrous septa are visible as high signal bands whereas the liver tissue and the HCC nodules show intermediate signal. Some areas with increased Lipiodol retention show low signal.

blood supply and allows high local concentrations of the drug for a longer period of time. In the phase-contrast images (5B, 5D) the fibrous septa are visible as high signal bands whereas the liver tissue and the HCC nodules show intermediate signal. Some areas with increased Lipiodol retention show low signal. Again the windowing is set to the visual optimum of each signal, which is marked in the histograms (5F).

Figure 6 presents the tomographic slices of a subcapsular hematoma after bilateral filtering. The contrast between the liver tissue in the upper right part of the images and the subcapsular hematoma in the lower left part is considerably lower in the absorption images (6A and 6D) compared to the phase-contrast images (6B and 6E), where the hematoma shows a high signal.

The last specimen was a metastasis of a mucinous adenocarcinoma of the colon. The corresponding filtered tomographic slices are shown in Figure 7. The phase-contrast images (7B, 7E) show a significantly higher soft-tissue contrast with low signal in the mucinous areas, intermediate signal in the liver tissue and higher signal for the tumor tissue and necrotic/hemorrhagic areas. In the absorption images (7A, 7C) only the mucinous parts of the metastasis are clearly visible as areas with low density. The other structures in the absorption images are barely visible since the contrast after filtering is in the same order of magnitude as the remaining low-frequency artifacts. Nevertheless, sharp edges are visible, which have been reliably detected in the phase-contrast image.

Discussion

Our results clearly demonstrate that the tumor boundary and the soft-tissue in general can be visualized with a lab-based imaging setup. The effective pixel sizes of 100 μm are one magnitude larger than the previously reported experimental results on human liver tissue [29] and on other tissue types gained at brilliant synchrotron sources [25,30]. This is not yet in the range of clinically relevant spatial resolution (i.e. 500 μm instead of 100 μm in our study) required to meet the stringent dose requirements for in-vivo applications [31], but it is the first experimental demonstration of the still present information gain when using PCCT in combination with polychromatic radiation and low spatial resolution for ex vivo human liver samples.

By the use of joined bilateral filtering, the CNR in both images was improved substantially. In the present study, most of the originally reconstructed phase-contrast images showed a much better CNR than the absorption-contrast images. Therefore, there was less mutual benefit but more a unidirectional one, viz. the absorption-contrast image gained much more than the phase-contrast image: Edges, which were completely invisible in the original FBP images were made visible thanks to their visibility in the phase-contrast image. However, we also found some high-contrast regions in the absorption-contrast image having a better CNR and in this region, the differential phase-contrast image profited from the joined processing. With regard to the different visible structures inside the liver specimens, especially the

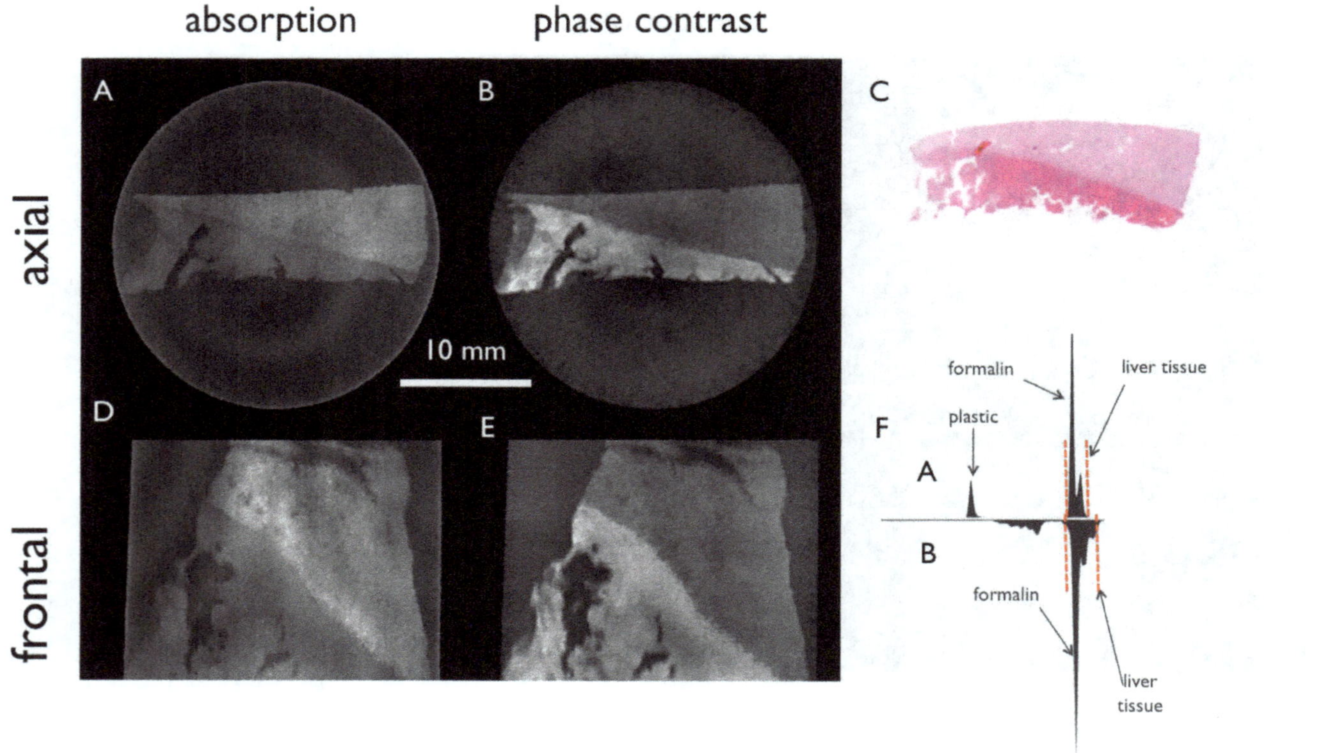

Figure 6. Filtered tomographic slices of a subcapsular hematoma. Conventional absorption- based (A, D) and phase-contrast (B, E) CT images of the liver specimen in two different planes. H&E stain (C) corresponds to image A and B, respectively, and the histogram (F) of the absorption (top) and the phase-contrast image (bottom) show the window level as red dashed lines. In the absorption images (A, D) the contrast between the liver tissue in the upper right part of the image (A, D) and the subcapsular hematoma in the lower left part is considerably lower compared to the phase-contrast image (B, E) where the hematoma shows a high signal.

combination of both information has the potential to improve the diagnostics without any use of contrast agents in future.

The low-frequency noise (rings), which can be observed in the attenuation images, is a combination of a beam-hardening effect and remaining fringes in the background, which are not removed by the normalization with a flat-field image. We did not apply any corrections for these effects to our data.

Our system has some limitations, which need to be discussed in more detail. One of the limitations of our study concerns the formalin fixation of the specimens. Especially this fact might change the contrast for different tissue types compared to in-vivo imaging of the tissue surrounded by circulating blood. Further studies are required to investigate the influence of formalin fixation on the contrast compared to fresh tissue in both, absorption and phase-contrast data.

The second important limitation is related to the fact that our laboratory setup is still in an experimental state. This means that it was not optimized for fast measurements, which makes it comparable to MRI with a microscopy coil in terms of scanning times, but allowing better spatial resolution. Optimization of other parameters, which are important for the phase-contrast imaging (as for example filtering of the spectrum or setup geometry) are subject of ongoing studies, and are non-trivial in combination with a polychromatic source of a limited flux. These parameters strongly influence the quality of the interferometer and its sensitivity, but at the same time can reduce the number of photons, which downgrades the image quality. Thus, our measurements do also not meet any dose requirements for in-vivo applications.

The applied dose can be roughly estimated from the number of the photons recorded by the detector. Approximately 600 photons were collected per image, per second and detector pixel. Taking into account the absorption of photons by the analyzer grating (50%), the quantum efficiency of the Pilatus detector (8% @ 35 keV and 25% @ 22 keV) and the effective source spectrum, we can estimate that the total applied dose to the sample was in the order of several Gy for a full tomography scan. Due to a non-optimized setup only a small fraction of the total applied dose really contributed to the signal formation and detection. Nevertheless, the comparison of the presented images of both signals - absorption and phase-contrast - is fair, since both were obtained simultaneously and at exact the same dose.

Various optimization steps applied to our system can bring the applied dose per scan into the range of conventional micro CT systems (e.g. small-animal micro CT systems), which have comparably high spatial resolution and apply several hundreds of mGy for a full tomography scan.

Optimization can be done from the detector side improving the detection efficiency of X-rays in the used energy range. The relatively low detector efficiency of our experimental system results in low photon statistic, which especially becomes apparent in the absorption images, where the image quality is worse than expected from measurements with an applied dose of several Gy. Modern detectors used in clinical systems can reach a quantum efficiency of up to 60% [32], which brings us already into the ball park of several hundreds mGy used in small animal scanning systems. A doubling of the visibility allows a dose reduction to a quarter at constant image quality [33]. Thus, raising visibility from currently

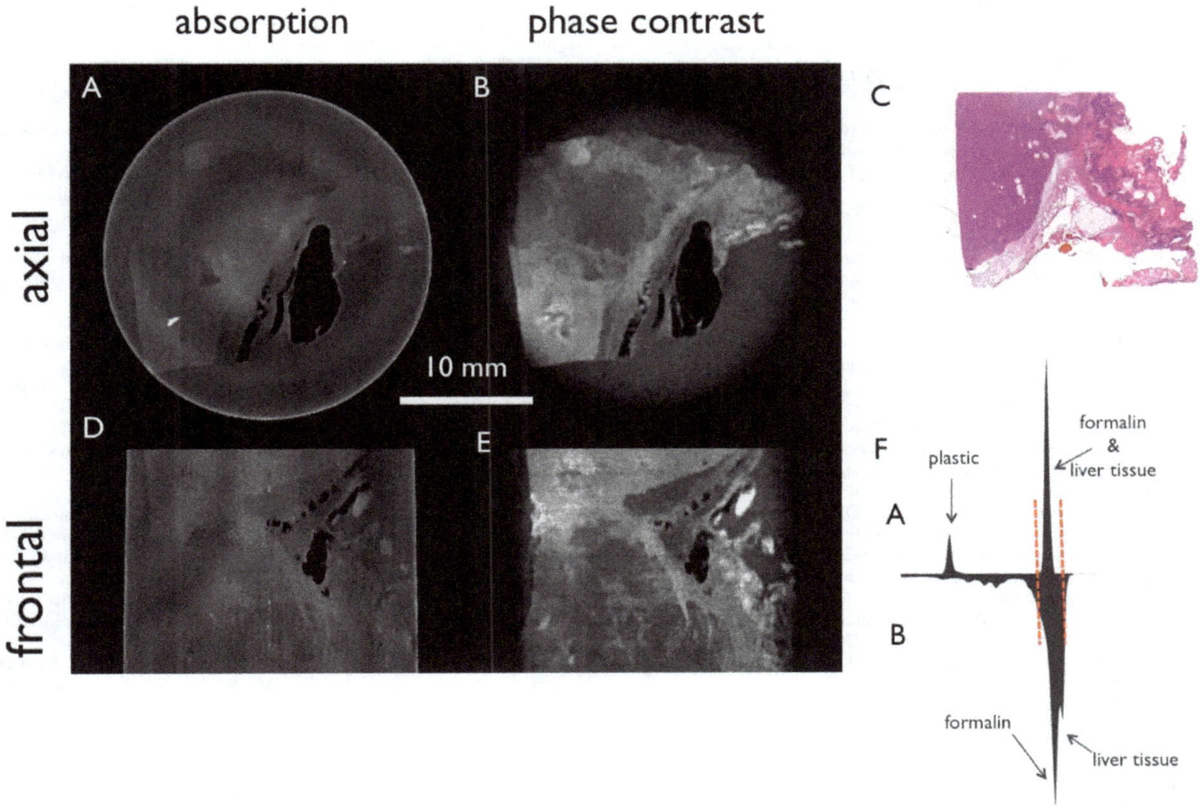

Figure 7. Filtered tomographic slices of a liver metastasis of a mucinous adenocarcinoma of the colon. Conventional absorption-based (A, D) and phase-contrast (B, E) CT images of the liver specimen in two different planes. H&E stain (C) corresponds to image A and B, respectively, and (F) shows the histograms of both signals with red dashed lines marking the window level. In the absorption images (A, C) only the mucinous parts of the metastasis are visible as areas with low density. The phase-contrast images (B, E) show a significantly higher soft-tissue contrast with low signal in the mucinous areas, intermediate signal in the liver tissue and higher signal for the tumor tissue and necrotic/hemorrhagic areas.

10% to 30% by optimization of gratings and setup geometry would reduce dose to 1/9 of the current value.

Advanced acquisition protocols can also reduce the acquisition time and the applied dose, which has been successfully demonstrated for grating-based imaging either theoretically or experimentally at synchrotron sources (low-dose grating-based phase-contrast imaging [34] and advanced stepping methods [35]). We also anticipate further possibilities to maintain the current CNRs at reduced dose and thus at reduced scan time by using iterative reconstruction techniques. In our experimental study the acquisition parameters like number of projections, number of phase steps, and acquisition time were arbitrarily chosen. Optimizing these parameters can significantly reduce the dose, e.g. utilizing a single-shot technique will allow a reduction of dose and acquisition time by a factor of 11 (as we have used 11 steps in the phase-stepping scan in our study) [36]. Furthermore, recently published results demonstrate that novel reconstruction methods can reduce dose and scanning time in phase-contrast CT of breast tissue by up to 74% [37].

The field-of-view of the grating-based imaging method is currently limited by the size of the available grating structures. Different efforts were made to overcome this limitation, by e.g. bending the wafer of large-area grating structures to account for the cone beam used for large field-of-views [38]. Recently, we could demonstrate that the grating-based method is able to work at high X-ray energies (up to 82 keV [39]), which brings it already in the range of clinically relevant X-ray energies. Further investigations are required to demonstrate the ability of the imaging method to image large objects in the range of the human body (20–40 cm diameter), which might lead to a degradation of image quality due to the non-negligible amount of scattering by large objects.

In conclusion, with our work we demonstrate the feasibility to assess the potential of phase-contrast imaging for different kind of liver diseases on ex vivo samples using laboratory-based X-ray generators. Our method provides a three-dimensional map of the attenuation coefficients and the electron density distribution of the specimen at the same time and the joined filtering combines the information to improve the image quality.

Author Contributions

Conceived and designed the experiments: JH MSW AAF PBN TK EJR FP. Performed the experiments: JH MSW AAF PBN. Analyzed the data: JH MSW AAF PBN TK. Contributed reagents/materials/analysis tools: MSW AAF PBN ED. Wrote the paper: JH.

References

1. Lanitis S, Zacharioudakis C, Zafeiriadou P, Armoutides V, Karaliotas C, et al. (2012) Incidental findings in trauma patients during focused assessment with sonography for trauma. American Surgeon 78: 366–372.

2. Seitz K, Greis C, Schuler A, Bernatik T, Blank W, et al. (2011) Frequency of tumor entities among liver tumors of unclear etiology initially detected by sonography in the noncirrhotic or cirrhotic livers of 1349 patients. Results of the

DEGUM multicenter study. Ultraschall in der Medizin (Stuttgart, Germany : 1980) 32: 598–603.
3. Völk M, Strotzer M, Lenhart M, Techert J, Seitz J, et al. (2001) Frequency of benign hepatic lesions incidentally detected with contrast-enhanced thin-section portal venous phase spiral CT. Acta radiologica (Stockholm, Sweden : 1987) 42: 172–5.
4. Berland LL, Silverman SG, Gore RM, Mayo-Smith WW, Megibow AJ, et al. (2010) Managing incidental findings on abdominal CT: white paper of the ACR incidental findings committee. Journal of the American College of Radiology : JACR 7: 754–73.
5. Sahani DV, Kalva SP (2004) Imaging the liver. Nursing Standard Official Newspaper Of The Royal College Of Nursing 10: 55–56.
6. Oudkerk M, Torres CG, Song B, König M, Grimm J, et al. (2002) Characterization of liver lesions with mangafodipir trisodium-enhanced MR imaging: multicenter study comparing MR and dualphase spiral CT. Radiology 223: 517–524.
7. Stacul F, van der Molen AJ, Reimer P, Webb JAW, Thomsen HS, et al. (2011) Contrast induced nephropathy: updated ESUR Contrast Media Safety Committee guidelines. European radiology 21: 2527–41.
8. Der Molen AJV, Thomsen HS, Morcos SK (2004) Effect of iodinated contrast media on thyroid function in adults. European Radiology 14: 902–907.
9. Thomsen HS, Morcos SK, Almén T, Aspelin P, Bellin MF, et al. (2010) Metformin and contrast media. Radiology 256: 672–3; author reply 673.
10. Cochran ST, Bomyea K, Sayre JW (2001) Trends in adverse events after IV administration of contrast media. Ajr American Journal Of Roentgenology 176.
11. Eiber M, Fingerle AA, Brügel M, Gaa J, Rummeny EJ, et al. (2012) Detection and classification of focal liver lesions in patients with colorectal cancer: retrospective comparison of diffusion-weighted MR imaging and multi-slice CT. European journal of radiology 81: 683–91.
12. Holzapfel K, Eiber MJ, Fingerle AA, Bruegel M, Rummeny EJ, et al. (2012) Detection, classification, and characterization of focal liver lesions: Value of diffusion-weighted MR imaging, gadoxetic acid-enhanced MR imaging and the combination of both methods. Abdominal imaging 37: 74–82.
13. Momose A (2005) Recent advances in X-ray phase imaging. Japanese Journal of Applied Physics 44: 6355–6367.
14. Bonse U, Hart M (1965) An X-Ray Interferometer. Appl Phys Lett 6: 155–156.
15. Beckmann F, Heise K, Kölsch B, Bonse U, Rajewsky MF, et al. (1999) Three-Dimensional Imaging of Nerve Tissue by X-Ray Phase-Contrast Microtomography. Biophysical Journal 76: 98–102.
16. Cloetens P, Ludwig W, Baruchel J, van Dyck D, van Landuyt J, et al. (1999) Holotomography: Quantitative phase tomography with micrometer resolution using hard synchrotron radiation x rays. Applied Physics Letters 75: 2912–2914.
17. Davis TJ, Gureyev TE, Gao D, Stevenson AW, Wilkins SW (1995) X-ray Image Contrast from a Simple Phase Object. Physical Review Letters 74(16): 3173–3177.
18. Dilmanian FA, Zhong Z, Ren B, Wu XY, Chapman LD, et al. (2000) Computed tomography of x-ray index of refraction using the diffraction enhanced imaging method. Physics in Medicine and Biology 45: 933–946.
19. Weitkamp T, Diaz A, David C, Pfeiffer F, Stampanoni M, et al. (2005) X-ray phase imaging with a grating interferometer. Optics Express 13: 6296–6304.
20. Momose A, Yashiro W, Takeda Y, Suzuki Y, Hattori T (2006) Phase Tomography by X-ray Talbot Interferometry for Biological Imaging. Japanese Journal of Applied Physics 45: 5254–5262.
21. Pfeiffer F, Kottler C, Bunk O, David C (2007) Hard X-Ray Phase Tomography with Low-Brilliance Sources. Physical Review Letters 98: 108105.
22. Bech M, Bunk O, David C, Ruth R, Rifkin J, et al. (2009) Hard X-ray phase-contrast imaging with the Compact Light Source based on inverse Compton X-rays. Journal of Synchrotron Radiation 16: 43–47.
23. Donath T, Pfeiffer F, Bunk O, Gruenzweig C, Hempel E, et al. (2010) Toward Clinical X-ray Phase-Contrast CT Demonstration of Enhanced Soft-Tissue Contrast in Human Specimen. Investigative Radiology 45: 445–452.
24. Jensen TH, Bech M, Bunk O, Donath T, David C, et al. (2010) Directional x-ray dark-field imaging. Physics in Medicine and Biology 55: 3317–3323.
25. Schulz G, Weitkamp T, Zanette I, Pfeiffer F, Beckmann F, et al. (2010) High-resolution tomographic imaging of a human cerebellum: comparison of absorption and grating-based phase contrast. Journal of The Royal Society Interface.
26. David C, Bruder J, Rohbeck T, Grünzweig C, Kottler C, et al. (2007) Fabrication of diffraction gratings for hard X-ray phase contrast imaging. Microelectronic Engineering 84: 1172–1177.
27. Reznikova E, Mohr J, Boerner M, Nazmov V, Jakobs PJ (2008) Soft X-ray lithography of high aspect ratio SU8 submicron structures. Microsystem Technologies 14: 1683–1688.
28. Koehler T, Roessl E (2012) Simultaneous de-noising in phase contrast tomography. AIP Conference Proceedings 1466: 78–83.
29. Noël PB, Herzen J, Fingerle AA, Willner M, Stockmar MK, et al. (2013) (Not yet published) Evaluation of the potential of phase-contrast computed tomography for improved visualization of cancerous human liver tissue. Zeitschrift fur medizinische Physik.
30. Sztrókay A, Herzen J, Auweter S, Liebhardt S, Mayr D, et al. (2012) Assessment of grating-based X-ray phase-contrast CT for differentiation of invasive ductal carcinoma and ductal carcinoma in situ in an experimental ex vivo set-up. European Radiology : 1–7.
31. Raupach R, Flohr T (2012) Performance evaluation of x-ray differential phase contrast computed tomography (PCT) with respect to medical imaging. Medical Physics 39: 4761–4774.
32. Ghetti C, Borrini A, Ortenzia O, Rossi R, Ordóñez PL (2008) Physical characteristics of GE Senographe Essential and DS digital mammography detectors. Medical physics 35: 456–63.
33. Köhler T, Jürgen Engel K, Roessl E (2011) Noise properties of grating-based x-ray phase contrast computed tomography. Medical physics 38 Suppl 1: S106.
34. Zanette I, Bech M, Rack A, Le Duc G, Tafforeau P, et al. (2012) Trimodal low-dose X-ray tomography. Proceedings of the National Academy of Sciences 109: 10199–10204.
35. Zanette I, Bech M, Pfeiffer F, Weitkamp T (2011) Interlaced phase stepping in phase-contrast x-ray tomography. Applied Physics Letters 98: 94101.
36. Bevins N, Zambelli J, Li K, Qi Z, Chen GH (2012) Multicontrast x-ray computed tomography imaging using Talbot-Lau interferometry without phase stepping. Medical physics 39: 424–8.
37. Zhao Y, Brun E, Coan P, Huang Z, Sztrókay A, et al. (2012) High-resolution, low-dose phase contrast X-ray tomography for 3D diagnosis of human breast cancers. Proceedings of the National Academy of Sciences of the United States of America 109: 18290–4.
38. Danielsson M, Cederwall B, Carlson P, Bohm C, Revol V, et al. (2011) X-ray interferometer with bent gratings: Towards larger fields of view. Nuclear Instruments and Methods in Physics Research Section A: Accelerators, Spectrometers, Detectors and Associated Equipment 648: S302–S305.
39. Willner M, Bech M, Herzen J, Zanette I, Hahn D, et al. (2013) Quantitative X-ray phase-contrast computed tomography at 82 keV. Opt Express 21: 4155–4166.

9

Early-Life Exposure to Bisphenol A Induces Liver Injury in Rats Involvement of Mitochondria-Mediated Apoptosis

Wei Xia*[⚬], Ying Jiang[⚬], Yuanyuan Li, Yanjian Wan, Juan Liu, Yue Ma, Zhenxing Mao, Huailong Chang, Gengqi Li, Bing Xu, Xi Chen, Shunqing Xu*

Key Laboratory of Environment and Health, Ministry of Education and Ministry of Environmental Protection, and State Key Laboratory of Environmental Health (Incubating), School of Public Health, Tongji Medical College, Huazhong University of Science and Technology, Wuhan, China

Abstract

Exposure to bisphenol A (BPA), a monomer widely used to manufacture polycarbonate plastics, has been reported to be associated with abnormalities of liver function and hepatic damage. However, the molecular mechanism under the pathogenesis of hepatic injury is unclear. In this study, the effect of perinatal exposure to BPA at the reference dose of 50 μg/kg/day on the apoptotic index in the liver of rat offspring was investigated. Increased levels of ALT and enhanced cell apoptosis were observed in the liver of rat offspring at 15 and 21 weeks, and significantly increased activity of caspase-3 and caspase-9 and elevated levels of cytochrome c were also confirmed. In addition, significant change in the expression levels of Bcl-2 and Bax were found in BPA-treated offspring at 21 weeks. For *in vitro* experiments, liver mitochondria were isolated from neonatal rats and were treated with BPA. BPA treatment led to a significant increase in mitochondrial permeability transition. Moreover, the supernatant from BPA-treated mitochondria significantly increased apoptotic changes in nuclei isolated from liver tissue. In conclusion, the study demonstrates that BPA induces mitochondria-mediated apoptosis in hepatic cells, which may contribute to long-term hepatotoxicity induced by early-life exposure to BPA.

Editor: Angel Nadal, Universidad Miguel Hernández de Elche, Spain

Funding: This work was supported by the National Program on Key Basic Research Project of China (973 Program) (2012CB722401), the National Natural Science Foundation of China (81030051, 21177046), the R&D Special Fund for Public Welfare Industry (Environment) (201309048), the National Basic Research Development Program of China (2008CB418206), the Fundamental Research Funds for the Central Universities, HUST (2012QN240, 2012TS072), and the Doctoral Fund of Ministry of Education of China (20120142120017). The funders had no role in study design, data collection and analysis, decision to publish, or preparation of the manuscript.

Competing Interests: The authors have declared that no competing interests exist.

* E-mail: xust@hust.edu.cn (SX); xiawei@hust.edu.cn (WX)

⚬ These authors contributed equally to this work.

Introduction

Bisphenol A (BPA) is an environmental chemical that has been widely used in the manufacture of polycarbonate plastics and epoxy resins for many years. Due to its major applications in the production of plastic food or beverage containers and the coating of food cans, people of different ages are inevitably exposed to BPA in daily life. BPA has been detected in human placenta [1], cord blood [2], amitotic fluid [3,4], fetal liver [5] and breast milk [6], making exposure of human neonates and infants a very real concern. A number of studies have revealed that maternal exposure to BPA during gestation and/or lactation induced adverse effects in offspring, such as affecting the development of reproductive organ [7,8] and metabolic function [9–12].

In humans and animals, the liver is the primary organ responsible for BPA metabolism to its glucurono-conjugated form [13]. From epidemiological studies, higher urinary concentration of BPA is associated with serum markers of abnormal liver function in human adults [14]. *In vivo* animal data suggest that BPA is able to induce reactive oxygen species generation and disturb enzyme activity in liver of rats [15,16], and induce some degree of fat infiltration in mice liver [17,18]. *In vitro*, BPA is known to induce cytotoxic effect on cultured rat hepatocytes at high doses [19,20]. However, whether perinatal exposure to BPA at environmentally relevant doses may exert these effects on liver and the pathogenesis of hepatoxicity induced by BPA remains to be determined.

Although there has been a focus on BPA as an endocrine disruptor due to its estrogenic activity, there might be other mechanisms that explain the effects of BPA. Mitochondrial dysfunction induced by BPA, including decrease in mitochondrial transmembrane potential and altered cellular oxidation-reduction, have been reported in the isolated rat hepatocytes [19], and in human HepG2 cell [21], suggesting mitochondria are a target of BPA at organelle level. It's known that mitochondria play a crucial role in apoptosis by releasing the intermembrane space proteins, such as cytochrome c (Cyt c), which is a key mediator of apoptosis for activation of caspase in the cytosol [22,23]. Additionally, an alteration in the ratio of pro-apoptotic to anti-apoptotic proteins of the Bcl-2 family, resided on the outer membrane of mitochondria, may modulate the release of apoptogenic proteins [24]. Recently, BPA-induced apoptosis has been demonstrated in cultured liver cells [19,25]. However, the mechanism of action of BPA on mitochondria during this process is unknown.

The U.S. Environmental Protection Agency and the European Food Safety Authority have established tolerable daily intake (TDI), or reference dose, of 50 μg/kg/day for BPA as a 'safe dose'. However, many researchers have suggested that BPA at such dose

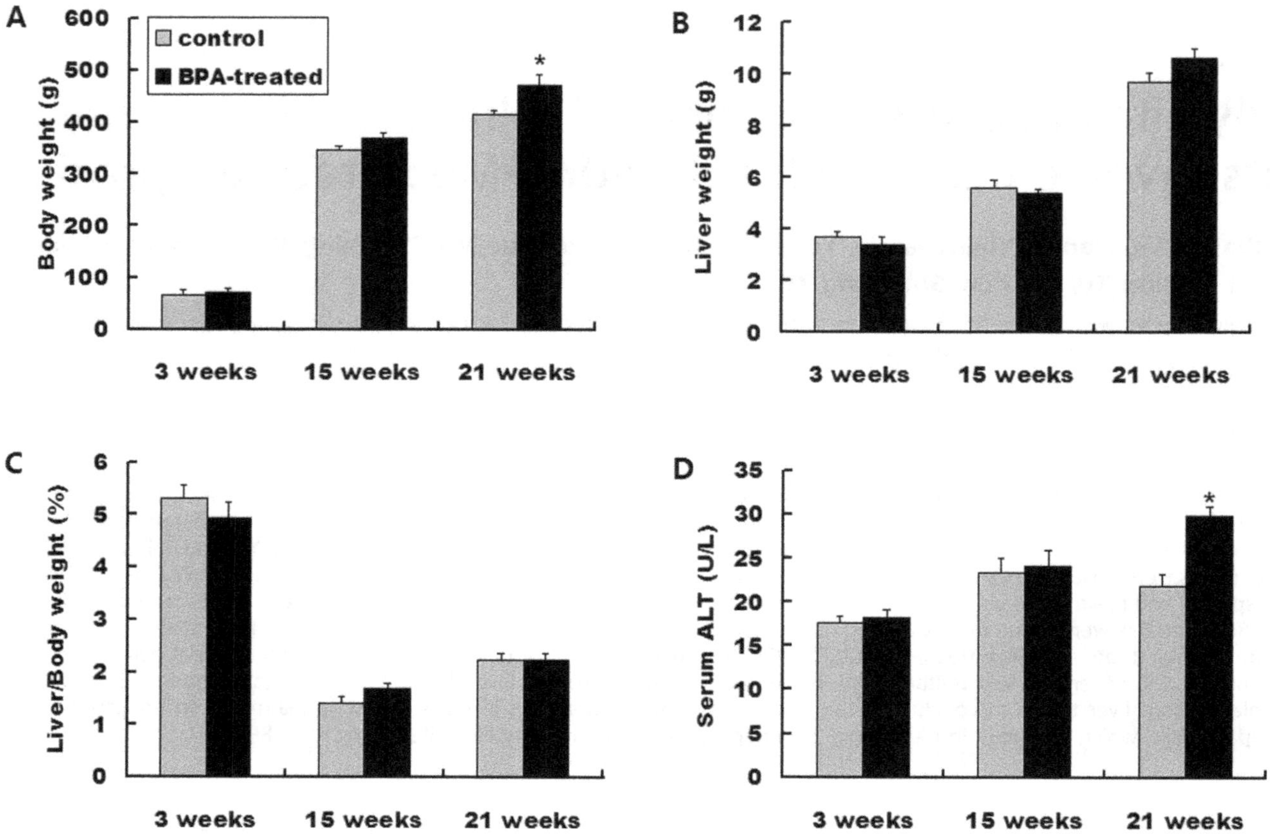

Figure 1. Body weight, liver weight, liver/body weight ratio and serum ALT of the rat offspring at 3, 15 and 21 weeks. (A) Body weight. (B) Liver weight. (C) Live/body weight ratio. (D) Serum ALT levels. Data represent as means ± S.E.M. (n = 6 rats per group, only 1 offspring was selected per litter). **P*<0.05 denotes significant difference compared with controls.

cause a variety of adverse effects [26]. Fetuses or newborns are more sensitive than adults, and exposure to chemicals during critical stages of development may cause irreversible long-lasting consequences [27]. In this study, we investigated the effect of perinatal exposure to BPA at TDI on the apoptotic index in the liver of rat offspring. In addition, the direct effect of BPA on the hepatic mitochondria was studied by using an *in vitro* apoptotic system.

Materials and Methods

In vivo Studies

Animals and treatments. All rats used in this study were treated humanely and with regard for alleviation of suffering, and the experimental protocols were approved by the Ethics Committee of Tongji Medical College (Permit Number: 2011-s2456). Virgin female (270–300 g) and male (350–400 g) genitor Wistar rats were purchased from Hubei Research Center of Laboratory Animal (Wuhan, China) and then housed in special pathogen-free conditions of 25±2°C temperature, 60–70% humidity and a controlled 12-h light/dark cycle. All animals were fed standard rodent chow [10] (ABSL-3 Lab of Wuhan University, Wuhan, China) and water *ad libitum*. Polypropylene plastic cages and glass water bottles were used in this study.

The day sperm-positive smear was determined as gestational day (GD) 0. Pregnant females were housed individually and randomly assigned to two groups that received either corn oil (Sigma-Aldrich, St. Louis, MO, USA) as the control or 50 μg/kg/day of BPA (Sigma-Aldrich, St. Louis, MO, USA) dissolved in corn oil by oral gravage from GD 0 to the end of lactation at postnatal day 21. The pups were given normal drinking water and fed standard rodent chow after weaning. At 3, 15 and 21 weeks, perinatally BPA-treated and control pups (n = 6 male rats in each group, belonging to different litters) were randomly selected, weighted and killed by decapitation.

Determination of BPA concentration in liver. Liver samples were removed from pups of the BPA-treated group and the control at birth day for analysis of BPA internal exposure levels. Details of sample pretreatments of the solid-phase extracts and the analysis of total BPA concentration by liquid chromatography–tandem mass spectrometry (LC-MS/MS) were in accordance with a previous study [28].

Liver sample collection and serum assays. Liver samples were removed from the pups and weighed, and then the samples were snap frozen at approximately −80°C until processing for analysis. Liver triglyceride (TG) was measured using a TG assay kit (Applygen Technologies Co. Ltd, Beijing, China), and the values were normalized to protein concentrations using the BCA protein quantitative assay kit (Thermo-Fisher, Waltham, MA, USA). Serum alanine aminotransferase (ALT) was measured using standard biochemical kits (BioVision, Milpitas, USA) according to the manufacturer's instructions.

Histological analysis. Terminal deoxynucleotide transferase-mediated deoxy-UTP nick end labeling (TUNEL) assay was used to identify double-stranded DNA fragmentation and the characteristics of DNA degradation by apoptosis. For the TUNEL staining, the standard protocol for paraffin sections was performed

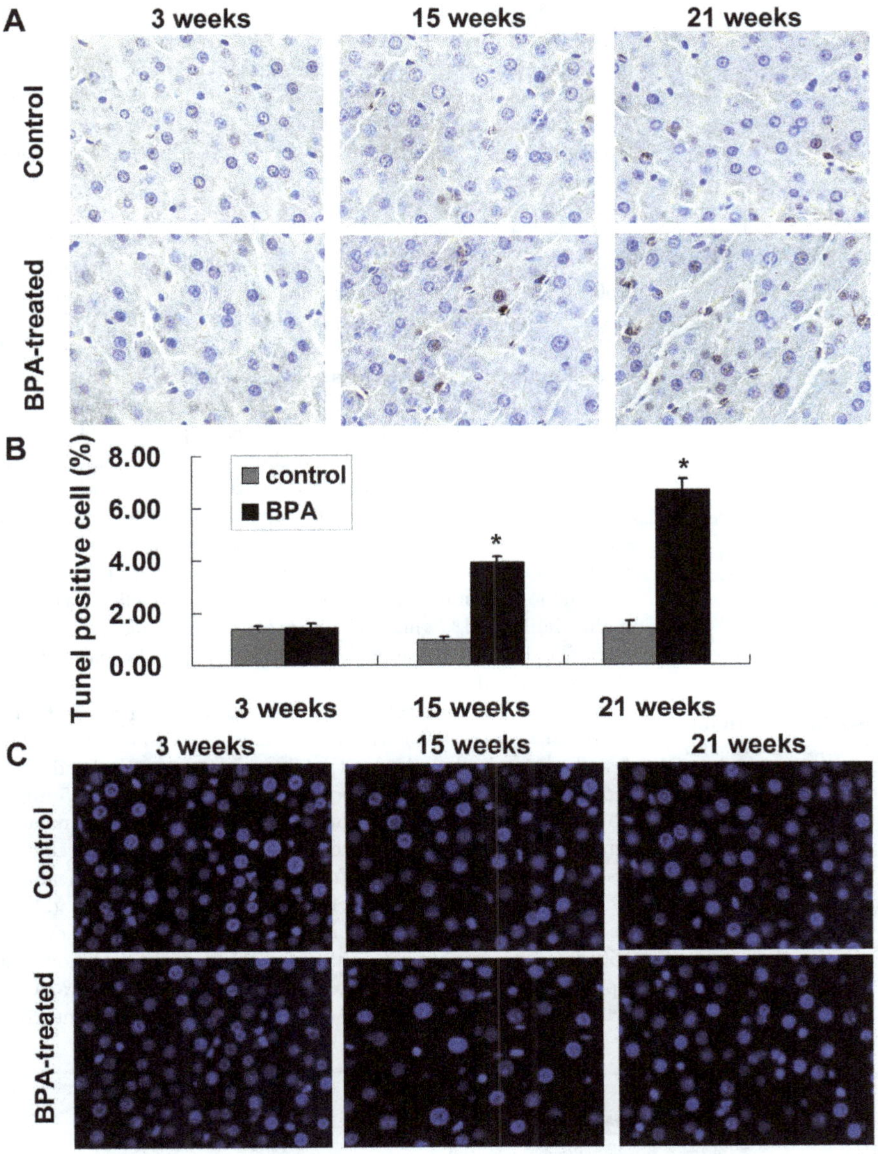

Figure 2. Perinatal exposure to BPA increases hepatocyte apoptosis of rat offspring. (A) Representative images of the TUNEL assay on liver tissue of the control and BPA-treated offspring at 3, 15 and 21 weeks. The TUNEL positive cells increased in the liver of BPA-treated offspring at 21 weeks (magnification, 400×). (B) Percentages of apoptotic cells in the livers from the control group and BPA-treated offspring. Percentages of apoptotic cells were quantified by counting TUNEL-positive cells in 1000 cells in a selected microscopic field per liver section. Data are means ± S.E.M. (n = 6 rats per group; only 1 offspring was selected per litter). $^*P<0.05$ compared with controls. (C) Representative images of Hoechst 33258-stained sections of liver tissue from rats of respective group (magnification, 400×).

according to the manufacturers' instructions (Roche Applied Science, IN, USA). Apoptotic cells were counted in a selected microscopic field per liver section by an experienced pathologist blind to the experimental protocol. The apoptosis index was expressed as a percentage of TUNEL-positive cells in 1000 cells counted in the same section [29]. Nuclear condensation and fragmentation typical of apoptotic cells were further assessed by using 33258 staining kit (Beyotime Institute of Biotechnology, Shanghai, China). DNA staining was viewed by fluorescence microscopy. In addition, liver sections were stained with Oil-Red-O to visualize lipid accumulation.

Measurement of caspase-3 and -9 activities. Activities of casase-3 and -9 of liver cells were determined using the caspase-3 and caspase-9 activity kits (Beyotime, Beijing, China) according to the manufacturer's instructions.

Immunoblotting for Bax, Bcl-2 and the release of Cytc. Total cytosolic proteins for analysis of the levels of Bax and Bcl-2, and the cytosolic proteins without mitochondrial fraction for analysis of the release of Cytc were prepared as previously described [30]. Protein samples (40 μg per lane) were subjected to 10% sodium dodecyl sulfate-Polyacrylamide gel electrophoresis and transferred onto polyvinylidene fluoride membranes (Bio-Rad, Hercules, CA, USA). Membranes were incubated with specific primary antibodies Bax, Bcl-2, Cytc (1:1000 diluted, Cell Signaling Technology, MA, USA) followed by incubation with horseradish peroxidase-conjugated secondary antibody. The intensity range of immunostaining was detected

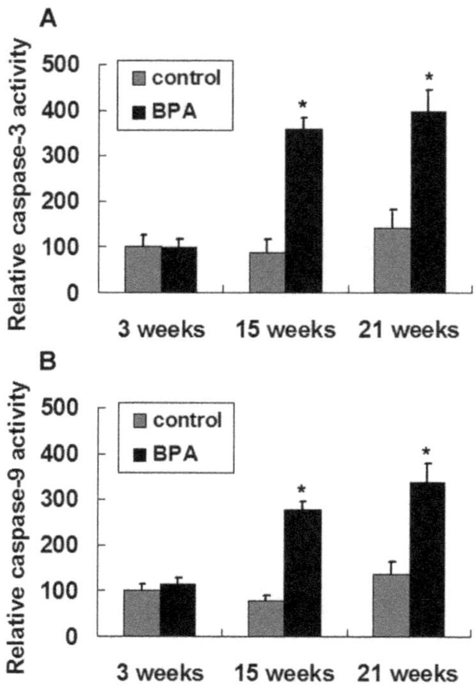

Figure 3. Activity of caspase-3 and caspase-9 in liver tissue after perinatal exposure to BPA. Activity of caspase-3 (A) and caspase-9 (B) in the liver of 3-week, 15-week and 21-week rat offspring were measured. Values are means ± S.E.M. (n = 6 rats per group; only 1 offspring was selected per litter). *$P<0.05$ compared with controls.

using the ECL chemiluminescence system (Thermo Fisher Scientific inc., Waltham, MA, USA).

In vitro Studies

Isolation of mitochondria and BPA treatment. To study the direct effect of BPA on mitochondria, liver mitochondria were isolated from untreated neonatal rats as described previously [30]. The mitochondria were purified by differential centrifugation and separation on a sucrose gradient (1.0 M/1.5 M). Then, the mitochondria were resuspended in a buffer (5 mg/mL bovine serum albumin, KH_2PO_4, 400 mM Mannitol, and 50 mM Tris HCl, pH 7.4) and kept on ice for up to 4 hr. The mitochondria were treated with 3% ethanol as the control, 1.47 ng/mL BPA or 2.60 ng/mL BPA β-d-glucuronide (Santa Cruz Biotechnology, CA, USA) dissolved in 3% ethanol.

Electron microscopy of isolated mitochondria and mitochondrial swelling assay. For mitochondrial swelling assay, mitochondria were washed and then resuspended with 0.025 M Tris HCl containing 0.175 M KCl (pH 7.4). Mitochondrial swelling, an indicator of mitochondrial permeability transition (PT), was measured by the decrease in the absorbance at 520 nm using a spectrophotometer after different time intervals in a temperature-controlled cell. To examine whether a change in MPT results in structural alterations, electron microscopic assessment was undertaken. The mitochondrial pellet was fixed in PBS-buffered 1% gluataraldehyde/1% paraformaldehyde, and examined by transmission electron microscopy (Tecnai G2 12, FEI, Netherland).

Isolation of nuclei and the morphologic features determination. Rat liver nuclei were isolated using a previously described standard method [31]. After mitochondria isolated from neonatal rat liver were treated with BPA at 30°C for 55 mins, reaction mixtures were centrifuged and then supernatants containing proteins released from mitochondria were collected as described previously [30]. For nuclear morphologic features assessment, 6 μl of liver nuclei, 1 mM $MgCl_2$, 1 mM dATP (deoxyadenosine 5′-triphosphate) and 50 μl of HeLa cytosol (250 g) were incubated with the BPA-treated mitochondrial supernatant at 37°C for 2 hr. Cyt c (Sigma, Santa Clara, CA, USA) was used as the positive control, and the supernatant from

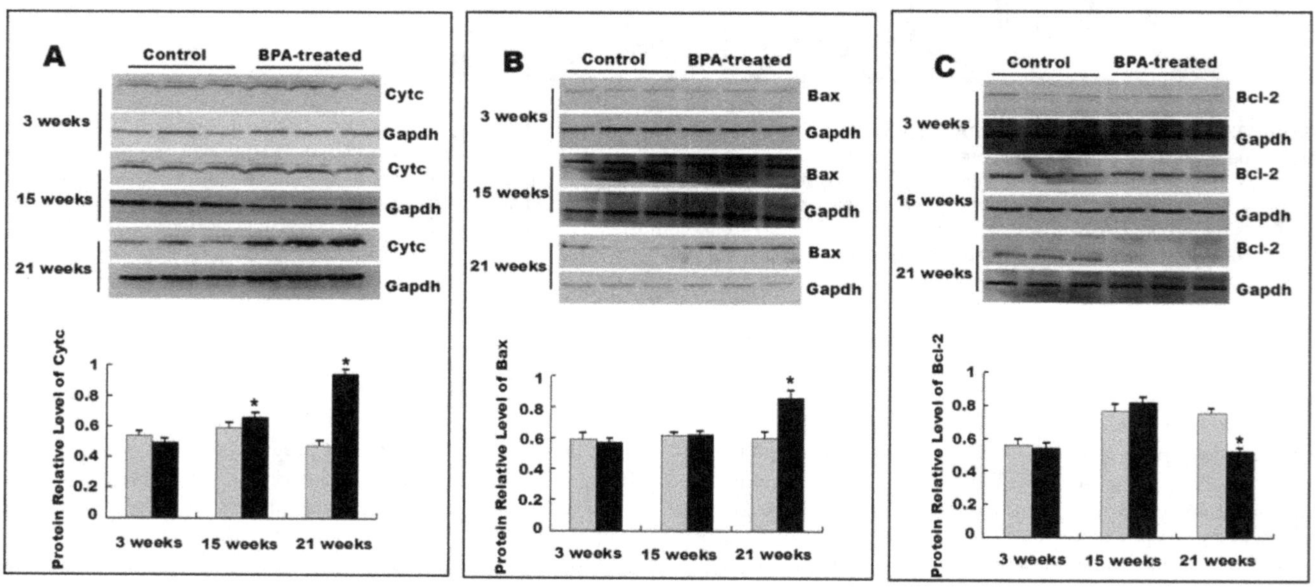

Figure 4. Perinatal exposure to BPA alters the levels of Cyt c, Bcl-2 and Bax. (A) Western blot analysis of the Cyt c release from mitochondria into the cytosol in rat livers at 3 and 21 weeks. Western blotting analysis of Bax (B) and Bcl-2 (C) in rat offspring liver at 3, 15 and 21 weeks. The protein expression levels were estimated by densitometry with Gapdh as an internal control. Data are expressed as means ± S.E.M. for three independent experiments (n = 6 rats per group; only 1 offspring was selected per litter).). *$P<0.05$ compared with controls.

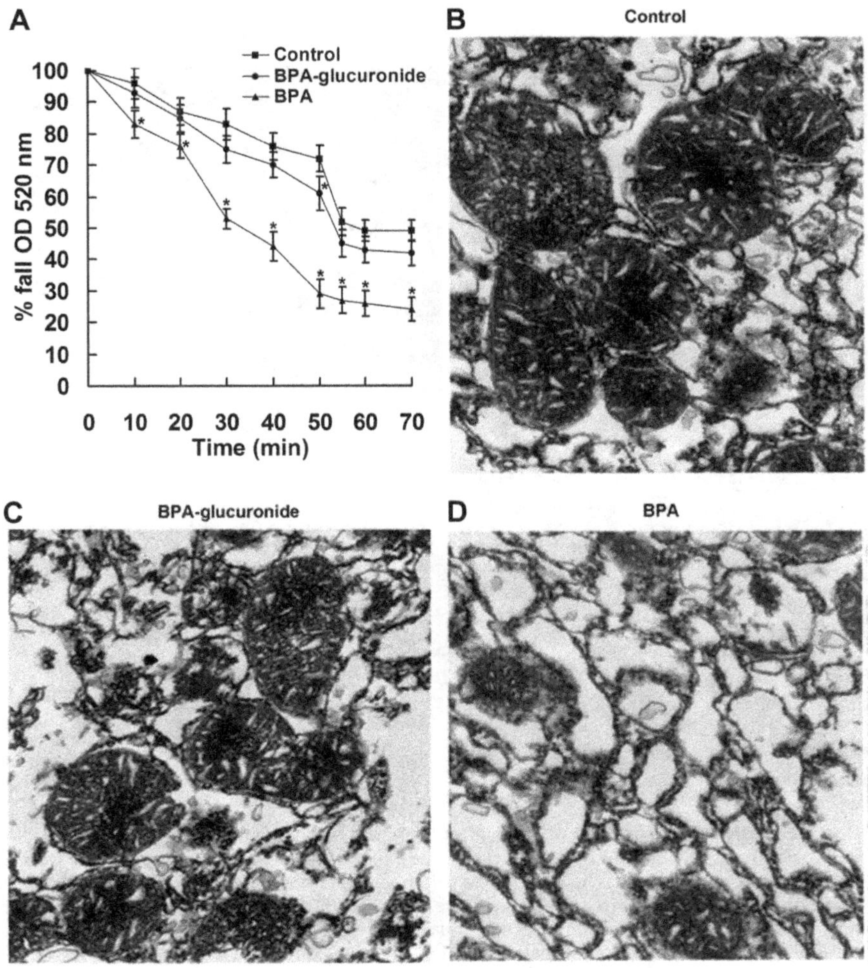

Figure 5. Effect of BPA on mitochondrial permeability transition (PT) and morphologic features of isolated liver mitochondria. (A) Changes of PT in the isolated mitochondria with time. Mitochondria isolated from neonatal rat liver were treated with BPA (0 and 1.47 ng/mL) or BPA-glucuronide (2.60 ng/mL). The decrease in optical density measured at 520 nm with time was normalized to 100. Data are shown of three independent experiments. Ultrastructural features of mitochondria treated with the control (B), BPA-glucuronide (C) and BPA (D). Representative images of transmission electron microscopy were shown (magnification, 10,000×).

untreated mitochondira was the negative control. The direct effect of BPA (1.47 ng/mL) on the isolated liver nuclei was also examined. After nuclei were stained with propidium iodide (PI), nuclear morphologic features were examined with a fluorescence microscope (Invitrogen, F14942, Carlsbad, CA, US).

Statistical Analysis

Data are expressed as means ± SEM and analyzed using SPSS 13.0 (SPSS, Chicago, IL). The changes over time were analyzed by repeated measures analysis of variance (ANOVA), and comparisons between the control and BPA-treated group at each time studied were analyzed using multivariate analysis of variance (MANOVA) followed by Bonferroni t-tests. The other data were analyzed with ANOVA. A *P*-value of <0.05 was considered statically significant.

Results

In vivo Studies

Perinatal exposure to BPA increases liver apoptosis in rat offspring. After perinatal exposure to BPA at the TDI, body weight gain of the pregnant rats, litter size and sex ratio showed no significant change compared to controls. The mean concentration of total BPA in the liver of the BPA-treated neonatal rats was 1.47 ± 0.39 ng/g, while BPA was detected under the detection limit in the control rats.

Body weight in the BPA-treated offspring and the control were increased in time trend and perinatal exposure to BPA significantly increased body weight at 21 weeks compared with the control group ($P<0.05$) (Fig. 1A). The liver weight were also increased over time, and there're no significant changes between the two groups at each age studied (Fig. 1B). The relative liver/body weight of the BPA-treated and control offspring remained similar throughout all ages studied (Fig. 1C). Liver injury was assessed by determining serum ALT, and time-course of BPA-increased serum ALT levels was observed. Perinatal exposure to BPA only resulted in a minor increase in serum ALT levels at 3 and 15 weeks but a significant increase at 21 weeks compared to the control ($P<0.05$) (Fig. 1D).

Hepatocyte apoptosis in liver tissue samples was examined using TUNEL assay. Perinatal exposure to BPA increased liver TUNEL-positive cells in the offspring with time, while a significant increase was observed only at 15 and 21 weeks compared with controls ($P<0.05$) (Fig. 2A, B). Hoechst stained liver sections also

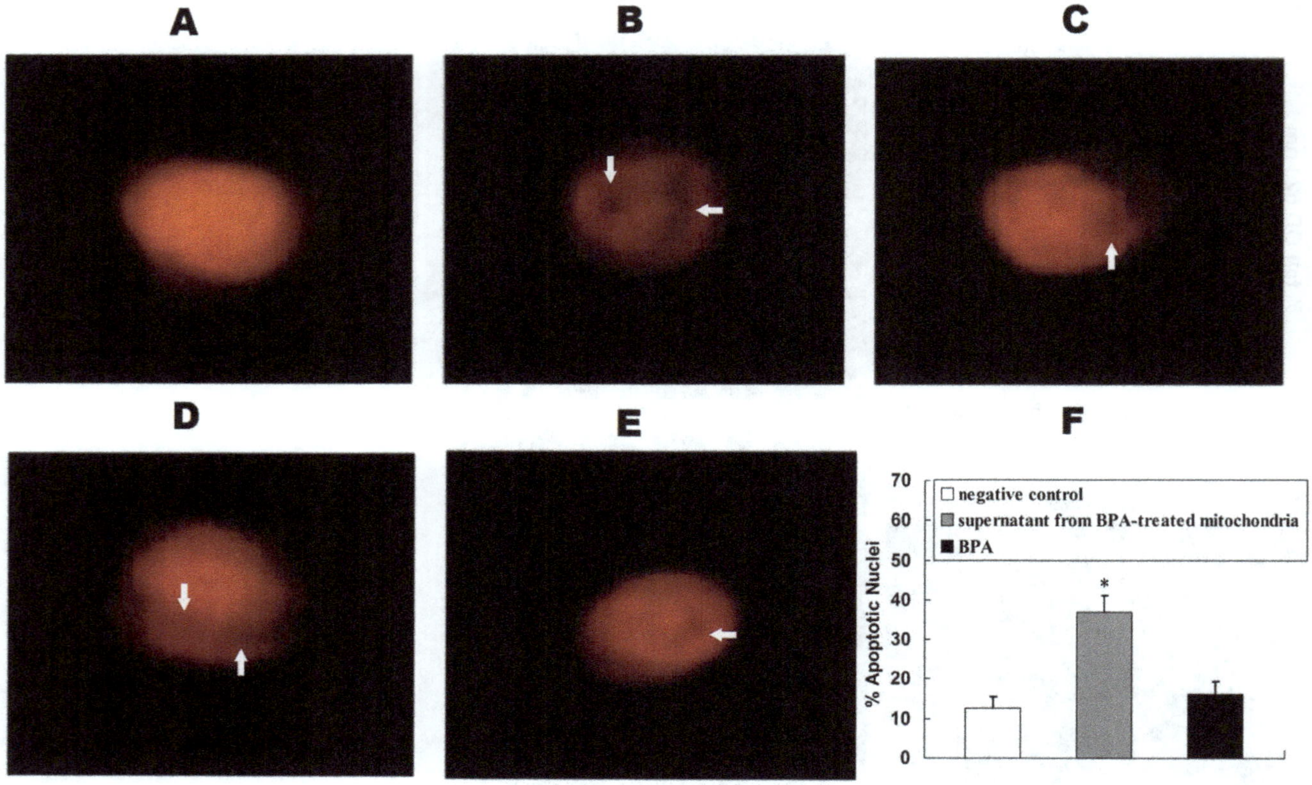

Figure 6. BPA-induced release of proteins and the initiation of apoptosis *in vitro*. After liver nuclei were incubated with the supernatant from the mitochondria treated with BPA, negative control, positive control or BPA, nuclear morphologic features were assessed. (A) Normal morphologic features; (B) Positive control; (C–E) Various stages of apoptosis in liver nuclei after incubation with BPA-treated mitochondrial supernatant, showing condensation or fragmentation of chromatin in nuclei (arrow); Representative images of three separate experiments are shown (magnification, 400×). (F) Changes of apoptotic nuclei. The percentage of apoptotic nuclei was counted in five different fields of view. The results are expressed as means±S.E.M. The experiment was repeated three times. *$P<0.05$ compared with the negative control.

revealed more apoptosis and chromatin condensation in the BPA-treated rats compared with the control at 15 and 21 weeks (Fig. 2C). Moreover, the BPA-treated rats exhibited a greater accumulation of lipids in the liver and significantly elevated hepatic TG at 27 weeks compared with the control; however, significant hepatic lipid accumulation was not present in 21-week-old BPA-treated rats (Figure S1).

Perinatal exposure to BPA activates caspase-3 and -9 in liver tissue. As capase-3 is the main effector caspase that is involved in apoptosis, we examined caspase-3 activity in the rat liver. Consistent with the TUNEL results, the BPA-treated offspring showed significantly higher activity of caspase-3 than the corresponding control group at 15 and 21 weeks ($P<0.05$) (Fig. 3A).

Due to the alteration in mitochondrial function caused by BPA was reported previously [19,21], the elevated caspase-3 activity observed in this study suggests that the initiator caspase-9 is activated via the mitochondrial pathway. Accordingly, we tested caspase-9 activity and found significant higher levels of caspase-9 activity in BPA-treated group at 15 and 21 weeks compared to the corresponding control group at each age ($P<0.05$) (Fig. 3B).

Perinatal exposure to BPA alters protein levels of Cyt c and the Bcl-2 family in rat liver. Activation of caspase-9 in liver cells of BPA-treated rat offspring suggests an involvement of mitochondria-dependent apoptotic pathway. Leakage of Cyt c from mitochondria is considered as a major event in cell apoptosis and may be accompanied by expression changes of pro- and anti-apoptotic members of the Bcl-2 family [24]. We evaluated the leakage of Cyt c from the mitochondria and the protein levels of Bax and Bcl-2 in the liver by Western blotting. Significantly increased leakage of Cyt c from the mitochondria was observed in liver from 15-weeks and 21-weeks rats with perinatal exposure to BPA compared to the corresponding control group at each age ($P<0.05$) (Fig. 4A). The levels of pro-apoptotic protein Bax were significantly increased in the liver of the BPA-treated rats at 21 weeks ($P<0.05$) (Fig. 4B), and the levels of anti-apoptotic protein Bcl-2 were significantly decreased in the BPA group at 21 weeks ($P<0.05$) (Fig. 4C).

In vitro Studies

Activation of caspases and the leakage of Cyc from mitochondria strongly implicate an impact of BPA on mitochondria to initiate hepatocyte apoptosis. To explore whether there was a cause-and-effect relationship, an *in vitro* study was performed. Liver mitochondria were isolated from untreated neonatal rats and then exposed to BPA at the dose which is equivalent to the internal exposure level of BPA detected in animal model.

BPA induces changes in mitochondrial PT and morphologic features. As the PT is associated with swelling of the mitochondrial matrix, to determine whether BPA induces PT, we determined the changes in volume of the isolated liver mitochondria by measuring the change of optical absorbance. BPA treatment (1.47 ng/mL) led to slow swelling of isolated liver mitochondria with time and induced a significant decrease in optical density from 20 min compared with the control ($P<0.05$) (Fig. 5A). After incubation of BPA for 55 min, swelling was sustained there-after. In addition, to examine whether BPA-glucuronide, the majority of conjugated BPA form, also has the similar effect on mitochondria PT, we used the same molar concentration of BPA-glucuronide (2.60 ng/mL) to test. BPA-glucuronide only induced a mild decrease in the optical density compared to the control (Fig. 5A).

From electron microscopic assessment, the control mitochondria showed regular cristae and integrated morphologic features (Fig. 5B), most of the mitochondria treated BPA-glucuronide were also normal (Fig. 5C). However, mitochondria treated with BPA were swollen, and outer membranes were enlarged and ruptured (Fig. 5D). BPA significantly increased mitochondria with abnormal morphologic features (50±4.6%) compared with the control (15±2.9%) ($P<0.05$), while BPA-glucuronide only induced 19±3.2% abnormal mitochondria.

BPA-induced release of proteins from the mitochondria initiates apoptosis in nuclei. The induction of PT induced by BPA suggests that possible apoptogenic proteins are released from the damaged mitochondria. In order to investigate if those proteins could initiates apoptosis in nuclei, the liver nuclei were isolated and incubated with proteins released from the mitochondria that had been treated with BPA, and apoptotic morphologic features stained with PI were assessed by a florescence microscope. The effect of BPA alone on nuclei was also investigated. The negative control showed normal morphologic features of liver nuclei with evenly distributed chromatin (Fig. 6A) and the positive control showed irregular condensations of chromatin in nuclei (Fig. 6B). After the liver nuclei were incubated with BPA-treated mitochondrial supernatant, condensed or fragmented nuclei characteristic of apoptosis were observed (Fig. 6C–E). The supernatant from BPA-treated mitochondria significantly increased the percentage of apoptotic nuclei (37.0%±4.2%) compared to the negative control (12.8%±2.6%) (Fig. 6F), while BPA only induced a mild increase in apoptotic nuclei (16.4%±3.3%).

Discussion

Many studies have investigated the long-lasting effects of BPA exposure at early development stages on the reproductive tract [7,8,32,33], neural behaviors [34,35] and metabolic function [9,10,12]. However, little data on the long-term effects of early BPA exposure at environmentally relevant dose on liver tissue were available. Although the dose of BPA we chosen in this study (50 μg/kg/day) is higher than human daily intake, the average total BPA concentration in the liver of BPA-treated rats (1.47 ng/g) was in the range of that reported in human fetal livers [5]. This is may be due to the fact that BPA metabolism in rodents differs from that in humans [36]. Thus, the dose we used in this study can be considered environmentally relevant. Here, we provide experimental evidence that early BPA exposure at environmentally relevant dose induces long-term injury on liver, and the activation of mitochondrial pathway of hepatocyte apoptosis may be involved in this process.

In the present study, we observed that perinatal exposure to BPA significantly increased the body weight of pups at adulthood, and the results are in accordance with some previous studies demonstrating increased postnatal growth in rodents prenatally or perinatally exposed to BPA at low doses [11,37]. Although the liver weight and liver/body weight ratio of BPA-treated pups didn't differ from controls, the significant increase in serum ALT levels at 21 weeks indicated that liver injury induced by BPA. Then, we assessed liver cell apoptosis and found an extremely significant increase in TUNEL positive cells in BPA-treated rats at 15 and 21 weeks, which accompanied by a modest increased level of serum ALT observed at 21 weeks. Serum ALT value has long been used as a marker of liver injury. However, actually, in some chronic liver injury, there is no apparent change in ALT observed. Some studies have demonstrated that the serum ALT values do not correlate with the severity of the histopathological changes and the parameters of apoptosis in liver disease, and suggest histological assessment can more accurately determine the disease severity [38].

Hepatic homeostasis is achieved through a regular cell turnover involving apoptosis of hepatocytes, and increased apoptosis of hepatocytes is considered to be an important mechanism contributing to various kinds of liver diseases [39]. The induction of apoptosis is correlated with the activation of caspases, which have proteolytic activity and are able to cleave proteins to result in cell shrinkage, chromatin condensation and DNA fragmentation [40]. We observed the significant increases in the activity of caspase-3 in BPA-treated offspring at 15 and 21 weeks compared to the corresponding control group, suggesting that apoptosis is caspase dependent. Caspase-3, a key molecular marker of apoptotic signaling, is activated by either mitochondria dependent or death receptor dependent apoptotic pathways. Previous researches reported that BPA induced mitochondria dysfunction in the isolated rat hepatocytes [19] and human HepG2 cell [21], which led us to study the role of mitochondria played in liver cell apoptosis induced by BPA. Consistent with the change of caspase-3 activity, the further findings of elevated levels of caspase-9 activity and cytosolic Cyt c in hepatocytes of BPA-treated pups at 15 and 21 weeks indicated an involvement of a mitochondrial pathway of apoptosis.

The Bcl-2 family of proteins, containing both pro-apoptotic and anti-apoptotic members, are known to regulate mitochondrial-mediated apoptosis [41]. However, we only found significant change in the expression of antiapoptotic Bcl-2 proteins and the proapoptotic Bax proteins in BPA-treated group at 21 weeks. It has been reported that some drug or hormone can enforce or inhibit mitochondrial PT and then induce or prevent apoptosis [30,42]. The induction of the PT, an important indicator of mitochondrial integrity and function, can result in mitochondrial swelling and the release of apoptogenic proteins from mitochondria [43]. The so-called PT is due to the opening of a regulated proteaceous pore, also called PT pore. The PT pore complex, which has been proposed located with inner/outer membrane contact sites, are viewed as an integrator that senses metabolic perturbations [42]. Perinatal exposure to BPA may act on the liver mitochondria in a direct or an indirect fashion to provoke PT first, causing release of apoptogenic proteins and activation of caspase.

Because the mechanism of BPA impacts on liver cells *in vivo* is complicated, an *in vitro* system was used to study the direct effect of BPA on liver mitochondria to minimize the systemic effects. We found that BPA induced a significant increase in mitochondrial PT coupled with ultrastructural changes in morphologic mitochondrial features, indicating a direct effect of BPA on mitochondria. In addition, the release of apoptogenic proteins from the mitochondria induced by BPA was further demonstrated to cause condensed chromatin in isolated liver nuclei.

We also investigated whether BPA-glucuronide has the similar effect of BPA on the isolated mitochondria, since BPA is metabolized into its glucurono-conjugated form *in vivo* [13] and glucuronidation is considered to be a detoxification mechanism [44]. Our results showed that the toxic effects of BPA are greater than those of its glucuronide metabolite. Thus, determination of both free and conjugated BPA may be more appropriate for risk assessment, but there is limited data currently since the quantification method continues to present challenges [45].

It's worth noting that the increased apoptosis induced by BPA took several weeks to become visible *in vivo*, but the *in vitro* results demonstrated that BPA had a direct effect on mitochondria. There are two reasons may explain the discrepancy. *In vivo*, the apoptotic cells will soon be phagocytized by the neighboring macrophage [46]. When the injury induced by low dose of BPA was not serious, we could not observe a significant increase in apoptosis cells. But it did not mean there was no potential injury. Some studies reported that early environmental stress during the initial stages of development could set a precedent for "priming" of the mitochondria to cause changes in mitochondria observed in adulthood [47,48]. Although the rat pups in our study were not treated with BPA after weaning and the metabolic clearance rate of BPA is only several hours [49], the cell apoptosis in liver and associated markers of mitochondria-dependent pathway become more serious with increasing age, demonstrating BPA has a long lasting effect through a direct or an indirect way. Thus, more early sensitive markers associated with mitochondrial injury should be explored in the future studies for better understanding the effect of BPA on mitochondrial *in vivo*.

Alterations in mitochondrial function have been implicated in the pathogenesis of hepatic steatosis which is also associated with hepatocyte apoptosis, and a recent *in vitro* study reported that BPA-induced lipid accumulation in HepG2 cells by disturbing mitochondrial function [21]. Therefore, we assessed hepatic lipid accumulation by Oil-Red-O staining and measuring hepatic TG. Significantly higher hepatic TG accumulation was observed in BPA-treated rats at the age of 27 weeks compared to the control group. The novel finding suggests that mitochondrial injury induced by perinatal exposure to BPA may also contribute to the later onset of hepatic steatosis, which needs further investigation.

In conclusion, this study demonstrates that BPA induces mitochondria-mediated apoptosis in hepatic cells, providing an explanation for long-term liver injury associated with early-life BPA exposure. In addition, our *in vitro* data indicate that BPA acts directly on mitochondria, altering mitochondrial ultrastructure, inducing PT and releasing proteins that lead to activation of apoptosis.

Supporting Information

Figure S1 Effect of perinatal exposure to BPA on lipid accumulation in the livers. (A) Representative images of Oil-Red-O staining of neutral lipids presented on sections of livers from the control and BPA-treated rats at 21 and 27 weeks. Neutral lipids appear in red (magnification, ×400). (B) Quantified analysis of TG in liver. Data are means ± S.E.M. (n = 6 rats per group; only 1 offspring was selected per litter). *$P<0.05$ compared with controls.

Author Contributions

Conceived and designed the experiments: WX YJ YL SX. Performed the experiments: WX YJ JL YM ZM HC GL. Analyzed the data: WX YJ YW BX XC. Contributed reagents/materials/analysis tools: SX WX. Wrote the paper: WX YJ YW.

References

1. Schonfelder G, Wittfoht W, Hopp H, Talsness CE, Paul M, et al. (2002) Parent bisphenol A accumulation in the human maternal-fetal-placental unit. Environ Health Perspect 110: A703–707.
2. Wan Y, Choi K, Kim S, Ji K, Chang H, et al. (2010) Hydroxylated polybrominated diphenyl ethers and bisphenol A in pregnant women and their matching fetuses: placental transfer and potential risks. Environ Sci Technol 44: 5233–5239.
3. Ikezuki Y, Tsutsumi O, Takai Y, Kamei Y, Taketani Y (2002) Determination of bisphenol A concentrations in human biological fluids reveals significant early prenatal exposure. Hum Reprod 17: 2839–2841.
4. Yamada H, Furuta I, Kato EH, Kataoka S, Usuki Y, et al. (2002) Maternal serum and amniotic fluid bisphenol A concentrations in the early second trimester. Reprod Toxicol 16: 735–739.
5. Cao XL, Zhang J, Goodyer CG, Hayward S, Cooke GM, et al. (2012) Bisphenol A in human placental and fetal liver tissues collected from Greater Montreal area (Quebec) during 1998–2008. Chemosphere 89: 505–511.
6. Sun Y, Irie M, Kishikawa N, Wada M, Kuroda N, et al. (2004) Determination of bisphenol A in human breast milk by HPLC with column-switching and fluorescence detection. Biomed Chromatogr 18: 501–507.
7. Prins GS, Birch L, Tang WY, Ho SM (2007) Developmental estrogen exposures predispose to prostate carcinogenesis with aging. Reprod Toxicol 23: 374–382.
8. Suzuki A, Sugihara A, Uchida K, Sato T, Ohta Y, et al. (2002) Developmental effects of perinatal exposure to bisphenol-A and diethylstilbestrol on reproductive organs in female mice. Reprod Toxicol 16: 107–116.
9. Alonso-Magdalena P, Vieira E, Soriano S, Menes L, Burks D, et al. (2010) Bisphenol A exposure during pregnancy disrupts glucose homeostasis in mothers and adult male offspring. Environ Health Perspect 118: 1243–1250.
10. Wei J, Lin Y, Li Y, Ying C, Chen J, et al. (2011) Perinatal exposure to bisphenol A at reference dose predisposes offspring to metabolic syndrome in adult rats on a high-fat diet. Endocrinology 152: 3049–3061.
11. Somm E, Schwitzgebel VM, Toulotte A, Cederroth CR, Combescure C, et al. (2009) Perinatal exposure to bisphenol a alters early adipogenesis in the rat. Environ Health Perspect 117: 1549–1555.
12. Liu J, Yu P, Qian W, Li Y, Zhao J, et al. (2013) Perinatal bisphenol A exposure and adult glucose homeostasis: identifying critical windows of exposure. PLoS One 8: e64143.
13. Pottenger LH, Domoradzki JY, Markham DA, Hansen SC, Cagen SZ, et al. (2000) The relative bioavailability and metabolism of bisphenol A in rats is dependent upon the route of administration. Toxicol Sci 54: 3–18.
14. Lang IA, Galloway TS, Scarlett A, Henley WE, Depledge M, et al. (2008) Association of urinary bisphenol A concentration with medical disorders and laboratory abnormalities in adults. Jama 300: 1303–1310.
15. Bindhumol V, Chitra KC, Mathur PP (2003) Bisphenol A induces reactive oxygen species generation in the liver of male rats. Toxicology 188: 117–124.
16. Hanioka N, Jinno H, Nishimura T, Ando M (1998) Suppression of male-specific cytochrome P450 isoforms by bisphenol A in rat liver. Arch Toxicol 72: 387–394.
17. Marmugi A, Ducheix S, Lasserre F, Polizzi A, Paris A, et al. (2012) Low doses of bisphenol A induce gene expression related to lipid synthesis and trigger triglyceride accumulation in adult mouse liver. Hepatology 55: 395–407.
18. Ronn M, Kullberg J, Karlsson H, Berglund J, Malmberg F, et al. (2013) Bisphenol A exposure increases liver fat in juvenile fructose-fed Fischer 344 rats. Toxicology 303: 125–132.
19. Nakagawa Y, Tayama S (2000) Metabolism and cytotoxicity of bisphenol A and other bisphenols in isolated rat hepatocytes. Arch Toxicol 74: 99–105.
20. Ooe H, Taira T, Iguchi-Ariga SM, Ariga H (2005) Induction of reactive oxygen species by bisphenol A and abrogation of bisphenol A-induced cell injury by DJ-1. Toxicol Sci 88: 114–126.
21. Huc L, Lemarie A, Gueraud F, Helies-Toussaint C (2012) Low concentrations of bisphenol A induce lipid accumulation mediated by the production of reactive oxygen species in the mitochondria of HepG2 cells. Toxicol In Vitro 26: 709–717.
22. Vaux DL (2011) Apoptogenic factors released from mitochondria. Biochim Biophys Acta 1813: 546–550.
23. Kroemer G, Galluzzi L, Brenner C (2007) Mitochondrial membrane permeabilization in cell death. Physiol Rev 87: 99–163.
24. Kluck RM, Bossy-Wetzel E, Green DR, Newmeyer DD (1997) The release of cytochrome c from mitochondria: a primary site for Bcl-2 regulation of apoptosis. Science 275: 1132–1136.
25. Asahi J, Kamo H, Baba R, Doi Y, Yamashita A, et al. (2010) Bisphenol A induces endoplasmic reticulum stress-associated apoptosis in mouse non-parenchymal hepatocytes. Life Sci 87: 431–438.
26. vom Saal FS, Hughes C (2005) An extensive new literature concerning low-dose effects of bisphenol A shows the need for a new risk assessment. Environ Health Perspect 113: 926–933.
27. Newbold RR (2004) Lessons learned from perinatal exposure to diethylstilbestrol. Toxicol Appl Pharmacol 199: 142–150.
28. Shao B, Zhao R, Meng J, Xue Y, Wu GH, et al. (2005) Simultaneous determination of residual hormonal chemicals in meat, kidney, liver tissues and milk by liquid chromatography-tamdem mass spectrometry. Analytica Chimica Acta 584: 41–50.
29. Chen T, Zhang L, Yue JQ, Lv ZQ, Xia W, et al. (2012) Prenatal PFOS exposure induces oxidative stress and apoptosis in the lung of rat off-spring. Reprod Toxicol 33: 538–545.

30. Upadhyay G, Singh R, Kumar A, Kumar S, Kapoor A, et al. (2004) Severe hyperthyroidism induces mitochondria-mediated apoptosis in rat liver. Hepatology 39: 1120–1130.
31. Blobel G, Potter VR (1966) Nuclei from rat liver: isolation method that combines purity with high yield. Science 154: 1662–1665.
32. Newbold RR, Jefferson WN, Padilla-Banks E (2007) Long-term adverse effects of neonatal exposure to bisphenol A on the murine female reproductive tract. Reprod Toxicol 24: 253–258.
33. Markey CM, Wadia PR, Rubin BS, Sonnenschein C, Soto AM (2005) Long-term effects of fetal exposure to low doses of the xenoestrogen bisphenol-A in the female mouse genital tract. Biol Reprod 72: 1344–1351.
34. Fujimoto T, Kubo K, Aou S (2006) Prenatal exposure to bisphenol A impairs sexual differentiation of exploratory behavior and increases depression-like behavior in rats. Brain Res 1068: 49–55.
35. Kundakovic M, Gudsnuk K, Franks B, Madrid J, Miller RL, et al. (2013) Sex-specific epigenetic disruption and behavioral changes following low-dose in utero bisphenol A exposure. Proc Natl Acad Sci U S A 110: 9956–9961.
36. Vandenberg LN, Maffini MV, Sonnenschein C, Rubin BS, Soto AM (2009) Bisphenol-A and the great divide: a review of controversies in the field of endocrine disruption. Endocr Rev 30: 75–95.
37. Patel BB, Raad M, Sebag IA, Chalifour LE (2013) Lifelong exposure to bisphenol a alters cardiac structure/function, protein expression, and DNA methylation in adult mice. Toxicol Sci 133: 174–185.
38. Canbakan B, Senturk H, Canbakan M, Toptas T, Tabak O, et al. (2010) Is alanine aminotransferase level a surrogate biomarker of hepatic apoptosis in nonalcoholic fatty liver disease? Biomarkers in medicine 4: 205–214.
39. Guicciardi ME, Gores GJ (2005) Apoptosis: a mechanism of acute and chronic liver injury. Gut 54: 1024–1033.
40. Elmore S (2007) Apoptosis: a review of programmed cell death. Toxicologic pathology 35: 495–516.
41. Shimizu S, Narita M, Tsujimoto Y (1999) Bcl-2 family proteins regulate the release of apoptogenic cytochrome c by the mitochondrial channel VDAC. Nature 399: 483–487.
42. Susin SA, Zamzami N, Kroemer G (1998) Mitochondria as regulators of apoptosis: doubt no more. Biochim Biophys Acta 1366: 151–165.
43. Green DR, Reed JC (1998) Mitochondria and apoptosis. Science 281: 1309–1312.
44. Snyder RW, Maness SC, Gaido KW, Welsch F, Sumner SC, et al. (2000) Metabolism and disposition of bisphenol A in female rats. Toxicol Appl Pharmacol 168: 225–234.
45. Kosarac I, Kubwabo C, Lalonde K, Foster W (2012) A novel method for the quantitative determination of free and conjugated bisphenol A in human maternal and umbilical cord blood serum using a two-step solid phase extraction and gas chromatography/tandem mass spectrometry. J Chromatogr B Analyt Technol Biomed Life Sci 898: 90–94.
46. Dini L, Pagliara P, Carla EC (2002) Phagocytosis of apoptotic cells by liver: a morphological study. Microsc Res Tech 57: 530–540.
47. Cotney J, McKay SE, Shadel GS (2009) Elucidation of separate, but collaborative functions of the rRNA methyltransferase-related human mitochondrial transcription factors B1 and B2 in mitochondrial biogenesis reveals new insight into maternally inherited deafness. Hum Mol Genet 18: 2670–2682.
48. Dillin A, Hsu AL, Arantes-Oliveira N, Lehrer-Graiwer J, Hsin H, et al. (2002) Rates of behavior and aging specified by mitochondrial function during development. Science 298: 2398–2401.
49. Volkel W, Colnot T, Csanady GA, Filser JG, Dekant W (2002) Metabolism and kinetics of bisphenol a in humans at low doses following oral administration. Chem Res Toxicol 15: 1281–1287.

10

Liver-Targeting of Interferon-Alpha with Tissue-Specific Domain Antibodies

Edward Coulstock[1], Jane Sosabowski[2], Milan Ovečka[1], Rob Prince[1], Laura Goodall[1], Clare Mudd[1¤], Armin Sepp[1], Marie Davies[1], Julie Foster[2], Jerome Burnet[2], Gráinne Dunlevy[1], Adam Walker[1*]

1 Innovation Biopharm Discovery Unit, Biopharm R&D, GlaxoSmithKline, Cambridge, United Kingdom, **2** Centre for Molecular Oncology, Barts Cancer Institute, Queen Mary University of London, London, United Kingdom

Abstract

Interferon alpha (IFNα) is used for the treatment of hepatitis C infection and whilst efficacious it is associated with multiple adverse events including reduced leukocyte, erythrocyte, and platelet counts, fatigue, and depression. These events are most likely caused by systemic exposure to interferon. We therefore hypothesise that targeting the therapeutic directly to the intended site of action in the liver would reduce exposure in blood and peripheral tissue and hence improve the safety and tolerability of IFNα therapy. We genetically fused IFN to a domain antibody (dAb) specific to a hepatocyte restricted antigen, asialoglycoprotein receptor (ASGPR). Our results show that the murine IFNα2 homolog (mIFNα2) fused to an ASGPR specific dAb, termed DOM26h-196-61, could be expressed in mammalian tissue culture systems and retains the desirable biophysical properties and activity of both fusion partners when measured *in vitro*. Furthermore a clear increase in *in vivo* targeting of the liver by mIFNα2-ASGPR dAb fusion protein, compared to that observed with either unfused mIFNα2 or mIFNα2 fused to an isotype control dAb V_HD2 (which does not bind ASGPR) was demonstrated using microSPECT imaging. We suggest that these findings may be applicable in the development of a liver-targeted human IFN molecule with improved safety and patient compliance in comparison to the current standard of care, which could ultimately be used as a treatment for human hepatitis virus infections.

Editor: C. Andrew Boswell, Genentech, United States of America

Funding: These authors have no support or funding to report.

Competing Interests: The authors have read the journal's policy and have the following conflicts: All authors (except JS, JF, and JB) were employees of GlaxoSmithKline at the time this work was carried out. JS, JF, and JB are researchers at Queen Mary University of London whose work on this project was funded by GlaxoSmithKline. All relevant patents have been declared, and there are no products in development or marketed products to declare.

* E-mail: adam.z.walker@gsk.com

¤ Current address: Horizon Discovery Ltd., Cambridge, United Kingdom

Introduction

The current standard of care for hepatitis C virus (HCV) infection is treatment with pegylated IFN alpha, (Pegasys® and Pegintron®) in combination with the nucleoside analogue Ribavirin [1,2]. The potent anti-viral, anti-proliferative and immunomodulatory mechanisms of the type I interferons, a class of cytokines to which IFNα belongs, are well documented [3]. Whilst clearly efficacious, the systemic delivery of IFNα not only generates an anti-viral response in the liver, but also results in leukocyte activation in the blood leading to adverse responses to the therapy including cytokine release, flu-like symptoms and depression. These side-effects can be severe which leads to a significant proportion of patients discontinuing treatment [4,5,6].

The targeting of bioactive molecules to tissues is an attractive concept and in particular may offer multiple benefits in the treatment of HCV with IFNα. The perceived benefits are two-fold, namely increasing the local concentration of a therapeutic compound at the required site of action, potentially retaining efficacy with a reduced dose, and reducing undesired activity of a therapeutic in non-target tissues, potentially improving safety and tolerability. The application of this concept in multiple disease indications has been investigated using a wide range of methodologies, for example site-specific delivery of cytotoxic drugs for cancer therapy [7,8], liposomal delivery of antigens in vaccine development [9] and the targeting of blood-brain barrier (BBB) receptors to facilitate transfer of biopharmaceuticals from the blood into the brain parenchyma [10].

Viral replication in HCV infection occurs predominantly in the liver. Asialoglycoprotein receptor (ASGPR) is a cell surface receptor expressed exclusively in hepatic parenchymal cells [11]. ASGPR is a C-type (calcium dependent) lectin composed of two transmembrane glycoprotein subunits, termed H1 and H2. The aglycosyl H1 and H2 subunits are approximately 35 and 33 kDa in size respectively, though purified ASGPR protein subunits are significantly larger due to post-translational modification. ASGPR mediates endocytosis of plasma glycoproteins that have exposed terminal galactose residues from which terminal sialic residues have been removed [12]. In addition, ASGPR has also been linked to the entry of HCV into hepatocytes [13]. Despite reports of potential extra hepatic expression in human kidney [14], thyroid [15] and activated T cells [16], ASGPR has been exploited in the targeting of therapeutic molecules to the liver. For example, ASGPR-targeted nanoparticles loaded with cytotoxic agents such as paclitaxel result in enhanced cell killing activity against ASGPR-positive cell lines when compared with free paclitaxel [17]. ASGPR-directed nanoparticles have also been used to deliver transgenes and antisense oligonucleotides to ASGPR-expressing primary hepatocytes and cell lines [18,19]. *In vivo* radioiodinated copolymers with ASGPR binding activity accumulate in the liver following intravenous administration in rats [20]. In a study conducted by Peng *et al.*, systemic delivery of the apoptin gene, which selectively induces apoptosis in malignant cells, linked to asialoglycoprotein resulted in specific delivery to ASGPR-positive HepG2 derived tumors xenografted in SCID mice and significant tumour regression. By contrast ASGPR-apoptin transgene conjugates were not able to induce tumour regression in non-hepatocyte derived A549 xenografted animals [21].

Compelling evidence for the potential application of ASGPR-mediated hepatic delivery in improving antiviral efficacy of type I interferons is provided in a study by Eto and Takahashi. Following enzymatic removal of terminal sialic acid residues from the N-linked oligosaccharide chain of human interferon beta (IFNβ), the investigators were able to demonstrate enhanced interferon signaling activity and inhibition of viral replication in HBV transfected HepG2 cells compared to the unmodified form of the protein [22]. This enhanced antiviral activity was presumably due to ASGPR binding, as it could be partially inhibited by natural ASGPR ligands such as asialofetuin. Significantly enhanced *in vivo* antiviral efficacy of murine asialo-IFNβ, compared with that of the unmodified protein, was also shown in HBV transfected BALB/c athymic nude mice.

In this study, using phage display technology we generated a dAb specific for ASGPR and genetically fused it to IFNα. The small size of dAbs (11–15 kDa) coupled with their high affinity for their respective antigen can help preserve the activity of fusion partners so makes their use attractive [23,24,25]. We show that the IFNα-ASGPR dAb fusion protein can be expressed in mammalian cells, that it binds to ASGPR expressed on liver cell lines and retains cytokine activity. Furthermore, using SPECT imaging we show that the fusion specifically targets the liver suggesting that this approach may have therapeutic application and ultimately lead to a reduction in adverse events associated with systemic delivery of IFNα.

Materials and Methods

Antigen and mIFNα2 protein generation

Human and murine ASGPR-H1 ectodomains and mIFNα2 were generated as $His_{(6)}$-tagged inserts via PCR and cloned into pDOM50, a derivative of the pTT5 HEK293E expression vector (National Research Council, Canada) using BamHI/HindIII restriction sites. Protein was expressed in HEK293 cells and secreted into the culture supernatant [26]. Expressed protein was then purified on Ni-NTA resin (Qiagen) according to manufacturer's instructions. Purified proteins were dialysed into Dulbecco's PBS.

Selection and Isolation of ASGPR specific dAbs by phage display

Human ASGPR antigen was passively coated on immunotubes (Nunc) overnight at 1 mg/ml in Tris-HCl buffered saline (TBS; 50 mM Tris-HCl, 150 mM NaCl, pH 8) supplemented with 5 mM $CaCl_2$ (TBS/Ca^{2+}). After coating with antigen, tubes were blocked by addition of 2% (w/v) Marvel non-fat milk in TBS supplemented with 5 mM $CaCl_2$ ($MTBS/Ca^{2+}$). Selections were carried out using phage libraries displaying antibody single variable domains. Library aliquots were incubated with antigen-coated immunotubes in $MTBS/Ca^{2+}$ before washing tubes with TBS/Ca^{2+}. Bound phage was then eluted with 1 mg/ml trypsin. Following selection, eluted phage was used to infect log phase TG1 *E.coli* and then infected cells were plated onto LB agar supplemented with 15 μg/ml tetracycline. Cells infected with the phage were then grown up in 2× yeast tryptone (2× YT) medium (supplemented with tetracycline) overnight at 37°C before precipitation of phage from the culture supernatant using chilled PEG-NaCl (20% (v/v) polyethylene glycol 8000, 2.5 M NaCl) and used in a second round of selection as above, using antigen coated at 0.2 mg/ml. Precipitated phage from this second round of selection was subsequently used in a third round of selection using antigen coated at 0.04 mg/ml.

Screening selection outputs for ASGPR specific dAbs

After three rounds of selection, dAb genes from each library pool were subcloned from the phage vector using the restriction enzymes SalI and NotI. The enriched dAb genes were ligated into the corresponding sites in pDOM10, a pUC119-based vector, in order to facilitate soluble expression of dAb proteins with a C-terminal FLAG epitope tag into the periplasm and culture supernatant of *E. coli* TOP10 cells (Invitrogen) transformed with the dAb expression construct. Transformants were grown overnight on LB agar plates supplemented with 100 μg/ml carbenicillin and 5% (w/v) glucose.

Individual colonies were then picked into 96-well plates containing 100 μl/well 2× YT medium supplemented with 100 μg/ml carbenicillin and grown at 37°C for 4 hours with shaking at 250 rpm. Protein expression was induced by addition of 100 μl per well 2× YT medium supplemented with 100 μg/ml carbenicillin and 0.1 mM IPTG, with overnight incubation using the same conditions.

The antigen binding of individual dAb clones was assessed by ELISA. Human ASGPR antigen was coated at 1 μg/ml onto a Maxisorp (NUNC) plate overnight at 4°C. The plate was then blocked with 2% (v/v) Tween 20 in TBS/Ca^{2+}, followed by incubation with dAb supernatant diluted 1:1 with 0.1% (v/v) Tween 20-TBS/Ca^{2+}, followed by detection with 1:5000 anti-FLAG (M2)-HRP (Sigma-Aldrich). All steps after blocking were carried out at room temperature. The binding of the dAb supernatant to a $His_{(6)}$-tagged glycosylated irrelevant control antigen was also analysed.

Expression and purification of dAb proteins

FLAG-tagged dAbs were expressed in TOP10 *E. coli* following growth in TB OnEx auto induction medium (Novagen) supplemented with 100 μg/ml carbenicillin at 30°C for 72 hrs. Expressed protein was purified from clarified culture supernatant using protein A coupled to NHS streamline resin (GE Healthcare). Briefly, proteins were batch-bound to resin for 4 hrs at room temperature before washing with 10 column volumes of 25 mM Na Acetate, pH 6. Bound protein was eluted with 4 CV 25 mM Na Acetate, pH 3, and then subsequently neutralised with $1/10^{th}$ vol. 1 M Na Acetate, pH 6.

Emulsion Based Affinity maturation of ASGPR specific dAb DOM26h-196

Affinity maturation of dAb clone DOM26h-196 was carried out by diversification of CDR regions using doped oligos where the diversified positions contained 85% parent base and an equimolar mix of the remaining three bases. Briefly the amplification products for individual CDR libraries were purified by gel electrophoresis, mixed in equal ratios, spliced by 'splicing of overlapping extension' (SOE) PCR and re-amplified by PCR.

Spliced and amplified libraries were thereafter cut with SalI and NotI enzymes and ligated into pIE2a2A vector. The *in vitro* expression construct was PCR amplified from the ligation and the libraries for CDR1, CDR2 and CDR3 were thereafter pooled for selection. Nine rounds of selection were carried out in total. In the first round of selection 2.5×10^9 molecules of library were compartmentalised in 1 ml of emulsion, in the subsequent eight rounds 5×10^8 DNA molecules per reaction were used. Affinity capture of protein-DNA complexes was carried out using human ASGPR antigen biotinylated with NHS-LC-biotin (Pierce, according to manufacturer's protocol). M280 Streptavidin Dynabeads at 3×10^7 beads per reaction (Invitrogen) were used throughout to capture ligand-dAb-DNA complexes. Following the final round of selection, the amplified DNA was cut with SalI/NotI enzymes, cloned into pDOM10 vector and transformed into Mach1 Chemically competent cells (Invitrogen). Selection outputs were expressed as described above and assayed for antigen-binding activity by BIAcore using both human and mouse ASGPR. Affinity maturation screening identified beneficial mutations in all three CDRs of clone DOM26h-196, suggesting the possibility of further improvement by CDR shuffling and screening. CDR1, 2 and 3 sequences from several improved clones were amplified by PCR before purifying by gel electrophoresis, mixing in equal ratios and splicing by SOE PCR. Spliced PCR fragments were cloned into pDOM10 expression vector and transformed into Mach1 Chemically competent cells (Invitrogen). 96 transformants were picked and used to express/purify dAb protein as described above. All 96 clones were assayed for antigen-binding activity by BIAcore, and from this screen clone DOM26h-196-61 was identified.

Flow cytometry

Flow cytometry data was generated using the ASGPR positive human hepatocarcinoma derived cell line Huh7, primary human hepatocytes (Celsis IVT) and the ASGPR negative monocyte derived cell line U937 (American Type Culture Collection, ATCC number CRL-1593.2). Adherent Huh7 cells were harvested using an enzyme-free cell dissociation buffer (Gibco) and washed in PBS containing Ca2+ and Mg2+ supplemented with 10% (v/v) pooled human serum (Sigma) (FACS buffer). U937 cells were harvested from culture & washed in FACS buffer & frozen primary hepatocytes were revived from storage immediately prior to the assay. All cells were seeded into 96 well v- bottomed microtitre plates (Nunc) at a concentration of 1×10^5 cells per well and incubated for 45 minutes at 4°C with the appropriate concentration of dAb or V_HD2 isotype control molecule. The cells were then washed with FACS buffer and incubated for one hour at 4°C with a mouse monoclonal antibody specific to human V_H domains (anti-V_H) for 45 minutes at 4°C. Following the incubation, cells were washed as before and were then incubated with an Alexa-647 conjugated goat anti-mouse pAb (Molecular Probes). Cells were then washed as before and resuspended in 100 μl PBS containing 1 μM Sytox®Blue dead cell exclusion dye (Molecular Probes). Fluorescence intensity in the APC channel was determined using a BD FACS Canto II flow cytometer.

Cloning and expression of mIFNα2-dAb fusion proteins

mIFNα2-dAb fusions were generated by SOE PCR and the inserts cloned into pDOM50, again using BamHI/HindIII. The mIFNα2-dAb fusions were expressed in HEK293 cells as previously described and then purified on protein A streamline or NiNTA resins as described above.

Surface plasmon resonance assay

BIAcore™ SA chip (Series S Sensor Chip SA Certified, GE Healthcare Bio-Sciences AB) was coated with biotinylated recombinant mouse ASGPR1. One flow cell (Fc1) was used as a reference flow cell. HBS-P+ buffer (10 mM HEPES, 150 mM NaCl, 0.05% Surfactant P20, pH 7.4) was used as running buffer. The sample compartment of the instrument was kept at 4°C throughout the experiment. The data collection rate was 10 Hz. A concentration series of molecules under investigation, prepared in running buffer, were injected over the surface of the chip at 50 μl/min flow rate at 25°C. The injection time was 90 s and the dissociation time was 120 s. Regeneration of the chip surface between injections (back to baseline) was carried out using 10 mM glycine pH 2.0 solution.

B16-Blue™ interferon activity assay

To confirm activity of the mIFNα2 arm of the fusion protein, B16-Blue™ IFNα/β cells (InvivoGen), stably transfected with a SEAP reporter gene under the control of the ISG54 promoter enhanced by a multimeric ISRE, were seeded at 5×10^4 cells/well in 50 μl of assay media (RPMI1640 supplemented with 10% FBS (v/v)) in 96-well microtitre plates. Test molecules, over a dose range up to 300 nM, were added in a 50 μl volume of assay media to the plates in quadruplicate and the plates incubated in a 5% CO_2 humidified atmosphere at 37°C. After 20 hours 40 μl of the culture supernatant was then transferred to fresh 96-well microtitre plate and 160 μl of QUANTI-Blue™ SEAP visualization reagent (made according to manufacturer's instructions) was added to each well. The plates were left at room temperature until an absorbance at 640 nm of 1.0–1.5 for the mIFNα2 control had been reached. The absorbance was read using an M5e plate reader (Spectramax). Data was analysed using GraphPad Prism software (Graphpad Software Inc.).

Conjugation of V_HD2 isotype control dAb with maleimide-DOTA

All buffers used for preparation, purification and radiolabelling of dAb/mIFNα2 conjugates were pre-treated with Chelex-100 resin (Bio-Rad). V_HD2 isotype control dAb was dialysed into 0.25 M HEPES, pH 7. The dialysed solution was treated with TCEP at a final concentration of 5 mM for 30 min followed by the addition of a 30-fold excess of maleimide-DOTA (Macrocyclics, Inc.). The reaction mixture was then left at room temperature overnight in the dark and then applied to protein A streamline resin equilibrated in HEPES, pH 7 before washing with 30 ml HEPES, pH 7 and elution in 0.25 ml fractions of 0.1 M glycine/HCl pH 2) into tubes containing ammonium acetate (final concentration and pH of fractions was 0.46 M ammonium acetate, pH 5). The conjugated protein was analysed by ESI-MS to confirm conjugation.

Conjugation of DOM26h-196-61, mIFNα2 and mIFNα2-dAbs with NHS-DOTA

DOM26h-196-61 and mIFNα2 were dialysed into PBS (PAA Laboratories GmbH, Pasching, Austria) while the mIFNα2-dAb fusions were dialysed into 25 mM Na Acetate solution, pH 8. NHS-DOTA (Macrocyclics, Inc.) was then added in a 4-fold molar excess and reacted overnight at room temperature. Conjugation solutions (except for mIFNα2) were then applied to protein A columns equilibrated in, pH 7.4, before washing with PBS, pH 7.4 and elution in 0.5 ml fractions of 0.1 M glycine/HCl, pH 2, into tubes containing ammonium acetate (final formulation of fractions was 0.46 M ammonium acetate, pH 5).

A

Kabat Residue	'	'	'	'	5	'	'	'	'	10	'	'	'	'	15	'	'	'	'	20
V_HD2 isotype	E	V	Q	L	L	E	S	G	G	G	L	V	Q	P	G	G	S	L	R	L
DOM26h-196-61	.	.	.	.	.	.	.	.	.	.	.	.	.	.	.	.	.	.	.	.

Kabat Residue	'	'	'	'	25	'	'	'	'	30	'	'	'	'	35	'	'	'	'	40
V_HD2 isotype	S	C	A	A	S	G	V	N	V	S	**H**	**D**	**S**	**M**	**T**	W	V	R	Q	A
DOM26h-196-61	.	.	.	.	.	.	F	T	F	E	**K**	**Y**	**A**	**.**	**A**	.	.	.	.	.

Kabat Residue	'	'	'	'	45	'	'	'	'	50	'	'	'	'	54	'	'	'	'	59
V_HD2 isotype	P	G	K	G	L	E	W	V	S	**A**	**I**	**R**	**G**	**P**	**N**	**G**	**S**	**T**	**Y**	**Y**
DOM26h-196-61	.	.	.	.	.	.	.	.	.	**R**	**.**	**S**	**A**	**R**	**G**	**V**	**T**	**.**	**.**	**.**

Kabat Residue	'	'	'	'	64	'	'	'	'	69	'	'	'	'	74	'	'	'	'	79
V_HD2 isotype	**A**	**D**	**S**	**V**	**K**	**G**	R	F	T	I	S	R	D	N	S	K	N	T	L	Y
DOM26h-196-61	**.**	**.**	**.**	**.**	**.**	**.**	.	.	.	.	.	.	.	.	.	.	.	.	.	.

Kabat Residue	'	'	'	'	82b	'	'	'	'	86	'	'	'	'	91	'	'	'	'	96
V_HD2 isotype	L	Q	M	N	S	L	R	A	E	D	T	A	V	Y	Y	C	A	S	**G**	**A**
DOM26h-196-61	.	.	.	.	.	.	.	.	.	.	.	.	.	.	.	.	.	.	**H**	**K**

Kabat Residue	'	'	'	'	100a'	'	'	'	'	100f'	'	'	'	'	101	'	'	'	'	106
V_HD2 isotype	**R**	**H**	**A**	**D**	**T**	**E**	**R**	**P**	**P**	**S**	**Q**	**Q**	**T**	**M**	**P**	**F**	W	G	Q	G
DOM26h-196-61	**.**	**.**	**E**	**H**	**.**	**R**	**F**	**D**	**S**	~	~	~	~	~	~	~	.	.	.	.

Kabat Residue	'	'	'	'	111	'	'
V_HD2 isotype	T	L	V	T	V	S	S
DOM26h-196-61	.	.	.	.	.	.	.

B

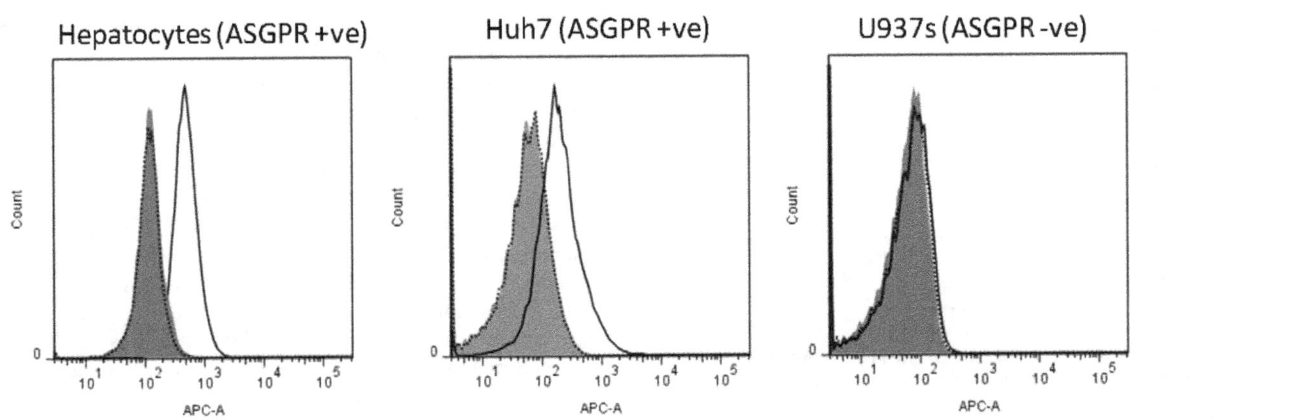

Figure 1. A – Sequence of DOM26h-196-61. Alignment of the primary sequence of the ASGPR specific dAb DOM26h-196-61 and the V_HD2 isotype control sequence. DOM26h-196-61 residues identical to the V_HD2 isotype control sequence are represented by '.' Residue numbering was determined by the method of Kabat [34], with the residues contained within the three complementary determining regions (CDRs) underlined and in bold. In CDR3 of DOM26h-196-61, the symbol '~' has been used to facilitate alignment but does not represent a residue. **B** – Flow cytometry of liver targeting dAbs. ASGPR specific DOM26h-196-61 dAb (solid line) and V_HD2 isotype control dAb (dotted line) were tested for binding to ASGPR positive primary human hepatocytes and the human hepatocarcinoma-derived cell line Huh7 by flow cytometry. Binding of DOM26h-196-61 to the ASGPR negative human cell line U937 is also shown for comparison. Detection of bound dAbs was demonstrated using a mouse monoclonal antibody specific for human V_H domains and an Alexa 647 conjugated goat anti-mouse pAb. Staining of cells in the absence of dAb is also shown for comparison (shaded histograms).

In the case of mIFNα2, the conjugation reaction was purified by dialysis against 0.2 M ammonium acetate, pH 5.5. Conjugated proteins were analysed by ESI-MS to confirm conjugation. Surface plasmon resonance and B16-Blue^{TM} assays were performed to assess ASGPR binding and mIFNα2 activity, respectively.

Radiolabelling of DOTA-protein conjugates and radiochemical analysis

The general radiolabelling protocol was as follows; 40–60 µl (26–50 MBq) of $^{111}InCl_3$ in 0.05 M HCl, 8–12 µl (1/5th the volume) of 1 M ammonium acetate, pH 4.5–5.5 (or in the case of IFN-DOM26h-196-61, 120 µl 0.1 M MES, pH 5.1) and 12.5–92.5 µg of protein was added to a low protein binding 1.5 ml polypropylene tube. The solution was heated to 40°C for 1.5–2.5 h and quenched with 0.1 M EDTA solution (1/20th reaction volume). Radiochemical purity was determined using size exclusion HPLC (SEC) using a YMC-Pack Diol-60 column (YMC Europe GmbH, Germany), 300×8.0 mm i.d., S-5 µm with a mobile phase of 200 mM phosphate buffer, pH 6.8 and thin layer chromatography (TLC), iTLC-SG (Varian Inc., CA) eluted with 0.1 M ammonium acetate, 50 mM EDTA, pH 5.5 or iTLC-SG (pre-soaked in 2% (w/v) BSA in water and dried at 37°C) eluted with 1:2:5 35% ammonia:ethanol:water. The reaction mixture was then diluted with 0.1% (w/v) bovine serum albumin in PBS (BSA/PBS) followed by filtration through a 0.22 µm filter.

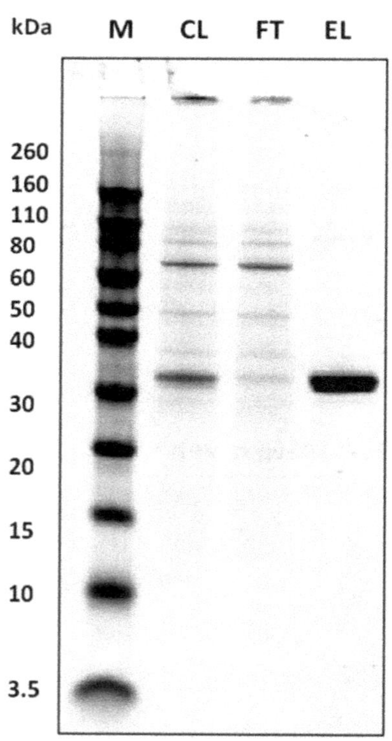

Figure 2. SDS-PAGE analysis of mIFNα2-dAb fusion protein purification. Purification on protein A Streamline resin from clarified cell culture supernatant results in a single band of the expected molecular mass of approximately 33 KDa. CL = clarified supernatant, FT = flowthrough fraction, EL = eluted fraction.

MicroSPECT/CT imaging

Radiolabeled dAb or mIFNα2-dAb fusion proteins diluted with BSA/PBS (10–17 MBq) were injected intravenously via the tail vein into a single female BALB/c mouse (except in the case of ^{111}In-DOTA-mIFNα2 where a female beige SCID was used). Whole body SPECT images were obtained under isoflurane anaesthesia at 3, 24 and 72-hrs (45-min each) using a Bioscan NanoSPECT/CT four-head camera (Bioscan Inc. Washington) fitted with 2 mm pinhole collimators in helical scanning mode (20 projections, 45-min scan) and CT images with a 45 kVP X-ray source. Images were reconstructed using InVivoScope software (Bioscan Inc).

Biodistribution studies in BALB/c mice

Radiolabel dAbs or mIFNα2-dAb fusion proteins diluted with BSA/PBS (0.15–0.5 MBq, radiolabelling efficiency corrected dose) were injected into female BALB/c mice ($n = 4$) via the tail vein. After 3 hours, the animals were terminated and tissues and organs of interest were collected, weighed and counted along with appropriate standards in a gamma counter (1282 Compugamma CS, LKB Wallac).

Results

Selections and affinity maturation

A series of ASGPR specific dAbs were selected from phage libraries using recombinant ASGPR H1 subunit purified from HEK293 culture supernatant. One clone, DOM26h-196, was chosen for further affinity improvements based on expression, selectivity/affinity for antigen and solution state properties (namely monomeric in solution as determined by size exclusion chromatography and melting temperature >55°C as determined by differential scanning calorimetry). Following affinity maturation, several DOM26h-196 derived dAbs were obtained that showed specific binding to ASGPR H1 subunit by surface plasmon resonance and ELISA (data not shown). DOM26h-196-61 dAb (amino acid sequence shown in Figure 1A) showed high affinity binding to the human ASGPR-H1 subunit ($K_D = 1$ nM), as well as high affinity binding to the murine antigen ($K_D = 4$ nM). Due to its human/mouse cross-reactivity this dAb was chosen as the targeting fusion partner for the IFN payload. The isotype control dAb, V_HD2, in contrast demonstrated no binding activity to human or murine ASGPR-H1.

When tested by flow cytometry for binding to ASGPR positive and negative cell lines DOM26h-196-61 bound to the ASGPR

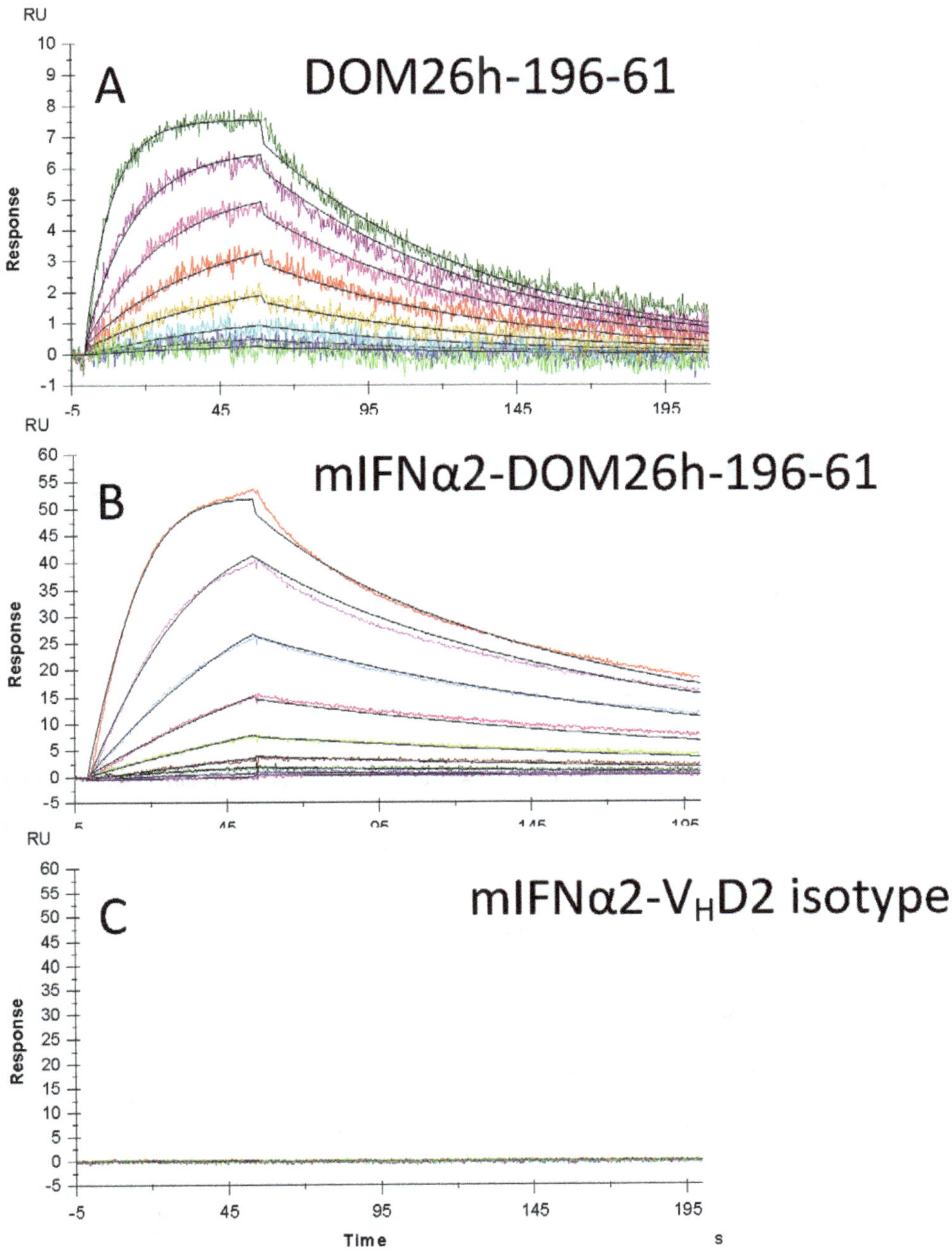

Figure 3. Surface plasmon resonance analysis of ASGPR specific dAbs and mIFNα2-dAb fusion proteins. Murine ASGPR H1 antigen immobilised on CM5 chip surface was used to analyse binding kinetics of DOM26h-196-61 and mIFNα2-DOM26h-196-61 injected over the chip surface at a constant flow rate of 50 μl.min^{-1}. mIFNα2-V_HD2 isotype control was also injected over the chip surface as a negative control for antigen binding.

positive cell line Huh7, with negligible binding to ASGPR negative U937 cell line observed. In addition to binding ASGPR positive cell lines DOM26h-196-61 also bound to primary human hepatocytes (Figure 1B). This strongly suggests that the ASGPR specific dAb DOM26h-196-61 specifically binds to native ASGPR expressed on the surface of hepatocytes and hepatocyte derived cell lines. As expected the V_HD2 isotype control dAb did not bind to any of the cells tested.

Expression and purification of mIFNα2-dAb fusion proteins

The mIFNα2-dAb fusion proteins were expressed in the pTT5/HEK293 mammalian expression system with expression levels comparable to those of hIFNα2b- AlbudAb^{TM} fusions described previously [28]. A simple, one step purification procedure using protein A streamline resin provided pure material, as determined by SDS-PAGE (Figure 2), with typical yields of 20 mg protein obtained per litre of culture supernatant.

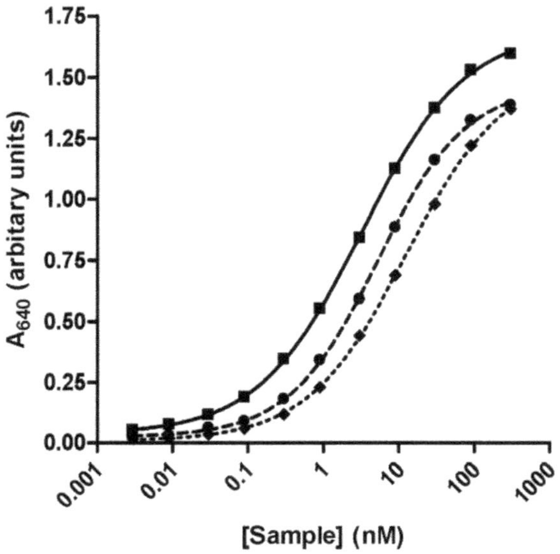

Molecule	EC_{50} (nM)
mIFNα2	3.2
mIFNα2-DOM26h-196-61	5.2
mIFNα2-DOM26h-V_HD2 isotype	12.4

Figure 4. ***In vitro* activity of mIFNα2 formatted as dAb fusions.** Activity of the mIFNα2-dAb fusion proteins was tested in the B16-Blue™ assay and compared to unfused mIFNα2 standard. Error bars are not visible as they are smaller than the data points, but represent standard error of the mean of 3 independent experiments. mIFNα2-DOM26h-196-61 (dashed line, closed circles) and mIFNα2-V_HD2 isotype control (dotted line, closed diamonds) showed comparable activity to the H_6-mIFNα2 standard (solid line, closed squares), with only minor increases in the EC_{50}.

When expressed as a genetic fusion to the C-terminus of mIFNα2, the DOM26h-196-61 dAb showed no reduction in affinity for ASGPR H1 as determined by surface plasmon resonance assays. K_D of the unmodified dAb was determined to be 1 nM for the human antigen (data not shown) and 4 nM for the mouse antigen (Figure 3). K_D of the mIFNα2-DOM26h-196-61 fusion protein for mouse ASGPR H1 was 0.6 nM indicating no detrimental effect on affinity of the dAb following fusion to mIFNα2.

B16-Blue™ IFNα/β reporter cell assay

The potency of mIFNα2 and mIFNα2-dAb fusion proteins was measured in the B16-Blue™ IFNα/β reporter gene assay (Figure 4). The potency of the DOM26h-196-61 and V_HD2 isotype control mIFNα2-dAb fusions ($EC_{50} = 5.2$ and 12.4 nM, respectively) is similar in this assay to that of non-dAb fused mIFNα2 ($EC_{50} = 3.2$ nM). These data therefore show that dAb fusion to the C-terminus of mIFNα2 results in only a modest decrease in potency of the IFN fusion partner, in the range 1.6–3.9 fold in our experiments.

Biodistribution and imaging of ^{111}In-DOTA-DOM26h-196-61 and ^{111}In-DOTA-V_HD2

DOTA conjugated dAbs were purified on protein A Streamline resin as described above, which provides a measure of protein functionality following conjugation. In addition DOTA conjugated DOM26h-196-61 was shown to be functional by BIAcore analysis of ASGPR binding activity (data not shown). Thin layer chromatography (TLC) analysis of the radiolabeled DOTA-DOM26h-196-61 and V_HD2 isotype control dAbs showed efficient labelling of both antibodies, with minimal amounts (<1%) of insoluble particulates present after filtration (data not shown). Following tail vein injection of radiolabeled antibodies biodistribution studies showed that 19.1±0.6% of the injected dose (ID) of ^{111}In-DOTA-DOM26h-196-61 remained in liver after three hours compared to only 0.55±0.07% ID/organ of the ^{111}In-DOTA-V_HD2 isotype control (Figure 5A). MicroSPECT/CT imaging studies of ^{111}In-DOTA-DOM26h-196-61 confirmed uptake in liver with significant levels also observed in the kidneys, most likely due to renal clearance of the antibody (Figure 5B). No uptake was observed in any other tissue apart from bladder, consistent with renal clearance of radiolabeled DOM26h-196-61. In contrast, there was no visible uptake in liver of the V_HD2 isotype control antibody. These data are therefore indicative of specific hepatic uptake of DOM26h-196-61 as a result of ASGPR binding *in vivo*.

Biodistribution and Imaging of ^{111}In-DOTA-mIFNα2, ^{111}In-DOTA-mIFNα2-DOM26h-196-61 and ^{111}In-DOTA-mIFNα2- V_HD2 isotype control

DOTA conjugated mIFNα2 and mIFNα2-dAb fusions proteins were shown to be functional in the B16 assay, with DOTA conjugation apparently having minimal impact on EC_{50} values obtained in this assay. In addition DOTA conjugated mIFNα2-DOM26h-196-61 was shown to be functional by BIAcore analysis of ASGPR binding activity (data not shown). TLC analysis of radiolabeled DOTA-mIFNα2, DOTA-mIFNα2-DOM26h-196-61 and DOTA-mIFNα2-V_HD2 isotype control showed efficient labelling of all three molecules, with minimal amounts (<1%) of insoluble particulates present after filtration (data not shown).

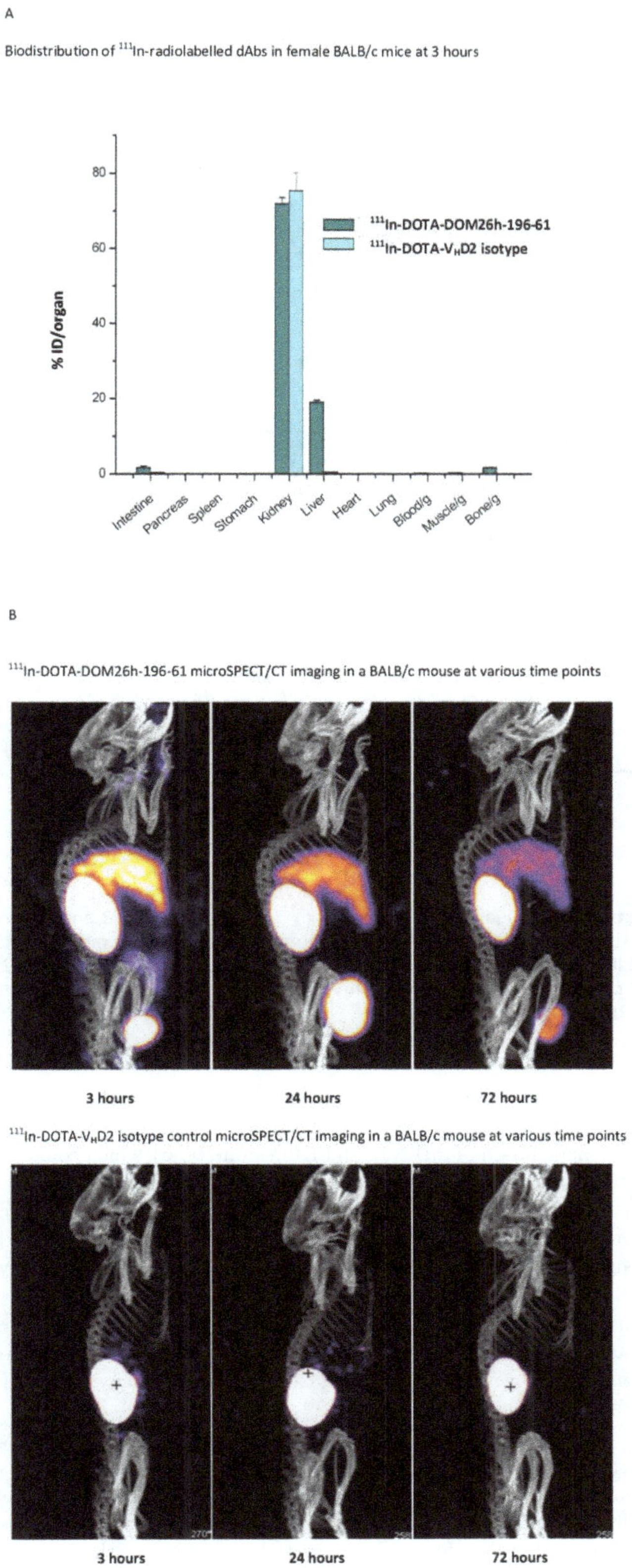

Figure 5. A – Quantitative analysis of ASGPR dAb biodistribution. Quantitative analysis of ^{111}In labelled dAb levels was carried out 3 hours after intravenous administration in BALB/c mice via tail vein injection of approximately 0.5 MBq radiolabelled dAb. Results show accumulation of radiolabeled ASGPR dAb DOM26h-196-61 in mouse liver is considerably higher than that observed with isotype control dAb. By contrast minimal uptake of either ASGPR dAb DOM26h-196-61 or V_HD2 isotype control dAb was observed in any other organ besides kidney. Error bars shown represent standard deviation of the mean, n = 4. **B**– *In vivo* imaging of ASGPR specific dAbs. Localisation of ^{111}In labelled dAbs in BALB/c mice at 3, 24 and 72 hours post injection. Images were captured following intravenous administration of 14–15 MBq of radiolabeled dAb via tail vein injection in BALB/c mice. Images show that signal is observed in kidney and bladder with both dAb molecules, whereas liver localisation is only observed with anti ASGPR V_H dAb DOM26h-196-61.

When tested in the B16-Blue^{TM} IFNα/β reporter gene assay the DOTA-conjugated mIFNα2, mIFNα2-DOM26h-196-61 and mIFNα2-V_HD2 isotype control molecules were shown to retain interferon activity at levels comparable to the unconjugated proteins (data not shown). Similarly, SPR analysis of DOTA-mIFNα2-DOM26h-196-61 showed that the conjugate retained mouse and human ASGPR binding activity comparable to the unconjugated protein (data not shown) indicating minimal impact of DOTA conjugation on the affinity for antigen.

Following intravenous administration of radiolabeled compounds biodistribution studies showed that at 3 hours after injection significant hepatic uptake of both mIFNα2 and mIFNα2-V_HD2 isotype control was observed, with 24.9±0.7% and 49.3±1.4% of the injected dose accumulating in liver respectively (figure 6). This is presumably due in part to binding of interferon receptor *in vivo* or hepatic clearance of mIFNα2, as the effect was observed in the absence of a dAb fusion partner. ^{111}In labelled DOTA-mIFNα2-DOM26h-196-61 shows extremely high hepatic uptake, with 73.1±3.0% of the injected dose observed in liver at 3 hours after intravenous administration. Increased hepatic uptake of mIFNα2-dAb fusions compared to mIFNα2 alone may be due in part to the increased molecular mass of the fusion proteins, resulting in increased systemic exposure and delayed clearance, whereas the increased hepatic uptake of ^{111}In-DOTA-mIFNα2-DOM26h-196-61 compared to that of ^{111}In-DOTA-mIFNα2-V_HD2 isotype control is most likely due to ASGPR binding of the fusion protein *in vivo*.

MicroSPECT/CT imaging studies confirm uptake of ^{111}In-DOTA-mIFNα2 in liver, with high levels in kidney and minimal uptake in all other tissues (figure 7A) which is interesting considering the ubiquity of IFNAR expression. By contrast the images obtained following ^{111}In-DOTA-mIFNα2-DOM26h-196-61 administration shows higher signal in liver compared to kidney, reflecting the increased hepatic targeting properties of this molecule. It is clear, in agreement with the biodistribution data in figure 6, from comparison of the images of animals injected with ^{111}In-DOTA-mIFNα2-DOM26h-196-61 and ^{111}In-DOTA-mIFNα2-V_HD2 isotype control that the liver-to-kidney ratio is higher in animals injected with the liver-targeted fusion protein (figure 7B), most likely as a direct result of ^{111}In-DOTA-mIFNα2-DOM26h-196-61 binding to ASGPR expressed on the surface of hepatocytes.

Discussion

Targeting of therapeutic payloads to specific cells or tissues is an attractive concept in terms of improving the safety and efficacy of the therapeutic. Antibody based methods for payload delivery have been described. For example, ASGPR single chain variable fragments (scFvs) conjugated to immunotoxins show increased cell killing in ASGPR expressing cell lines HepG2 and Huh7 compared to non-conjugated immunotoxin scFv fragments [27]. Here we demonstrate that domain antibodies specific to ASGPR

Biodistribution of ^{111}In-radiolabelled mIFNα2-196-61, mIFNα2-V_HD2 isotype control and mIFNα2 in female BALB/c mice at 3 hours.

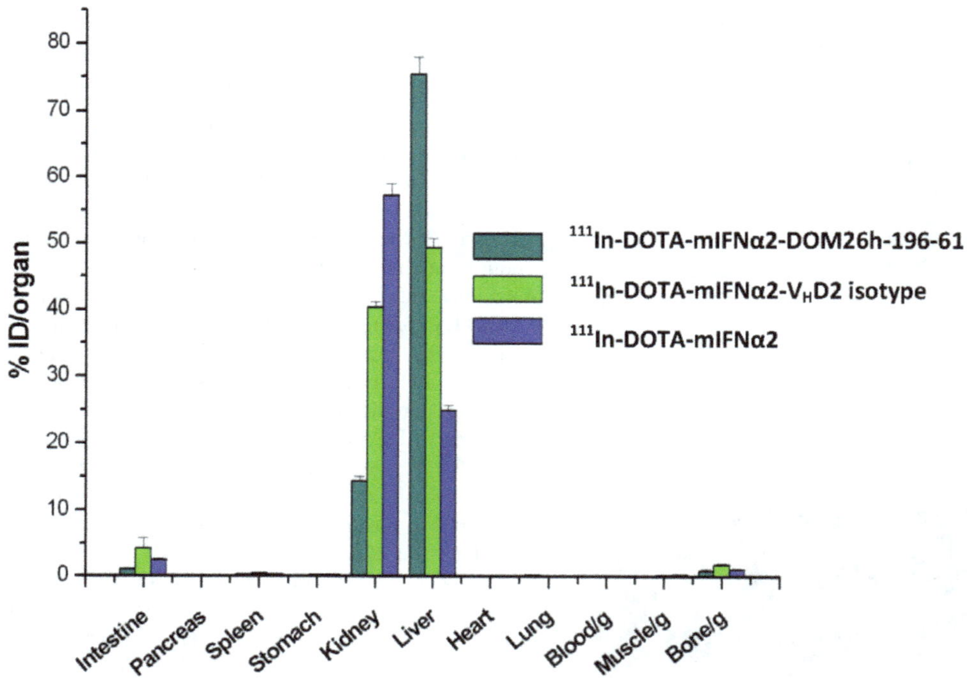

Figure 6. Quantitative analysis of mIFNα2 and mIFNα2-dAb biodistribution. Quantitative analyses of ^{111}In labelled mIFNα2 and fusion protein levels were carried out 3 hours after intravenous administration in BALB/c mice via tail vein injection of approximately 0.5 MBq radiolabeled compound. Results show accumulation of radiolabelled mIFNα2-dAb fusions in mouse liver is considerably higher than that observed with mIFNα2. Data also shows increased hepatic accumulation of mIFNα2-DOM26h-196-61 compared to mIFNα2-DOM26h-V_HD2 isotype control. Error bars shown represent standard deviation of the mean, n = 4 (n = 3 in the case of mIFNα2).

expressed exclusively on hepatocytes can be used to target delivery of IFN to the liver.

Selection of ASGPR specific dAbs from phage libraries resulted in a number of distinct and sequence diverse dAbs with a wide range of affinities to the antigen. Following affinity maturation of ASGPR dAbs, clone DOM26h-196-61 was found to have high affinity for both human and mouse antigens, with 1 nM and 4 nM equilibrium dissociation constants observed when binding the human and mouse antigens respectively.

In order to assess binding to native ASGPR, which consists of H1 homodimers, H1/H2 heterodimers and tetrameric H1 complexes, flow cytometry assays were carried out using detection antibodies specific to human immunoglobulin heavy chain variable domains. We show that the ASGPR specific clone DOM26h-196-61 binds to primary human hepatocytes and the human hepatoma derived cell line Huh7, which has been shown to express ASGPR H1 subunit [29]. By contrast this antibody did not bind to non ASGPR expressing cell lines such as U937, and the V_HD2 isotype control antibody did not bind to ASGPR positive cell lines including Huh7. Taken together these data provide evidence that DOM26h-196-61 binds specifically to cell surface expressed ASGPR H1 subunits, though it is not clear whether the antibody binds preferentially to distinct forms of ASGPR, for example the heterodimeric H1/H2 complex.

Given that our aim of developing ASGPR specific dAbs was to target therapeutically relevant payloads to the liver, we generated a genetic fusion of mIFNα2 and DOM26h-196-61 which could be easily expressed using the pTT-HEK mammalian cell culture system and purified by employing a simple affinity based capture method which utilises protein A coupled resins. The purified mIFNα2- DOM26h-196-61 fusion protein was subsequently shown to retain high levels of interferon activity in reporter gene assays and affinity for ASGPR in surface plasmon resonance analysis. ASGPR dAbs are therefore amenable to genetic fusion to interferon, without significantly affecting the activity of either fusion partner *in vitro*.

Natural ASGPR ligands have been shown to specifically accumulate in liver *in vivo* following, for example, intravenous administration of radio-iodinated asialorosomucoid in rats [30], ^{111}In labelled asialofetuin in mice and rats [31] and liposomes decorated with asialofetuin in mice [32]. Here we show, using microSPECT/CT imaging and biodistribution studies, striking differences between the distribution of the ASGPR specific dAb DOM26h-196-61 and the V_HD2 isotype control dAb following radio labelling with ^{111}In, with up to 20% of the injected dose of DOM26h-196-61 distributing to the liver 3 hours after intravenous administration. By contrast the V_HD2 isotype control dAb shows minimal uptake in liver, with an apparent 40 fold reduction in liver uptake compared to animals injected with DOM26h-196-

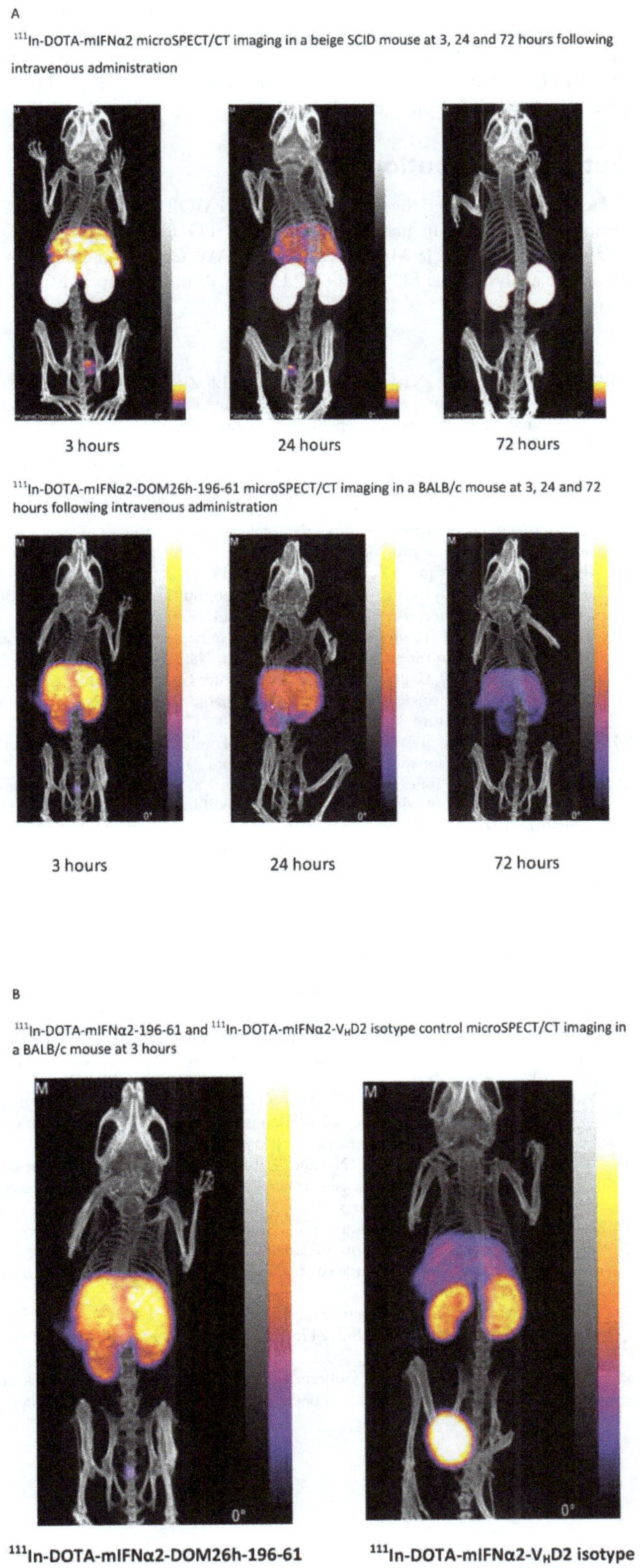

Figure 7. A– *In vivo* imaging of mIFNα2 and mIFNα2-DOM26h-196-61. Localisation of ^{111}In labelled mIFNα2 in beige SCID mouse and ^{111}In labelled mIFNα2-DOM26h-196-61 in BALB/c mouse at 3, 24 and 72 hours post injection. Images were obtained following intravenous administration of 12–15 MBq of radiolabeled compound via tail vein injection in BALB/c mice. Images show that signal is observed in liver, kidney and bladder with IFN molecules. **B**– *In vivo* imaging of mIFNα2-V_HD2 and mIFNα2-DOM26h-196-61. Localisation of ^{111}In labelled mIFNα2-dAb fusions in BALB/c mice at 3, 24 and 72 hours post injection. Images were obtained following intravenous administration of 12–15 MBq of radiolabelled compound via tail vein injection in BALB/c mice. Images show that signal is observed in liver, kidney and bladder with both fusion proteins; however the extent of liver uptake is clearly higher in the animal injected with mIFNα2-DOM26h-196-61, in agreement with biodistribution data.

61. Levels of both antibodies were low in all other tissues assayed, with the exception of kidney and bladder. The significant amounts of radiolabelled DOM26h-196-61 and V_HD2 isotype control dAb present in these tissues are not unexpected, as both antibodies are significantly below the molecular mass of approximately 66 KDa required to prevent renal clearance. Using immunohistochemistry with well characterised monoclonal antibodies to human ASGPR we saw no detectable expression in kidney, thyroid tissue or peripheral blood mononuclear cells, whilst demonstrating high levels of ASGPR expression in normal human liver tissue samples (data not shown). Hence, these microSPECT/CT studies conclusively demonstrate the liver targeting properties of ASGPR specific dAbs following systemic intravenous administration.

Imaging and biodistribution studies show that murine interferon alpha shows some degree of uptake in the liver in the absence of any fusion partner, and is perhaps not unexpected as this may reflect hepatic interferon receptor engagement responsible for driving the antiviral activity of interferon alpha *in vivo*. Alternatively these results may also be explained by hepatic clearance and metabolism. Fusion of murine interferon alpha to the V_HD2 isotype control antibody resulted in elevated hepatic uptake compared to unfused interferon, which may in part be explained by the increased size leading to delayed clearance of the fusion protein, though detailed pharmacokinetic analysis will be required to confirm this. Fusion of murine interferon alpha to the liver-targeting dAb DOM26h-196-61 resulted in the highest level of hepatic uptake of any of the molecules studied in this example, approximately threefold greater than that observed with the unfused mIFNα2 protein. Despite the fact that the mIFNα2-V_HD2 isotype control dAb and mIFNα2-DOM26h-196-61 fusion proteins were of comparable size, the hepatic uptake of mIFNα2-DOM26h-196-61 was significantly higher, leading us to the conclusion that this effect was a direct result of ASGPR binding on the surface of hepatocytes, and that ASGPR specific domain antibodies can be used to affect the biodistribution of therapeutically relevant payloads such as type I interferons, increasing the level of uptake in target organs and tissues. We therefore suggest that targeting IFN to the liver for the treatment of hepatropic virus infections such as HCV may result in increased efficacy through delivering the dose to the site of action but also that the dose of IFN could be reduced and the level of efficacy would be similar to the current standard of care. Either way we predict there would be improved safety implications following treatment with IFN.

There are documented examples of domain antibodies in development to address a number of autoimmune and inflammatory indications which would require repeat administrations of subcutaneously administered drug, for example TNF specific domain antibody constructs [33]. These molecules are currently undergoing evaluation in phase II clinical trials, demonstrating the utility of systemically administered domain antibodies in the development of novel therapeutics with antagonist activity. However as the approach described in this paper rather involves use of domain antibodies targeted to a specific tissue type in order to alter the distribution of agonist molecules *in vivo* this would merit further studies being conducted to investigate detailed pharmacokinetics and efficacy in preclinical models.

Acknowledgments

The authors would like to thank Dr John Spaull and Mick Hurle for immunohistological analysis of tissue samples as well as Professor Steve Mather and Dr Elena DeAngelis for intellectual input. **Disclaimer:** All animal studies were carried out in accordance with the Animals (Scientific Procedures) Act 1986 and the GSK Policy on the Care, Welfare and Treatment of Laboratory Animals. All experiments (regulated procedures) performed were approved for the purposes of this study by the Queen Mary University of London Project Assessment Committee (PAC) which meets throughout each year and examines all requests from investigators for *in vivo* research. In addition, all animal research is strictly controlled by the UK Home Office who issue licences enabling competent researchers to perform *in vivo* studies on live animals.

Author Contributions

Conceived and designed the experiments: EC JS MO LG AS RP MD AW. Performed the experiments: EC JS MO RP LG CM AS JF JB GD. Analyzed the data: EC JS MO LG AS RP MD AW. Contributed reagents/materials/analysis tools: EC JS MO RP LG AS. Wrote the paper: EC AW.

References

1. Fried MW, Shiffman ML, Reddy KR, Smith C, Marinos G, et al. (2002) Peginterferon alfa-2a plus ribavirin for chronic hepatitis C virus infection. New Engl J Med 347: 975–982.
2. Fried MW, Hadziyannis SJ (2004) Treatment of chronic hepatitis C infection with peginterferons plus ribavirin. Semin Liver Dis 24: 47–54.
3. Platanias LC (2005) Mechanisms of type-I- and type-II-interferon-mediated signalling. Nat Rev Immunol 5: 375–386.
4. Dusheiko G (1997) Side effects of alpha interferon in chronic hepatitis C. Hepatology 26: 112S–121S.
5. Iorio R, Pensati P, Botta S, Moschella S, Impagliazzo N, et al. (1997) Side effects of alpha-interferon therapy and impact on health-related quality of life in children with chronic viral hepatitis. Pediatr Infect Dis J 16: 984–990.
6. Dieperink E, Ho SB, Thuras P, Willenbring ML (2003) A prospective study of neuropsychiatric symptoms associated with interferon-alpha-2b and ribavirin therapy for patients with chronic hepatitis C. Psychosomatics 44: 104–112.
7. Wu AM, Senter PD (2005) Arming antibodies: prospects and challenges for immunoconjugates. Nat Biotechnol 23: 1137–1146.
8. Iyer U, Kadambi VJ (2011) Antibody drug conjugates - Trojan horses in the war on cancer. J Pharmacol Toxicol Methods 64: 207–212.
9. Van Broekhoven CL, Parish CR, Demangel C, Britton WJ, Altin JG (2004) Targeting dendritic cells with antigen-containing liposomes: a highly effective procedure for induction of antitumor immunity and for tumor immunotherapy. Cancer Res 64: 4357–4365.
10. Pardridge WM (2010) Biopharmaceutical drug targeting to the brain. J Drug Targeting 18: 157–167.
11. Spiess M, Lodish HF (1985) Sequence of a second human asialoglycoprotein receptor: conservation of two receptor genes during evolution. Proc Natl Acad Sci USA 82: 6465–6469.
12. Deal KA, Cristel ME, Welch MJ (1998) Cellular distribution of 111In-LDTPA galactose BSA in normal and asialoglycoprotein receptor-deficient mouse liver. Nucl Med Biol 25: 379–385.
13. Saunier B, Triyatni M, Ulianich L, Maruvada P, Yen Pet al. (2003) Role of the asialoglycoprotein receptor in binding and entry of hepatitis C virus structural proteins in cultured human hepatocytes. J Virol 77: 546–559.
14. Seow YY, Tan MG, Woo KT (2002) Expression of a functional asialoglycoprotein receptor in human renal proximal tubular epithelial cells. Nephron 91: 431–438.
15. Pacifico F, Montuori N, Mellone S, Liguoro D, Ulianich L, et al. (2003) The RHL-1 subunit of the asialoglycoprotein receptor of thyroid cells: cellular localization and its role in thyroglobulin endocytosis. Mol Cell Endocrinol 208: 51–59.
16. Park JH, Cho EW, Shin SY, Lee YJ, Kim KL (1998) Detection of the asialoglycoprotein receptor on cell lines of extrahepatic origin. Biochem Biophys Res Commun 244: 304–311.
17. Jeong YI, Seo SJ, Park IK, Lee HC, Kang IC, et al. (2005) Cellular recognition of paclitaxel-loaded polymeric nanoparticles composed of poly(gamma-benzyl L-glutamate) and poly(ethylene glycol) diblock copolymer endcapped with galactose moiety. Int J Pharm 296: 151–161.
18. Zhang XQ, Wang XL, Zhang PC, Liu ZL, Zhuo RX, et al. (2005) Galactosylated ternary DNA/polyphosphoramidate nanoparticles mediate high gene transfection efficiency in hepatocytes. J Controlled Release 102: 749–763.
19. Zhang Y, Qi XR, Gao Y, Wei L, Maitani Y, et al. (2007) Mechanisms of co-modified liver-targeting liposomes as gene delivery carriers based on cellular uptake and antigens inhibition effect. J Controlled Release 117: 281–290.
20. Duncan R, Seymour LCW, Scarlett L (1986) Fate of N-(2-hydroxypropyl)-methacrylamide copolymers with pendent galactosamine residues after intravenous administration to rats. Biochim Biophys Acta Gen Subj 880: 62–71.
21. Peng DJ, Sun J, Wang YZ, Tian J, Zhang YH, et al. (2007) Inhibition of hepatocarcinoma by systemic delivery of Apoptin gene via the hepatic asialoglycoprotein receptor. Cancer Gene Ther 14: 66–73.
22. Eto T, Takahashi H (1999) Enhanced inhibition of hepatitis B virus production by asialoglycoprotein receptor-directed interferon. Nat Med 5: 577–581.
23. Ward ES, Gussow D, Griffiths AD, Jones PT, Winter G (1989) Binding activities of a repertoire of single immunoglobulin variable domains secreted from Escherichia coli. Nature 341: 544–546.
24. Holt LJ, Herring C, Jespers LS, Woolven BP, Tomlinson IM (2003) Domain antibodies: proteins for therapy. Trends Biotechnol 21: 484–490.
25. Holt LJ, Basran A, Jones K, Chorlton J, Jespers LS, et al. (2008) Anti-serum albumin domain antibodies for extending the half-lives of short lived drugs. Protein Eng Des Sel 21: 283–288.
26. Loignon M, Perret S, Kelly J, Boulais D, Cass B, et al. (2008) Stable high volumetric production of glycosylated human recombinant IFNalpha2b in HEK293 cells. BMC Biotechnology 8:65.
27. Trahtenherts A, Benhar I (2009) An internalizing antibody specific for the human asialoglycoprotein receptor. Hybridoma 28: 225–233.
28. Walker A, Dunlevy G, Rycroft D, Topley P, Holt L, et al. (2010) Anti-serum albumin domain antibodies in the development of highly potent, efficacious and long-acting interferon. Protein Eng Des Sel 23: 271–8.
29. Treichel U, Meyer zum Büschenfelde KH, Stockert R, Poralla T, Gerken G (1994) The asialoglycoprotein receptor mediates hepatic binding and uptake of natural hepatitis B virus particles derived from viraemic carriers. J Gen Virol 75: 3021–3029.
30. Yang DY, Ouyang CH, Lu FG, Liu XW, Huang LQ (2007) Targeting specificity and pharmacokinetics of asialoorosomucoid, a specific ligand for asialglycoprotein receptor on hepatocyte. J Dig Dis 8: 89–95.
31. Abe M, Lai J, Kortylewicz ZP, Nagata H, Fox IJ, et al. (2003) Radiolabeled constructs for evaluation of the asialoglycoprotein receptor status and hepatic functional reserves. Bioconjugate Chem. 14: 997–1006.
32. Kallinteri P, Liao WY, Antimisiaris SG, Hwang KHJ (2001) Characterization, stability and in-vivo distribution of asialofetuin glycopeptide incorporating DSPC/CHOL liposomes prepared by mild cholate incubation. J Drug Targeting 9: 155–168.
33. Gay R, Clarke A, Elgundi Z, Domagala T, Simpson R, et al. (2010) Anti-TNFα domain antibody construct CEP-37247: Full antibody functionality at half the size. MAbs 2: 625–638.
34. Kabat EA, Wu TT, Perry H, Gottesman K (1991) Sequences of Proteins of Immunological Interest, 5th edition. Bethesda, MD: United States Department of Health and Human Services.

Detailed Analysis of Temporal Features on Contrast Enhanced Ultrasound may Help Differentiate Intrahepatic Cholangiocarcinoma from Hepatocellular Carcinoma in Cirrhosis

Rui Li[1]*, Meng-Xia Yuan[1], Kuan-sheng Ma[2], Xiao-Wu Li[2], Chun-Lin Tang[1], Xiao-Hang Zhang[1], De-Yu Guo[3], Xiao-Chu Yan[3]

1 Department of Ultrasound, Southwest Hospital Affiliated to Third Military Medical University, Chongqing, China, **2** Department of Hepato-biliary-Pancreatic Surgery, Southwest Hospital Affiliated to Third Military Medical University, Chongqing, China, **3** Department of Pathology, Southwest Hospital Affiliated to Third Military Medical University, Chongqing, China

Abstract

Aim: To verify if detailed analysis of temporal enhancement patterns on contrast enhanced ultrasound (CEUS) may help differentiate intrahepatic cholangiocarcinoma (ICC) from hepatocellular carcinoma (HCC) in cirrhosis.

Methods: Thirty three ICC and fifty HCC in cirrhosis were enrolled in this study. The contrast kinetics of ICC and HCC was analyzed and compared.

Results: Statistical analysis did not reveal significant difference between ICC and HCC in the time of contrast first appearance and arterial peak maximum time. ICC displayed much earlier washout than that of HCC (47.93±26.45 seconds vs 90.86±31.26 seconds) in the portal phase, and most ICC (87.9%) showed washout before 60 seconds than HCC (16.0%). Much more ICC (78.8%) revealed marked washout than HCC (12.0%) while most HCC (88.0%) showed mild washout or no washout in late part of the portal phase (90–120 seconds). Twenty six out of thirty three ICC (78.8%) demonstrated both early washout(<60seconds) and marked washout in late part of the portal phase, whereas, only six of fifty HCC (12.0%)showed these temporal enhancement features ($p = 0.000$).When both early washout and marked washout in the portal phase are taken as diagnostic criterion for ICC, the diagnostic sensitivity, specificity, positive predictive value, negative predictive value and accuracy were 78.8%,88.0%,81.3%,86.3%,and 84.3% respectively by CEUS.

Conclusions: Analysis of detailed temporal enhancement features on CEUS is helpful differentiate ICC from HCC in cirrhosis.If a nodule in cirrhotic liver displays hyper-enhancement in the arterial phase followed by early and marked washout in the portal phase, the nodule is highly suspicious of ICC rather than HCC.

Editor: Ming-Lung Yu, Kaohsiung Medical University Hospital, Kaohsiung Medical University, Taiwan

Funding: The authors have no support or funding to report.

Competing Interests: The authors have declared that no competing interests exist.

* E-mail: raylee7991@163.com

Introduction

Intrahepatic peripheral cholangiocarcirnoma (ICC) constitutes the second most common primary liver malignant tumor in cirrhotic patients, accounting for 1%–3% of newly developed tumors[1,2],and the incidence of ICC appears raising,especially in Western countries [3]. Cirrhotic patients may undergo surveillance for hepatocellular carcinoma (HCC) by ultrasound every 3–6 months [4,5].When a focal liver lesion is detected by ultrasound in a cirrhotic patient, a high suspicion of HCC arises. However, not all malignant tumors in cirrhosis are HCC, theoretically, ICC also may be found in cirrhosis. Differentiation between them is essential for surgical planning and prognosis assessment because ICC and HCC have different biological behaviour and prognosis[6,7].The European Federation of Societies for Ultrasound in Medicine and Biology (EFSUMB)defined typical contrast enhanced ultrasound (CEUS) vascular pattern of ICC as rim-like enhancement/non-enhancement in arterial phase followed by hypo/non-enhancement during the portal and late phases [8], but these recommendations are based on studies in which most patients did not have underlying cirrhosis. There is little information regarding the CEUS pattern of ICC in cirrhosis. Up to now, only three retrospective studies including a relatively limited number of patients have described the ICC enhancement pattern at CEUS and the associated risk of misdiagnosis with HCC [9,10,11]. These studies showed that CEUS was at risk of misdiagnosis of ICC for HCC in about 47.6%-68.8% patients. However, some CEUS features may help suspect ICC, especially in some cases with inconclusive CT or MRI [11,12] and this topic remains of high interest. Hence, the principle aim of our study was

Table 1. Demographics of patients with ICC and HCC in cirrhosis.

	ICC	HCC	*P*
Age			
mean (year)	49.21±8.99	53.24±11.39	0.077
Median (year)	32–75, 48	31–76, 53.5	
Male/female (n)	29/4	43/7	0.805
AFP (ng/ml)			
<20	23	23	
20–200	6	8	
>200	4	19	0.032
Child-pugh classification			
A	29	44	0.987
B	4	6	
C	0	0	
Nodule size (mm)			
mean±SD	49.91±27.07	59.14±23.09	0.890
Median(range)	40 (17–114)	42.5 (17–103)	
Number of nodules (n)			
1	27	37	0.640
2	4	8	
3	0	2	
>3	2	3	
Etiology of cirrhosis			
Hepatitis B	28	46	0.305
Hepatitis C	0	0	
Hepatitis B and hepatitis C	0	0	
Others	5	4	
Echogenicity of nodules			
hypoechoic	17	24	0.941
isoechoic	1	1	
hyperechoic	5	10	
mixed	10	15	

to compare CEUS imaging features of ICC and HCC in cirrhotic patients, to verify if detailed analysis of temporal enhancement patterns on CEUS may help differentiate ICC from HCC in this compelling clinical situation.

Methods

Patients

We retrospectively analyzed patients who were diagnosed with ICC and HCC on cirrhosis in which CEUS had been performed in our hospital between January 2005 and February 2014.The following inclusion criteria were applied:

(A) Histologically proven liver cirrhosis by representative resections or biopsies from the liver parenchyma;

(B) The diagnosis of ICC and HCC had to be pathologically proven (through assessment of surgical specimen or biopsy);

(C) Real-time CEUS was performed for diagnosis within less than a month before surgical operation or biopsy

Exclusion criteria were:

(A) Patients with mixed hepatocellular-cholangiocellular carcinoma.

(B) Systemic chemotherapy or targeted therapy prior to the CEUS.

(C) ICC and HCC without cirrhosis.

HCC sample cases were randomly selected to form the study group by using the sequence numbers created by the SPSS 13.0 software package (SPSS Inc, Chicago, IL).

The study protocol and consent procedure of the patients were approved by the institutional ethics board of Southwest Hospital. All patients signed their written informed consent to participate in this study after thorough explanation of the study protocol and procedure. Written informed consent according to the ethical guidelines from Declaration of Helsinki was obtained from each patient in this study. We performed a per-patient analysis. In a patient with more than one solid lesion in the liver, only the largest one was measured and investigated because CEUS could not scan multiple nodules simultaneously after one injection of contrast agent if the nodules are not at the same scan plane.

Table 2. Perfusion characteristics of ICC and HCC on CEUS in cirrhotic patients.

Characteristics	ICC	HCC	*P*
Arterial phase			
Contrast first appearance (s)			
mean±SD	12.63±4.71	12.46±3.82	0.852
Median(range)	5–24, 11	6–23, 12.5	
Arterial peak maximum (s)			
mean±SD	20.24±5.66	21.04±4.70	0.488
Median(range)	9–33, 20	13–34, 20	
Hyperenhancement			
Homogeneous	10 (30.3%)	24 (48.0%)	0.109
Heterogeneous	23 (69.7%)	26 (52.0%)	
Portal phase			0.000
Mild washout	6 (18.2%)	33 (66.0%)	
Marked washout	26 (78.8%)	6 (12.0%)	
No washout	1 (3.0%)	11 (22.0%)	
Late phase			0.000
Mild washout	3 (9.1%)	27 (54.0%)	
Marked washout	30 (90.9%)	22 (44.0%)	
No washout	0 (0%)	1 (2.0%)	
Washout first appearance (s)			
mean±SD	47.93±26.45	90.86±31.26	0.000
Median(range)	41 (21–153)	83(36–185)	
Emergence of washout			
<60S	29 (87.9%)	8 (16.0%)	0.000
61–120S	3 (9.1%)	36 (72.0%	
>120S	1 (3.0%)	6 (12.0%)	

Image acquisition

US examinations were performed by two experienced physicians with over 15 years of experience of liver ultrasound examination (R L, and XH Z) with an Acuson Sequoia 512 ultrasound unit (Siemens Medical Solutions, Santa Clara, Calif). Baseline US was performed with a multi-frequency 4C1 convex array probe. The gray-scale US characteristics of the lesion, including location, size, shape, and echogenicity were recorded. CEUS was performed by using contrast pulse sequencing (CPS) imaging. Split screen image was used to show the same scanning plane of gray scale ultrasound simultaneously. Real-time contrast imaging setting was used with a low mechanical index of <0.2 to avoid the microbubbles disruption. A volume of 2.4 mL of a second-generation US blood pool contrast agent (SonoVue, Bracco Imaging B.V, Geneva, Switzerland) was injected into cubital vein in bolus via a 20-gauge needle followed by a 5 mL saline flush. After contrast medium injection, hepatic lesion was scanned continuously for up to 4 min. The whole vascular phase was studied, consisting of the arterial phase (0–30 s from beginning of contrast agent bolus injection), portal phase (31–120 s after the injection), and delayed phase (121–240 s after the injection) according to EFSUMB recommendations [8]. In each case, the enhancing intensity and pattern of the target nodule during each vascular phase were recorded. For specified temporal analysis, the portal phase was divided into three parts, namely early part (31–60 s from beginning of contrast agent bolus injection), middle part (61–90 s after the injection) and late part (91–120 s after the injection) of the portal phase.

CEUS image analysis

The contrast vascular patterns on CEUS were defined by comparing the enhancement behaviour of the tumor with the surrounding liver parenchyma and were classified as:

(1) Peripheral hyper-enhancement—irregular rim-like hyper-enhancement at the peripheral part of the lesion with sparse filiform and punctiform internal enhancement.

(2) Heterogeneous hyper-enhancement—when the lesion displays mixed hyper-enhancement inhomogeneously at both the periphery and the central part of the lesion.

(3) homogeneous hyper-enhancement—when the whole lesion shows hyper-enhancement homogeneously.

(4) Hypo-enhancement—the lesion enhances in the less degree than that of the surrounding liver parenchyma.

(5) Iso-enhancement—the lesion enhances in the similar degree as the surrounding liver parenchyma.

(6) Non-enhancement—no appearance of contrast agent (microbubbles) at both the periphery and the central part of the lesion.

Wash-out appearance was considered as the presence of hypo-enhancement of the lesion in the portal or late phases preceded by

Table 3. Parametric measurements of ICC and HCC perfusion features on CEUS.

	ICC	HCC	*P*
Arterial phase			
Peak intensity of tumors (db)			
Mean±SD	97.29±36.81	121.97±28.77	0.001
Median(range)	101.90 (26.38–182.87)	122.82 (47.31–173.77)	
Tumor/tissue ratio of intensity			
Mean±SD	1.44±0.52	1.86±0.69	0.003
Median(range)	1.33 (0.43–2.69)	1.72 (0.99–3.65)	
Portal phase			
Lowest intensity of tumor(db)			
Mean ±SD	41.71±18.31	66.94±21.34	0.000
Median(range)	41.85 (8.19–105.54)	68.24(20.93–135.56)	
Lowest tumor/tissue ratio of intensity in late portal phase (90–120 s)			
Mean±SD	0.44±0.14	0.77±0.15	0.000
Median(range)	0.42 (0.26–0.94)	0.81 (0.34–0.99)	
Late phase			
Lowest intensity of tumor(db) in late phase (170–190 s)			
Mean±SD	33.42±14.49	51.72±15.69	0.000
Median(range)	32.75(6.37–83.7)	52.32 (21.84–81.88)	
Tumor/tissue ratio of intensity in late phase (170–190 s)			
Mean±SD	0.39±0.1	0.66±0.14	0.000
Median(range)	0.39 (0.21–0.61)	0.66 (0.36–0.94)	

hyper-enhancement in the arterial phase, a lesion lacking any enhancement in all phases was not defined as washout. When a nodule shows heterogeneous hyper-enhancement in the arterial phase, observation of washout was confined to the area showing hyper-enhancement in the arterial phase, and the area showing non-enhancement was excluded from the observation. The extent of washout was classified as:

(1) Marked washout—when the lesion displays obviously lower echogenicity than the surrounding liver parenchyma in the portal or late phases preceded by hyper-enhancement in the arterial phase.
(2) Mild washout —when the lesion shows slightly lower echogenicity than the surrounding liver parenchyma in the portal or late phases preceded by hyper-enhancement in the arterial phase.
(3) No washout—when the lesion enhances in the similar degree or higher degree as the surrounding liver parenchyma in the portal or late phases preceded by hyper-enhancement in the arterial phase.

The tumor contrast kinetics was analyzed by review on the recorded clips. The time of contrast first appearance, the time of peak maximum enhancement in the arterial phase, time of emergence of washout, in comparison to the surrounding liver tissue was documented. Intensity of peak maximum enhancement of tumor in the arterial phase, intensity of tumor enhancement in late part of the portal phase (still frames from the CEUS cine clips 90–120 seconds after contrast agent injection) and intensity of tumor enhancement of the late phase (still frames from the CEUS cine clips 170–190 seconds after contrast agent injection)were measured suing a Sonomath software (AMBITION BIOTRCH, Chongqing, China).A circular region of interest (ROI) with a size corresponding to that of the tumor and another ROI in the adjacent non-tumor liver parenchyma with similar depth were manually drawn.Tumor/tissue ratio of enhancement intensity was calculated by dividing enhancement intensity of tumor with enhancement intensity of adjacent liver parenchyma in the same still image.

CT scan

Abdomen CT was performed with multi-detector-row CT (MDCT, Definition, Siemens, Erlangen, Germany) using a 4 phase contras-enhanced protocol (unenhanced, hepatic arterial, portal venous, and delayed phases). First, an unenhanced scan was obtained through the liver. Next, after intravenous infusion of 2 ml/kg of a nonionic iodine-containing contrast agent (ultravist 370, Scherning AG, Berlin, Germany) using a power injector (Stellant CT Injection System, Medrad, Indianola, Pennsylvania) at a rate of 4.0 ml/sec. Contrast-enhanced scans were obtained in arterial with bolus test trigger for optimal characterization of focal hepatic lesions. Data acquisitions were obtained through the whole liver in a craniocaudal direction during a single breath-hold helical acquisition for 4–6 sec with 5 mm slice thickness and 0.5 s rotation time. The acquisition of the arterial phase was automatically started 5 s after contrast agent reaching the threshold in the aorta. The start of acquisition sequences was 60 s for the portal venous phase and 180 s for the delayed phase.

Categorization of enhancement patterns at CT

The enhancement through each of the different phases after intravenous contrast administration was registered as follows: (1) globally hyperdense: increased signal relative to the surrounding

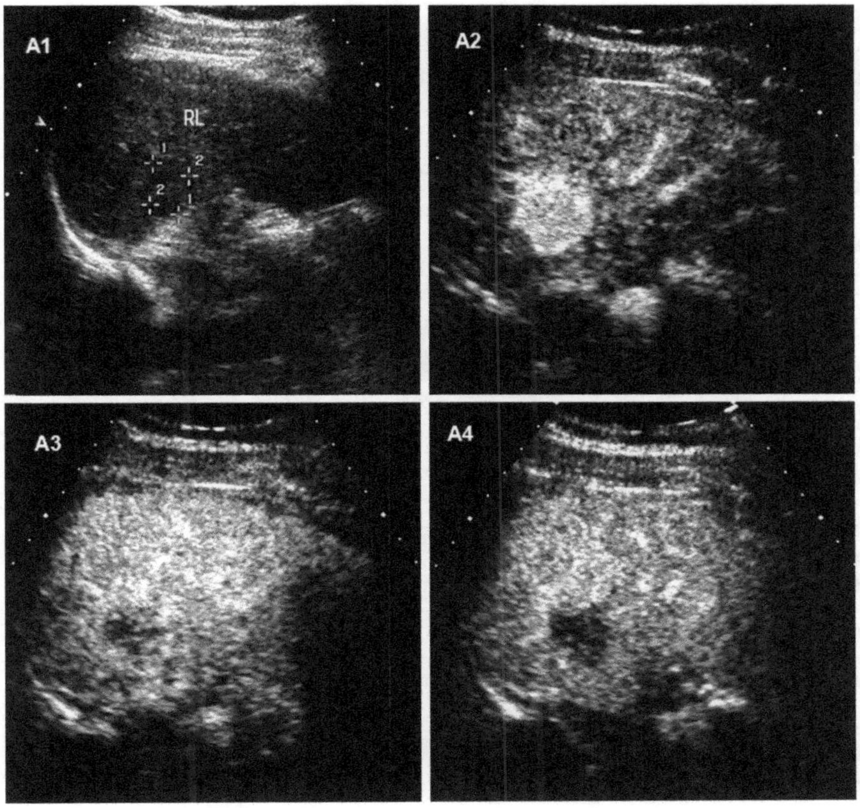

Figure 1. Intrahepatic cholangiocellular carcinoma (ICC) in a 48-year old man with cirrhosis. A1 Conventional ultrasound shows a hypoechoic nodule of 22 mm in diameter in the right lobe of liver. A2 On contrast-enhanced ultrasound, the lesion appears as homogeneous hyperenhancement 19 seconds after the administration of contrast agent. A3 The lesion shows first wash-out 38 seconds after the injection of contrast agent. A4 The lesion appears as marked wash-out at 50 seconds after the administration of contrast agent.

liver parenchyma, involving the totality of the lesion; (2) partially hyperdense: increased signal involving more than 25% of the lesion cross-section area with a non-homogeneous distribution; (3)peripherally hyperdense: increased signal limited to the periphery of the lesion, involving less than 25% of its area, resembling a rim-like pattern; (4) isodense: same density as the surrounding liver parenchyma; (5) hypodense: lower density compared to the liver parenchyma involving more than half of the cross-sectional area of the tumor. Dynamic pattern of enhancement was defined according to the analysis of the progression of contrast enhancement over the progressive different phases of the study, as follows: (1) stable persistent contrast enhancement: the nodule enhancement is unmodified from the arterial to the portal venous and delayed phases; (2) progressive contrast enhancement: the nodule enhances progressively over time, reaching maximal intensity in delayed phases; (3) 'wash-out' pattern: global/partial hyperdense of the lesion during the arterial phase followed by hypodense in portal and/or delayed venous phases; (4) all other cases. This classification was adopted from Rimola et al [13]and lavarone et al[14]

CT findings were evaluated in consensus by 2 abdominal radiologists (PC and SYD) with 14 and 22 years of experience in liver radiology who were blinded to the contrast-enhanced ultrasonographic findings and pathological results of the tumors.

Statistical analysis

We performed a per-patient analysis in this study. Baseline characteristics of the patients are expressed as median and range or count and proportion. Comparison of patients with ICC and patients with HCC was done by using the Student t test for continuous variables and Fisher, s exact test for categorical variables. A P value of less than 0.05 was considered statistically significant. Statistical analysis were performed using the SPSS 13.0 software package (SPSS Inc, Chicago, IL)

Results

Characteristics of the patients

Due to the inclusion–exclusion criteria of the study,some ICC patients were excluded because they had: (1) ICC without histological evidence for liver cirrhosis (n = 84); (2) mixed hepatocellular-cholangiocellular carcinomain in cirrhotic patients (n = 28).Finally, this retrospective search yielded a total 33 histologically proven ICC in cirrhotic patients. Twenty six cases of ICC were diagnosed histologically after resection (78.8%) and 7 cases after biopsy (21.2%). Some HCC patients were excluded because: (1) No histological evidence for liver cirrhosis (n = 392); (2)Transarterial chemoembolization therapy prior to CEUS (n = 140).Fifty histologically proven HCC (10 well differentiated HCC,25moderately differentiated HCC and 15 poorly differentiated HCC) were randomly selected from 897 HCC in cirrhotic patients to form the HCC study group. Forty eight cases of HCC were diagnosed histologically after resection (96%) and 2 cases after biopsy (4%). The characteristics of the cirrhotic patients with ICC and HCC are presented in Table 1. Patients with ICC and HCC showed no statistical difference in terms of age, sex, etiology, Child-Pugh class and tumor size. Patients with HCC had higher

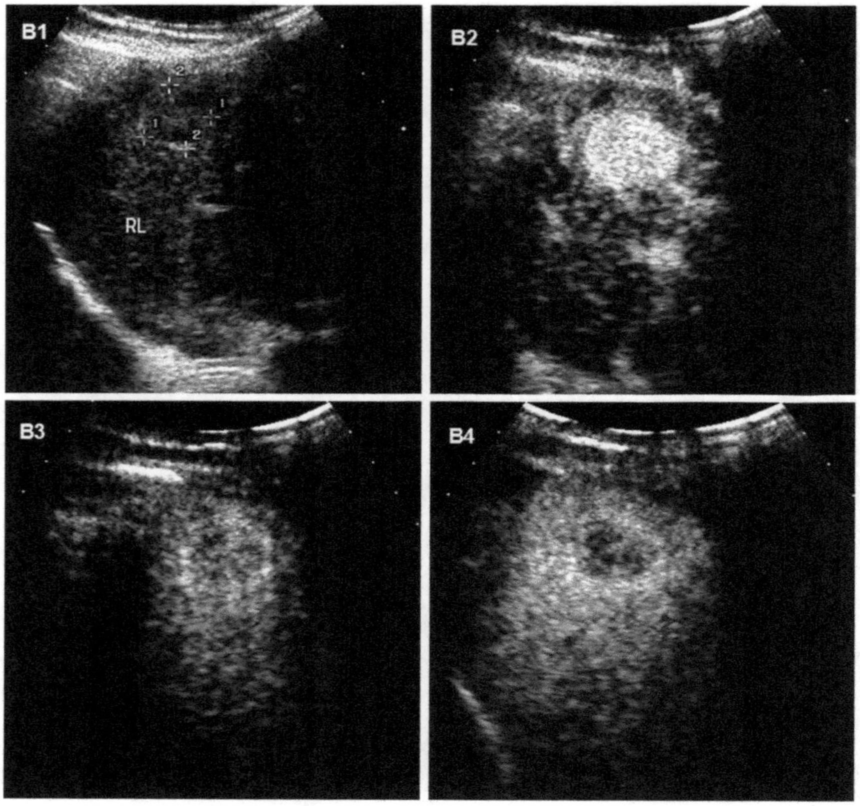

Figure 2. Hepatocellular carcinoma (HCC) with moderate differentiation in a 31-year old man with cirrhosis. B1 Conventional ultrasound displays a hypoechoic nodule of 20 mm in the right lobe of liver. B2 The lesion shows homogeneous hyperenhancement 16 seconds after the administration of contrast agent. B3 The lesion shows first wash-out appearance at 95 seconds after injection of contrast agent. B4 The lesion appears as mild wash-out 179 seconds after the administration of contrast agent.

AFP levels than those with ICC.AFP exceeded 200 ng/ml in more HCC patients (38.0%) than that in ICC patients (12.1%, $p=0.032$).The echogenicity patterns of ICC were similar to that of HCC on conventional ultrasound.

Characteristics of CEUS enhancement

The perfusion characteristics of ICC and HCC on CEUS are demonstrated in Table 2.The parametric measurement of ICC and HCC perfusion features at CEUS are presented in Table 3.

Arterial phase assessment

Statistical analysis did not reveal significant difference between ICC and HCC in the time of contrast first appearance of tumor, arterial peak maximum time of tumor, and the proportion of homogeneous hyper-enhancement and heterogeneous hyper-enhancement in the arterial phase. The results of software calculation indicated that the peak intensity of tumor and tumor/tissue ratio of intensity were lower in ICC than that in HCC in arterial phase ($p<0.05$).

Portal phase assessment

ICC displayed much earlier washout than that of HCC (47.9±26.45 seconds vs 90.9±31.26 seconds) in portal phase, and most ICC (87.9%) showed washout within 60 seconds post contrast agent injection (Fig 1) than HCC did while much more HCC (84.0%) revealed washout after 60 seconds (Fig 2). Under visual assessment by the operator, much more ICC (78.8%) revealed marked washout (Fig 3) than HCC (12.0%) while most HCC showed mild washout or no washout (Fig 4) in late part of the portal phase (90–120 seconds after contrast agent injection). In addition, the results of software calculation indicated that the extent of washout of tumor and tumor/tissue ratio of intensity were lower in ICC than that in HCC during late part of the portal phase ($p<0.05$). The onset of washout and peak extent of washout (tumor/tissue ratio of intensity) in portal phases were demonstrated in plotted graphs (Fig 5,Fig6). Measurement of tumor/tissue ratio of intensity rather than tumor intensity only was adopted to reflect peak extent of washout in the portal phase because washout was defined as when the lesion displays lower echogenicity than the surrounding liver parenchyma in the portal or late phases preceded by hyper-enhancement in the arterial phase.

Twenty six out of thirty three ICC (78.8%) demonstrated both early washout (<60seconds) and marked washout in late part of the portal phase, whereas, only six of fifty HCC (12.0%) showed this temporal enhancement features ($p=0.000$).

Late phase assessment

Marked washout was displayed in more ICC nodules than in HCC nodules (90.9% vs 44.0%) while more HCC nodules showed mild washout or no washout than ICC nodules did in the late phase (56.0% vs 9.1%). The results of software calculation demonstrated that the extent of washout of tumor and tumor/tissue ratio of intensity were lower in ICC than that in HCC during the late phase ($p<0.01$).

Typical dynamic vascular pattern for ICC on CEUS was considered both early washout(<60seconds) and marked washout

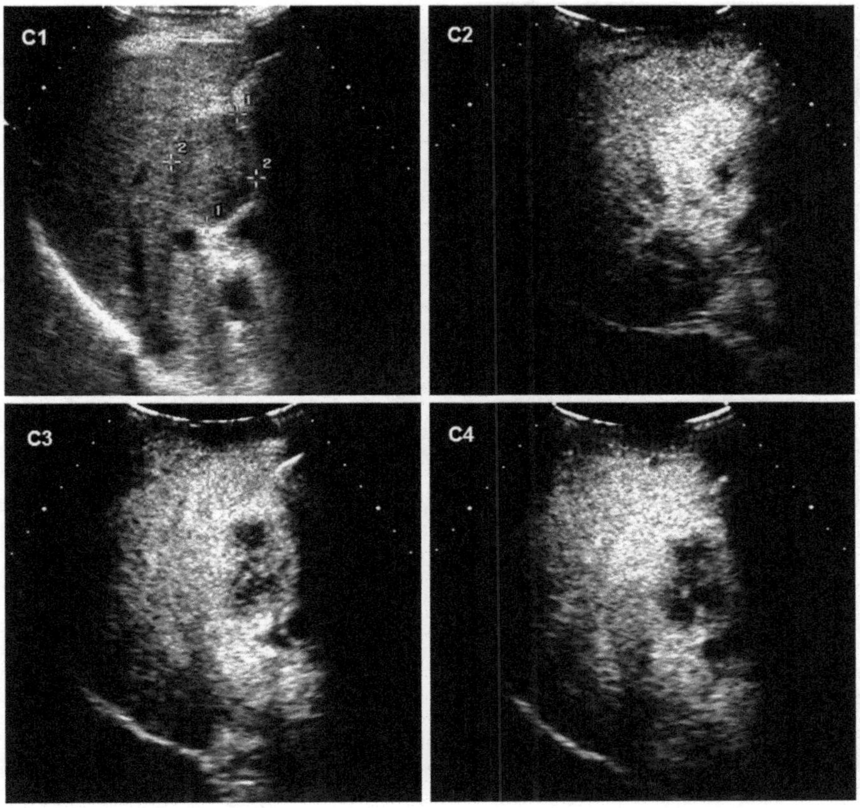

Figure 3. Intrahepatic cholangiocellular carcinoma (ICC) in a 42-year old man with cirrhosis. C1 Conventional ultrasound shows a hypoechoic nodule of 46 mm in diameter in the right lobe of liver. C2 The lesion displays heterogeneous hyperenhancement 23 seconds after the administration of contrast agent at CEUS. C3 The lesion shows first wash-out appearance 48 seconds after injection of contrast agent. C4 The lesion appears as marked wash-out 91 seconds after the administration of contrast agent.

during late part of the portal phase (90–120 seconds after contrast agent injection) in this study. When this criterion was applied, the diagnostic sensitivity, specificity, positive predictive value, negative predictive value and accuracy were 78.8%,88.0%,81.3%,86.3%,and 84.3% respectively by CEUS.

Of the ICC group, 31 cases had contras-enhanced CT scan and only 1case had MRI scan. Of the HCC group, 48 cases received contras-enhanced CT scan and no patient had MRI scan. Analysis of the dynamic enhancement pattern throughout the different vascular phases in 31 ICC patients showed 14 ICC (45.2%) had a progressive enhancement pattern, 6 ICC (19.4%) stable enhancement pattern, 9 ICC (29.0%) washout enhancement pattern, and 2 ICC (6.5%)other enhancement pattern (one ICC showed peripheral hyperdence in both arterial and portal phases followed by isodense in the delayed phase,the other ICC had isodense in the arterial phase, peripheral hyperdence in the portal phase and followed by hypodence in the delayed phase). The dynamic enhancement pattern throughout the different vascular phases in 48 HCC patients were as follow: 3 HCC (6.3%) had progressive enhancement pattern, 6 HCC (12.5%) stable enhancement pattern, 38 HCC (79.2%) washout enhancement pattern, and1 HCC (2.1%) other enhancement pattern (global hyperdence in both arterial and portal phases followed by isodense in the delayed phase).

Typical dynamic vascular pattern for ICC on contrast enhanced CT was considered either progressive enhancement pattern or stable enhancement pattern [14].When this criterion was adopted, the diagnostic sensitivity, specificity, positive predictive value, negative predictive value and accuracy were 64.5%,81.3%,69.0%,78.0%,and 74.7% respectively by contrast enhanced CT.

Statistical analysis showed no difference in the diagnostic sensitivity, specificity, positive predictive value, negative predictive value and accuracy between CEUS and contrast enhanced CT ($p>0.05$).

Discussion

CEUS has been introduced about 10 years ago for characterization of focal liver lesions, and its excellent diagnostic value established by many prospective studies including the German DEGUM-study with over 1000 patients [15] and the French multicentre study [16]. CEUS was proven able to characterize liver tumors with at least the same accuracy range as contrast enhanced computed tomography and contrast enhanced magnetic resonance imaging [17,18]. Therefore, CEUS has been included together with CT and MRI in the imaging techniques accepted for the non-invasive diagnosis of HCC in the guidelines from the American Association for the Study of Liver Diseases (AASLD) 2005[4]. However, in a retrospective series of 21 patients with histologically confirmed ICC on cirrhosis collected between 2003 and 2009, the Barcelona Clinic Liver Cancer (BCLC) group found that ten ICC had similar CEUS enhancement pattern considered diagnostic for HCC, consisting in homogeneous arterial hyperenhancement followed by washout [9].Based on the results of this study, CEUS has been dropped from the diagnostic techniques of nodules in cirrhosis in the updated AASLD guidelines 2011[19]

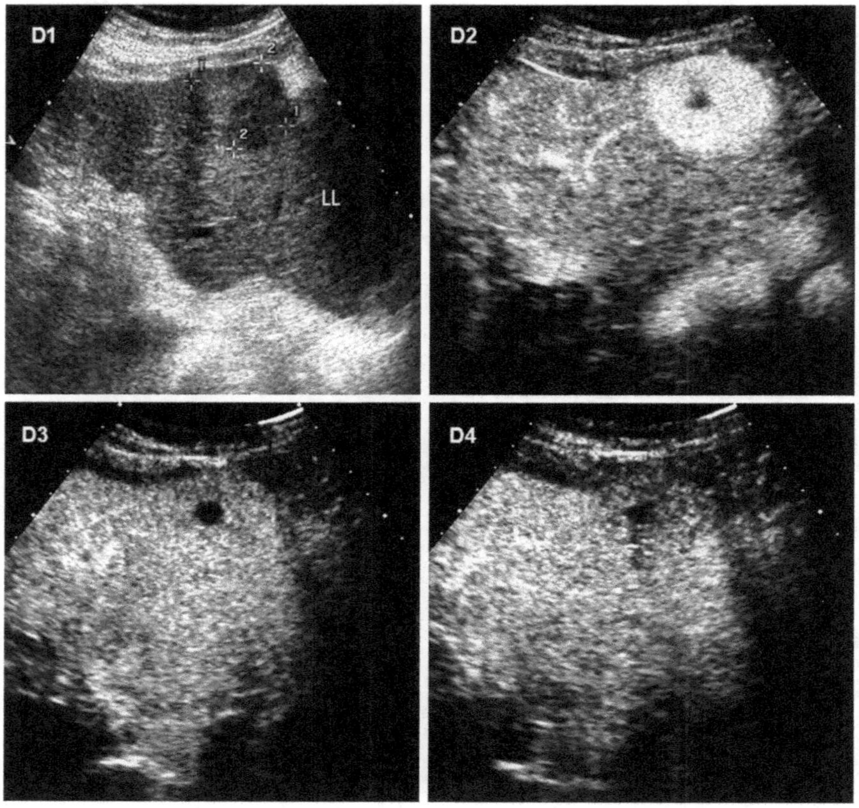

Figure 4. Hepatocellular carcinoma (HCC) with moderate differentiation in a 72-year old man with cirrhosis. D1 Conventional ultrasound shows a hypoechoic nodule of 41 mm in diameter in the left lobe (L L) of liver. D2 The lesion shows heterogeneous hyperenhancement 25 seconds after the administration of contrast agent at CEUS, the non-hyperenhancement area at the central part of the lesion indicating necrosis. D3 The lesion shows no wash-out appearance 60 second after injection of contrast agent. D4 The lesion displays mild wash-out 185 seconds after the administration of contrast agent.

and subsequently also from the guidelines of European Association for the study of the liver (EASL) [5].However, this removal has been raised much controversial arguments and was not well received in Europe and Asia[12].

The results of our study revealed arterial peak intensity of tumor and tumor/tissue ratio of intensity in the arterial phase were lower in ICC than that of HCC, and this was in agreement with a previous study [20].Our study demonstrated that 69.7% of ICC with heterogeneous hyper-enhancement and 30.3% of ICC with homogeneous hyper-enhancement in the arterial phase and 88% of ICC had early wash out in 60 seconds. The rate of ICC showing homogeneous hyper-enhancement in the arterial phase is lower than those of two previous studies (47.6% and 52% respectively) by Vilana et al [9] and Galassi [11].More ICC demonstrated early washout in our study than those reported by Vilana et al [9] which

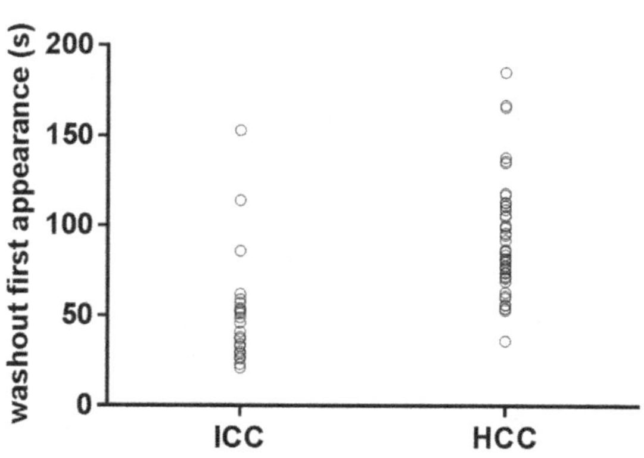

Figure 5. Frequency distribution of washout onset in portal phase (seconds). Washout onset is earlier in patients with intrahepatic cholangiocellular carcinoma (ICC) than in those with hepatocellular carcinoma (HCC).

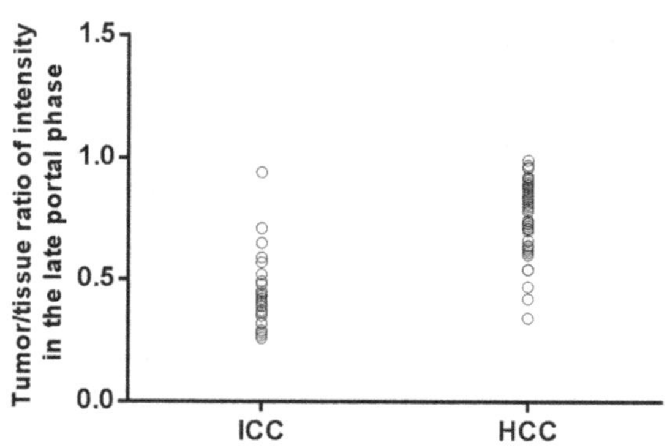

Figure 6. Frequency distribution of peak extent of washout in portal phase (Tumor/tissue ratio of intensity) in portal phase. The peak extent of washout is greater in patients with intrahepatic cholangiocellular carcinoma (ICC) than in those with hepatocellular carcinoma (HCC).

showed that 29% of ICC had washout beyond 120 seconds. An explanation of this difference could be the tumor size, which was larger in our study (median size of the tumors was 40 mm) as compared with the other two studies (median tumor size was 32 mm and 29 mm respectively).Another possible reason could be the etiology of cirrhosis. In the present study, 28 of the 33 (84.8%) patients with ICC were positive for HBsAg. In contrast, most patients with ICC (62.5% and 71.4% respectively) in cirrhotic liver were related to HCV infection in the two previous studies [9,11].The rate of hepatitis B infection in ICC of our study is really much higher than other countries. Actually, most HCC occur in patients with cirrhosis in Asia, especially in China. Patients with cirrhosis who undergo surveillance may have an earlier stage of HCC at diagnosis [21]. Unfortunately, surveillance for HCC in patients with cirrhosis is recommended but may not be successfully performed. Less than 20% of patients with cirrhosis who developed HCC received regular surveillance in the United States [22].HCC were detected during surveillance in the minority of patients even at major referral center[23].Surveillance for HCC is still not a consolidated practice as it should be[24]. Previous study also demonstrated that more than half of ICC (11/21, 52.4%) in cirrhosis were larger than 30 mm in size, and the largest one reached 70 mm [9].Therefore, differential diagnosis of large ICC from large HCC is still a more common clinical situation worldwide for the majority of liver tumors are found not at very early stage in cirrhotic patients. It is necessary to point out that large nodules showing heterogeneous hyper-enhancement in arterial phase followed by washout in the portal or late venous phase are also liable to the diagnosis of HCC, for CEUS definition of HCC was complete hypervascularity or partial hypervascularity (due to non-enhancing areas indicating necrosis) in arterial phase with a chaotic and irregular vascularisation followed by hypo-enhancing pattern in portal or late phase [8]. Therefore, typical enhancement pattern for HCC should not be confined to global hyper-enhancement in arterial phase followed by washout in the portal or late venous phase.

The present study demonstrated that most ICC (87.9%) showed washout before 60 seconds than HCC did (16.0%).Vilana et al also reported that half of ICC in cirrhosis showed washout before 60 seconds at CEUS [9]. Galassi et al found that more than half of ICC showed washout during portal phase though it was not specified the exact timing of first occurrence of washout [11].On the other hand, Boozari et al [25] reported in a prospective study in cirrhotic patients that even moderately or poorly differentiated HCC had a rather late onset of washout (120±71.8 seconds) and it is longer in well differentiated HCC (164±2.1seconds),indicating most HCC manifest much slower washout appearance in cirrhosis.

In this study, we found that much more ICC (78.8%) displayed marked washout than HCC did while most HCC (88%) showed mild washout or no washout in late part of the portal phase. Mild or moderate wash-out is considering as typical for HCC by the recent release of the EFSUMB liver CEUS guidelines [26].

Further analysis of our data revealed that most ICC (78.8%) demonstrated both early washout(<60seconds) and marked washout during late part of the portal phase, whereas, only few cases of HCC (12.0%) showed this temporal enhancement features. When these dynamic CEUS features were applied in differentiating ICC and HCC in cirrhosis, CEUS has similar diagnostic efficacy to contrast enhanced multi-detector-row CT. The possibility to grade the intensity of the wash-out in the late venous phase applies to all contrast imaging techniques (including CEUS,CT and MRI), whereas the possibility to establish an accurate temporal pattern of enhancement belongs to CEUS only, due to it's a real time imaging modality [26,27,28].

Therefore, our data are satisfactory to state that when a nodule displayed early washout (namely before 60 seconds post contrast agent injection) and marked washout in late part of the portal phase at CEUS in cirrhosis, it is no longer typical for HCC, but highly suspicious of ICC.

There were some limitations to our study. First, it was limited by its retrospective nature though we provide a relatively large series of pathologically proven ICC in cirrhosis seen at CEUS and contrast-enhanced multiphasic multi-detector CT. Our results need to be validated in prospective studies in the future though it is difficult because the low incidence of ICC in cirrhosis. Second, it is impossible for us to compare the diagnostic efficacy of CEUS and MRI because only one case out of 33 cases of ICC had MRI scan in our series, and this reflects the fact that in many countries worldwide, with a high incidence of HCC, the availability of MRI is very low.

In conclusion, the data of our study demonstrated that analysis of detailed temporal enhancement features on CEUS may help differentiate ICC from HCC in cirrhosis.If a nodule in cirrhotic liver displays hyper-enhancement in the arterial phase followed by early and marked washout in the portal phase, the nodule is highly suspicious of ICC rather than HCC. when considering a refinement of CEUS diagnosis by more detailed temporal features, namely, timing of washout emergence and degree of intensity of washout in the portal phase, the proportion of ICC cases at risk of misdiagnosis with HCC would decreased in cirrhotic patients.

Author Contributions

Conceived and designed the experiments: RL. Performed the experiments: X-HZ K-sM X-WL M-XY C-LT D-YG X-CY. Analyzed the data: M-XY C-LT. Contributed reagents/materials/analysis tools: D-YG X-CY. Wrote the paper: RL. Interpretation of Contrast-Enhanced Ultrasound: RL X-HZ. Collection of Contrast-Enhanced Ultrasound Data: M-XY C-lT. Analysis of Contrast-Enhanced Ultrasound Data: M-XY C-lT. Interpretation of clinical data, liver surgery. K-sM X-WL. Interpretation of pathology: D-YG X-CY.

References

1. Rimola J, Forner A, Tremosini S, Reig M, Vilana R, et al. (2012) Non-invasive diagnosis of hepatocellular carcinoma 2 cm in cirrhosis. Diagnostic accuracy assessing fat, capsule and signal intensity at dynamic MRI. J Hepatol 56:1317–1323.
2. Serste T, Barrau V, Ozenne V, Vullierme MP, Bedossa P, et al. (2012) Accuracy and disagreement of computed tomography and magnetic resonance imaging for the diagnosis of small hepatocellular carcinoma and dysplastic nodules: role of biopsy. Hepatology 55:800–806.
3. Shaib Y, El-Serag HB (2004) The epidemiology of cholangiocarcinoma. Semin Liver Dis 24: 115–125.
4. Bruix J, Sherman M (2005) Management of hepatocellular carcinoma. Hepatology 42: 1208–1236.
5. EASL-EORTC (2012) Clinical practice guidelines Management of hepatocellular carcinoma. J Hepatol 56: 908–943.
6. Khan SA, Thomas HC, Davidson BR, Taylor-Robinson SD (2005) Cholangiocarcinoma. Lancet 366:1303–1314.
7. Blechacz B, GoresGJ (2008) Cholangiocarcinoma: Advances in Pathogenesis, Diagnosis, and Treatment. Hepatology 48:308–319.
8. Claudon M, Cosgrove D, Albrecht T, Bolondi L, Bosio M, et al. (2008) Guidelines and good clinical practice recommendations for contrast enhanced ultrasound (CEUS) - update 2008. Ultraschall Med 29: 28–44.
9. Vilana R, Forner A, Bianchi L, Garcia-Criado A, Rimola J, et al. (2010) Intrahepatic peripheral cholangiocarcinoma in cirrhosis patients may display a vascular pattern similar to hepatocellular carcinoma on contrast-enhanced ultrasound. Hepatology 51:2020–2029.
10. Li R, Zhang XH, Ma KS, Li XW, Xia F, et al. (2013) Dynamic enhancing vascular pattern of intrahepatic peripheral cholangiocarcinoma on contrast-enhanced ultrasound: the influence of chronic hepatitis and cirrhosis. Abdom Imaging 38: 112–119.

11. GalassiM, Iavarone M, Rossi S, Bota S, Vavassori S, et al. (2013) Patterns of appearance and risk of misdiagnosis of intrahepatic cholangiocarcinoma in cirrhosis at contrast enhanced ultrasound. Liver International 33:771–779.
12. Barreiros AP, Piscaglia F, Dietrich CF (2012) Contrast enhanced ultrasound for the diagnosis of hepatocellular carcinoma(HCC): comments on AASLD guidelines. J Hepatol 57:930–932.
13. Rimola J, Forner A, Reig M, Vilana R, Rodríguez-Lope C, et al. (2009) Cholangiocarcinoma in cirrhosis: absence of contrast washout in delayed phases by magnetic resonance imaging avoids misdiagnosis of hepatocellular carcinoma. Hepatology 50:791–798.
14. Iavarone M, Piscaglia F, Vavassori S, Galassi M, Sangiovanni A, et al. (2013) Contrast enhanced CT-scan to diagnose intrahepatic cholangiocarcinoma in patients with cirrhosis. J Hepatol 58:1188–1193.
15. Strobel D, Seitz K, Blank W, Schuler A, Dietrich C, et al. (2008) Contrast-enhanced ultrasound for the characterization of focal liver lesions diagnostic accuracy in clinical practice (DEGUM multicentre trial). Ultraschall Med 29: 499–505.
16. Tranquart F, Correas JM, Ladam Marcus V, Manzoni P, Vilqrain V, et al. (2009) Real time contrast-enhanced ultrasound in the evaluation of focal liver lesions: diagnostic efficacy and economical issues from a French multicentric study. J Radiol 90:109–22.
17. Dietrich CF, Kratzer W, Strobe D, Danse E, Fessl R, et al. (2006) Assessment of metastatic liver disease in patients with primary extrahepatic tumors by contrast-enhanced sonography versus CT and MRI. World J Gastroenterol 12:1699–1705.
18. Sangiovanni A, Manini MA, Iavarone M, Romeo R,Forzenigo LV, et al. (2010) The diagnostic and economic impact of contrast imaging techniques in the diagnosis of small hepatocellular carcinoma in cirrhosis. Gut 59:638–644.
19. Bruix J, Sherman M (2011) Management of hepatocellular carcinoma: an update. Hepatology 53:1020–1022.
20. Chen LD, Xu HX, Xie XY, Xie XH, Xu ZF, et al. (2010) Intrahepatic cholangiocarcinoma and hepatocellular carcinoma: differential diagnosis with contrast-enhanced ultrasound. Eue Radiol 20:743–753.
21. Bolondi L, Sofia S, Siringo S, Gaiani S, Casali A, et al. (2001) Surveillance program of cirrhotic patients for early diagnosis and treatment of hepatocellular carcinoma: a cost effectiveness analysis. Gut 48:251–259.
22. Davila JA, Morgan RO, Richardson PA, Du XL, McGlynn KA, et al. (2010) Use of surveillance for hepatocellular carcinoma among patients with cirrhosis in the United States. Hepatology 52:132–141.
23. Yang JD, Harmsen WS, Slettedahl SW, Chaiteerakij R, Enders FT, et al. (2011) Factors that affect risk for hepatocellular carcinomaand effects of surveillance. Clin Gastroenterology Hepatology 9: 617–623.
24. Editorial (2011) Surveillance for hepatocellular carcinoma: a standard of care, not a clinical option. Hepatology 54: 1898–1900.
25. Boozari B, Soudah B, Rifai K, Schneidewind S, Vogel A, et al. (2011) Grading of hypervascular hepatocellular carcinoma using late phase of contrast enhanced sonography - a prospective study. Dig Liver Dis43: 484–90.
26. Claudon M, Dietrich CF, Choi BI, Cosgrove DO, Kudo M, et al. (2013) Guidelines and Good Clinical Practice Recommendations for Contrast Enhanced Ultrasound (CEUS) in the Liver-Update 2012. Ultraschall Med 34: 11–29.
27. Bolondi L, Correas JM, Lencioni R, Weskott HP, Piscaglia F (2007) New perspectives for the use of contrast-enhanced liver ultrasound in clinical practice. Dig Liver Dis 39:187–195.
28. Lencioni R, Piscaglia F, Bolondi L (2008) Contrast-enhanced ultrasound in the diagnosis of hepatocellular carcinoma. J Hepatol 48:848–857.

12

Demonstration of Metabolic and Cellular Effects of Portal Vein Ligation using Multi-Modal PET/MRI Measurements in Healthy Rat Liver

András Fülöp[1*◑], Attila Szijártó[1◑], László Harsányi[1], András Budai[1], Damján Pekli[1], Diána Korsós[1], Ildikó Horváth[2], Noémi Kovács[3], Kinga Karlinger[4], Domokos Máthé[3¶], Krisztián Szigeti[2¶]

1 1st Department of Surgery, Semmelweis University, Budapest, Hungary, **2** Department of Biophysics and Radiation Biology, Semmelweis University, Budapest, Hungary, **3** CROmed Translational Research Centers, Budapest, Hungary, **4** Department of Radiology and Oncotherapy, Semmelweis University, Budapest, Hungary

Abstract

Objectives: In the early recognition of portal vein ligation (PVL) induced tumor progression, positron emission tomography and magnetic resonance imaging (PET/MRI) could improve diagnostic accuracy of conventionally used methods. It is unknown how PVL affects metabolic patterns of tumor free hepatic tissues. The aim of this preliminary study is to evaluate the effect of PVL on glucose metabolism, using PET/MRI imaging in healthy rat liver.

Materials and Methods: Male Wistar rats (n = 30) underwent PVL. 2-deoxy-2-(^{18}F)fluoro-D-glucose (FDG) PET/MRI imaging (nanoScan PET/MRI) and morphological/histological examination were performed before (Day 0) and 1, 2, 3, and 7 days after PVL. Dynamic PET data were collected and the standardized uptake values (SUV) for ligated and non-ligated liver lobes were calculated in relation to cardiac left ventricle (SUV_{VOI}/SUV_{CLV}) and mean liver SUV (SUV_{VOI}/SUV_{Liver}).

Results: PVL induced atrophy of ligated lobes, while non-ligated liver tissue showed compensatory hypertrophy. Dynamic PET scan revealed altered FDG kinetics in both ligated and non-ligated liver lobes. SUV_{VOI}/SUV_{CLV} significantly increased in both groups of lobes, with a maximal value at the 2nd postoperative day and returned near to the baseline 7 days after the ligation. After PVL, ligated liver lobes showed significantly higher tracer uptake compared to the non-ligated lobes (significantly higher SUV_{VOI}/SUV_{Liver} values were observed at postoperative day 1, 2 and 3). The homogenous tracer biodistribution observed before PVL reappeared by 7th postoperative day.

Conclusion: The observed alterations in FDG uptake dynamics should be taken into account during the assessment of PET data until the PVL induced atrophic and regenerative processes are completed.

Editor: Vincent Wong, The Chinese University of Hong Kong, Hong Kong

Funding: The work leading to this invention has received funding from the European Union's Seventh Framework Program (FP7/2007-2013) under grant agreement n° HEALTH-F2-2011-278850 (INMiND). This study was supported in part by the European Community FP7 Transnational Access grant QNANO. The funders had no role in study design, data collection and analysis, decision to publish, or preparation of the manuscript. No other current funding sources were involved in this study.

Competing Interests: Domokos Ma´the´ and Noe´mi Kova´cs are employees of CROmed. CROmed does not have any financial, or non-financial interest in the subject matter or materials discussed in this manuscript. The other authors declare that they have no conflict of interest.

* E-mail: fulop.andras2@gmail.com

◑ These authors contributed equally to this work.

¶ These authors also contributed equally to this work.

Introduction

Despite advances in chemotherapy regimens and ablative techniques, extended hepatectomy is considered as a gold standard for the treatment of primary and secondary liver cancers. [1–3] Nevertheless, surgical resection can be accomplished only in 20–30% of the cases, due to insufficient amount of remaining liver mass after hepatectomy (future remnant liver volume; FRLV). [4] It is known for decades that occlusion of the portal vein results in atrophy of the occluded liver lobe, while owing to the unique regeneration capacity, the unoccluded liver tissue shows compensatory hypertrophy. [5] Based on this observation portal vein occlusion techniques, such as portal vein ligation (PVL) or embolization (PVE), have been introduced to increase the future volume of the remnant liver before major liver resection. [6] Considering that at the time of diagnosis most liver malignancies show multiple bilateral patterns, a two-stage resection with portal vein occlusion has recently been developed. During the first stage of this novel treatment procedure, small metastasectomies in the potential future remnant liver in combination with the occlusion of the contralateral portal vein are performed with or without chemotherapy. In the second curative stage, after compensatory hypertrophy of cleared unoccluded lobes, the portal-deprived liver lobes with residual tumors are removed. [7].

Although, the above detailed two-stage procedure is more widely used, there is increasing evidence that PVL/PVE-induced changes have a strong stimulatory effect on tumor growth as well. Thus, there might be an increased risk, that portal vein occlusion could stimulate not only the growth of future remnant liver, but also significantly affects tumor size and tumor spread in both occluded and non-occluded liver segments. [8] Several clinical and preclinical studies have demonstrated the increased proliferative activity of malignant cells after preoperative portal vein occlusion. [9–11] Tumor progression in the liver between the time of PVL/PVE and the next phase of hepatectomy is responsible for the majority of changes into irresectable state which occurs in approximately 20% of the cases of planned for two-stage surgeries. [12,13].

The average time to achieve optimal FRLV (optimal time of the second, curative operation) is approximately 1 month after PVL/PVE. [14] During this waiting period, the monitoring of regenerative process and tumor progression are essential. In a clinical scenario, computed tomography (CT) is currently the gold-standard method of assessing the increase in FRLV. [15] However, CT volumetry may not be reliable in the detection of residual tumor growth, because the accuracy of CT is poor for smaller (<0.2–1 cm) tumor sizes. [16] MRI, especially with liver-specific contrast agents, could improve the sensitivity by providing better soft-tissue contrast, but is not sufficiently specific leading to number of false positive lesions. [17] These drawbacks of morphological imaging techniques indicate the importance of additional functional imaging assays, which could more specifically recognize tumor progression during two-stage hepatectomy combined with portal vein ligation.

In clinical oncology positron emission tomography (PET) is an extremely valuable tool for tumor diagnosis, staging, restaging and for treatment response follow-up. [18] To image hepatic neoplasia several PET radiopharmaceuticals are available, such as [^{11}C]-acetate, [^{11}C]-choline and 2-deoxy-2-(^{18}F)fluoro-D-glucose (FDG). In the oncologic use of PET, however, FDG is the most commonly used tracer, which is able to assess the typically enhanced glucose transport and metabolism in malignant tumors. FDG was found to be superior in detecting residual tumor growth and tumor recurrence compared to morphologic imaging procedures, furthermore, FDG-PET is the primary imaging modality for detection of distant (extrahepatic) metastasis. [19] Although, FDG is an excellent tracer in case of tumor localization, it is not tumor specific. [20] Increased FDG uptake was observed in several energy-intensive processes such as inflammation, as well as during regeneration. The regenerative and atrophic process induced by the ligation/embolization of portal vein is associated with not only volumetric, but also with hemodynamic and metabolic changes. [21] These complex alterations after PVL/PVE may also affect the FDG uptake patterns of tumor free hepatic tissues, which constitute a challenge in the differentiation of these processes from intrahepatic tumor spread. Therefore, unfolding the changes regarding FDG uptake after PVL/PVE in a tumor free, healthy liver is essential in the early recognition of tumor progression.

There is no study in the literature that assesses the changes in FDG uptake pattern of normal liver after PVL/PVE. Kinetic FDG data combined with volumetric information available from MR imaging of the liver, are more reliable than PET alone or PET/CT. Thus, the aim of our present study was to selectively evaluate dynamics of FDG uptake in occluded and non-occluded liver lobes by in vivo multimodal FDG PET-MRI (nanoScan PET/MRI) in a well-established rat model of portal vein ligation.

Materials and Methods

Portal Vein Ligation (PVL)

The experimental design was regulated in strict adherence to the National Institutes of Health guidelines for animal care and approved by Committee on Animal Experimentation of Semmelweis University (permit number: 22.1/2408/3/2011 and XIV-I-001/29-7/2012). 200–250 g male Wistar rats (Charles River Hungary Ltd., Budapest, Hungary) were kept on standard chow and water *ad libitum* in specific, pathogen-free conditions at 22–24°C with a 12-hour light-dark cycles. Animals were allowed to acclimatize for 1 week before starting experiments. After intraperitoneal injection of ketamine (75 mg/kg) and xylazine (7.5 mg/kg), animals were placed in a supine position and median laparotomy was performed. The median and left lateral lobes were gently mobilized to reveal the portal pedicels. Under operating microscope (Zeiss Opmi Surgical Microscope, Carl Zeiss Meditec AG, Jena, Germany) the portal branches feeding the median, left lateral and caudate lobes (approximately 80% of total liver mass) were dissected and completely ligated with 6–0 silk. Great care was taken to avoid damaging the vulnerable hepatic artery and bile duct. At the end of the procedure the liver lobes were gently repositioned anatomically, the peritoneal cavity was closed in two layers by running suture (4–0) and the animals were returned to their cages until further examination. Before (0 day) and 1, 2, 3, 7 days after portal vein ligation, rats were sacrificed by exsanguination for histological analysis. The liver was removed and the ligated and non-ligated lobes were weighted separately after expulsion of blood by gentle compression with gauze. Liver specimens were taken from the excised left lateral lobe (ligated lobe) and the superior right lobe (non-ligated lobe). Samples were fixed in 4% neutral-buffered formalin and embedded in paraffin for further histological and immunohistochemical examination (see below). At each time point, six animals were used (n = 6; in all n = 30).

Positron Emission Tomography/Magnetic Resonance Imaging (PET/MRI)

In a separate study additional 6 animals underwent imaging 12 hours before and 1, 2, 3 and 7 days after portal vein ligation. Images were acquired with a PET/MRI (nanoScan PET/MRI, Mediso Ltd., Hungary) sequential animal imaging system. Blood glucose levels were confirmed to be within the normal range before injection of the radioactive tracer and throughout the study. In the PET experiment 6.5±1.0 MBq of FDG in 0.2 mL volume was injected into the tail vein, under anesthesia (2% isoflurane in 100% O_2 gas). To prevent movement, the animals were fixed to a rat chamber (MultiCell Imaging Chamber, Mediso Ltd., Hungary) and positioned in the center of field of view (FOV). Dynamic list-mode PET data were collected in three-dimensional acquisition mode. The MRI images (matrix size 140×140; 0.5 mm; 30 slices; 1.3 mm; gap 0.5 mm) were acquired for 50 minutes (25 minutes for each imaging) with T1-weighted (SE2D; TR/TE 800/10 ms; FOV 70 mm; NEX 4), T2-weighted (FSE2D; TR/TE 4733/60 ms; FOV 70 mm; NEX 2) sequences. PET volumes were reconstructed using a three-dimensional Ordered Subsets Expectation Maximization (3D-OSEM) algorithm (Tera-Tomo, Mediso Ltd., Hungary) into dynamic frames of 10×30 s, 10×60 s, 10×270 s (total 60 min, 30 frames) for all scans with a voxel size of 0.3 mm. Static images were generated based on frame 21 (15th to 19th minutes were integrated after tracer injection). PET and MRI images were automatically coregistered by the PET/MRI instrument's acquisition software. Reconstructed, reoriented and coregistered images were further analyzed with Fusion (Mediso

Ltd., Hungary) and VivoQuant (inviCRO LLC, US) dedicated image analysis softwares by placing appropriate Volume of Interests (VOI) on the organs. Two volume of interests were delineated manually slice by slice on each T1 weighted scans. One VOI consisted of the ligated liver lobes and the other of the non-ligated liver lobes. For volumetric analysis the built-in VOI statistics of the VivoQuant software was used, which determines the volume from voxel size and number of voxels in the VOIs. In order to get more precise values of the volumes, the T1 weighted slices were interpolated through the slice direction to create an isovoxel data set. For FGD uptake, the standardized uptake value (SUV) was calculated by dividing the mean radioactivity concentration (MBq/mL) by injected dose per body weight (MBq/g). The mean SUV for ligated and for non-ligated liver lobes were selectively recorded. The mean SUV of corresponding liver lobes was expressed in relation to a reference tissue SUV (cardiac left ventricle; SUV_{VOI}/SUV_{CLV}) and to the mean liver SUV (SUV_{VOI}/SUV_{Liver}).

Evaluation of Liver Regeneration and Atrophy

Liver lobe wet weight was measured separately after exsanguinations using a laboratory scale (Mettler Toledo AG 245, Mettler-Toledo LLC, Columbus, OH, readability: 0.01 mg/0.1 mg). The relative weight of ligated and non-ligated lobes to the body weight (BW) was then calculated and expressed as follows: liver weight (g)/100 g BW. The liver volume change was measured by MRI and the relative liver volume was expressed as mm^3/100 g BW. The change in liver volume calculated from PET/MRI was compared with the results derived from autopsy.

Histological and Immunohistochemical Examination

After liver weight measurement, one slice was removed for pathological examination from the same anatomic position in each animal. The formalin fixed, paraffin embedded 3–5 micrometer thick sections underwent light microscopic observation after hematoxylin and eosin staining. *Necrosis* was assessed by morphological features (swollen cytoplasm, vacuolization, disrupted cell and organelle membranes and lytic nuclear changes) on each section. The extent of necrosis was graded on a scale of 0–4 described by Suzuki [22]: grade 0– absence of necrosis; grade 1– single cell necrosis; grade 2–30% lobular necrosis; grade 3–60% lobular necrosis; grade 4– more than 60% lobular necrosis. Hepatocyte *apoptotic cell death* was identified also by morphological criteria (cell shrinkage, chromatin condensation, margination and apoptotic bodies) and was counted in 10 consecutive high-power fields (HPF, x200) and expressed in absolute numbers.

For the detection of *mitotic activity* Ki-67 immunohistochemical staining was applied on formalin-fixed, paraffin-embedded tissues. Avidin–biotin–peroxidase complex immunohistochemical method was performed for antigen retrieval. [23] Primary antibodies were MIB-5 antibody against Ki-67 (DAKO, Glostrup, Denmark) of hepatocytes. Labeling index was defined as the mean number of Ki-67-positive cells per HPF (×200), respectively.

To determine *cellular glycogen content*, periodic acid and Schiff (PAS) staining was used. The intensity of PAS staining was graded on a five tier scale (0: no staining –5: highly intense). The level of glycogen content was determined by scoring at least three independent microscopic fields for each sample.

The above mentioned histological and immunohistochemical evaluations were performed in blinded fashion by two experienced pathologists.

Statistical Analysis

Mann–Whitney U test and two sample Student t-test were used to compare data between groups. Normality was tested by Kolmogorov-Smirnov test. Correlation between variables was tested by Spearman's method. All tests were performed using the Statistical Package for Social Sciences (IBM SPSS Statistics 20.0 software, IBM Corporation, Armonk, NY, USA). Values are expressed as means ± S.D. A $p<0.05$ confidence interval was considered as statistically significant.

Results

Liver Hypertrophy and Atrophy Induced by Portal Vein Ligation

The weight of the portal-deprived lobes decreased rapidly after the operation and reached approximately one-fourth its original weight on postoperative day 7. On the other hand the non-ligated liver lobes underwent compensatory gain in weight. By a balance of atrophy and hypertrophy, the weight of total liver was maintained near to the baseline throughout the entire experiment. The volume of liver lobes changed in parallel with the liver weights. The volume change, based on MRI volumetry, correlated well with the weight change derived from autopsy ($r = 0.842$; $p< 0.001$); (Figure 1.).

Histomorphological Characteristics of Ligated and Non-ligated Liver Lobes

Atrophy of portal-deprived liver lobes was mainly caused by the combination of necrosis and apoptosis. Extensive coagulation necrosis occurred in the central zone of liver lobules one day after the ligation. The necrotic areas became significantly reduced in size at postoperative day 2 and 3. At this time, a high number of macrophages were observed in the necrotic region. Seven days after the operation necrosis could not be observed, while the normal hepatic architecture recovered, with no signs of fibrosis. The number of apoptotic hepatocytes also increased rapidly after the operation and reached the peak on postoperative day 2. Apoptosis was most frequently present at the boundary between necrotic and non-necrotic areas and remained elevated until the 7th postoperative day. In contrast, in the non-ligated liver lobes, the presence of necrosis and apoptosis was not typical (Figure 2. A–B).

To examine proliferating capacity of the liver Ki-67 immunohistochemical staining was performed. Ki-67 is expressed by proliferating cells in late G1, S, G2 and M phases, however it is absent in the resting, G0 phase, therefore it is a reliable marker to detect mitotic activity. With this immunohistochemical staining, increased mitotic activity was found in non-ligated lobes with the peak response at 2nd days. Thereafter, the number of positive cells decreased and reached the baseline level at 7th postoperative day. However, in the ligated liver lobes the number of Ki-67 positive cells did not change significantly during the experiment (Figure 2. C–D).

Liver showed a moderate, homogeneous glycogen staining before (day 0) PVL. Day 1 after ligation, PAS positive glycogen granules almost completely disappeared in ligated lobes and the glycogen content of cells returned to baseline level just at day 7. In contrast, the PAS staining in non-ligated liver lobes did not show significant alterations compared to the baseline level (day 0) in any examined time point (Figure 3).

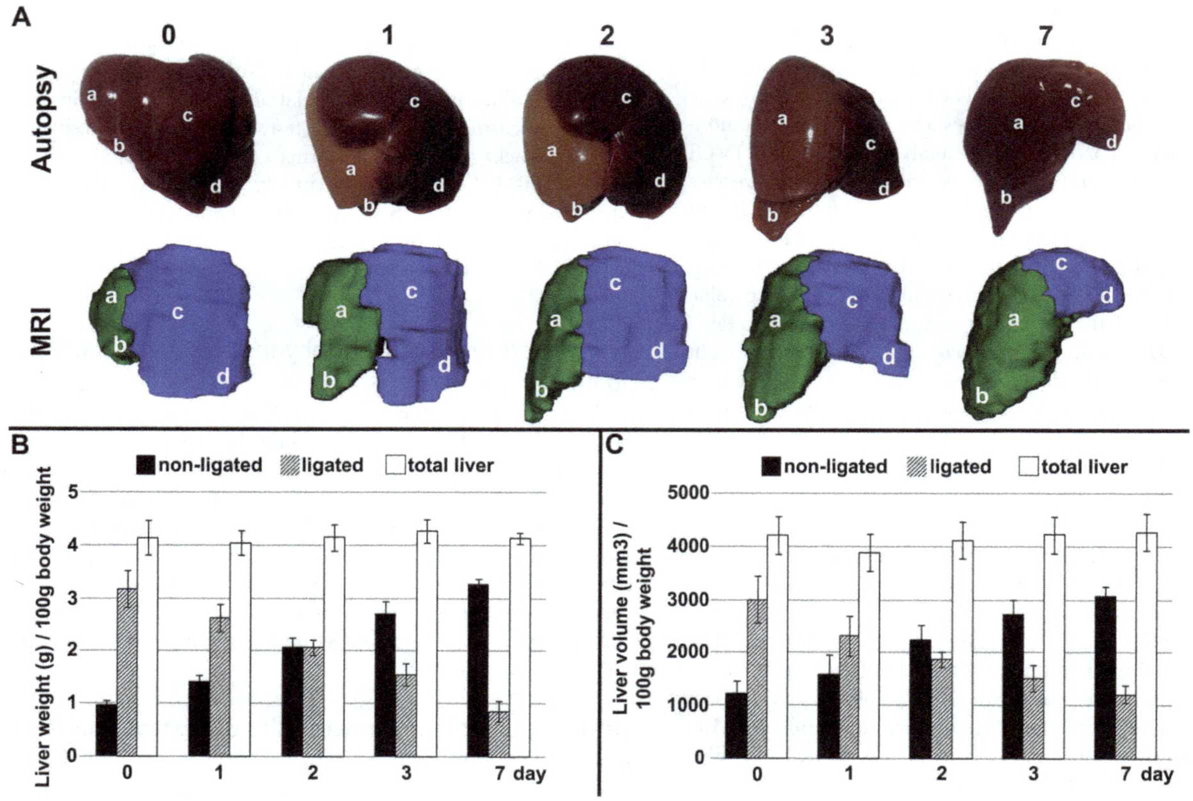

Figure 1. Changes in weight and volume of the liver after portal vein ligation. A: The macroscopic appearance of liver by post mortem examinations and three dimensional MRI reconstruction preoperatively (0), as well as 1, 2, 3 and 7 days after portal vein ligation (PVL). Changes in weight (B) and volume (C) of total liver, ligated and non-ligated liver lobes at the examined time points. The alteration in liver weight showed a significant positive correlation with the volume change ($r = 0.842$, $P < 0.001$; tested by Spearman's method). Values are expressed as mean ± S.D. Each column represents the average of 6 animals. a = superior right lateral lobe; b = inferior right lateral lobe; c = median lobe; d = left lateral lobe.

^{18}F-FDG Data Analysis

Dynamic PET scans revealed an altered FDG kinetics characterized by prolonged tracer elimination in both ligated and non-ligated liver lobes. The alterations in time activity curves of ligated lobes were more remarkable compared to the non-ligated lobes (Figure 4.). Before PVL the liver showed homogenous tracer biodistribution. After PVL, FDG uptake within the liver shifted towards the ligated lobes. The SUV_{VOI}/SUV_{CLV} showed a significantly increased FDG uptake in ligated liver lobes. That value was maximal on 2nd postoperative day and returned near to the baseline at the 7th day. In non-ligated lobes the SUV_{VOI}/SUV_{CLV} also increased, but in a significantly lower extent compared to the ligated lobes. The increment in FDG uptake of non-ligated lobes reached a statistically significant level on 2nd and 3rd postoperative day only, as compared to the baseline (Figure 5.). SUV_{VOI}/SUV_{Liver} in ligated lobes significantly increased compared to that in non-ligated liver lobes with the maximal level on 2nd postoperative day. Then at 7th postoperative day the SUV_{VOI}/SUV_{Liver} returned to baseline levels and the lobes of liver showed again similar FDG uptake pattern (Figure 6. A–B).

Discussion

In the recent years two-stage hepatectomy with portal vein ligation became widely used to surgically treat large primary or secondary liver tumors. However portal vein occlusion not only induces liver regeneration, but also potentially results in loco-regional or metastatic tumor spread, making liver resection difficult. [9] In the early recognition of postoperative tumor progression (regional and distant metastases alike), the anatomic information derived from conventional CT or MRI can be insufficient, thus the introduction of functional imaging assays is required to improve diagnostic accuracy. However, to draw adequate conclusion from PET studies, exploring the alteration in tracer kinetics in normal, tumor free liver tissues after PVL is necessary.

In our experiment PET/MRI was used to evaluate the PVL induced alterations in the FDG uptake in parallel with the change in volume of ligated and non-ligated liver lobes in healthy rats. In our study, PVL induced volume and weight changes in liver mass, that are typical in such cases. [5] The ligated liver lobes underwent a massive atrophic process, while the non-ligated lobes showed compensatory hyperplasia. As a result the total liver mass was unchanged throughout the entire experiment. This progressive volumetric alteration was completed by postoperative day 7.

In parallel to the volume changes, dynamic PET data revealed altered FDG kinetics in both the ligated and non-ligated liver lobes after PVL. To accurately determine the alteration in FDG uptake, mean SUV of liver lobes were compared to a reference image derived from the blood input of the left cardiac ventricle. SUV_{VOI}/SUV_{CLV} highly significantly increased in ligated lobes, while in the non-ligated lobes just a moderate increase was observed. The different FDG uptake of the ligated and non-ligated lobes was more obvious, when the SUV of corresponding lobes was compared to the whole liver radioactivity concentration. Before PVL, the liver showed homogenous FDG distribution.

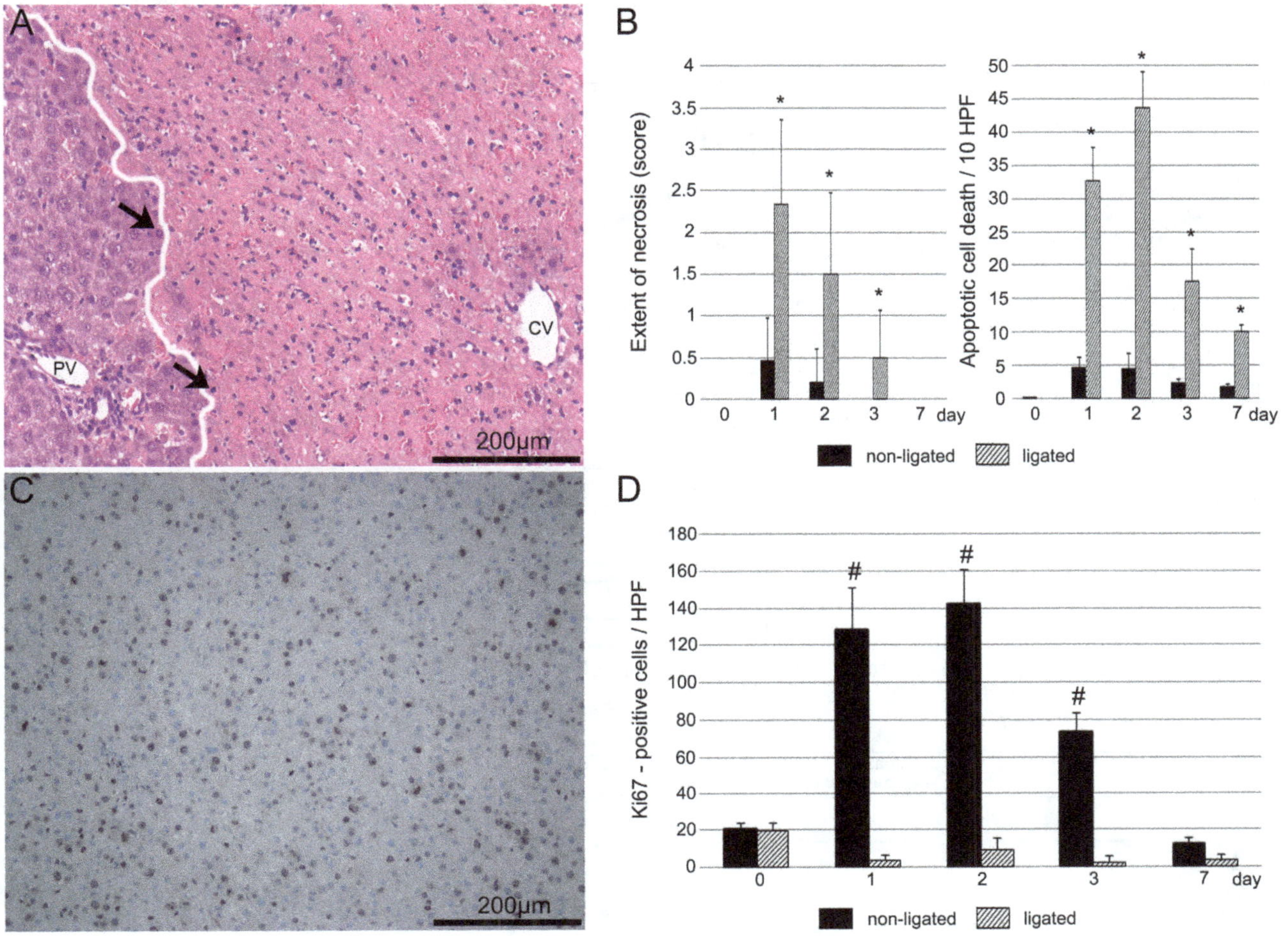

Figure 2. Histomorphological characteristics of the liver after portal vein ligation. A: Histomorphological characteristics of the ligated lobes 1 day after portal vein ligation (PVL). Wide necrotic areas were seen around the central vein. At the boundary between the necrotic and non-necrotic areas (white line) apoptosis was frequently present (black arrows). B: The extent of necrotic areas and the number of apoptotic cell death significantly increased in ligated lobes compared with that seen in non-ligated liver lobes. C: Ki-67 labeling in non-ligated lobes on 2nd day after surgery. Ki-67 antibody reacts with the nuclear structure present exclusively in the proliferative phase of the cell cycle. In the non-ligated liver lobes immunohistochemistry (brown stain) show a high expression level of Ki-67 in cell nuclei, which represent an increased mitotic activity of the hepatocytes. D: Mitotic activity of hepatocytes significantly increased in non-ligated liver lobes, with the peak response on day 2. In contrast, the Ki-67 positivity of ligated lobes did not change significantly throughout the experiment. Values are expressed as mean ± S.D. Each column presents the average of 6 animals. PV= portal vein; CV= central vein; *= $p<0.05$ versus non-ligated lobes; #= $p<0.05$ versus ligated lobes.

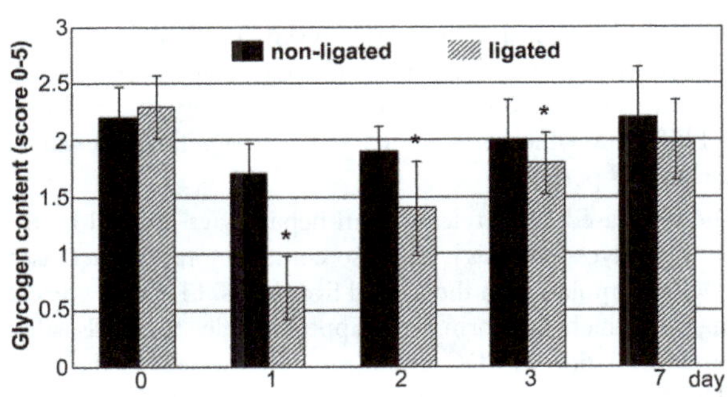

Figure 3. Glycogen content of cells. Glycogen content of ligated lobes (striped column) decreased markedly after portal vein ligation and it reached the baseline level at postoperative day 7. In non-ligated lobes (black column), the PAS staining did not show any significant alteration throughout the experiment. Values are expressed as mean ± S.D. Each column represents the average of 6 animals. *= $p<0.05$ versus the baseline level (0 day) of the corresponding lobes.

After PVL, the SUV_{VOI}/SUV_{Liver} significantly elevated in the ligated lobes compared to that in the non-ligated part of liver. The contrast between the lobes was the most significant at postoperative day 2. Thereafter, by the postoperative 7th day, when the PVL induced volumetric alterations were completed, the pre-PVL FDG uptake pattern returned and the lobes of liver showed again similar tracer biodistribution.

To explore the cause of these altered FDG uptake pattern, histological examinations were performed. Our results suggest that two main processes could be responsible for the remarkable elevated FDG accumulation in ligated lobes:

(1) The atrophy of portal deprived liver lobes is mainly caused by coagulation necrosis, as a result of the cessation of portal vascular inflow and the consequent hypoxic condition around the central vein. [24] The reduction in the numbers of the viable cells through necrosis should be reflected by decreased FDG uptake. [25] However, in the ligated lobes increased FDG accumulation was detected, for which some energy-intensive processes surrounding these necrotic lesions may

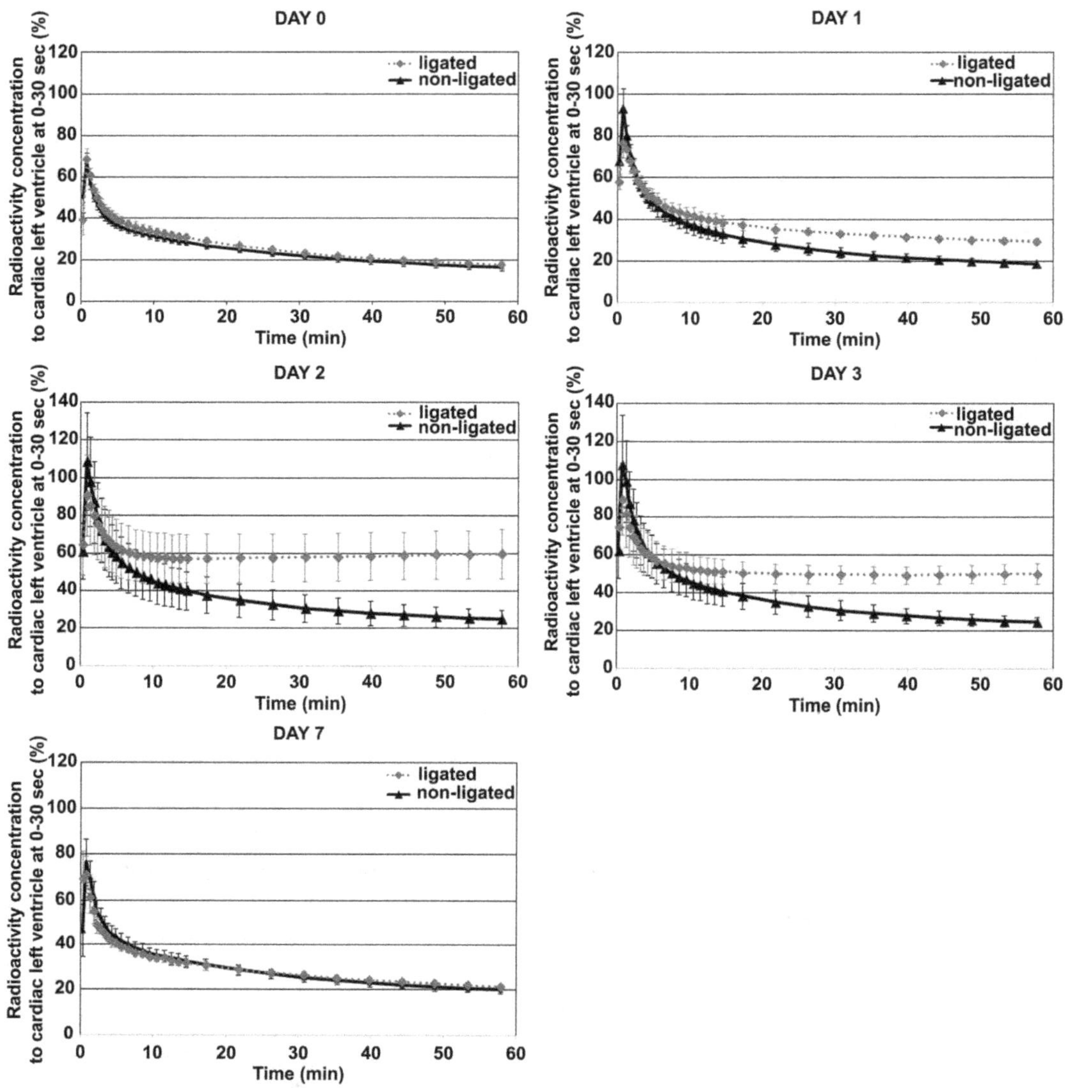

Figure 4. Time activity curves of ligated and non-ligated lobes at different time points. After portal vein ligation (PVL) the characteristics of curves showed altered tracer kinetics in both ligated (gray; dotted line) and non-ligated (black; solid line) liver lobes, but these changes in ligated lobes were more pronounced. The most significant alterations can be seen on 2nd postoperative day, then 7 days after the operation the curves characteristic showed similar appearance to the pre-PVL data.

responsible. (A) *Apoptosis:* At the boundary between necrotic and non-necrotic areas, a large number of apoptotic cells were found. It is well-documented, that apoptosis is an energy-intensive process, because adenosine-triphosphate (ATP) is required for the activation of the efferent molecules of caspase family. However, in these areas around the necrotic fields, a moderate degree of hypoxia is still present. [26] The limited ability of oxygen leads to anaerobic glycolysis, a less efficient use of glucose, with increased necessity of glucose extraction from blood, which consequently could lead to enhanced FDG uptake of the apoptotic cells, and could be reflected in the PET scan. [27–29] (B) *Inflammation*: Besides apoptosis, a massive inflammatory reaction was also present around the necrotic regions in the slides. At postoperative day one, macrophages appeared at the rim of the necrotic areas and began to remove the debris. Activated macrophages are characterized with high glucose turnover and consequently increased FDG uptake. [30] It should be noted that, the above detailed histological alterations showed considerable individual variation on first 3 postoperative days, when the atrophic process was the most intensive. This variability also reflected in PET data, which is characterized by a significant deviation during this period.

(2) The decreased FDG release from hepatocytes- caused by the elevated glycogenolysis – can also contribute to the increased FDG accumulation in the ligated liver lobes. FDG is a glucose analog, which is normally trapped inside the cells after phosphorylation as FDG-6-phosphate. However, in the liver, FDG-6-phosphate is dephosphorylated and rapidly released, presumably due to the high activity of glucose-6-phosphatase (G-6-Pase). [31] In our experiment an abrupt loss of liver glycogen was observed in the portal deprived liver lobes, which suggests that the ligated lobes may take part in maintaining blood glucose level by accelerated glycogenolysis after PVL. Although, the extent of glycogenolysis is elevated after PVL, the enzyme activity of G-6-Pase of ligated liver

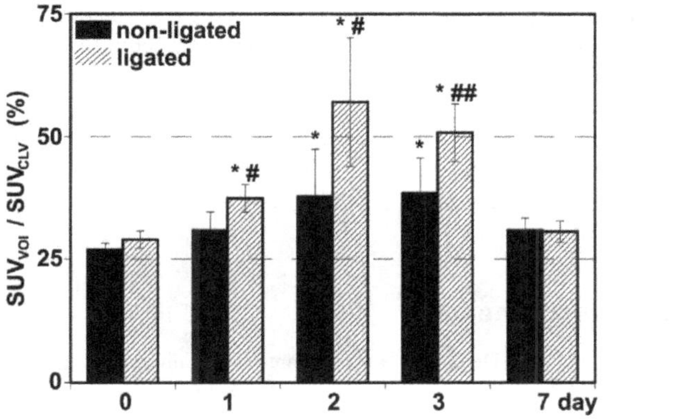

Figure 5. The ratio of mean SUV of ligated and non-ligated lobes to cardiac left ventricle SUV. The FDG uptake significantly increased in ligated (striped column) liver lobes, with maximal value on 2nd postoperative day and returned to near to the baseline 7 day after portal vein ligation. In non-ligated (black column) lobes the tracer uptake also increased, but significantly lower extent compared to the ligated lobes. Values are expressed as mean ± S.D. Each column represents the average of 6 animals. *= $p<0.05$ versus the baseline level (0 day) of the corresponding lobes; #= $p<0.05$ versus non-ligated lobes; ##= $p<0.01$ versus non-ligated lobes.

lobes are shown to be unaltered. [32][33] The elevated glycogenolysis and the unchanged G-6-Pase activity of the ligated liver lobes, might result in the intracellular accumulation of glucose-6-phosphate, which is capable to inhibit the dephosphorylation, thereby the release of FDG-6-phosphate by competing for the catalytic unit of G-6-Pase.

In non-ligated liver lobes FDG uptake also increased, but to a significantly lower extent than in ligated lobes, despite the presence of massive regeneration characterized by high mitotic activity of cells. Cell division would supposedly be associated with high glucose/FDG-uptake. [34] However, literature data demonstrated that glucose is not the primary energy source of regeneration in the liver. Already in early phase of regeneration the hepatic metabolism is shifted from carbohydrates utilization to the consumption of lipids. [35] Consistent with this, Brinkmann et al showed that after partial hepatectomy intracellular concentrations of glucokinase decreased to less than one third within the first 72 hours. [36] Given that the level of active glucokinase is a determining factor in FDG uptake, the altered glycolytic activity of hepatocytes during liver regeneration could explain why FDG uptake increased just moderate level in non-ligated liver lobes, despite the significant mitotic activity. Another explanation for moderate FDG uptake in the non-ligated lobes might lie in the high portal glucose supply of liver. Rocheleau et al showed a 230% increase in flow of non-ligated lobes after PVL and 96% of this flow is derived from the portal vein. [37] Taking into account that the portal vasculature receives three times more glucose per minute than the hepatic artery, the glucose supply of the regenerating liver mass is abundant. [38] However, the high plasma glucose levels can inhibit FDG uptake by competing for the binding site of the hepatic glucose transporter proteins. [39] This competition between plasma glucose and FDG could result in the moderate-level of FDG uptake observed in non-ligated, regenerating liver lobes by PET scan.

The above detailed alteration in FDG uptake pattern could have a significant impact on the evaluation of PET studies after PVL. The increased FDG accumulation, especially in the case of ligated lobes, could make difficult the assessment of tumor progression by increased background activity until the PVL induced alterations are completed. However, it also should be noted that, the alteration in FDG uptake of non-ligated lobes was moderate and reached significant level only at the 2nd and 3rd postoperative days. This lower-grade lobar FDG activity might make possible the early recognition of residual tumorous lesions in non-ligated liver shortly after the operation. Considering that, in terms of treatment decision, the critical points are the tumor progression in the future remnant liver (non-ligated lobes) or the formation of distant metastases, the use of FDG-PET/MRI could be beneficial in the early assessment of tumor response to PVL.

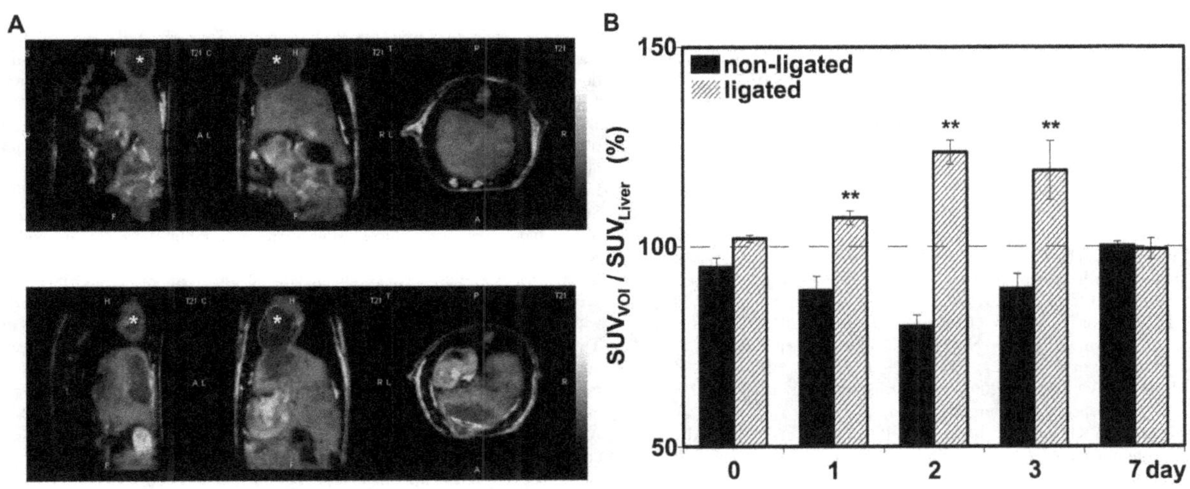

Figure 6. Tracer biodistribution in ligated and non-ligated liver lobes. A:Representative coregistered PET and MRI image of rat liver before (top) and 3 days after (bottom) portal vein ligation (PVL). The PET reconstruction is based on frame 21 (at 15–19 minutes). The top inset picture shows a homogeneous liver FDG uptake pattern in both liver lobes. The small inhomogeneity is related to the morphology of liver. After PVL the liver shows inhomogeneous tracer distribution with significantly increased FDG uptake in ligated lobes, while the tracer uptake in cardiac left ventricle (*) remain constant. B: The ratio of mean SUV of ligated (striped column) and non-ligated (black column) liver lobes to mean liver SUV. The SUV_{VOI}/SUV_{Liver} significantly increased in ligated liver lobes compared to the non-ligated lobes after PVL with the peak response on day 2. Values are expressed as mean ± S.D. Each column represents the average of 6 animals. **= $p<0.01$ versus non-ligated lobes.

Nevertheless, our study has some limitations. The main limitation is the use of normal, healthy liver. In a clinical scenario, the primary and secondary liver tumors usually appear in cirrhotic or fatty livers, in which circumstances the PVL induced alterations and consequently the imaging characteristics of liver lobes may vary. Furthermore, this study examined only tumor-free animals, however, the altered circumstances caused by PVL may result in alteration of tumor FDG uptake as well. Further research on tumor-bearing animals is needed to evaluate this potential tumor response regarding to FDG-uptake after PVL. Finally, it should be noted that FDG is appropriate for the diagnosis only of FDG positive tumors. However, some liver cancer, such as hepatocellular carcinoma is characterized by variable FDG uptake caused by the variation in the expression of G-6Pase. In such case, the results from FDG-PET/MRI could become uncertain, therefore more specific tracers, such as [^{11}C]-acetate should be used. [40].

Conclusion

The aim of the study was to evaluate the FDG uptake pattern in healthy liver after PVL in small animals. Our result showed an altered FDG uptake pattern in both ligated and non-ligated liver lobes after PVL. These alterations in FDG uptake should be taken into account during the assessment of PET data until the PVL induced atrophic and regenerative processes are completed. Because this initial study merely examined healthy animals, further preclinical and clinical studies are needed to define the impact of FDG-PET in therapeutic follow-up after a two stage-hepatectomy combined with PVL.

Acknowledgments

The authors thank Dr. Gábor Lotz (Semmelweis University, Budapest, Hungary) for the assessment of the histological slides.

Author Contributions

Conceived and designed the experiments: KS AS LH. Performed the experiments: AB DP DK IH NK. Analyzed the data: KS IH NK AF. Contributed reagents/materials/analysis tools: IH NK KK DM. Wrote the paper: AF KS DM AS.

References

1. Kawasaki S, Makuuchi M, Kakazu T, Miyagawa S, Takayama T, et al. (1994) Resection for multiple metastatic liver tumors after portal embolization. Surgery 115: 674–677.
2. Takayama T (2011) Surgical treatment for hepatocellular carcinoma. Jpn J Clin Oncol 41: 447–454.
3. Bengmark S, Ekberg H, Evander A, Klofver-Stahl B, Tranberg KG (1988) Major liver resection for hilar cholangiocarcinoma. Ann Surg 207: 120–125.
4. Gock M, Eipel C, Linnebacher M, Klar E, Vollmar B (2011) Impact of portal branch ligation on tissue regeneration, microcirculatory response and microarchitecture in portal blood-deprived and undeprived liver tissue. Microvasc Res 81: 274–280.
5. Rozga J, Jeppsson B, Bengmark S (1986) Portal branch ligation in the rat. Reevaluation of a model. Am J Pathol 125: 300–308.
6. Broering DC, Hillert C, Krupski G, Fischer L, Mueller L, et al. (2002) Portal vein embolization vs. portal vein ligation for induction of hypertrophy of the future liver remnant. J Gastrointest Surg 6: 905–913; discussion 913.
7. Clavien PA, Petrowsky H, DeOliveira ML, Graf R (2007) Strategies for safer liver surgery and partial liver transplantation. N Engl J Med 356: 1545–1559.
8. Kokudo N, Tada K, Seki M, Ohta H, Azekura K, et al. (2001) Proliferative activity of intrahepatic colorectal metastases after preoperative hemihepatic portal vein embolization. Hepatology 34: 267–272.
9. Barbaro B, Di Stasi C, Nuzzo G, Vellone M, Giuliante F, et al. (2003) Preoperative right portal vein embolization in patients with metastatic liver disease. Metastatic liver volumes after RPVE. Acta Radiol 44: 98–102.
10. Heinrich S, Jochum W, Graf R, Clavien PA (2006) Portal vein ligation and partial hepatectomy differentially influence growth of intrahepatic metastasis and liver regeneration in mice. J Hepatol 45: 35–42.
11. Elias D, De Baere T, Roche A, Mducreux, Leclere J, et al. (1999) During liver regeneration following right portal embolization the growth rate of liver metastases is more rapid than that of the liver parenchyma. Br J Surg 86: 784–788.
12. de Graaf W, van den Esschert JW, van Lienden KP, van Gulik TM (2009) Induction of tumor growth after preoperative portal vein embolization: is it a real problem? Ann Surg Oncol 16: 423–430.
13. Hahn O, Dudas I, Pajor P, Gyorke T, Korom C, et al. (2013) [ALPPS (Associated Liver Partition and Portal vein ligation for Staged hepatectomy) – faster and greater growth of liver]. Magy Seb 66: 21–26.
14. Abdalla EK, Hicks ME, Vauthey JN (2001) Portal vein embolization: rationale, technique and future prospects. Br J Surg 88: 165–175.
15. de Graaf W, van Lienden KP, van den Esschert JW, Bennink RJ, van Gulik TM (2011) Increase in future remnant liver function after preoperative portal vein embolization. Br J Surg 98: 825–834.
16. Hammerstingl R, Huppertz A, Breuer J, Balzer T, Blakeborough A, et al. (2008) Diagnostic efficacy of gadoxetic acid (Primovist)-enhanced MRI and spiral CT for a therapeutic strategy: comparison with intraoperative and histopathologic findings in focal liver lesions. Eur Radiol 18: 457–467.
17. Willatt JM, Hussain HK, Adusumilli S, Marrero JA (2008) MR Imaging of hepatocellular carcinoma in the cirrhotic liver: challenges and controversies. Radiology 247: 311–330.
18. Juweid ME, Cheson BD (2006) Positron-emission tomography and assessment of cancer therapy. N Engl J Med 354: 496–507.
19. Antoch G, Vogt FM, Veit P, Freudenberg LS, Blechschmid N, et al. (2005) Assessment of liver tissue after radiofrequency ablation: findings with different imaging procedures. J Nucl Med 46: 520–525.
20. Vogt FM, Antoch G, Veit P, Freudenberg LS, Blechschmid N, et al. (2007) Morphologic and functional changes in nontumorous liver tissue after radiofrequency ablation in an in vivo model: comparison of 18F-FDG PET/CT, MRI, ultrasound, and CT. J Nucl Med 48: 1836–1844.
21. Bennink RJ, Dinant S, Erdogan D, Heijnen BH, Straatsburg IH, et al. (2004) Preoperative assessment of postoperative remnant liver function using hepatobiliary scintigraphy. J Nucl Med 45: 965–971.
22. Suzuki S, Toledo-Pereyra LH, Rodriguez FJ, Cejalvo D (1993) Neutrophil infiltration as an important factor in liver ischemia and reperfusion injury. Modulating effects of FK506 and cyclosporine. Transplantation 55: 1265–1272.
23. Hsiao IT, Lin KJ, Chang SI, Yen TC, Chen TC, et al. (2010) Impaired liver regeneration of steatotic rats after portal vein ligation: a particular emphasis on (99m)Tc-DISIDA scintigraphy and adiponectin signaling. J Hepatol 52: 540–549.
24. Abdalla EK, Barnett CC, Doherty D, Curley SA, Vauthey JN (2002) Extended hepatectomy in patients with hepatobiliary malignancies with and without preoperative portal vein embolization. Arch Surg 137: 675–680; discussion 680–671.
25. Kubota K, Ishiwata K, Kubota R, Yamada S, Tada M, et al. (1991) Tracer feasibility for monitoring tumor radiotherapy: a quadruple tracer study with fluorine-18-fluorodeoxyglucose or fluorine-18-fluorodeoxyuridine, L-[methyl-14C]methionine, [6-3H]thymidine, and gallium-67. J Nucl Med 32: 2118–2123.
26. Ikeda K, Kinoshita H, Hirohashi K, Kubo S, Kaneda K (1995) The ultrastructure, kinetics and intralobular distribution of apoptotic hepatocytes after portal branch ligation with special reference to their relationship to necrotic hepatocytes. Arch Histol Cytol 58: 171–184.
27. Stewart EE, Chen X, Hadway J, Lee TY (2006) Correlation between hepatic tumor blood flow and glucose utilization in a rabbit liver tumor model. Radiology 239: 740–750.
28. Song S, Xiong C, Lu W, Ku G, Huang G, et al. (2013) Apoptosis imaging probe predicts early chemotherapy response in preclinical models: A comparative study with 18F-FDG PET. J Nucl Med 54: 104–110.
29. Takei T, Kuge Y, Zhao S, Sato M, Strauss HW, et al. (2005) Enhanced apoptotic reaction correlates with suppressed tumor glucose utilization after cytotoxic chemotherapy: use of 99mTc-Annexin V, 18F-FDG, and histologic evaluation. J Nucl Med 46: 794–799.
30. Abouzied MM, Crawford ES, Nabi HA (2005) 18F-FDG imaging: pitfalls and artifacts. J Nucl Med Technol 33: 145–155; quiz 162–143.
31. Caraco C, Aloj L, Chen LY, Chou JY, Eckelman WC (2000) Cellular release of [18F]2-fluoro-2-deoxyglucose as a function of the glucose-6-phosphatase enzyme system. J Biol Chem 275: 18489–18494.
32. Mueller L, Grotelueschen R, Meyer J, Vashist YK, Abdulgawad A, et al. (2003) Sustained function in atrophying liver tissue after portal branch ligation in the rat. J Surg Res 114: 146–155.
33. Zakko WF, Berg CL, Gollan JL, Green RM (1998) Hepatocellular expression of glucose-6-phosphatase is unaltered during hepatic regeneration. Am J Physiol 275: G717–722.
34. Pauwels EK, Ribeiro MJ, Stoot JH, McCready VR, Bourguignon M, et al. (1998) FDG accumulation and tumor biology. Nucl Med Biol 25: 317–322.

35. Rosa JL, Perez JX, Detheux M, Van Schaftingen E, Bartrons R (1997) Gene expression of glucokinase regulatory protein in regenerating rat liver. Hepatology 25: 324–328.
36. Brinkmann A, Katz N, Sasse D, Jungermann K (1978) Increase of the gluconeogenic and decrease of the glycolytic capacity of rat liver with a change of the metabolic zonation after partial hepatectomy. Hoppe Seylers Z Physiol Chem 359: 1561–1571.
37. Rocheleau B, Ethier C, Houle R, Huet PM, Bilodeau M (1999) Hepatic artery buffer response following left portal vein ligation: its role in liver tissue homeostasis. Am J Physiol 277: G1000–1007.
38. Alexander B, Rogers C, Naftalin R (2002) Hepatic arterial perfusion decreases intrahepatic shunting and maintains glucose uptake in the rat liver. Pflugers Arch 444: 291–298.
39. Pauwels EK, Sturm EJ, Bombardieri E, Cleton FJ, Stokkel MP (2000) Positron-emission tomography with [18F]fluorodeoxyglucose. Part I. Biochemical uptake mechanism and its implication for clinical studies. J Cancer Res Clin Oncol 126: 549–559.
40. Ho CL, Yu SC, Yeung DW (2003) 11C-acetate PET imaging in hepatocellular carcinoma and other liver masses. J Nucl Med 44: 213–221.

13

Liver Fibrosis in Type I Gaucher Disease: Magnetic Resonance Imaging, Transient Elastography and Parameters of Iron Storage

Anneloes E. Bohte[1]⑨, Laura van Dussen[2*]⑨, Erik M. Akkerman[1], Aart J. Nederveen[1], Ralph Sinkus[3], Peter L. M. Jansen[4], Jaap Stoker[1], Carla E. M. Hollak[2]

1 Department of Radiology, Academic Medical Center, University of Amsterdam, Amsterdam, The Netherlands, **2** Department of Endocrinology and Metabolism, Academic Medical Center, University of Amsterdam, Amsterdam, The Netherlands, **3** CRB3, UMR 773, Inserm, Université Paris Diderot, Sorbonne Paris Cité, Clichy, France, **4** Department of Gastroenterology and Hepatology, Academic Medical Center, University of Amsterdam, Amsterdam, The Netherlands

Abstract

Long term liver-related complications of type-1 Gaucher disease (GD), a lysosomal storage disorder, include fibrosis and an increased incidence of hepatocellular carcinoma. Splenectomy has been implicated as a risk factor for the development of liver pathology in GD. High ferritin concentrations are a feature of GD and iron storage in Gaucher cells has been described, but iron storage in the liver in relation to liver fibrosis has not been studied. Alternatively, iron storage in GD may be the result of iron supplementation therapy or regular blood transfusions in patients with severe cytopenia. In this pilot study, comprising 14 type-1 GD patients (7 splenectomized, 7 non-splenectomized) and 7 healthy controls, we demonstrate that liver stiffness values, measured by Transient Elastography and MR-Elastography, are significantly higher in splenectomized GD patients when compared with non-splenectomized GD patients ($p=0.03$ and $p=0.01$, respectively). Liver iron concentration was elevated (>60±30 µmol/g) in 4 GD patients of whom 3 were splenectomized. No relationship was found between liver stiffness and liver iron concentration. HFE gene mutations were more frequent in splenectomized (6/7) than in non-splenectomized (2/7) participants ($p=0.10$). Liver disease appeared more advanced in splenectomized than in non-splenectomized patients. We hypothesize a relationship with excessive hepatic iron accumulation in splenectomized patients. We recommend that all splenectomized patients, especially those with evidence of substantial liver fibrosis undergo regular screening for HCC, according to current guidelines.

Editor: Andrea Dardis, University Hospital S. Maria della Misericordia, Italy

Funding: The authors have no support or funding to report.

Competing Interests: The authors have read the journal's policy and have the following conflicts: A.E.B., E.M.A., A.J.N., R.S., and J.S. report no potential conflicts of interest. L.V.D. has received travel reimbursements for participation in meetings on lysosomal storage disorders from Genzyme corp. and Protalix Biotherapeutics. C.E.M.H. has received travel reimbursements and speaker/consultancy fees for participation in meetings on lysosomal storage disorders from Genzyme corp., Shire HGT and Protalix Biotherapeutics. All fees are donated to the Gaucher Stichting, a non-profit fund stimulating research on lysosomal storage disorders. P.L.M.J. has received travel reimbursement to various liver conferences unrelated to this work paid from research funds or companies.

* E-mail: l.vandussen@amc.uva.nl

⑨ These authors contributed equally to this work.

Introduction

Gaucher disease (GD) is one of the most prevalent lysosomal storage disorders, currently treatable with enzyme replacement therapy (ERT) and substrate reduction therapy (SRT) [1–5]. Long term liver complications that have been associated with GD include fibrosis and cirrhosis [6]. In addition, several studies have reported on the occurrence of hepatocellular carcinoma (HCC) among GD patients [7–13] and one cohort study reported that the risk of developing HCC was increased in GD patients, suggesting that splenectomy – formerly the only treatment option – could be a risk factor for the development of HCC in GD patients as a result of advanced hepatic involvement after splenectomy [8]. The pathophysiology, however, has not been fully elucidated. Immunological abnormalities such as T-cell dysfunction or chronic stimulation of the immune system have been implicated in the pathophysiology of the elevated cancer risk in GD patients [14,15]. An alternative hypothesis is the relationship with increased iron storage in the liver, in which iron promotes the formation of reactive oxygen species, causing hepatocellular injury. Raised serum ferritin concentrations are a well-known laboratory feature of GD, and can be used to monitor response to treatment [16–21]. These high ferritin concentrations have been suggested to reflect an altered iron metabolism in GD [22].

Both ERT and SRT have been shown to be highly effective in reversing cytopenia and reducing organ volumes. Splenectomies are now rarely necessary [23–25]. However, a substantial number of GD patients currently on treatment have had a splenectomy in the past. These patients may suffer from residual disease, which may cause partial unresponsiveness to treatment [26–28]. As this cohort ages, particular care should be taken to ensure proper monitoring with respect to the occurrence of long term complications, including HCC. Since liver fibrosis and hepatic iron storage are known risk factor for the development of HCC, screening for both entities could therefore be of additional value in the management of GD patients [29,30].

Liver biopsy is not a desirable procedure to evaluate the presence of fibrosis and iron accumulation in GD, given the patients' increased bleeding tendency. Lately however, new non-invasive and accurate quantitative imaging methods have become available by which a number of liver parameters can be evaluated. Transient Elastography (TE) and magnetic resonance elastography (MRE) both measure tissue stiffness of the liver, which is associated with the presence of fibrosis [31–33]. The techniques can predict the presence of cirrhosis and related complications such as portal hypertension and both techniques have shown to be of value for the non-invasive detection of liver fibrosis in patients with chronic liver disease [34,35]. Liver iron concentration (LIC) can also be measured non-invasively using MRI, as iron shortens T1, T2, and T2* relaxation times, leading to a lower signal intensity of the hepatic parenchyma, representing total body iron stores [36–38].

We speculate that the increased HCC risk in splenectomized GD patients is related to the presence of fibrosis and iron. Our objective therefore was to investigate whether GD patients with and without splenectomy (Sx) differed with respect to liver stiffness and iron content.

Materials and Methods

Ethics Statement

This study was approved by the institutional review board of the Academic Medical Center, Amsterdam, The Netherlands. All clinical investigations were conducted according to the principles expressed in the Declaration of Helsinki. Written informed consent was obtained from all participants.

Study Design and Participants

Between April 2010 and March 2012 we prospectively included 23 adult participants: eight splenectomized (Sx) GD patients, eight non-splenectomized (non-Sx) GD patients and seven healthy controls, matched for age and sex with the non-Sx GD group.

GD patients were eligible if they had been on treatment for at least two years (either ERT or SRT). Exclusion criteria for all participants were: known chronic liver disease (viral hepatitis, HIV, primary biliary cirrhosis, primary sclerosing cholangitis, autoimmune hepatitis, Wilson's disease, a-1-antitripsinedeficiency, abetalipoproteinemia), type 2 diabetes, use of drugs with known steatogenic effects on the liver (with the exception of oral contraceptives), alcohol consumption of >3 units/day for males and >2 units/day for females or contra-indications for MRI. History of iron intake and blood transfusion were recorded for all GD patients.

Study Procedures

A flow-chart of the study procedures is shown in Figure 1. Most GD patients visit the outpatient clinic two to four times a year. All study procedures were therefore performed on the same day as the scheduled regular appointment. If we were unable to complete all procedures on this single day, this was done at the next scheduled appointment.

Quantitative Imaging (All Participants)

Liver Iron Concentration (LIC). LIC measurements were performed at 1.5 Tesla MR system (Siemens, Magnetom Avanto, Germany). Two accepted methods were applied in all participants during a single MR session:

(1) LIC measurement according to Gandon et al. [39], in which an online quantification algorithm was used (http://www.radio.univ-rennes1.fr). Signal intensity values were measured manually in regions of interest (ROI) in the liver and paraspinous muscle on five scans, which were each acquired using a gradient echo sequence with varying echo times and flip angles (FA), resulting in T1, proton density and increasing T2 weighting. The Gandon method consisted of 5 breath hold scans of 20 seconds each. Signal intensity values were entered online, and a mean LIC ±95% confidence interval (CI) in μmol/g was returned. A LIC value is significantly elevated when the lower limit of the returned 95% CI equals 36 μmol/g or above. This corresponds to a mean LIC value of approximately >60 μmol/g, as the magnitude of the 95% CIs is usually ±20 μmol/g or greater [39].

(2) T2* measurement: Gradient echo sequence with repetition time 300 ms, 12 echoes with echo times from 0.99 to 16.5 ms in steps of 1.41 ms, number of slices 3, slice thickness 10 mm, voxel size 3×3 mm, FA 20° and field of view 380×380 mm. T2* relaxation times, which are inversely proportional to LIC, were calculated from the obtained images. T2* anatomical maps were created for both the liver and, if present, the spleen, giving an impression of the heterogeneity of iron distribution. Reference values for T2* relaxation times were derived from St. Pierre et al: approximately >22 ms [36,37]. The T2* acquisition comprised a single breath hold scan of 15 seconds.

Transient Elastography (TE). TE (Fibroscan©, Echosens, France) measures the propagation speed of a shear wave using ultrasound. The shear waves are generated by a small vibrating device that is positioned on the top of the ultrasound transducer. The velocity of the propagating shear waves correlates with tissue stiffness. TE can measure liver stiffness in a cylinder of approximately 1 cm in diameter and 4 cm in length [40].

TE was performed by three examiners, one expert (>500 measurements) and two less experienced examiners (<100 measurements), who were trained by the expert. Measurements were carried out at three different locations, taking into account the often heterogeneous liver morphology in GD patients.

(1) At the intersection between the xyphoid line and the median axillary line (reference location).

(2) 2–3 cm anterior of the reference position in the same intercostal space (anterior location).

(3) 2–3 cm posterior to the reference position in the next intercostal space on the same xyphoid line as the reference position (posterior location).

A minimum of 10 measurements were performed. Median liver stiffness (mLS), success rate (SR) and interquartile range (IQR) was recorded. The following reliability criteria for TE were applied [41]:

- very reliable: IQR/mLS ≤0.10;
- reliable: IQR/mLS between 0.10 and 0.30, or IQR/mLS >0.30 with mLS <7.1 kPa;
- poorly reliable: IQR/mLS >0.30 with mLS ≥7.1 kPa

MR Elastography (MRE). The principle of MRE is comparable to that of TE. Low frequency mechanical waves are sent into the liver by a portable transducer, inducing shear stresses while propagating. A motion-sensitive MRI sequence measures the resulting displacement fields (Figure 2 B), in three orthogonal

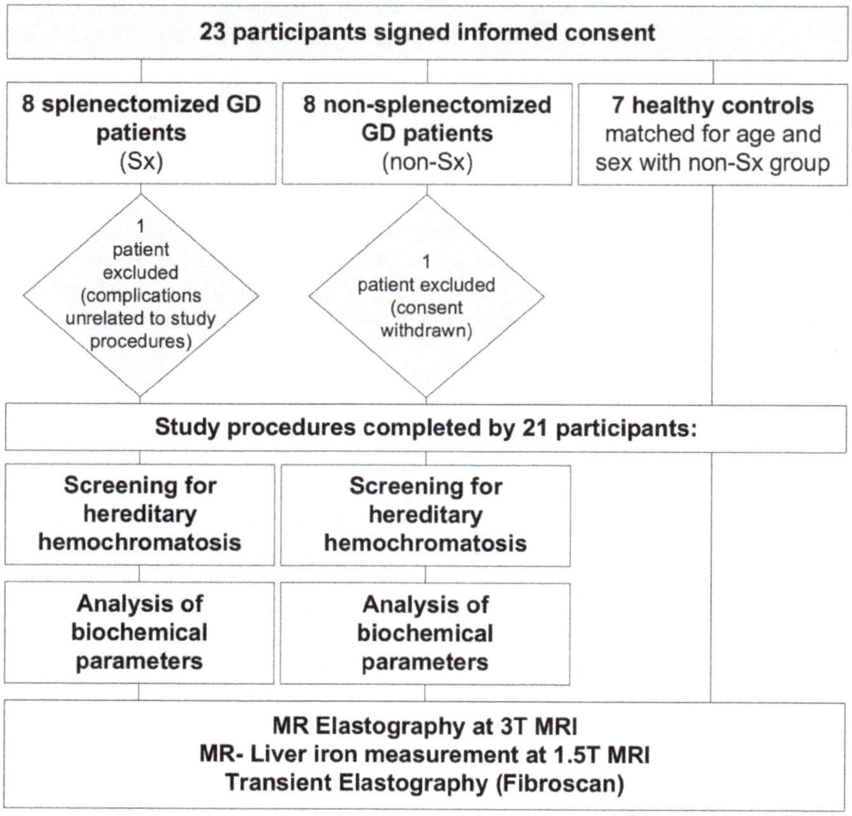

Figure 1. Study flow chart.

directions. From these 3D- displacement fields, the *shear modulus G** is analyzed. The real part of G* is the *storage modulus G′*. This storage modulus G′ can be referred to as *elasticity* [42,43]. The elasticity with MRE is, like TE, expressed in kPa. Its magnitude is by rule 1/3 of the stiffness value measured with TE [32]. In practice, however, this 1/3 rule does not apply exactly.

For the acquisition of MR elastograms of the liver, mechanical waves of 50 Hz were applied to the liver by a portable transducer, which was placed against the right side of the chest. MRE was performed on a 3.0 Tesla MR system (Intera, Philips Healthcare, The Netherlands). Transverse slices were obtained through the mid-level (feet-head direction) of the liver using a motion sensitive 2D spin-echo based echo-planar imaging sequence with the

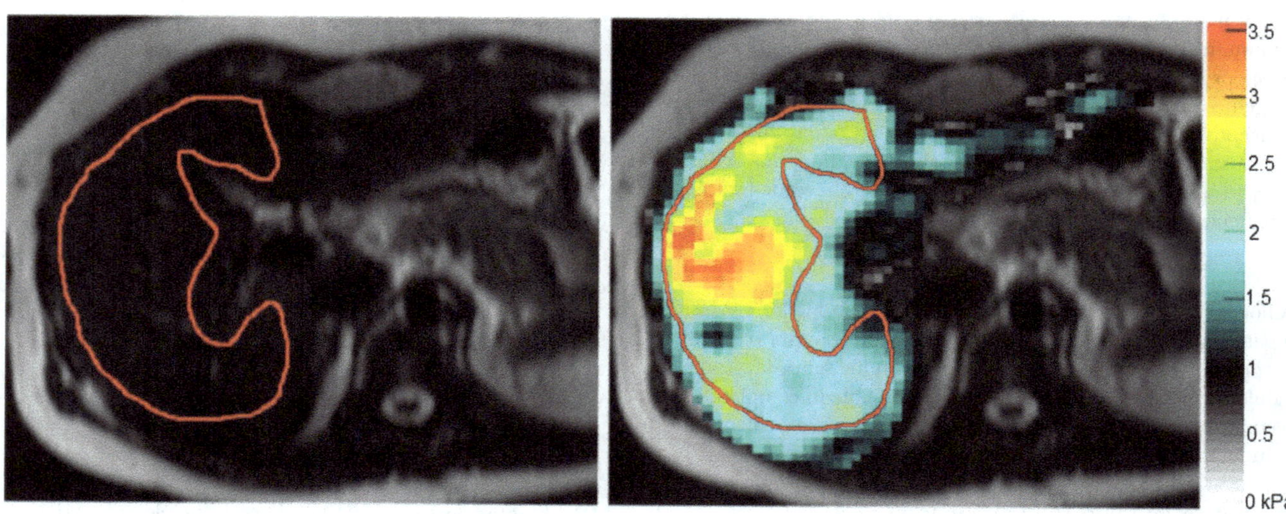

Figure 2. MRE: selection of region of interest (ROI) in the liver. ROIs are drawn manually on the elastograms, in the lateral part of the right liver lobe while avoiding liver margins and large hepatic vessels. The mean elasticity value within the ROI in this example (Sx GD patient) is 2.3 kPa (colored bar represents kPa). The corresponding stiffness measured with TE was 7.2 kPa.
doi:10.1371/journal.pone.0057507.g002

following acquisition parameters: repetition time 560 ms, echo time 40 ms, FA 90°, number of slices 7, slice thickness 4 mm; field of view 320×320 mm and matrix size 80×80. MRE acquisition time was 78 seconds, divided over 6 breath holds on expiration. Elastograms of the liver were reconstructed using dedicated post-processing software (provided by R. Sinkus, Clichy, France) [43]. A region of interest was manually drawn in the right liver lobe, avoiding liver margins and major blood vessels (Figure 2). Elasticity measured inside this region of interest was used for analysis.

Laboratory Parameters of GD Severity, Iron Metabolism and Hemochromatosis Mutation Analysis (GD Patients Only)

Concentrations of chitotriosidase, angiotensin-converting enzyme (ACE), ferritin, plasma iron, total iron binding capacity (TIBC), iron saturation, and transferrin and hemoglobin are determined regularly as standard-of-care in our GD patients. Chitotriosidase activity was measured using the 4MU-deoxychitobioside substrate, as described by Aguilera et al. and slightly modified by Schoonhoven et al [44,45]. Genotyping for the chitotriosidase 24-bp duplication was performed by PCR [46]. Chitotriosidase values of patients who were heterozygous for this chitotriosidase mutation were multiplied by 2. Both ACE and Ferritin were measured as markers of GD activity. Plasma iron, TIBC, iron saturation and transferrin were included to assess iron metabolism.

HFE mutations are relatively common in the Northern European population; 3.5–15% is heterozygous for the C282Y mutation and 20% is heterozygous for the H63D mutation [29,47]. As high ferritin levels are a common feature in both GD and hemochromatosis, it has been suggested that the possibility of concurrent genetic hemochromatosis should be excluded in GD patients [48]. Therefore all GD patients in this study were tested for the common C282Y and H63D mutations in the HFE gene to investigate the presence or absence of hereditary hemochromatosis/carriership.

Statistical Analysis

For quantitative imaging, results of non-Sx GD patients were compared with those of the matched controls. Comparisons between non-Sx and Sx GD patients were made for all study parameters. Non-parametric, two-tailed tests were employed on all statistical analyses. For correlations, Spearman's rho was calculated. For comparison of means and proportions, Mann Whitney U and Fisher's exact test was used. A p-value of less than 0.05 was considered statistically significant. All analyses were performed with PASW statistics 18 (SPSS, Chicago, Ill, USA) and GraphPad Prism 5 (GraphPad Software, INC, La Jolla, CA, USA).

Results

Participants

Of the 23 included participants (16 GD and 7 controls), 21 completed all study procedures. Two patients were excluded after inclusion: one Sx GD patient was unable to participate due to complications unrelated to the study procedures; one non-Sx GD patient withdrew consent before study procedures were completed. One patient was included shortly after undergoing a partial liver resection of segment IV because of a HCC.

MR-LIC measurement was technically unsuccessful initially in one patient, but was repeated successfully six months later. Due to prolonged technical problems with our TE system, examinations could not be performed in six participants during the visit in which MRI was performed and biochemical data were collected. The TE examinations were completed three to twelve months later.

Anthropometric data of all participants and disease characteristics of GD patients, including age at Sx, age at start of treatment, history of iron supplementation and/or blood transfusions and GD genotype, are summarized in Table 1 and 2.

Quantitative Imaging (All Participants)

Liver iron concentration. LIC values calculated using the method of Gandon showed excellent correlation with T2* measurements (rho = 0.85, $p<0.01$). LIC was elevated (>60±30 μmol/g with the Gandon method) in four GD patients of whom 3 were splenectomized. There were no significant differences between non-Sx GD and Sx GD patients, or between non-Sx and controls (Figure 3 A, Table 3). Reconstruction of T2* anatomical maps of the liver (Figure 4) visualizes distinct differences in LIC between participants.

Transient Elastography. TE measurements of both the anterior and posterior locations were difficult to perform, with very low success rates. Results are therefore only reported for the reference location. Of note is that TE results at the reference locations were *poorly reliable* according to the criteria by Boursier et al [35]: in two participants: one non-Sx GD patient (TE 7.2 kPa, IQR 35%) and one Sx GD patient (TE 16.0 kPa, IQR 64%). For the latter patient, liver cirrhosis was also confirmed histologically. Using a cutoff of 7.0 kPa for the presence of substantial fibrosis (stage F2 or higher) with TE, seven GD patients would be classified as having substantial fibrosis (1 non-Sx, 6 Sx), versus none of the healthy controls [43].

Sx GD patients had significantly higher stiffness values compared with non-Sx GD patients (p = 0.03), as shown in Figure 3 B and Table 3. There were no significant differences between non-Sx and controls.

MR elastography. In three Sx GD patients, acquisition of MRE was not possible due to high liver iron concentrations, causing complete MR signal loss. The four successful MRE acquisitions in the Sx GD group were significantly higher than the non-Sx GD group (p = 0.01), as shown in Figure 3 C. Again, there were no significant differences between non-Sx and controls (Table 3).

Laboratory Parameters of GD Severity, Iron Metabolism and Hemochromatosis Mutation Analysis (GD Patients Only)

Sx GD patients had significantly higher ACE concentrations ($p<0.01$) compared with non-Sx GD patients. The difference in chitotriosidase activity showed a trend ($p = 0.07$). There was no significant difference in ferritin concentration or any of the other parameters of iron metabolism (Table 4). Although 9 of 14 GD patients had an elevated ferritin concentration, only one Sx patient showed signs of increased iron storage, which is defined as a ferritin concentration above the upper limit of normal combined with an iron saturation >45% [44]. This patient was heterozygous for the H63D mutation.

HFE mutations were present in 8 of 14 GD patients (57%): two C282Y heterozygotes, two H63D homozygotes and four H63D heterozygotes. Six out of 7 Sx GD patients and two out of 7 non-Sx GD patients carried a mutation ($p = 0.10$). Figures 3 A–C show the distribution of HFE mutations between Sx and non-Sx groups in relation to LIC-Gandon, TE and MRE.

Table 1. Participant characteristics.

	Controls ($n=7$) median (range)	Non-Sx GD ($n=7$) median (range)	Sx GD ($n=7$) median (range)
Sex (m/f)	6/1	6/1	4/3
Age (y)	44 (26–59)	46 (24–61)	55 (39–70)
BMI (kg/m2)	22.7 (20.8–28.6)	23.1 (21.1–27.4)	24.8 (21.0–27.7)
Age Sx (y)			20 (4–32)
Age start treatment (y)		37 (17–45)	43 (29–59)
Treatment (ERT:SRT)		6:1	6:1
Genotype			
N370S/N370S		0	1
N370S/L444P		4	2
N370S/other or unknown		3	4

Relationships between Study Parameters

Liver iron concentration. Besides a significant correlation between LIC-Gandon and T2* (rho = 0.85, p<0.01), we observed a strong correlation between LIC-Gandon and ferritin concentration (rho = 0.84, p<0.01), and between LIC-Gandon and transferrin concentration (rho = −0.62, p = 0.02), Figure 5 A–C. LIC-Gandon did not correlate with the remaining biochemical parameters, or with TE (rho = 0.10, p = 0.73) or MRE (rho = −0.40, p = 0.23). Correlations of T2* with the aforementioned parameters were similar to those observed for LIC-Gandon (data not shown).

Of 4 patients with elevated LIC, the 3 splenectomized patients (no 9, 12, 14, table 2) had received blood transfusion in their past, although the number of transfusions varied. The fourth, non-splenectomized patient (no 6) had not received blood transfusions, but was treated with iron supplementation for a few months as an adolescent. Conversely, 3 patients with a history of multiple blood transfusions (no 1, 10, 11) had normal LIC.

Transient elastography. TE measurements correlated significantly with MRE (rho = 0.67, p = 0.02), with chitotriosidase activity (rho = 0.62, p = 0.02) and with ACE (rho = 0.60, p = 0.03), Figure 5 D–F. Correlations between TE measurements and plasma iron concentration (rho = 0.50, p 0.07) and iron saturation (rho = 0.47, p 0.09) showed a trend. There was no significant correlation with ferritin, total iron binding capacity or transferrin.

Discussion

This study is the first to demonstrate that liver stiffness values are significantly higher in splenectomized GD patients when compared with GD patients with an intact spleen, as measured by TE and MRE. TE and MRE techniques can be used to identify and monitor GD patients to assess the presence of liver fibrosis. We also showed that liver stiffness parameters and liver iron content in non-Sx GD patients were not different from their matched healthy controls. Considering our hypothesis that splenectomized patients are particularly at risk for the develop-

Table 2. Iron status GD patients.

Case no	Age	Sx*	HFE genotype	Blood transfusions	Iron suplementation	LIC (SD) (Gandon)	TE (kPa)
1	43	No	wt/wt	Yes, 5–6 age 8; donor age 19–21	Yes, not in the last 12 years	25 (20)	4.4
2	46	No	wt/wt	No	Yes, briefly age 10	60 (30)	4.8
3	43	No	wt/wt	No, donor age 17–20	No	40 (20)	6.1
4	24	No	wt/wt	No	No	35 (20)	6.6
5	61	No	H63D/H63D	No	Yes, age 15–20	30 (20)	7.2
6	49	No	C282Y/wt	No, donor age 25–29	Yes, age 15	**90 (30)**	3.4
7	59	No	wt/wt	No, donor age 25–40	No	20 (20)	4.2
8	39	Yes	wt/wt	Yes, 1× age 20	Yes, several months, not recently	28 (20)	7.2
9	55	Yes	H63D/H63D	Yes, >40× until age 36	Yes, childh./adol.	**95 (30)**	3.5
10	48	Yes	H63D/wt	Yes, 5–10× childhood	Yes, childh./adol.,briefly age 41	35 (20)	10.5
11	70	Yes	H63D/wt	Yes, >80× age 48, 1× age 56	Yes, childhood	10 (20)	8.7
12	66	Yes	C282Y/wt	Yes, 4× age 17–50	Yes, several days age 17–50	**170 (50)**	9.9
13	55	Yes	H63D/wt	Yes, 1× age 26	Yes, age 15–16	30 (20)	8.8
14	63	Yes	H63D/wt	Yes, 40 units until age 45	No	**250 (50)**	16

*Sx = splenectomy.

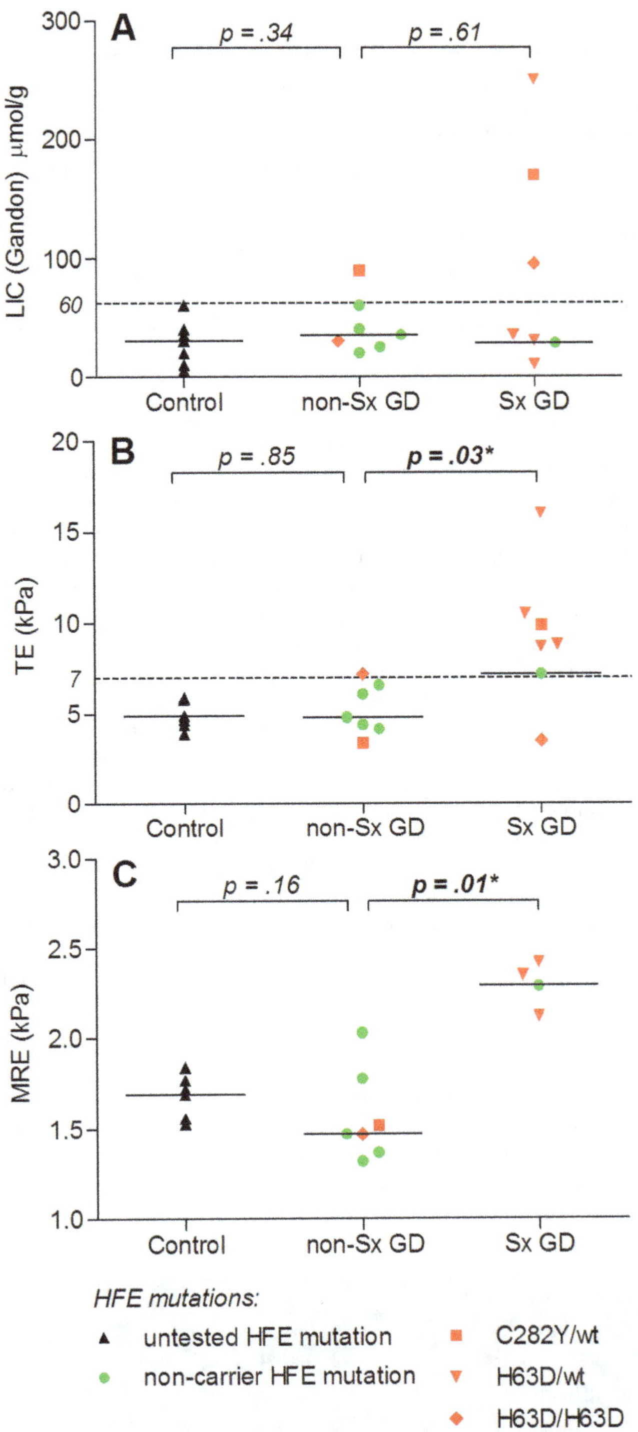

Figure 3. Comparison of quantitative imaging results and distribution of HFE mutations. Solid black horizontal lines represent median values. Presence and distribution of HFE mutations in GD patients are shown in red and green. (A) MR-liver iron concentration (Gandon). Dashed line represents upper limit of normal (60 μmol/g). Median (range) in μmol/g: controls ($n = 7$) 30 (5–66); non-Sx GD ($n = 7$) 35 (20–90); Sx GD ($n = 7$) 35 (10–250). (B) Transient elastography results. Dashed line represents cutoff value for the presence of substantial liver fibrosis (Metavir ≥ F2). Median (range) in kPa: controls ($n = 7$) 4.9 (3.9–5.9); non-Sx GD ($n = 7$) 4.8 (3.4–7.2); Sx GD ($n = 7$) 8.8 (3.5–16.0). (C) MR elastography results. Median (range) in kPa: controls ($n = 7$) 1.69 (1.53–1.84); non-Sx GD ($n = 7$) 1.47 (1.32–2.03); Sx GD ($n = 4$) 2.32 (2.12–2.42).

ment of HCC, we suggest that this risk is related to the presence of fibrosis in the liver.

We did not add a splenectomized control group as fibrosis is not caused by splenectomy, but rather splenectomy indicates advanced Gaucher disease. A similar relationship between risk for bone complications and splenectomy has previously been shown [23,49,50].

One patient was included shortly after undergoing a resection of a liver segment because of HCC. He had a history of severe GD including a splenectomy, bone complications and anemia despite splenectomy, requiring transfusions (approximately 40 units of packed red blood cells) before the start of enzyme replacement therapy (ERT). PCR testing for hepatitis B and C was negative in this patient. Interestingly, we found this patient to have both the highest concentration of liver iron (250±50 μmol/g), as well as the highest liver stiffness value with TE: 16.0 kPa, a value being suggestive of the presence of severe liver fibrosis and probable cirrhosis [51]. Histopathological analysis of resected liver parenchyma that surrounded the tumor confirmed both liver cirrhosis and severe iron overload. HFE mutation analysis showed heterozygosity for the H63D mutation. MRE was unsuccessful due to the high iron load. This patient started ERT 18 years ago with quick and complete recovery of blood counts but with remaining high chitotriosidase activities, indicative of residual Gaucher cell burden.

Although not previously used in GD, numerous studies have demonstrated the ability of TE to predict liver fibrosis, cirrhosis and cirrhosis-related complications in various chronic liver diseases [31,51,52]. The European Association for the study of the Liver (EASL) have recently included TE in their guidelines for assessing disease severity in hepatitis C [53]. MRE is still under development and is at this point mainly used as a research tool. The technique also has a good diagnostic accuracy for non-invasive fibrosis assessment [54]. A head-to-head study comparing the accuracies of MRE and TE was in favor of MRE [32]. However, the fact that MRE measurements were unsuccessful in three of seven Sx GD patients due to high liver iron load – while TE was successful - highlights an important limitation of this technique at present. TE identified high stiffness of the liver in two of these three cases, which suggests that these patients were at risk, and illustrates that this subgroup should not be missed. A technical solution for this limitation of MRE is already being developed, making use of short echo times and fractional encoding [42].

This study also revealed a difference in the frequency of mutations in the HFE gene between splenectomized and non-splenectomized patients. This difference was found by chance, since screening was performed primarily to exclude hereditary hemochromatosis as a cause for iron accumulation. The majority (6 of 8) involved H63D mutations, which have not been associated with clinically significant iron storage, unless present in combination with the C282Y mutation [55]. Although this finding might be suggestive of a relationship between mutations in the HFE gene and GD, further evaluation - in a larger cohort - is warranted regarding the relationship between HFE mutations and other parameters of GD severity.

Stein et al investigated the occurrence of iron overload in GD type I patients and found signs of iron overload in only 3 of 114 patients, 2 of whom carried the H63D mutation (1 homozygous, 1 heterozygous) in de HFE gene - as compared with 38/114 in the total cohort [48]. In contrast, our study revealed signs of iron overload, albeit to varying extent, in 4 of 14 GD patients. This difference might be explained by the difference in the populations that were studied: 53% of the population studied by Stein et al. was homozygous for the N370S mutation, which is generally

Table 3. Quantitative imaging results.

	Controls ($n=7$) median (range)	Non-Sx GD ($n=7$) median (range)	Sx GD ($n=7$) median (range)	*p*	
				Controls vs. non-Sx	Non-Sx vs. Sx
LIC-Gandon (μmol/g) ref <60±30 μmol/g	30 (5–60)	35 (20–90)	35 (10–250)	0.34	0.61
LIC T2* (ms) ref >22 ms	26 (16–33)	19.0 (8.7–27.0)	23.0 (3.2–32.0)	0.07	0.95
TE (kPa) ref <7.0 kPa for<F2	4.9 (3.9–5.9)	4.8 (3.4–7.2)	8.8 (3.5–16.0)	0.85	**0.03**
MR Elastography (kPa) ref unknown	1.69 (1.53–1.84)	1.47 (1.32–2.03)	2.32 (2.12–2.42); $n=4$	0.16	**0.01**

associated with milder disease manifestations, whereas we had only one such patient in our cohort.

We did not find a relationship between LIC and fibrosis in our study. First of all, patients with increased liver stiffness did not always have an elevated LIC, suggesting that other factors than iron storage must be involved as well. Four patients had iron overload (>60±30 μmol/g), of whom two had moderately elevated LIC values of 170±50 and 250±50 μmol/g, and liver stiffness values indicating the presence of substantial fibrosis: 9.9 and 16.0 kPa, respectively (TE). In the other two patients, with mildly elevated LIC values of 90 and 95 μmol/g, TE values were normal. Bassett et al described fibrosis and cirrhosis in patients with hereditary hemochromatosis only at hepatic iron concentrations exceeding 400 μmol/g [56]. Guyader et al did not confirm these results, but in their cohort comprising 197 patients with homozygous C282Y hemochromatosis, median LIC of patients with no or moderate fibrosis (F0–F2) was 250 μmol/g versus 461 μmol/g in those with severe fibrosis and cirrhosis (F3–F4) [57]. The previously stated example of our patient who developed HCC further illustrates the complexity of an analysis of the relationship between LIC and fibrosis, which may be confounded by HFE mutation status and history of transfusions. Nevertheless, HCC risk in GD patients is perhaps best explained as the result of a combination of local effects of GD storage cells and these (GD associated) factors.

Based on the MRI technique used, we are unable to differentiate between iron stored in Gaucher cells and iron stored in hepatocytes. The pattern of iron deposition may influence toxicity. While iron deposits have been described in Gaucher cells, parenchymal iron storage has been observed in GD patients who developed HCC as well (personal observations).

A limitation of this study is that we did not perform laboratory assessments of iron storage and screening for HFE mutations in our control group, since we wanted to focus on the novel imaging techniques and limit the invasiveness of participation in this study. In the GD groups, biochemical parameters were assessed for routine clinical practice, so only additional consent had to be given for the HFE mutation screening. However, none of the controls had signs of hemochromatosis based upon LIC data.

Furthermore, the high IQRs associated with some of the liver stiffness measurements using TE. A common recommendation for validation of successful measurements is that the interquartile range should be less than 30% of the median liver stiffness measurement value. A study by Lucidarme et al identified IQR as a factor of overestimation of liver fibrosis and suggested an even stricter cutoff value of 0.21 [58]. Castera et al identified an operator experience fewer than 500 examinations as a reason for unreliable results, which is a factor that may have influenced the current study results [31]. However, repeating TE analyses while excluding the three participants in whom IQR exceeded 30% did not change statistical significance (data not shown).

All GD patients were treated with either enzyme replacement therapy or substrate reduction therapy. Whether this has influenced the parameters of liver stiffness or iron content cannot be concluded from this study. The differences between splenectomized and non-splenectomized GD patients and the observation that splenectomy can be avoided by ERT suggests that ERT may

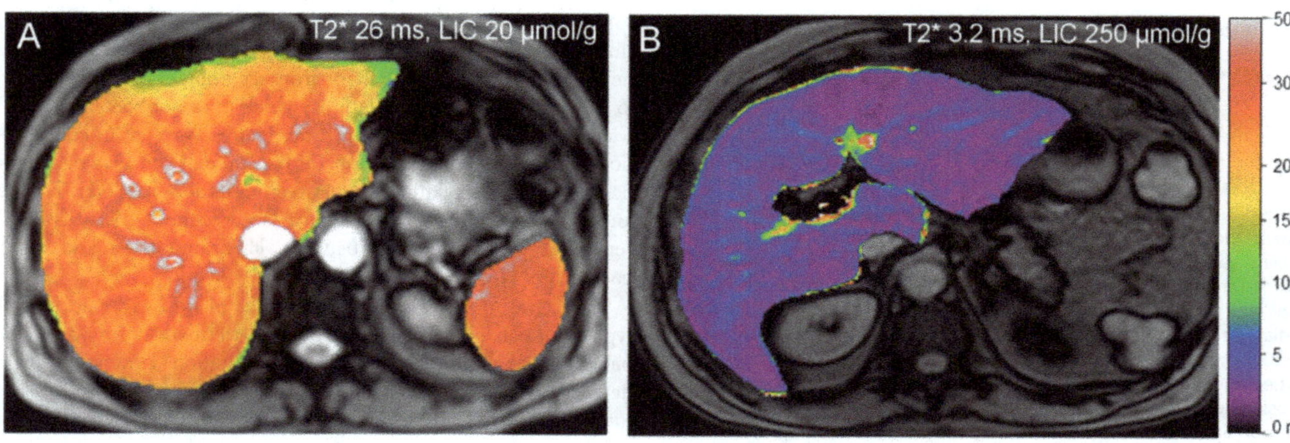

Figure 4. T2* maps of the liver. (A) Healthy control with a normal liver T2* value of 26 ms (LIC-Gandon: 20±20 μmol/g). (B) Sx-GD patient with severe iron overload: T2* value in the liver is short: 3.2 ms; the corresponding LIC measured with the Gandon method was high: 250±50 μmol/g.

Table 4. Biochemical assessment.

	Non-Sx GD ($n=7$) median (range)	Sx GD ($n=7$) median (range)	p
Chitotriosidase activity (nmol/ml.h) *ref 10–190 nmol/ml.h*	3,318 (1,269–16,177)	9,160 (4,175–31,021); $n=6$	0.07
ACE (U/L) *ref 20–70 U/L*	65 (53–100)	124 (85–150); $n=6$	**<0.01**
Hemoglobin level (mmol/L) *ref ♂ 8.5–10.5 mmol/l ♀7.5–10 mmol/L*	9.4 (8.8–9.8)	8.4 (6.8–9.2)	**<0.01**
Ferritin (μg/L) *ref ♂ 25–300 μg/L, ♂premenopausal 15–200, ♀ postmenopausal 20–250*	315 (85–802)	475 (219–3,109)	0.13
Transferrin (g/L) *ref 2–3.6 g/L*	2.22 (1.95–2.72)	2.05 (1.72–3.43)	0.70
Iron (μmol/L) *ref ♂ 11–32 μmol/L, ♀ 11–27 μmol/L*	15.6 (11.9–16.1)	21.6 (10.6–30.9)	0.16
TIBC (μmol/L) *ref 50–91 μmol/L*	55.9 (49.1–68.5)	51.7 (43.3–86.4)	0.70
Iron saturation *ref 0.20–0.55*	0.25 (0.22–0.31)	0.31 (0.24–0.65)	0.10

decrease the risk for development of hepatic fibrosis and cirrhosis-related complications in the future.

In conclusion, TE and MRE can be used to detect and monitor liver fibrosis in patients with GD. We hypothesize a relationship with excessive hepatic iron accumulation in splenectomized patients. However, the role of iron storage needs further study. Since the splenectomized GD group showed more advanced liver disease than the non-splenectomized GD group, we recommend

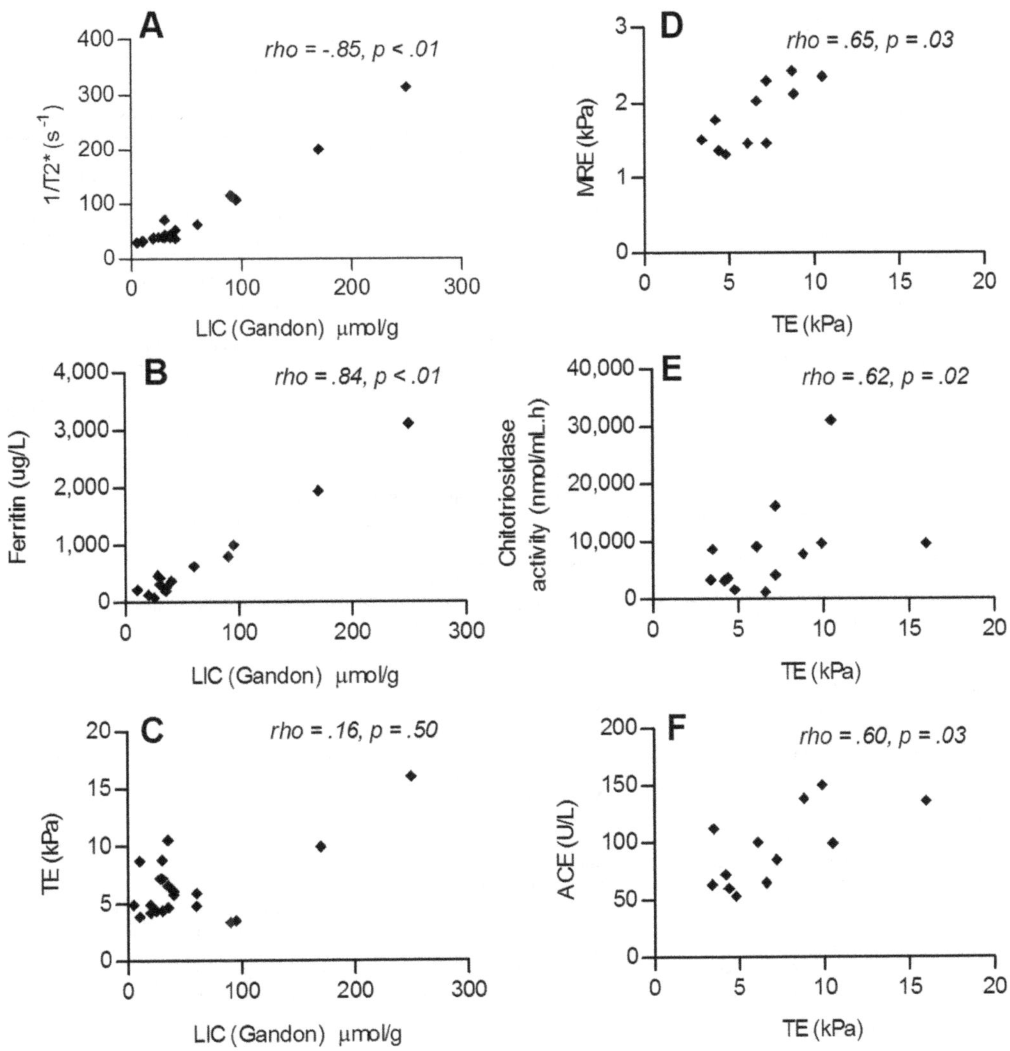

Figure 5. Correlations between study parameters. A–C: correlations between MR-LIC and 1/T2* ($n=21$), TE ($n=21$) and ferritin concentration ($n=14$). D–F: correlations between TE and MRE ($n=18$), Chitotriosidase activity ($n=14$) and ACE ($n=14$).

that all splenectomized patients, especially those with evidence of substantial liver fibrosis undergo regular screening for HCC, according to current guidelines.

Acknowledgments

The authors acknowledge the Dutch Gaucher patients for their willingness to participate in this study, and Prof. dr. J.M.F.G Aerts (Dept of Medical Biochemistry, Academic Medical Center, Amsterdam, The Netherlands) for providing the chitotriosidase assay, the helpful discussions and review of the manuscript.

Author Contributions

Read and reviewed the manuscript: AEB LVD EMA AJN RS PLMJ JS CEMH. Conceived and designed the experiments: AEB LVD EMA JS CEMH. Performed the experiments: AEB LVD EMA. Analyzed the data: AEB LVD EMA. Contributed reagents/materials/analysis tools: EMA AJN PLMJ RS. Wrote the paper: AEB LVD JS CEMH.

References

1. Beutler E, Grabowski GA (2001) Gaucher Disease. In: Scriver CR, Beaudet AL, Sly WS, Valle D, editors. The Metabolic and Molecular Bases of Inherited Disease. 8 ed. New York: McGraw-Hill. 3636.
2. Brady RO, Pentchev PG, Gal AE, Hibbert SR, Dekaban AS (1974) Replacement therapy for inherited enzyme deficiency. Use of purified glucocerebrosidase in Gaucher's disease. N Engl J Med 291: 989–993.
3. Cox T, Lachmann R, Hollak C, Aerts J, van Weely S, et al. (2000) Novel oral treatment of Gaucher's disease with N-butyldeoxynojirimycin (OGT 918) to decrease substrate biosynthesis. Lancet 355: 1481–1485.
4. Grabowski GA, Barton NW, Pastores G, Dambrosia JM, Banerjee TK, et al. (1995) Enzyme therapy in type 1 Gaucher disease: comparative efficacy of mannose-terminated glucocerebrosidase from natural and recombinant sources. Ann Intern Med 122: 33–39.
5. Poorthuis BJ, Wevers RA, Kleijer WJ, Groener JE, de Jong JG, et al. (1999) The frequency of lysosomal storage diseases in The Netherlands. Hum Genet 105: 151–156.
6. Lachmann RH, Wight DG, Lomas DJ, Fisher NC, Schofield JP, et al. (2000) Massive hepatic fibrosis in Gaucher's disease: clinico-pathological and radiological features. QJM 93: 237–244.
7. Breiden-Langen CM, Buchsel R, Brambs HJ, Oehlert M, Matern S (1991) Coincidence of Gaucher disease with primary hepatocellular carcinoma. Leber Magen Darm 21: 126, 129–126, 130.
8. de Fost M., vom Dahl S, Weverling GJ, Brill N, Brett S, et al. (2006) Increased incidence of cancer in adult Gaucher disease in Western Europe. Blood Cells Mol Dis 36: 53–58.
9. Erjavec Z, Hollak CE, de Vries EG (1999) Hepatocellular carcinoma in a patient with Gaucher disease on enzyme supplementation therapy. Ann Oncol 10: 243.
10. Lee RE (1982) The pathology of Gaucher disease. Prog Clin Biol Res 95: 177–217.
11. Taddei TH, Kacena KA, Yang M, Yang R, Malhotra A, et al. (2009) The underrecognized progressive nature of N370S Gaucher disease and assessment of cancer risk in 403 patients. Am J Hematol 84: 208–214.
12. Xu R, Mistry P, McKenna G, Emre S, Schiano T, et al. (2005) Hepatocellular carcinoma in type 1 Gaucher disease: a case report with review of the literature. Semin Liver Dis 25: 226–229.
13. Zimran A, Liphshitz I, Barchana M, Abrahamov A, Elstein D (2005) Incidence of malignancies among patients with type I Gaucher disease from a single referral clinic. Blood Cells Mol Dis 34: 197–200.
14. Shoenfeld Y, Gallant LA, Shaklai M, Livni E, Djaldetti M, et al. (1982) Gaucher's disease: a disease with chronic stimulation of the immune system. Arch Pathol Lab Med 106: 388–391.
15. Bassan R, Montanelli A, Barbui T (1985) Interaction between a serum factor and T lymphocytes in Gaucher disease. Am J Hematol 18: 381–384.
16. Brill NE, Mandlebaum FS, Libman E (1905) Primary splenomegaly - Gaucher type. Report on one of four cases occurring in a single generation of one family. Am J Med Sci : 491.
17. Lee RE, Balcerzak SP, Westerman MP (1967) Gaucher's disease. A morphologic study and measurements of iron metabolism. Am J Med 42: 891–898.
18. Lorber M (1960) The occurrence of intracellular iron in Gaucher's disease. Ann Intern Med. 53[2], 293.
19. Lorber M, Nemes JL (1967) Identification of ferritin within Gaucher cells. An electron microscopic and immunofluorescent study. Acta Haematol 37: 189–197.
20. Morgan MA, Hoffbrand AV, Laulicht M, Luck W, Knowles S (1983) Serum ferritin concentration in Gaucher's disease. Br Med J (Clin Res Ed) 286: 1864.
21. Weisberger J, Emmons F, Gorczyca W (2004) Cytochemical diagnosis of Gaucher's disease by iron stain. Br J Haematol 124: 696.
22. Lorber M (1970) Adult-type Gaucher's disease: a secondary disorder of iron metabolism. Mt Sinai J Med 37: 404–417.
23. Cox TM, Aerts JM, Belmatoug N, Cappellini MD, vom Dahl S, et al. (2008) Management of non-neuronopathic Gaucher disease with special reference to pregnancy, splenectomy, bisphosphonate therapy, use of biomarkers and bone disease monitoring. J Inherit Metab Dis 31: 319–336.
24. Krasnewich D, Dietrich K, Bauer L, Ginns EI, Sidransky E, et al. (1998) Splenectomy in Gaucher disease: new management dilemmas. Blood 91: 3085–3087.
25. Ponce E, Moskovitz J, Grabowski G (1997) Enzyme therapy in Gaucher disease type 1: effect of neutralizing antibodies to acid beta-glucosidase. Blood 90: 43–48.
26. de Fost M., van Noesel CJ, Aerts JM, Maas M, Poll RG, et al. (2008) Persistent bone disease in adult type 1 Gaucher disease despite increasing doses of enzyme replacement therapy. Haematologica 93: 1119–1120.
27. Hollak CE, Belmatoug N, Cole JA, vom Dahl S, Deegan PB, et al. (2012) Characteristics of type I Gaucher disease associated with persistent thrombocytopenia after treatment with imiglucerase for 4–5 years. Br J Haematol 158: 528–538.
28. Perel Y, Bioulac-Sage P, Chateil JF, Trillaud H, Carles J, et al. (2002) Gaucher's disease and fatal hepatic fibrosis despite prolonged enzyme replacement therapy. Pediatrics 109: 1170–1173.
29. EASL clinical practice guidelines for HFE hemochromatosis (2010) J Hepatol 53: 3–22.
30. EASL-EORTC clinical practice guidelines: management of hepatocellular carcinoma. (2012) J Hepatol 56: 908–943.
31. Castera L, Foucher J, Bernard PH, Carvalho F, Allaix D, et al. (2010) Pitfalls of liver stiffness measurement: a 5-year prospective study of 13,369 examinations. Hepatology 51: 828–835.
32. Huwart L, Sempoux C, Vicaut E, Salameh N, Annet L, et al. (2008) Magnetic resonance elastography for the noninvasive staging of liver fibrosis. Gastroenterology 135: 32–40.
33. Yin M, Talwalkar JA, Glaser KJ, Manduca A, Grimm RC, et al. (2007) Assessment of hepatic fibrosis with magnetic resonance elastography. Clin Gastroenterol Hepatol 5: 1207–1213.
34. Castera L (2012) Noninvasive methods to assess liver disease in patients with hepatitis B or C. Gastroenterology 142: 1293–1302.
35. Poca M, Puente A, Graupera I, Villanueva C (2011) Prognostic markers in patients with cirrhosis and portal hypertension who have not bled. Dis Markers 31: 147–154.
36. St Pierre TG, Clark PR, Chua-Anusorn W (2005) Measurement and mapping of liver iron concentrations using magnetic resonance imaging. Ann N Y Acad Sci 1054: 379–385.
37. St Pierre TG, Clark PR, Chua-Anusorn W, Fleming AJ, Jeffrey GP, et al. (2005) Noninvasive measurement and imaging of liver iron concentrations using proton magnetic resonance. Blood 105: 855–861.
38. Wood JC, Enriquez C, Ghugre N, Tyzka JM, Carson S, et al. (2005) MRI R2 and R2* mapping accurately estimates hepatic iron concentration in transfusion-dependent thalassemia and sickle cell disease patients. Blood 106: 1460–1465.
39. Gandon Y, Olivie D, Guyader D, Aube C, Oberti F, et al. (2004) Non-invasive assessment of hepatic iron stores by MRI. Lancet 363: 357–362.
40. Sandrin L, Fourquet B, Hasquenoph JM, Yon S, Fournier C, et al. (2003) Transient elastography: a new noninvasive method for assessment of hepatic fibrosis. Ultrasound Med Biol 29: 1705–1713.
41. Boursier J, Zarski JP, de Ledinghen, V, Rousselet MC, Sturm N, et al. (2012) Determination of reliability criteria of liver stiffness evaluation by transient elastography. Hepatology.
42. Garteiser P, Sahebjavaher RS, Ter Beek L, van Beers BE, Salcudean SE, et al. (2012) Rapid 3D motion-encoding using steady-state FFE pulse sequence: application towards multifrequency MR rheology. Proc Intl Soc Mag Reson Med 20: 3423.
43. Sinkus R, Siegmann K, Xydeas T, Tanter M, Claussen C, et al. (2007) MR elastography of breast lesions: understanding the solid/liquid duality can improve the specificity of contrast-enhanced MR mammography. Magn Reson Med 58: 1135–1144.
44. Aguilera B, Ghauharali-van der Vlugt K, Helmond MT, Out JM, Donker-Koopman WE, et al. (2003) Transglycosidase activity of chitotriosidase: improved enzymatic assay for the human macrophage chitinase. J Biol Chem 278: 40911–40916.
45. Schoonhoven A, Rudensky B, Elstein D, Zimran A, Hollak CE, et al. (2007) Monitoring of Gaucher patients with a novel chitotriosidase assay. Clin Chim Acta 381: 136–139.
46. Boot RG, Renkema GH, Verhoek M, Strijland A, Bliek J, et al. (1998) The human chitotriosidase gene. Nature of inherited enzyme deficiency. J Biol Chem 273: 25680–25685.
47. Nederlandse Internisten Vereniging, Nederlandse Vereniging voor Klinische Chemie en Laboratoriumgeneeskunde, Vereniging Artsen Laboratoriumdiagnostiek (2007) Dutch Guideline Hereditary Hemochromatosis.
48. Hughes D, Cappellini MD, Berger M, Van Droogenbroeck J, de Fost M, et al. (2007) Recommendations for the management of the haematological and onco-haematological aspects of Gaucher disease. Br J Haematol 138: 676–686.

49. Deegan PB, Pavlova E, Tindall J, Stein PE, Bearcroft P, et al. (2011) Osseous manifestations of adult Gaucher disease in the era of enzyme replacement therapy. Medicine (Baltimore) 90: 52–60.
50. Rodrigue SW, Rosenthal DI, Barton NW, Zurakowski D, Mankin HJ (1999) Risk factors for osteonecrosis in patients with type 1 Gaucher's disease. Clin Orthop Relat Res : 201–207.
51. Tsochatzis EA, Gurusamy KS, Ntaoula S, Cholongitas E, Davidson BR, et al. (2011) Elastography for the diagnosis of severity of fibrosis in chronic liver disease: a meta-analysis of diagnostic accuracy. J Hepatol 54: 650–659.
52. Castera L, Vergniol J, Foucher J, Le BB, Chanteloup E, et al. (2005) Prospective comparison of transient elastography, Fibrotest, APRI, and liver biopsy for the assessment of fibrosis in chronic hepatitis C. Gastroenterology 128: 343–350.
53. European Association of the Study of the Liver hepatitis C virus clinical practice guidelines (2012) Liver Int 32 Suppl 1: 2–8.
54. Wang QB, Zhu H, Liu HL, Zhang B (2012) Performance of magnetic resonance elastography and diffusion-weighted imaging for the staging of hepatic fibrosis: A meta-analysis. Hepatology.
55. Bacon BR, Adams PC, Kowdley KV, Powell LW, Tavill AS (2011) Diagnosis and management of hemochromatosis: 2011 practice guideline by the American Association for the Study of Liver Diseases. Hepatology 54: 328–343.
56. Bassett ML, Halliday JW, Powell LW (1986) Value of hepatic iron measurements in early hemochromatosis and determination of the critical iron level associated with fibrosis. Hepatology 6: 24–29.
57. Guyader D, Jacquelinet C, Moirand R, Turlin B, Mendler MH, et al. (1998) Noninvasive prediction of fibrosis in C282Y homozygous hemochromatosis. Gastroenterology 115: 929–936.
58. Lucidarme D, Foucher J, Le BB, Vergniol J, Castera L, et al. (2009) Factors of accuracy of transient elastography (fibroscan) for the diagnosis of liver fibrosis in chronic hepatitis C. Hepatology 49: 1083–1089.

14

Superficial Nephrons in BALB/c and C57BL/6 Mice Facilitate *In Vivo* Multiphoton Microscopy of the Kidney

Ina Maria Schießl[1], Sophia Bardehle[2,3], Hayo Castrop[1]*

1 Institute of Physiology, University of Regensburg, Regensburg, Germany, **2** Institute of Physiology, Department of Physiological Genomics, Ludwig-Maximilians-University, Munich, Germany, **3** Institute for Stem Cell Research, Helmholtz Zentrum, Munich, Germany

Abstract

Multiphoton microscopy (MPM) offers a unique approach for addressing both the function and structure of an organ in near-real time in the live animal. The method however is limited by the tissue-specific penetration depth of the excitation laser. In the kidney, structures in the range of 100 µm from the surface are accessible for MPM. This limitation of MPM aggravates the investigation of the function of structures located deeper in the renal cortex, like the glomerulus and the juxtaglomerular apparatus. In view of the relevance of gene-targeted mice for investigating the function of these structures, we aimed to identify a mouse strain with a high percentage of superficially located glomeruli. The mean distance of the 30 most superficial glomeruli from the kidney surface was determined in 10 commonly used mouse strains. The mean depth of glomeruli was 118.4±3.4, 123.0±2.7, 133.7±3.0, 132.3±2.6, 141.0±4.0, 145.3±4.3, 148.9±4.2, 151.6±2.7, 167.7±3.9, and 207.8±3.2 µm in kidney sections from 4-week-old C3H/HeN, BALB/cAnN, SJL/J, C57BL/6N, DBA/2N, CD1 (CRI), 129S2/SvPas, CB6F1, FVB/N and NMRI (Han) mice, respectively (n = 5 animals from each strain). The mean distance from the kidney surface of the most superficial glomeruli was significantly lower in the strains C3H/HeN Crl, BALB/cAnN, DBA/2NCrl, and C57BL/6N when compared to a peer group consisting of all the other strains ($p<.0001$). In 10-week-old mice, the most superficial glomeruli were located deeper in the cortex when compared to 4-week-old animals, with BALB/cAnN and C57BL/6N being the strains with the highest percentage of superficial glomeruli (25% percentile 116.7 and 121.9 µm, respectively). In summary, due to significantly more superficial glomeruli compared to other commonly used strains, BALB/cAnN and C57BL/6N mice appear to be particularly suitable for the investigation of glomerular function using MPM.

Editor: Robert A. Fenton, Aarhus University, Denmark

Funding: The expert support provided by Uwe deVries, Institute of Anatomy, University of Regensburg, is gratefully acknowledged. The microscope used in this study was financed in part by funding from the Deutsche Forschungsgemeinschaft (SFB699). No additional external funding was received for this study. The funders had no role in study design, data collection and analysis, decision to publish, or preparation of the manuscript.

Competing Interests: The authors have declared that no competing interests exist.

* E-mail: hayo@castrop.com

Introduction

The key functional determinates of renal function in vivo, such as renal blood flow, capillary blood flow, glomerular filtration rate, and tubular reabsorption, are usually assessed at the whole organ level. In turn, the structural basis of renal function, such as the structure of the filtration barrier or the tubular system, is classically investigated ex vivo by microscopic evaluation of fixed or frozen tissue. In contrast to conventional approaches, multiphoton microscopy (MPM) is a unique method for addressing both renal function and structure in near-real time in the live animal [1]. However, the use of MPM in kidney research limits imaging of functionally relevant structures located deep within the organ, such as the renal medulla. These structures are beyond the reach of the current excitation MPM lasers for in vivo applications [2]. As a consequence, MPM is limited to the renal cortex, where imaging with reasonable resolution is only possible in the most superficial tissues. The limited range of MPM imaging in the kidney is related to high light scattering and absorption by the heterogeneous renal tissue, and this range is markedly more restricted than in other organs with optically clear parenchyma, such as the brain [3,4].

Although the aforementioned technical limitation is of minor relevance for imaging superficially located structures such as the proximal tubule, the distal convoluted tubule, and the most superficially located cortical collecting duct, it hinders the investigation of other functionally highly relevant structures, such as the glomerulus and the juxtaglomerular apparatus (JGA). Therefore, MPM imaging of the glomerulus and the JGA has primarily been performed in Munich-Wistar-Froemter (MWF) rats, a rat strain that features many superficially located glomeruli [5,6]. However, the use of MWF rats in kidney research is problematic, because this rat strain suffers from progressive deterioration of kidney function, due to the development of proteinuria, glomerulosclerosis, and hypertension [5,6,7,8,9]. In mice, MPM imaging of superficially located glomeruli has been reported in intact BL/6 mouse kidneys, but imaging has been preferentially performed in the kidneys of young animals because the number of glomeruli close to the kidney surface decreases considerably as the organ grows [10]. At present, no systematic data are available in terms of glomerular depth in different mouse strains. Consequently, we aimed to identify a mouse strain that features close-to-surface glomeruli, similar to those observed in MWF rats. Such a mouse strain would be preferable for all MPM evaluations of the glomerulus and would allow back-crossing of relevant transgenic strains into the identified ideal genetic background. For this purpose, 10 commonly used mouse strains were evaluated in terms of the depth of their most superficially located glomeruli. In addition, we determined the influence of growth and age on the distance of glomeruli from the kidney surface.

We found substantial differences in the number and average depth of the most superficially located glomeruli in the various mouse strains. In adult mice, BALB/c and C57BL/6 appear to be the most suitable strains for MPM imaging. However, when imaging the kidneys of young animals, the preferred strains are BALB/c, C3H/N, and DBA/2. Despite marked strain differences, MWF rats exhibited superior imaging conditions than all mouse strains evaluated in the current study.

Methods

Animals

Mice 4 and 10 weeks of age (n = 5 from each age group) of the following 10 commonly used strains were analyzed: 129 [129S2/SvPas], BL/6 [C57BL/6N], CB6F1 [CB6F1], C3H/N [C3H/HeN], NMRI [NMRI (Han)], SJL [SJL/J], DBA/2 [DBA/2N], BALB/c [BALB/cAnN], FVB/N [FVB/N] and CD-1 [CD1 (CRI)]. The abbreviated versions of the strain names will be used throughout the manuscript. Both male and female mice were used in this study (Charles River Laboratories International, Inc.). Animal care and experimentation were approved by the local government, *Regierung der Oberpfalz* (54-2532.1-11/12), and carried out in accordance with National Institutes of Health principles as outlined in the *Guide for the Care and Use of Laboratory Animals.* All animal surgery was performed under ketamine/xylazine anesthesia, and anesthetized animals were sacrificed by cervical dislocation at the end of the experiments. Animals were not treated with any drug or intervention before anesthesia.

Histology

Animals were perfused with 40 ml of 3% paraformaldehyde solution in phosphate buffered saline (pH 7.2) at a constant perfusion pressure of 120 mm Hg. After embedding in paraffin, areas from the middle of the kidney were sliced (6 μm) and stained with hematoxylin and eosin stain (H&E). The depth of all glomeruli within one section of the cortex was measured using Fijii Image J and arranged according to the distance from the organ's surface. To measure the depth of the glomeruli, the length of the

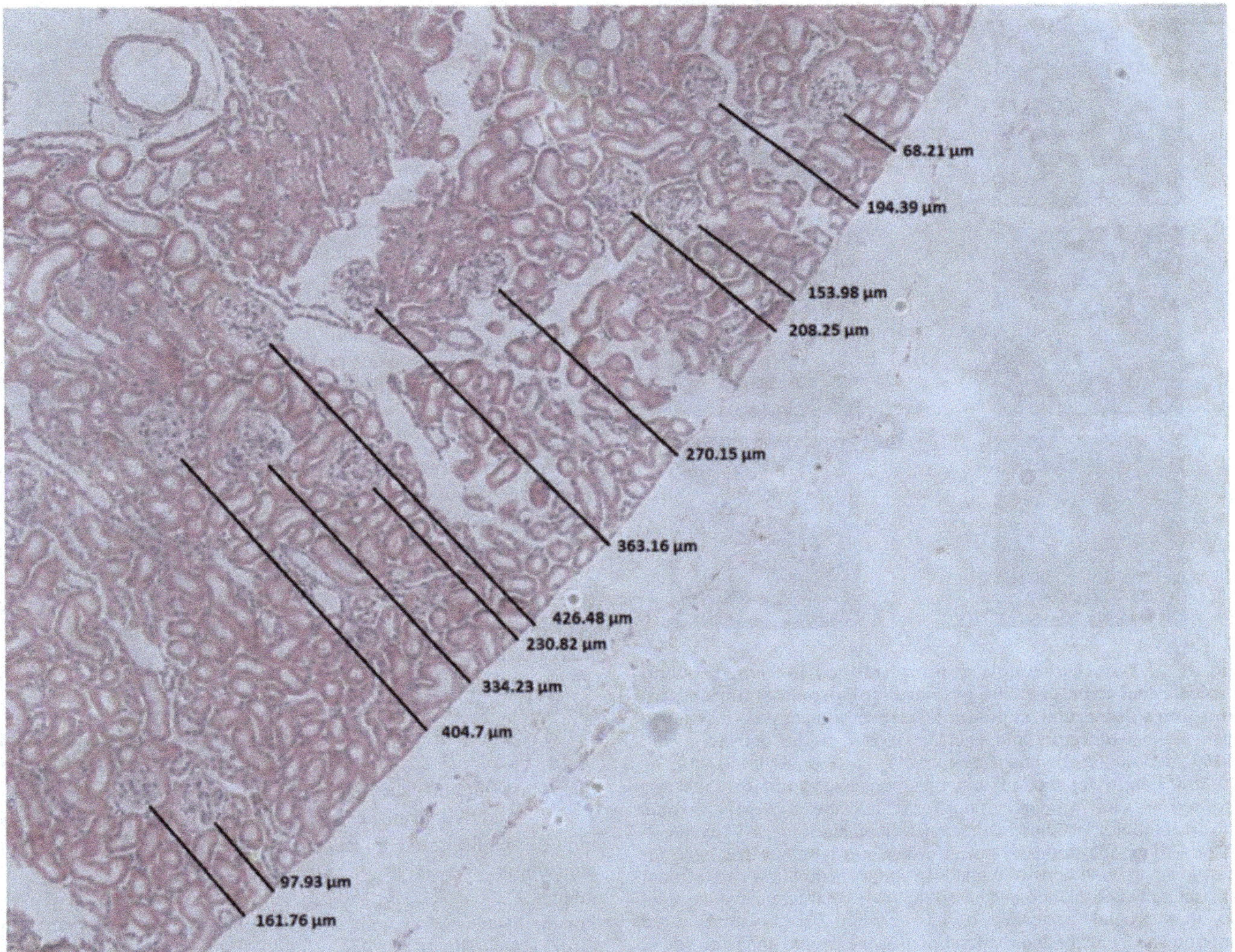

Figure 1. Determination of the depth of glomeruli from the kidney surface of a mouse. The length of the shortest vertical line from the kidney surface to the closest aspect of the glomerulus was determined.

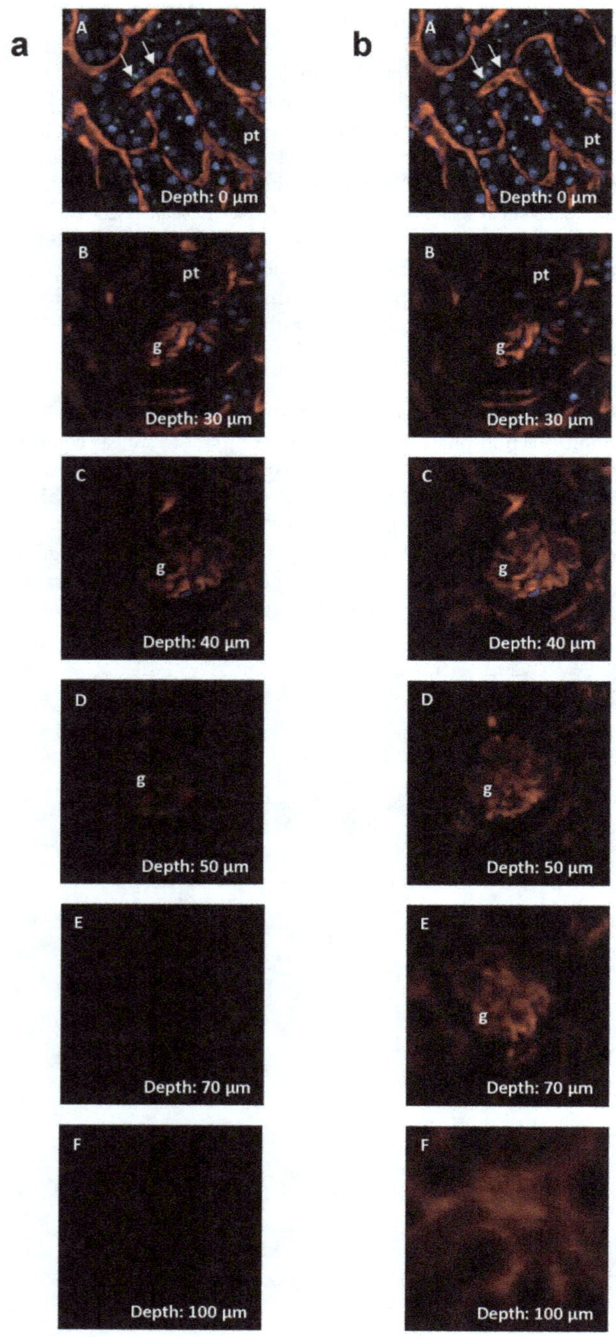

Figure 2. Z-stack through a mouse kidney in vivo, showing typical renal structures like glomeruli (g), proximal tubules (pt) and extraglomerular capillaries (arrows). Images were acquired with internal detectors and gain and offset of the detectors were maintained during the imaging process. (A) – (F) show layers in 0, 30, 40, 50, 70, and 100 µm depth underneath the kidney surface. Capillaries (arrows) are shown in red using Texas Red-labeled 70 kDa dextran. Proximal tubules (pt) showed green autofluorescence. a, left column: Z-stack without adjusted laser power, which was set at 15% of 3.2 W for best imaging conditions of the kidney surface. Without an adjustment of laser power, resolution decreased rapidly so that tissue in a depth of 50 µm was barely accessible. b, right column: Z-stack with adjusted laser power. By increasing the laser power, the limited image quality in deeper layers could be partly compensated. In a depth of 100 µm, maximum laser power produced a bright image, which however was blurry and of low resolution due to light scattering and absorption.

shortest connecting line from the kidney surface to the closest aspect of the glomerulus was determined (fig. 1). The 30 most superficial glomeruli of each section were used for further analysis. The total number of glomeruli analyzed per section was between 89 and 182.

Multiphoton Microscopy

Animals were anesthetized by i.p. injections of ketamine/xylazine (100/10 mg/kg of body weight). Polyethylene tubing was inserted into the trachea to facilitate breathing, and the jugular vein was cannulated for dye injections. For imaging of the kidney, the left kidney was exposed by a small flank incision. For the liver a horizontal incision right under the sternum was performed and the organ was exteriorized by gently applied pressure on the abdomen. For in vivo live imaging in the adult mouse brain a chronic cranial window was prepared as previously described [18]. After unilateral craniotomy of 3 mm in diameter above the somatosensory cortex, a glas cover slip (5 mm in diameter) was permanently sealed with dental acrylic. The animal was then placed upon an inverse Zeiss LSM 710 NLO confocal fluorescence microscope (Carl Zeiss Jena GmbH, Jena, Germany), which was equipped with an applicable warming plate to maintain the animal's body temperature at 37°C. Excitation was achieved using a Chameleon Ultra-II MP laser (Coherent Deutschland GmbH, Dieburg, Germany) at 860 nm with a laser power of 3200 mW. Emission was collected using external detectors (nondescanned detectors with filterset 1: beamsplitter 500–550, longpass (LP) 555 and filterset 2: beamsplitter P 565–610 including mirror) or internal (descanned) detectors. For internal detectors the following filters and beamsplitters were used to visualize different colors: a) blue channel: 404–499/main beamsplitter (MBS) 458; b) green channel: 503–590/MBS 760+; and c) red channel: 596–685/filter wheel (FW)1: rear. The pinhole was opened to the maximum. Images were acquired using a 40× long distance (LD) C-Apochromat 40/1.1 water objective. Second harmonic generation microscopy was used (excitation at 860 nm, emission at 430 nm) for visualization of collagen. Vasculature was labeled by Texas Red conjugated with 70 kDa dextran (20 mg/ml stock solution purified by PD-10 Sephadex G-25M columns [GE Healthcare, Buckinghamshire, UK]). The purified solution (50 µl) was injected i.v., and nuclei were stained using Hoechst 33342 (25 µl of a 10 mg/ml solution). Both dyes were purchased from Invitrogen (Life Technologies Corporation). For the generation of z-stacks, images at various depths of the kidney tissue were acquired, beginning from the very top of the organ, where collagen fibers of the kidney capsule were visible. The gain and offset of the detectors were kept constant, while the laser power was adjusted to keep the light intensity of the images slightly below saturation. Twelve-bit 1024×1024 pixel images were obtained using a pixel dwell time of 3.15 µs and a line average of 5. For acquisition of z-stacks without adjustment of the laser power, the laser power was set to 15%, which gave the best light intensity for the first image of the z-stack in kidney, liver and brain. A z-stack to a tissue depth of 100, 40, and 300 µm for kidney, liver, and brain, respectively was built by acquiring one image/µm. For acquisition of z-stacks with adjustment of laser power, images of the kidney capsule and images 0, 30, 50, 60 and 100 µm below the capsule were acquired. For the liver, were imaging conditions appeared to be worse than in the kidney, images in depths of 0, 10, 20, 30 and 40 µm below the collagen fibers were acquired. In the brain tissue layers in depths of 5, 60, 120, 200 and 300 µm below the surface were investigated. To increase the resolution in deeper areas, the laser power was adjusted to the optimum for each image.

A

B

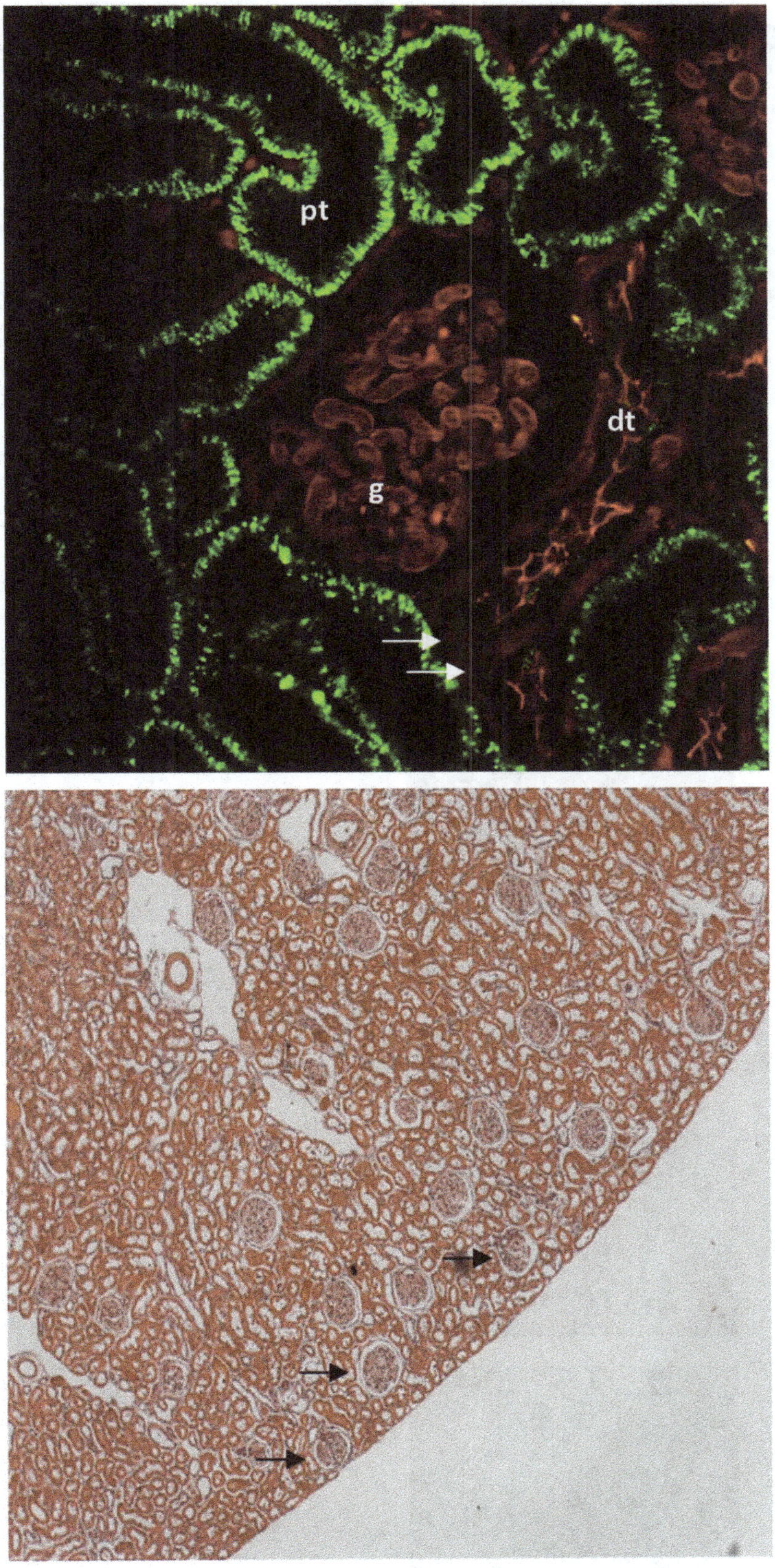

Figure 3. MPM imaging conditions in a kidney of a MWF rat in vivo. (A) Image of a superficial glomerulus (g) and a distal tubule (dt) in the kidney of a MWF rat. Proximal tubules (pt) showed green autofluorescence. Intra- and extraglomerular capillaries (arrows) were visualized with Texas Red-labeled 70 kDa dextran. The glomerulus was located directly underneath the renal capsule allowing high resolution imaging. (B) Histology of a MWF rat kidney section with many superficial glomeruli (arrows).

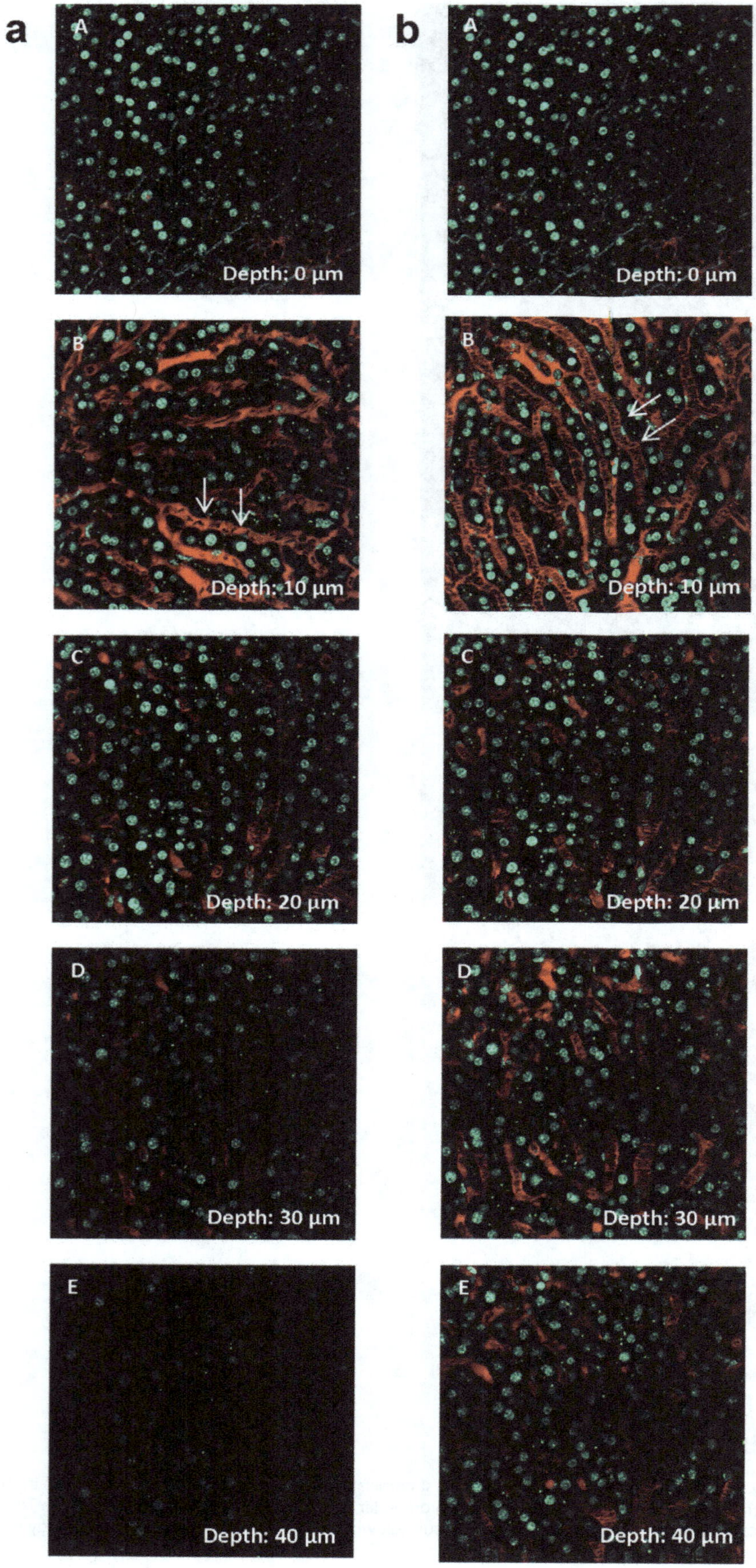
a
A
Depth: 0 µm
B
Depth: 10 µm
C
Depth: 20 µm
D
Depth: 30 µm
E
Depth: 40 µm
b
A
Depth: 0 µm
B
Depth: 10 µm
C
Depth: 20 µm
D
Depth: 30 µm
E
Depth: 40 µm

Figure 4. Z-stack through a mouse liver in vivo. Liver images were acquired with internal detectors and gain and offset of the detectors were maintained during the imaging process. (A) – (E) show layers in 0, 10, 20, 30 and 40 µm depth underneath the liver surface. The sinusoids (arrows) were labeled with Texas Red 70 kDa Dextran, the nuclei in cyan by Hoechst 33342. MPM imaging of the liver was highly limited by the light scattering properties of the liver tissue. a, left column: Z-stack without an adjustment of laser power. Image brightness rapidly decreased and imaging was limited to a depth of 40 µm from the organ's surface. b, right column: Z-stack with adjusted laser power. By increasing the laser output the loss of brightness and resolution can be partly compensated, so that a depth of 40 µm underneath the surface became accessible.

Statistics

Column statistics were performed using Graph Pad Prism 5. A One-Way ANOVA test was conducted to determine differences in glomeruli depth between the strains. In addition, strains with the most superficial glomeruli were compared to a peer group containing all other strains using an unpaired t-test.

Results

Assessment of Excitation-laser Tissue Penetrance in Kidney, Liver, and Brain

To assess the imaging conditions of the kidney compared to other organs, we compared in a first experiment the MPM imaging suitability of the kidney, liver, and brain of BL/6 mice under identical imaging conditions, including the same excitation laser, microscope, and acquisition software. MPM imaging was performed in kidneys of BL/6 mice to assess the brightness and image quality as a function of the image's distance from the kidney's surface. As shown in fig. 2a, when the laser output power was kept constant, the accessibility of the mouse kidney tissue for MPM imaging decreased rapidly when moving from the kidney surface to deeper layers. Thus, structures located 60 µm from the kidney surface were barely accessible. The image quality, however, could be considerably improved by increasing the laser power for the assessment of structures located deeper in the kidney. By increasing the laser power, structures in the range of 100 µm from the kidney surface became accessible, such as the glomerulus shown in fig. 2b. Although the overall accessibility of mouse and rat kidneys for MPM imaging was similar, the image quality of rat glomeruli at a given depth from the organ's surface tended to be superior to that of mice (data not shown). In contrast to BL/6 mice, kidneys of MWF rats showed many glomeruli just underneath the renal capsule, allowing high quality imaging of the glomerular structure and of functional features, such as glomerular capillary flow (fig. 3).

Like for MPM of the kidney, the quality of in vivo MPM imaging of liver structures decreased rapidly with increasing distance from the organ's surface. For example, a depth of 40 µm was determined as the limit for reliable assessment of vascular blood flow after adjustment of laser output power (fig. 4). Overall, the accessibility of structures located distant from the liver's surface was markedly more compromised than those in the kidney.

In contrast to the kidney and liver, imaging of the mouse brain allowed high quality imaging of structures located as deep as 300 µm from the brain surface (fig. 5). Even depths up to 600 µm were accessible for the brain, as previously shown [3].

Depth of Glomeruli in 4-week-old Mice of Various Strains

To identify mouse strains with superficial glomeruli and ideal MPM imaging conditions similar to those observed in MWF rats, 4-week-old juvenile mice of 10 different strains were evaluated in a first set of experiments. Mice of both genders were analyzed as one data set because no gender differences were detected. For MPM, suitable glomeruli are located randomly within the tissue and only the most superficial ones are usually used for imaging. Thus we measured the depth of all glomeruli within one section and only analyzed the depth of the 30 most superficial glomeruli per kidney section. The mean distances from the kidney surface of the 30 most superficial glomeruli were 118.4±3.4, 123.0±2.7, 133.7±3.0, 132.3±2.6, 141.0±4.0, 145.3±4.3, 148.9±4.2, 151.6±2.7, 167.7±3.9, and 207.8±3.2 µm for the C3H/N, BALB/c, SJL, BL/6, DBA/2, CD-1, 129, CB6F1, FVB/N, and NMRI strains, respectively (n = 5 animals from each strain) (fig. 6A). In parallel with the mean distance of glomeruli from the kidney surface, the 25th percentile of the most superficial glomeruli differed markedly between the strains. The most superficial glomeruli were observed in a depth of less than 100.4 and 107.0 µm in C3H/N and BALB/c mice, respectively. The deepest glomeruli occurred in FVB/N and NMRI mice, in which the 25% most superficial glomeruli were located 142.1 and 185.1 µm, respectively, from the kidney's surface. In summary, the average depth of the most superficial glomeruli was significantly lower in the strains C3H/N, BALB/c, DBA/2, and BL/6 when compared to a peer group consisting of all the other strains ($p<.0001$; fig. 6B).

Depth of Glomeruli in 10-week-old Mice of Various Strains

The same analysis of glomerular depth was repeated in adult mice 10 weeks of age. The average kidney weight of all strains was 161.2±2.1 mg in adult 10-week-old mice compared to 112.9±3.8 mg in 4-week-old juvenile animals. As a consequence of kidney growth, the average depth of the 30 most superficial glomeruli in each kidney section increased from 147.0±4.2 µm in 4-week-old mice to 170.1±5.4 µm in 10-week-old mice ($p<.001$). In adult mice, the average distances from the kidney surface of the 30 most superficial glomeruli were 136.5±3.8, 151.9±3.1, 162.0±3.4, 164.8±4.1, 170.0±4.8, 171.0±3.4, 171.8±3.6, 182.3±5.8, 193.0±5.2, and 197.3±3.4 µm for BL/6, BALB/c, FVB/N, DBA/2, CD-1, SJL, NMRI, 129, C3H/N, and CB6F1 strains, respectively (fig. 7A). The mean distance of the glomeruli from the kidney surface was generally paralleled by the number representing the 25% most superficially located glomeruli, which ranged from 116.7 µm in BL/6 to 175.4 µm in CB6F1 mice (fig. 7A).

Although the 25th percentile of glomeruli depth from the kidney surface was in the borderline range (for BL/6 and BALB/c strains) or out of range (for all other strains) of in vivo MPM, we found single glomeruli that were as close as 15 and 50 µm from the renal surface in the BL/6 and BALB/c strains, respectively. In summary, adult mice from the BL/6 and BALB/c strains showed significantly more superficially located glomeruli when compared to the average of all other strains ($p<.0001$; fig.7B).

Discussion

The conditions for in vivo MPM differ in various tissues depending on their optical density and heterogeneity. These tissue-specific conditions limit the penetration depth of the excitation laser at a given wavelength and impact the image quality due to various light scattering phenomena. Although deeper structures can be made accessible by increasing the output power of the

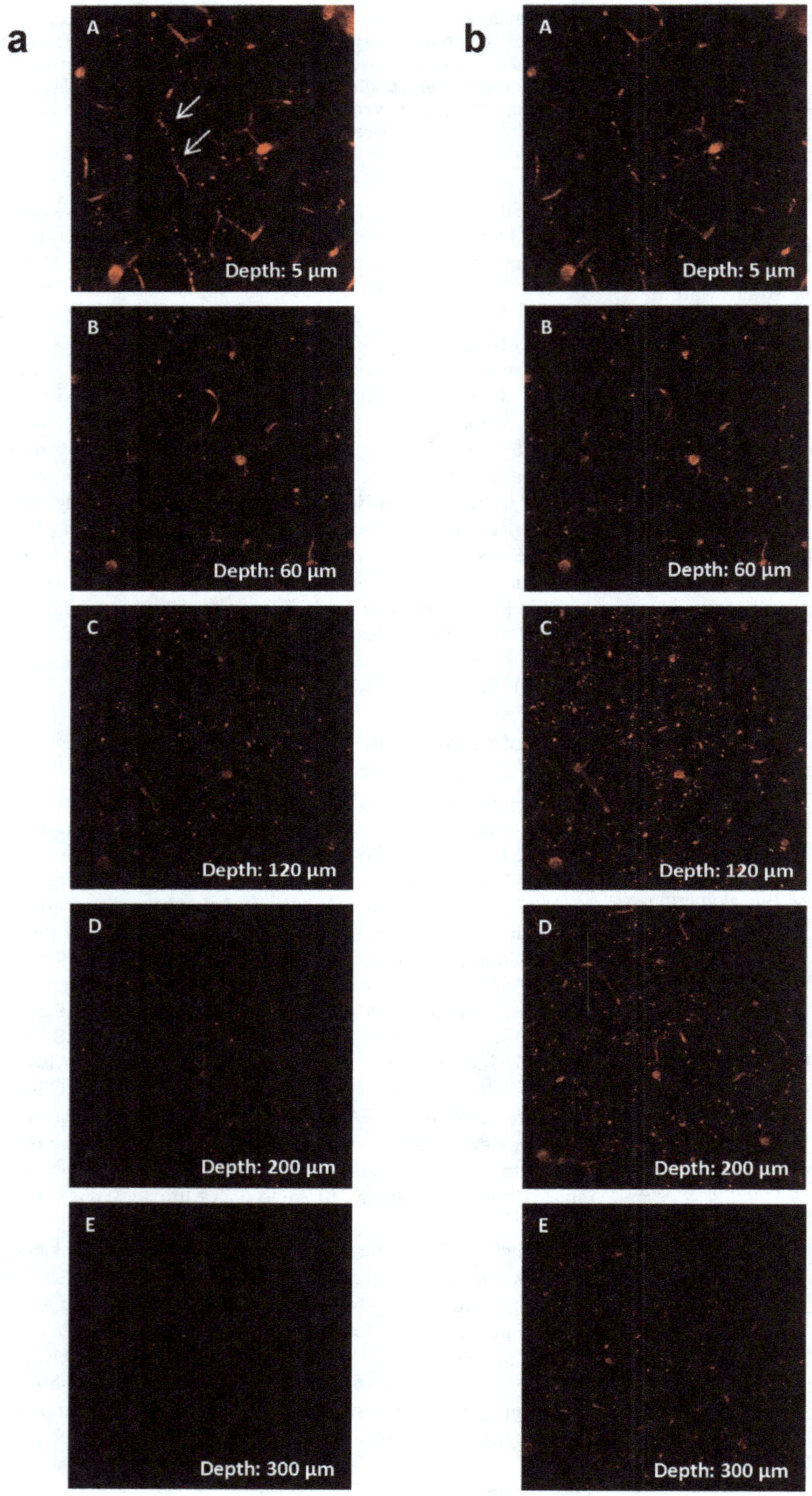

Figure 5. z-stack of the postcentral gyrus of the mouse brain in vivo. (A)–(E) show blood vessels (arrows), stained by Texas Red 70 kDa Dextran in 5, 60, 120, 200 and 300 µm underneath the brain surface. Internal detectors were used with maintained settings for gain and offset. a, left column: Without laser adjustment all blood vessels within the 300 µm range were visible, but appeared darker and blurry below a depth of 200 µm. b, right column: the same region acquired with adjustment of the laser power. In contrast to the liver and kidney a much deeper penetration into the tissue was possible.

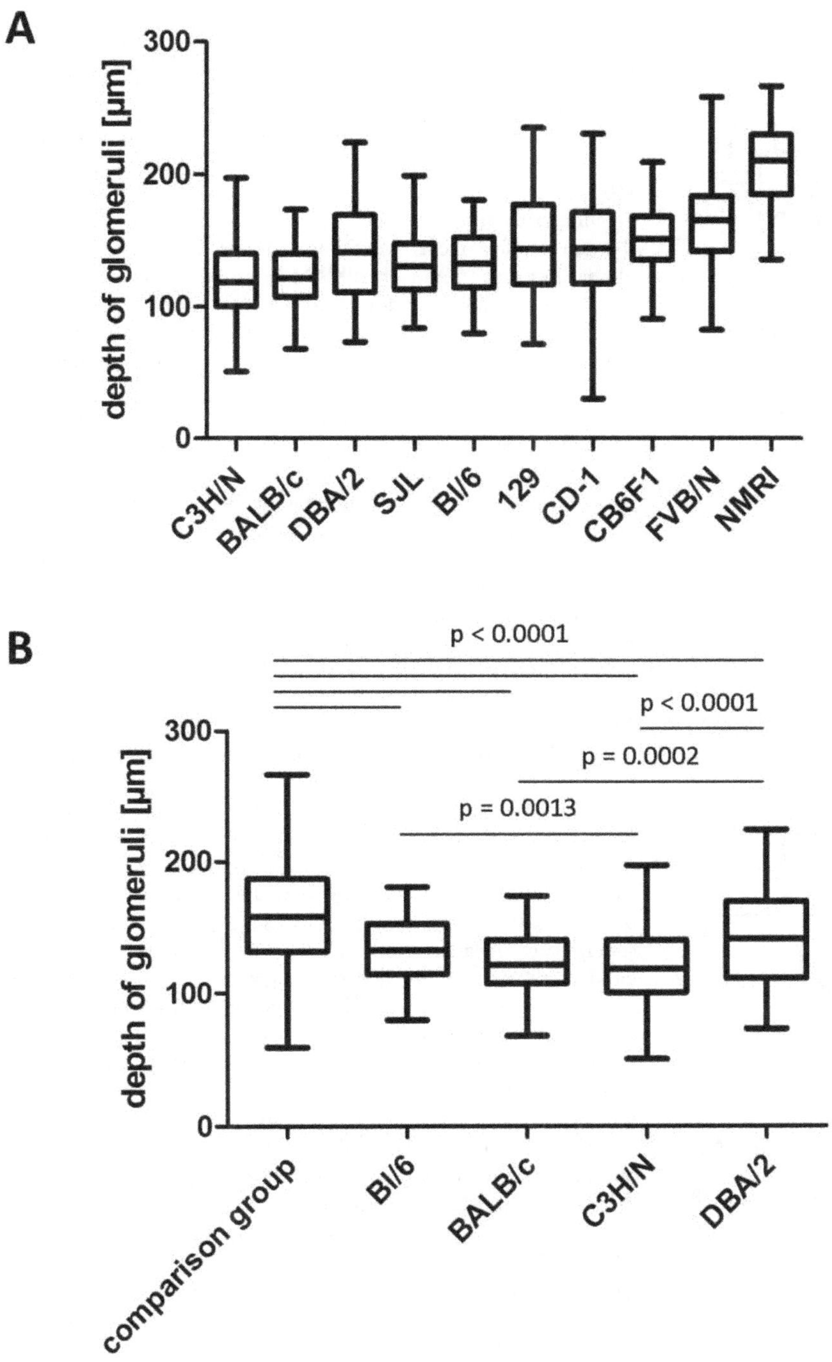

Figure 6. Depth of glomeruli in 4-week-old juvenile mice. Box-plot shows mean±25% (boxes) and the 5–95% percentile (whiskers). (A) Box-plot of all ten strains arranged according to the 25% percentile. (B) Box-plot of the peer group (129, CB6F1, NMRI, SJL, FVB, CD-1) vs. Bl/6, BALB/c, C3H/N and DBA/2.

excitation laser, the quality of the images is compromised by increased light scattering, which leads to the capitation of bright pictures with low resolution. Furthermore, high excitation laser power results in local phototoxicity, which may compromise the functional features of interest. In this study for the first time we performed a direct comparison for the MPM accessibility of different organs using the same microscope, excitation laser, software and imaging settings. In accordance with previous studies, our comparison of imaging conditions for mouse brain, liver, and kidney tissue revealed that the brain offers excellent imaging conditions compared to other organs, allowing imaging of structures 300 µm and deeper below the pial surface [4,11]. MPM imaging of the liver, in comparison, was markedly more difficult because structures deeper than 40 µm were barely accessible. This difficulty may be related to specific anatomic features of the liver, such as dense capillaries and sinusoids. In terms of accessibility for

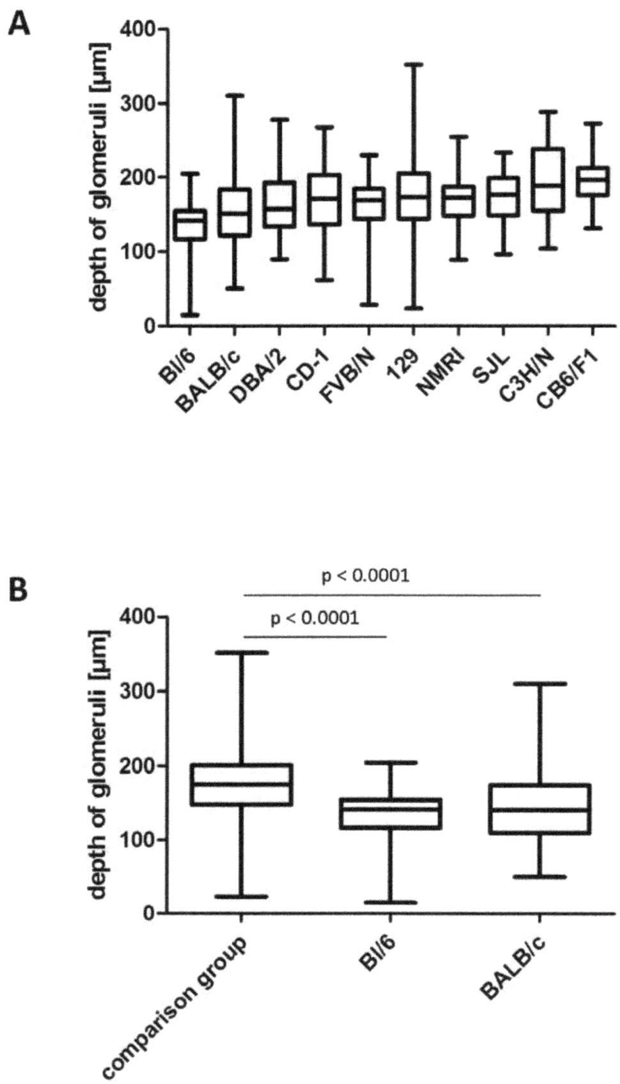

Figure 7. Depth of glomeruli in 10-week-old adult mice. Box-plot shows mean±25% (boxes) and the 5–95% percentile (whiskers). (A) Box-plot of all ten strains arranged according to the 25% percentile. (B) Box-plot of the peer group (129, CB6F1, C3H/N, NMRI, SJL, DBA/2, FVB, CD-1) vs. Bl/6 and BALB/c.

MPM the kidney was between the brain and liver. Structures in the kidneys located up to 100 µm from the organ's surface were accessible. However, depending on the setup, the quality of the pictures in terms of brightness and resolution decreased substantially as a function of the depth of the section. Similar like in most MPM studies of living tissues, we used a water immersion objective. This provides the best optical beam pathway conditions for the in vivo approach, because, first, the kidney was embedded into a 0.9% saline solution for the imaging session and, secondly, the kidney tissue consists mostly of water. Therefore the refraction index of the kidney is more similar to saline than for example glycerol. By using a water immersion objective we minimized the discrepancy between the optical and geometrical depth. All depth measurements in this study are based on the mechanical movement of the stage along the z-axis, which we defined as the penetration depth. It should be noted that in all our MPM imaging, the penetration depth was lower than the free working distance of the applied objective.

The imaging range that we observed for the kidney has also been reported by other groups and might be problematic if assessment of the structure and function of the glomerulus and JGA is desired [2]. As a consequence, most in vivo MPM studies of the glomerulus have been conducted with MWF rats [10,12,13,14], which are characterized by a high concentration of glomeruli just underneath the renal capsule. MWF rats therefore offer ideal conditions for MPM imaging of the glomerulus and JGA. Before MPM became available, MWF rats were traditionally used for micropuncture studies [15,16], and their renal function has been well documented. One drawback, however, is that MWF rats not only have a desirable high percentage of superficially located glomeruli, they also show a reduced nephron number when compared to other commonly used strains such as Sprague Dawley or Wistar rats [17]. As a model of low nephron number, ageing MWF rats develop hypertension, progressive glomerulosclerosis, proteinuria, and, eventually, deterioration of renal function [6,7,17]. For reasons that are not entirely clear, the renal phenotype of MWF rats is more pronounced in male than female rats, making females more suitable for use in studies assessing the structure and function of the kidney and, more specifically, of the glomerulus [8]. These issues could be in part circumvented by the use of the closely related MW Simonsen (MWS) strain. In contrast to MWF rats, MWS rats are less proteinuric and they rarely develop glomerulosclerosis. However, the number of superficial glomeruli in MWS rats is more limited compared to MWF rats [13].

In this study, our aim was to identify a mouse strain with favorable MPM imaging conditions of the kidney similar to those observed in MWF rats. Although imaging of the function and structure of the glomerulus has been done in mice, there are no data available regarding the most suitable strain in terms of superficially located glomeruli. Such a mouse strain may circumvent problems related to compromised kidney function in MWF rats and improve MPM imaging of the large pool of genetically altered mouse models by respective back-crossing into a favorable genetic background. Only few MPM studies of the kidney have been done in mice due to the limited accessibility of the glomeruli. Unilateral ureter obstruction was used in some experiments to move glomeruli to the kidney surface, however this apparently is associated with alteration in glomerular capillary blood flow and generalized inflammation of the kidney [18,19].

Ten commonly used mouse strains were included in the study, which differed markedly in the number of their most-superficial glomeruli. In general, juvenile mice (4 weeks of age) of all strains showed more superficial glomeruli compared to adult mice (10 weeks of age) and, consequently, appeared more suitable for use in MPM imaging. In this context, it should be noted that most studies using MPM of the mouse kidney were conducted with young animals [10]. The specific use of juvenile animals, however, imposes some critical drawbacks. First, it remains unclear if data on glomerular function obtained from juvenile animals are fully transferable to adult mice. Secondly, functional and structural alterations of glomerular capillaries, podocytes, and Bowman's capsule in chronic disease models usually become apparent only in the aging kidney. Thirdly, pharmacologic manipulation of glomerular function often requires drug administration over a given time period, which may be too lengthy for young animals. Despite these general limitations, we identified a significantly greater number of superficial glomeruli in the kidneys of young C3H/N, BALB/c, DBA/2, and BL/6 mice in comparison to all other strains, leaving them particularly suitable for MPM imaging of the kidney. The FVB and 129 strains are commonly used for the generation of transgenic mice by pronuclear injection and transgene transfection of embryonic stem cells for the generation of knockout models. These strains ranked in the middle to upper end compared to the other strains and displayed rather few superficial glomeruli. Therefore these standard backgrounds of genetically modified mice are not particularly suited for in vivo MPM of the glomerulus, and backcrossing to a BL/6 or BALB/c strain would be recommended if animals are intended for MPM imaging.

In adult mice (10 weeks of age) the strains BALB/c and BL/6 were preferable because they showed the highest percentage of superficial glomeruli within the range of good MPM imaging conditions. For all mouse strains, the distance of glomeruli from the kidney surface increased in parallel to kidney growth. Additionally, the width of the *cortex corticis*, the area of the cortex underneath the renal capsule that is free of glomeruli, expanded as the kidneys grew. Interestingly, there were striking differences in the relative broadening of the glomeruli-free area during growth between different strains. For example, we found a high number of superficially located glomeruli in the kidneys of 4-week-old C3H/N mice, but this particular strain showed few superficial glomeruli at 10 weeks of age. Thus, the overall suitability of adult C3H/N mice for MPM imaging of renal glomeruli was poor. These apparent differences in the growth of various part of the nephron that leads to the broadening of the subcapsular cortex, which is virtually free of glomeruli, appears to be both strain- and species-dependent. In contrast to some of the mouse strains used in this study, the distribution pattern of glomeruli in the renal cortex in humans and dogs was shown to be largely constant during postnatal growth of the kidney [20,21].

Although none of the evaluated mouse strains exhibited ideal conditions for MPM imaging similar to those of MWF rats, it should be noted that there was a substantial scatter of glomerular depth in mice. Even if the average depth of the 30 most superficial glomeruli per section was out of reach for MPM, we found scattered superficial glomeruli in many of the strains, with a particular high incidence in BALB/c and BL/6 mice. Given that a mouse kidney has somewhere in the range of 8.000–12.000 glomeruli [22], 5% of the most superficial glomeruli would be estimated at 200. With a surface area of approximately 150 mm^2, it should be possible to find at least one glomerulus within one mm^2 that can be easily accessed by MPM with optimal imaging quality.

In summary, the accessibility of renal glomeruli for MPM imaging in mice is highly strain- and age-dependent. Taking together both age groups of this study, the highest numbers of superficial glomeruli readily accessible for MPM were found in BALB/C and BL/6 mice. These strains are preferable for MPM imaging experiments of the kidney, particularly for those studies focused on structural and functional features of the glomerulus.

Acknowledgments

The expert support provided by Uwe deVries, Institute of Anatomy, University of Regensburg, is gratefully acknowledged.

Author Contributions

Conceived and designed the experiments: IMS HC. Performed the experiments: IMS SB HC. Analyzed the data: IMS SB HC. Contributed reagents/materials/analysis tools: SB HC. Wrote the paper: IMS HC.

References

1. Denk W, Strickler JH, Webb WW (1990) Two-photon laser scanning fluorescence microscopy. Science 248: 73–76.
2. Peti-Peterdi J, Burford JL, Hackl MJ (2011) The first decade of using multiphoton microscopy for high-power kidney imaging. Am J Physiol Renal Physiol 302: F227–233.
3. Kobat D, Horton NG, Xu C (2011) In vivo two-photon microscopy to 1.6-mm depth in mouse cortex. J Biomed Opt 16: 106014.
4. Stosiek C, Garaschuk O, Holthoff K, Konnerth A (2003) In vivo two-photon calcium imaging of neuronal networks. Proc Natl Acad Sci U S A 100: 7319–7324.
5. Hackbarth H, Buttner D, Jarck D, Pothmann M, Messow C, et al. (1983) Distribution of glomeruli in the renal cortex of Munich Wistar Fromter (MWF) rats. Ren Physiol 6: 63–71.
6. Hackbarth H, Gwinner W, Alt JM, Hagemann I, Thiemann A, et al. (1991) The Munich Wistar Fromter rat: proteinuria and blood pressure in correlation to the number of superficial glomeruli. Ren Physiol Biochem 14: 246–252.
7. Remuzzi A, Puntorieri S, Battaglia C, Bertani T, Remuzzi G (1990) Angiotensin converting enzyme inhibition ameliorates glomerular filtration of macromolecules and water and lessens glomerular injury in the rat. J Clin Invest 85: 541–549.
8. Remuzzi A, Puntorieri S, Mazzoleni A, Remuzzi G (1988) Sex related differences in glomerular ultrafiltration and proteinuria in Munich-Wistar rats. Kidney Int 34: 481–486.
9. Schulz A, Litfin A, Kossmehl P, Kreutz R (2002) Genetic dissection of increased urinary albumin excretion in the munich wistar fromter rat. J Am Soc Nephrol 13: 2706–2714.
10. Peti-Peterdi J, Sipos A (2010) A high-powered view of the filtration barrier. J Am Soc Nephrol 21: 1835–1841.
11. Rochefort NL, Jia H, Konnerth A (2008) Calcium imaging in the living brain: prospects for molecular medicine. Trends Mol Med 14: 389–399.
12. Russo LM, Sandoval RM, McKee M, Osicka TM, Collins AB, et al. (2007) The normal kidney filters nephrotic levels of albumin retrieved by proximal tubule cells: retrieval is disrupted in nephrotic states. Kidney Int 71: 504–513.
13. Sandoval RM, Wagner MC, Patel M, Campos-Bilderback SB, Rhodes GJ, et al. (2012) Multiple factors influence glomerular albumin permeability in rats. J Am Soc Nephrol 23: 447–457.
14. Tanner GA (2009) Glomerular sieving coefficient of serum albumin in the rat: a two-photon microscopy study. Am J Physiol Renal Physiol 296: F1258–1265.
15. Eisenbach GM, Liew JB, Boylan JW, Manz N, Muir P (1975) Effect of angiotensin on the filtration of protein in the rat kidney: a micropuncture study. Kidney Int 8: 80–87.
16. Thurau K, Schnermann J (1965) [the Sodium Concentration in the Macula Densa Cells as a Regulating Factor for Glomerular Filtration (Micropuncture Experiments)]. Klin Wochenschr 43: 410–413.
17. Rovira-Halbach G, Alt JM, Brunkhorst R, Frei U, Kuhn K, et al. (1986) Single nephron hyperfiltration and proteinuria in a newly selected rat strain with superficial glomeruli. Ren Physiol 9: 317–325.
18. Forbes MS, Thornhill BA, Chevalier RL (2011) Proximal tubular injury and rapid formation of atubular glomeruli in mice with unilateral ureteral obstruction: a new look at an old model. Am J Physiol Renal Physiol 301: F110–117.
19. Kuligowski MP, Kitching AR, Hickey MJ (2006) Leukocyte recruitment to the inflamed glomerulus: a critical role for platelet-derived P-selectin in the absence of rolling. J Immunol 176: 6991–6999.
20. Horster M, Kemler BJ, Valtin H (1971) Intracortical distribution of number and volume of glomeruli during postnatal maturation in the dog. J Clin Invest 50: 796–800.
21. Fetterman GH, Shuplock NA, Philipp FJ, Gregg HS (1965) The Growth and Maturation of Human Glomeruli and Proximal Convolutions from Term to Adulthood: Studies by Microdissection. Pediatrics 35: 601–619.
22. Bonvalet JP, Champion M, Courtalon A, Farman N, Vandewalle A, et al. (1977) Number of glomeruli in normal and hypertrophied kidneys of mice and guinea-pigs. J Physiol 269: 627–641.

Visualization of Acute Liver Damage Induced by Cycloheximide in Rats using PET with [^{18}F]FEDAC, a Radiotracer for Translocator Protein (18 kDa)

Akiko Hatori, Joji Yui, Lin Xie, Tomoteru Yamasaki, Katsushi Kumata, Masayuki Fujinaga, Hidekatsu Wakizaka, Masanao Ogawa, Nobuki Nengaki, Kazunori Kawamura, Ming-Rong Zhang*

Molecular Imaging Center, National Institute of Radiological Sciences, Chiba, Japan

Abstract

Liver damage induced by drug toxicity is an important concern for both medical doctors and patients. The aim of this study was to noninvasively visualize acute liver damage using positron emission tomography (PET) with *N*-benzyl-*N*-methyl-2-[7,8-dihydro-7-(2-[^{18}F]fluoroethyl)-8-oxo-2-phenyl-9*H*-purin-9-yl]acetamide ([^{18}F]FEDAC), a radiotracer specific for translocator protein (18 kDa, TSPO) as a biomarker for inflammation, and to determine cellular sources enriching TSPO expression in the liver. A mild acute liver damage model was prepared by a single intraperitoneal injection of cycloheximide (CHX) into rats. Treatment with CHX induced apoptosis and necrotic changes in hepatocytes with slight neutrophil infiltration. The uptake of radioactivity in the rat livers was measured with PET after injection of [^{18}F]FEDAC. The uptake of [^{18}F]FEDAC increased in livers damaged from treatment with CHX compared to the controls. Presence of TSPO was examined in the liver tissue using quantitative reverse transcriptase-polymerase chain reaction and immunohistochemical assays. mRNA expression of TSPO was elevated in the damaged livers compared to the controls, and the level was correlated with the [^{18}F]FEDAC uptake and severity of damage. TSPO expression in the damaged liver sections was mainly found in macrophages (Kupffer cells) and neutrophils, but not in hepatocytes. The elevation of TSPO mRNA expression was derived from the increase of the number of macrophages with TSPO and neutrophils with TSPO in damaged livers. From this study we considered that PET imaging with [^{18}F]FEDAC represented the mild liver damage through the enhanced TSPO signal in inflammatory cells. We conclude that this method may be a useful tool for diagnosis in early stage of acute liver damage.

Editor: Simon Afford, University of Birmingham, United Kingdom

Funding: The authors have no support or funding to report.

Competing Interests: The authors have declared that no competing interests exist.

* E-mail: zhang@nirs.go.jp

Introduction

Medical drugs and their metabolites are believed to have caused liver dysfunction in many cases [1]. Jaundice appears in cholestatic liver disease; however, accurate symptoms in real-time are not easy to observe in cases of hepatocellular injury-type drug-induced liver damage. Moreover, taking a drug continuously without noticing liver dysfunction sometimes causes hepatic failure [2]. In order to inhibit deterioration, early detection and a timely cure are required. At present, evaluation of serum levels of liver-associated enzymes such as alanine aminotransferase (ALT) and aspartate aminotransferase (AST) is important, but a histological evaluation of liver damage may be difficult solely on the basis of serum biomarker measurements [2–4]. Because of the limitations of liver biopsy and the currently available noninvasive imaging techniques, such as computed tomography (CT) and magnetic resonance imaging (MRI), new noninvasive modalities that accurately and rapidly distinguish liver damage and assess damage severity have become a requirement in hepatology [5]. Compared to serum tests and histological assessments, positron emission tomography (PET) imaging with a specific radiotracer enables direct, quantitative, and multispatial visualization of physiological and cellular processes at multiple time points and at the macroscopic level [6].

Researchers have investigated the pathophysiological mechanisms of liver failure in liver damage models, including inflammation, apoptosis, and fibrosis [7–9]. A single administration of protein synthesis inhibitor, cycloheximide(CHX) has been shown to induce apoptosis [10–12] and necrotic changes in hepatocytes with slight neutrophil infiltration in rats [12]. Kupffer cells are resident liver macrophages and can phagocytose apoptotic hepatocytes [13]. After the engulfment of apoptotic cells in pathophysiologic conditions, activated Kupffer cells may cause damage to hepatocytes by releasing inflammatory cytokines or by inducing neutrophil infiltration [14–16]. Kupffer cells also produce anti-inflammatory cytokines such as interleukin-10 and play an important role in counteracting the effect of proinflammatory cytokines and attenuating liver damage [17].

It has been found that translocator protein (18 kDa; TSPO) increases in inflammatory cells during the occurrence and progress of inflammation [18]. TSPO is a receptor complex primarily present in the mitochondria. TSPO has broad functions related to the regulation of cholesterol transport, steroid hormone synthesis, porphyrin and heme transport, apoptosis, cell proliferation, anion transport, mitochondrial function regulation, immunomodulations, and inflammation [18]. Steady-state mRNA levels of TSPO expression are low in the liver and brain, and high in the adrenal glands, kidneys, spleen, skeletal muscle, and lungs [19]. TSPO expression in blood cells has also been reported, in which phagocytic cells, such as monocytes and polymorphonuclear neutrophils, show significantly higher TSPO expression than lymphocytes [20]. Thus, TSPO has become a useful biomarker for monitoring inflammation using PET with a specific radiotracer [21]. We have used PET with *N*-benzyl-*N*-methyl-2-[7,8-dihydro-7-(2-[^{18}F]fluoroethyl)-8-oxo-2-phenyl-9*H*- purin-9-yl]acetamide ([^{18}F]FEDAC), a TSPO-specific radiotracer, to noninvasively monitor various inflammatory diseases, such as neuroinflammation [22], lung inflammation [23], and non-alcoholic fatty liver disease [24].

In the present study, we used PET with [^{18}F]FEDAC to visualize acute liver damage in a rat model prepared by injecting CHX into rats. We measured the liver uptake of [^{18}F]FEDAC with a small-animal PET scanner at several time points after CHX treatment. Presence of TSPO in the liver tissue was examined under the protein level and the relationship between TSPO expression and [^{18}F]FEDAC uptake was elucidated. The objective of this study was to determine the utility of [^{18}F]FEDAC-PET in monitoring the occurrence and progression of acute liver damage.

Materials and Methods

Production of [^{18}F]FEDAC

[^{18}F]FEDAC (n = 10) was prepared in-house by reaction of a precursor with [^{18}F]fluoroethyl bromide, with >98% radiochemical purity and 140–210 GBq/μmol specific activity [22].

Study Animals

Male Sprague-Dawley rats (6–7 weeks old) were purchased from Japan SLC (Shizuoka, Japan). All animals received humane care and all experiments were approved by the Animal Ethics Committee of the National Institute of Radiological Sciences (Permit Number: 10–1005, Chiba, Japan) and were carried out according to the recommendations of the Committee for the Care and Use of Laboratory Animals, National Institute of Radiological Sciences.

Preparation of a Rat Model of Liver Damage

After acclimation, 32 of 35 healthy rats were selected for the CHX treatment. The rats were anesthetized with 5% (v/v) isoflurane and injected intraperitoneally with 5 mg/kg of CHX (Sigma-Aldrich, St. Louis, MO) dissolved in 1.0 ml of physiological saline solution. They were divided into 4 groups of 8 rats each: CHX 1 h, 2 h, 4 h, and 6 h. For the control group, an additional 8 normal rats were used without CHX treatment. Four rats from each group were used to perform the small-animal PET study, and the others were sacrificed at each designated time point after CHX treatment for serum assessment and pathological examinations. Blood was drawn from the inferior vena cava of each anesthetized rat. A part of each rat liver was excised and fixed in 10% neutral buffered formalin for histopathological evaluation. The remaining liver samples were stored at -80°C for quantitative reverse-transcription polymerase chain reaction (qRT-PCR) assay and immunohistochemical examination.

Analysis of Liver Enzymes in Serum

Blood samples were kept at room temperature for 1 h, followed by centrifugation at 3000 rpm for 15 min to prepare sera. The serum activities of alanine aminotransferase (ALT) and aspartate aminotransferase (AST) were determined using the Japan Society of Clinical Chemistry reference method according to the manufacturer's instructions.

Histopathology

The fixed liver samples were embedded in paraffin and cut into 4-μm-thick sections for staining with hematoxylin-and-eosin (H&E) according to a standard protocol. Frozen liver samples were cut in-house into 6-μm-thick slices by a cryotome (HM560, Carl Zeiss, Oberkochen, Germany) for immunohistochemical examinations.

PET Study on Rats

PET scans were performed using a small-animal Inveon PET scanner (Siemens, Knoxville, TN), which provides 159 transaxial slices with 0.796 mm (center-to-center) spacing, a 10 cm transaxial field of view, and a 12.7 cm axial field of view. Before scanning, rats were anesthetized with 5% (v/v) isoflurane and maintained thereafter by 1–2% (v/v) isoflurane. Emission scans were acquired for 30 min in 3-dimensional (3D) list mode with an energy window of 350–750 keV, immediately after intravenously injecting [^{18}F]FEDAC (10 MBq/0.16–0.25 mL, 40–80 pmol) into the rats (n = 4 for each group). After the PET scans were finished, all rats were sacrificed and radioactivity concentrations in the liver and blood were measured using a 1480 Wizard Automatic Gamma Counter (PerkinElmer, Waltham, MA).

All list-mode acquisition data were sorted into 3D sinograms, which were then Fourier re-binned into 2D sinograms (frames × min: 2×0.5, 3×1, 8×2, 2×5). Dynamic images were reconstructed with filtered back-projection using a Hanning filter, and a Nyquist cutoff of 0.5 cycles/pixel. A region of interest was placed on the liver using ASIPro VM (Analysis Tools and System Setup/Diagnostics Tool, Siemens Medical Solutions USA). Regional uptake of radioactivity was decay-corrected to the injection time and expressed as the standardized uptake value (SUV), which was normalized to the injected radioactivity and body weight. SUV = (radioactivity per milliliter tissue/injected radioactivity) × gram body weight. The areas under the time-activity curves ($AUC_{0-30\ min}$, SUV × min) for liver were calculated from 0 min to 30 min after injection.

Immunohistochemical Staining Assay

Double staining with primary antibodies was performed using a rabbit anti-mouse TSPO antibody (NP155, 1:1000) [25] and either a monoclonal mouse anti-rat ED1 antibody (1:100; AbD Serotec, Raleigh, NC) for identifying Kupffer cells and macrophages in liver, or a monoclonal mouse anti-myeloperoxidase (MPO) antibody (1:10; Abcam, Cambridge, MA) for identifying neutrophils. The sections were incubated with the primary antibody overnight at 4°C.

After the first immunoreaction, the sections were incubated with fluorophore-conjugated (Alexa Fluor 546 nm) secondary antibody and biotin-conjugated secondary antibody followed by the method of tyramide signal amplification (TSA) using the Fluorescein System (PerkinElmer) for 1 h at room temperature. The sections were mounted with a DAPI-containing medium (Vector Laboratories, Burlingame, CA).

The number of ED1 with TSPO-positive cells or MPO with TSPO-positive cells was quantified by manual counting in an area of 0.14 mm^2 per field for 10 microscopic fields of the periportal or centrilobular regions in the hepatic lobule, respectively. Areas of the portal tract in the periportal region and areas of the central vein in the centrilobular region of each microscopic field were measured using Win ROOF software (Mitani, Tokyo, Japan) and counted out from each region. The results are represented as the

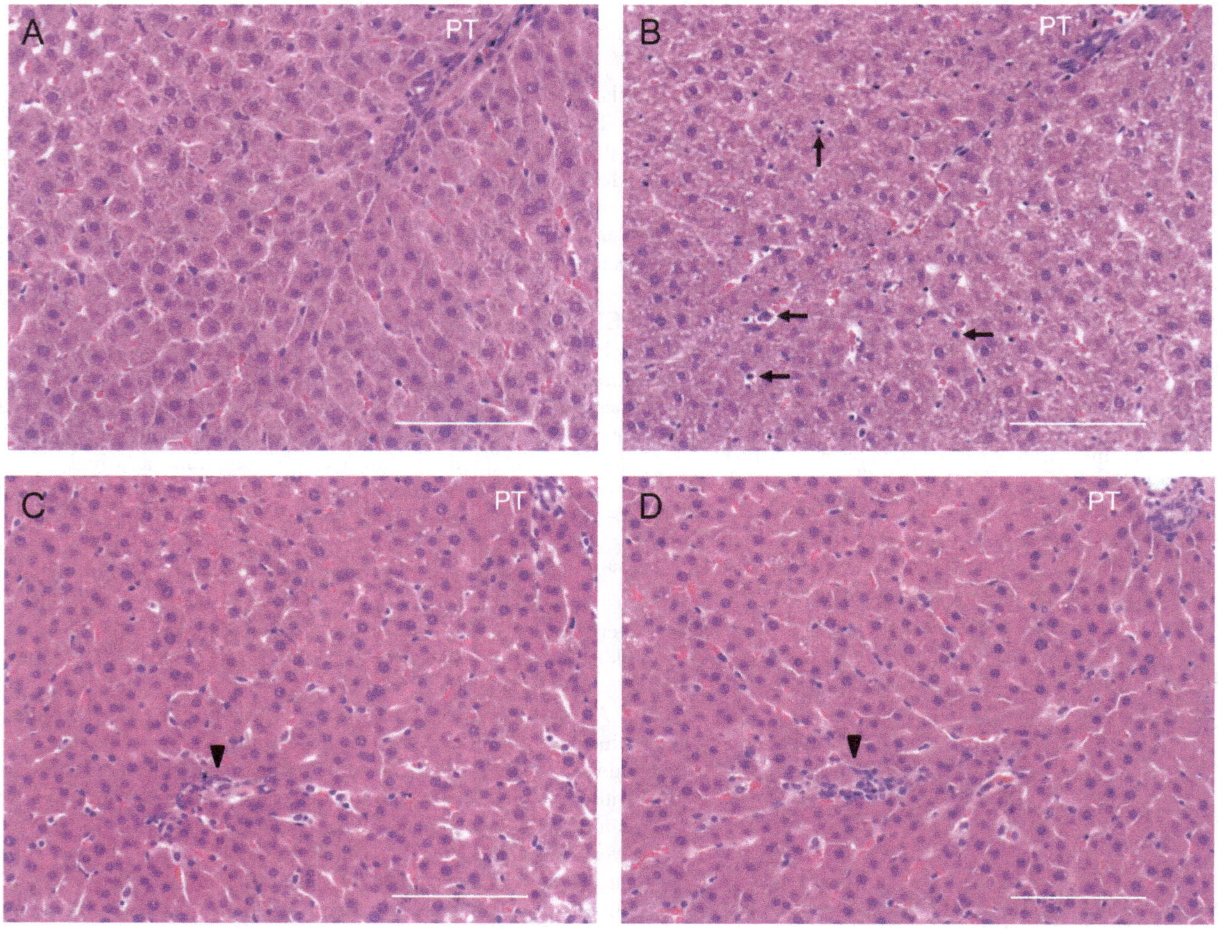

Figure 1. Effect of CHX treatment on histopathological images of rat livers. Hematoxylin and eosin stained sections of (A) control, (B) CHX 2 h, (C) 4 h and (D) 6 h. (B) At 2 h after CHX treatment, arrows show apoptotic cells showing marked condensation of cytoplasm and nuclear pyknosis. (C, D) Arrow heads show spotty hepatocellular necroses with mild neutrophil infiltration. Abbreviation: portal triad (PT). Scale bar: 100 μm.

number of ED1 with TSPO-positive cells or MPO with TSPO-positive cells per 1 mm^2.

RNA Preparation and Quantitative Reverse Transcriptase-polymerase Chain Reaction

Total RNA was extracted from frozen livers using Sepasol-RNA 1 Super (Nacalai Tesque, Kyoto, Japan) according to the manufacturer's protocol. The quality of total RNA was checked by the ratio of 260/280 nm with NanoDrop ND-1000 (LMS, Tokyo). qRT-PCR was performed using the TaqMan method on an Applied Biosystems StepOne system (Carlsbad, CA). Target-specific primers and probes for signal transducers and activators of TSPO and 18S ribosomal RNA (18S rRNA) were purchased from Applied Biosystems. The normalized Ct value of each gene was obtained by subtracting the Ct value of 18S rRNA. The fold change of each gene versus the controls was calculated.

Statistics

Data are expressed as the mean ± SE. Comparisons were made using a one-way analysis of variance followed by a Bonferroni post hoc test. The analysis was performed using GraphPad Prism 5 software (GraphPad Software, La Jolla, CA). Differences between groups were considered significant when the p-value was less than 0.05.

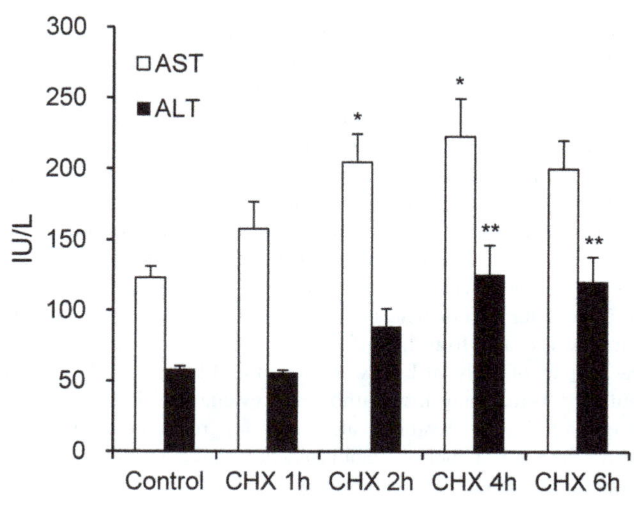

Figure 2. Serum ALT and AST activities. The AST and ALT activities (mean ± SE, n=4) at 4 h after CHX treatment were 1.8 and 2.2 fold higher than those in the control group, respectively. A significant difference ($p<0.05$) was seen for the following comparisons, *: AST, control versus CHX 2 h or 4 h; **: ALT, control versus CHX 4 h or 6 h.

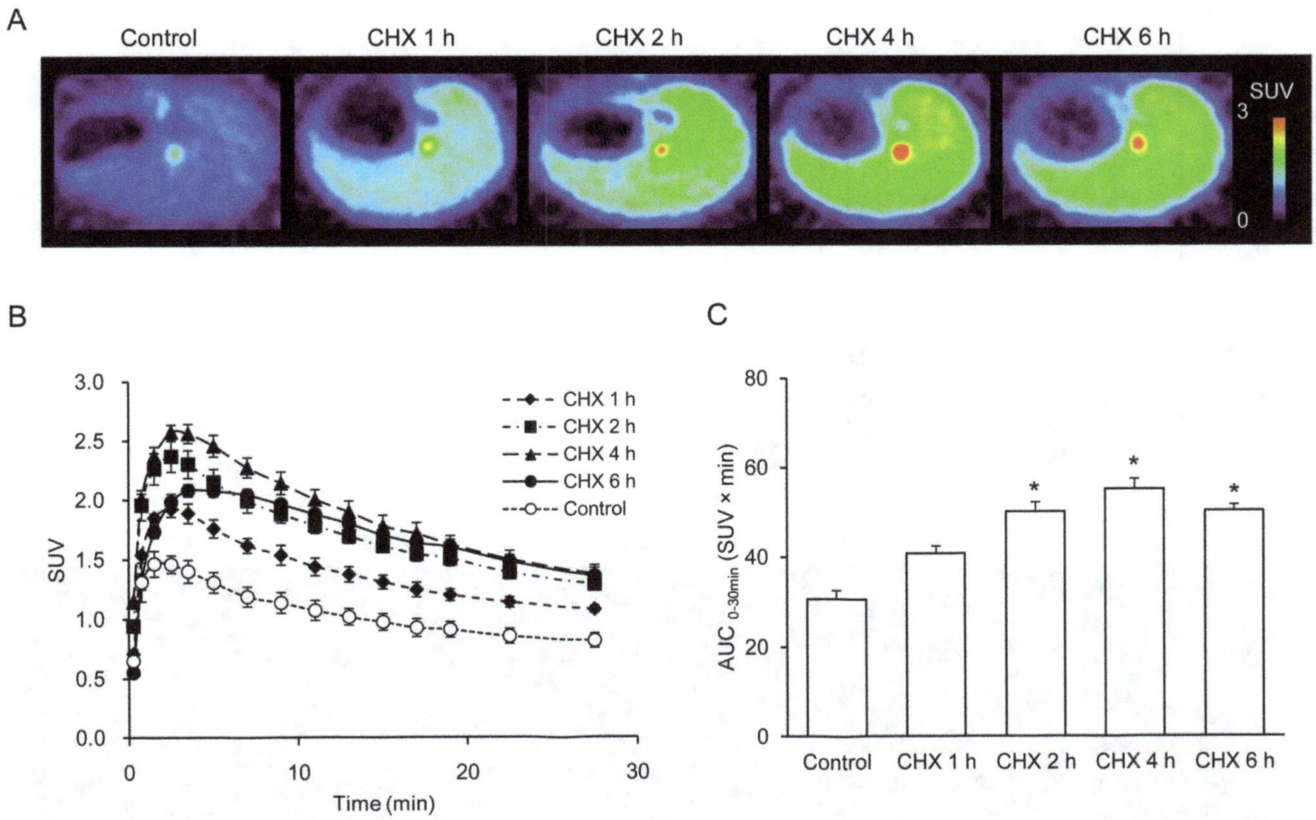

Figure 3. Radioactivity accumulating in the livers of the control and CHX-treated rats. (A) Representative transverse PET liver images acquired between 0 and 30 min after injection of [^{18}F]FEDAC. The pseudocolor bar represents the level of [^{18}F]FEDAC accumulation in the liver. The livers were more visible with time by 4 h after CHX treatment. (B) Time-activity curves of the livers. (n = 4 for each group). (C) Values of areas under the time-activity curves ($AUC_{0-30\ min}$; SUV × min, mean ± SE) were calculated from the time-activity curves between 0 and 30 min. The values were increased at 2 h (1.6 fold), 4 h (1.8 fold) and 6 h (1.6 fold) after CHX treatment compared with the control group. A significant difference ($p<0.05$) was seen in the following comparisons, *: control versus CHX 2 h, 4 h, or 6 h.

Results

Histopathology

Figure 1 shows H&E-stained images reflecting representative histological alterations in liver sections in the control (A), CHX 2 h (B), CHX 4 h (C), and CHX 6 h (D) groups. The control shows normal liver architecture. There was an unclear difference between the control group and 1 h of CHX treatment. After 2 h of CHX treatment, apoptotic cells showing marked condensation of the cytoplasm and nuclear pyknosis were observed in the hepatocytes. After 4 h of treatment, mild hepatocellular necroses and mild inflammatory cell infiltration were observed. Spotty hepatocellular necroses with inflammatory cells observed at 6 h were less than those seen at 4 h after treatment.

Analysis of Liver Enzymes in Serum

The results of serum ALT and AST activities are presented in Figure 2. The AST and ALT activities in the CHX group increased and showed the highest level at 4 h after the treatment. The AST level at 4 h, 222.8±26.7 IU/L, was 1.8 fold higher than that in the control group, 123.2±8.1 IU/L. Also, the ALT level at 4 h, 125.4±20.8 IU/L, was 2.2 fold higher than that in the control group, 58.2±2.3 IU/L. The AST and ALT activities at 6 h after CHX treatment, 200.0±19.9 and 120.3±17.7 IU/L, respectively, showed a tendency to decrease.

PET Study

To visualize liver damage in the CHX-treated model, PET scans were performed for 30 min after injection of [^{18}F]FEDAC. Figure 3A shows representative PET summation images between 0 and 30 min. Compared to the control image, radioactivity in the livers was increased 1 h, 2 h, 4 h, and 6 h after CHX treatment. The livers were more visible with time by 4 h after CHX treatment.

Table 1. Radioactivity in liver and blood 30 min after injection of [^{18}F]FEDAC.

	Radioactivity concentration (SUV)		
	Liver	Blood	Liver/Blood
Control	1.35±0.04	0.44±0.02	3.07±0.19
CHX 1 h	2.02±0.05a	0.49±0.04	4.16±0.41
CHX 2 h	2.15±0.10a	0.49±0.03	4.46±0.20b
CHX 4 h	2.13±0.08a	0.49±0.01	4.37±0.22b
CHX 6 h	2.17±0.07a	0.48±0.02	4.58±0.33b

Note. Data are presented as the mean ± SE. n = 4.
a Significantly different ($p<0.05$) from the control of Liver.
b Significantly different ($p<0.05$) from the control of Liver/Blood.

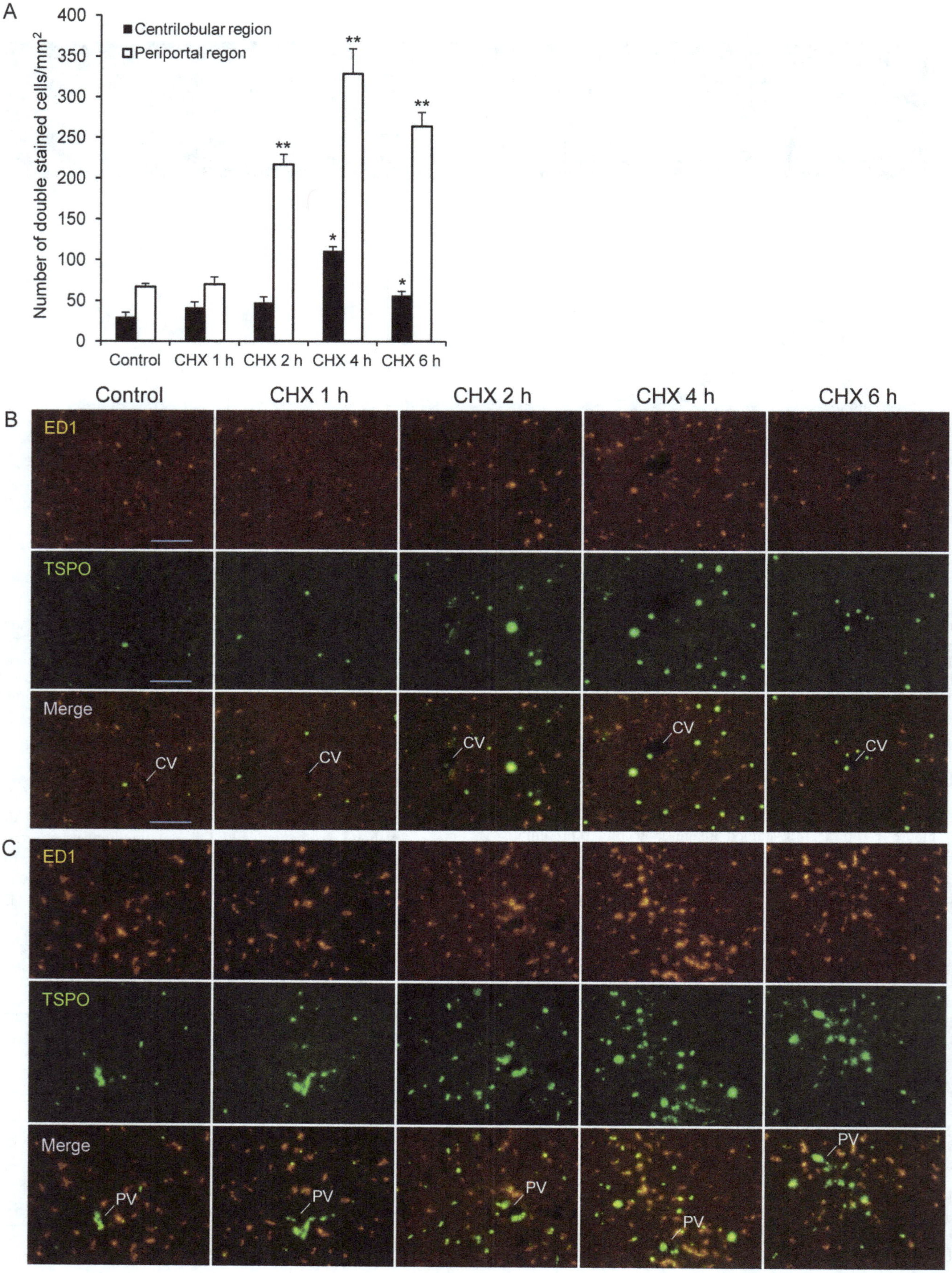
A
Number of double stained cells/mm²
400
350
300
250
200
150
100
50
0
Centrilobular region
Periportal region
**
**
**
*
*
Control
CHX 1 h
CHX 2 h
CHX 4 h
CHX 6 h
B
C
ED1
TSPO
Merge
CV
PV

Figure 4. Increased TSPO levels were expressed in macrophages in liver tissues after CHX treatment. (A) The number of double immunofluorescence staining cells of ED1 and TSPO in the centrilobular and periportal regions of hepatic lobules in the control and CHX-treated rats. A significant difference ($p<0.05$) was seen for the following comparisons, *: centrilobular region, control versus CHX 4 h or 6 h; **: periportal region, control versus CHX 2 h, 4 h, or 6 h. (B, C) Double immunofluorescence labeling of ED1 (red) and TSPO (green) in the centrilobular region (B) and the periportal region (C). Macrophages with TSPO expression increased after CHX treatment, and higher number of double stained cells was distributed in the periportal region than in the centrilobular region at all observed time points. Abbreviations: central vein (CV), portal vein (PV). Scale bar: 100 μm.

Figures 3B and C show the liver time-activity curves and uptake values, represented as $AUC_{0-30\ min}$. The uptake of radioactivity accumulating in the livers increased significantly 2 h after CHX treatment and reached a maximum at 4 h (Figure 3C). The values for 2 h, 4 h and 6 h treatment groups were 50.1±2.1 (1.6 fold), 55.2±2.2 (1.8 fold) and 50.3±1.3 (1.6 fold), respectively, compared with the control group (30.7±1.9).

Radioactivity concentrations in the liver and blood after the 30 min-PET scans were measured and are shown in Table 1. The liver uptake 1 h after CHX treatment increased significantly compared to that of the control group; however, the blood uptake was shown at a level similar to the controls. The ratio of radioactivity in the liver to that in the blood in the treated group was higher than that in the control group; 4.4±0.2 at 4 h after CHX treatment versus 3.1±0.2 in the control group, $p<0.05$. These results indicated that the present liver images are not largely confounded by the blood radioactivity.

Immunohistochemical Staining Assay

Double immunofluorescence stainings of ED1 (red) and TSPO (green) in the centrilobular and periportal regions of hepatic lobules in the control and CHX-treated livers are shown in Figures 4B and C, respectively. In the controls, hepatic macrophages expressing TSPO, mainly comprised of Kupffer cells, were observed in a small number of cells. TSPO expression in the hepatocytes was low. The double-stained cells increased after CHX treatment both in the centrilobular and periportal regions. As shown in Figure 4C, dense fluorescence representing TSPO expression was detected in the hepatic arteriole and the intra-lobular bile duct of the portal tract, with less fluorescence in fibrotic regions, and weak signals from the portal vein were observed for all time points, including the controls. The numbers of hepatic macrophages with TSPO expression in the centrilobular and periportal regions were calculated and are shown in Figure 4A. The areas of the portal tract and central vein were counted out from the microscopic fields of the periportal and centrilobular regions, respectively. More macrophages with TSPO were distributed in the periportal region than in the centrilobular region at all observed time points. The highest number of macrophages with TSPO at 4 h after treatment was 328.0±30.7 per mm^2 in the periportal region and 111.4±5.0 per mm^2 in the centrilobular region.

The results of MPO (red) and TSPO (green) double immunofluorescence stainings are shown in Figures 5B and C, as observed in the centrilobular and periportal regions, respectively. Neutrophils (MPO-positive cells) with and without TSPO were few in the control group. Neutrophils with TSPO expression increased after CHX treatment both in the centrilobular and periportal regions. In Figure 5C, TSPO expression in the portal tract was detected, similar to Figure 4C. The numbers of neutrophils with TSPO expression in the centrilobular and periportal regions were calculated and are shown in Figure 5A. More neutrophils with TSPO were distributed in the periportal region than in the centrilobular region after CHX treatment. The highest number of neutrophils with TSPO at 4 h after the treatment was 186.6±9.1 per mm^2 in the periportal region and 83.8±5.4 per mm^2 in the centrilobular region.

Gene Expression Associated with TSPO

mRNA expression of the TSPO functional macromolecular signaling complex was quantified by qRT-PCR (Figure 6). Hepatic TSPO mRNA expression was increased at 2 h (2.1 fold), 4 h (2.4 fold) and 6 h (2.1 fold) after CHX treatment compared with the control group. The TSPO mRNA levels increased correspondingly with the TSPO expression and liver damage severity.

Discussion

This study noninvasively visualized liver damage using PET with the TSPO-specific radiotracer [^{18}F]FEDAC. In the PET study for the rat model of mild acute liver damage, significant increases in radioactive signals from the liver corresponded with increases in TSPO expression. The qRT-PCR and immunohistochemical assays confirmed the correlation between the increase in TSPO expression and the severity of damage. The main cellular sources of [^{18}F]FEDAC uptake specific to TSPO were found to be macrophages (Kupffer cells) and neutrophils in the liver tissue.

The CHX-induced acute liver damage model was used in the present study to characterize liver changes in the early phase of liver damage. There is experimental evidence that CHX induces apoptosis and necrotic changes in hepatocytes with slight neutrophil infiltration [12]. Moreover, treatment with CHX accelerated phagocytosis of apoptotic hepatocytes by Kupffer cells and the subsequent release of inflammatory cytokines by activated Kupffer cells [13–16]. In addition to the histopathology experiment (Figure 1), serum chemistry assays of AST and ALT were examined in this model. Both transaminases increased to only 2-folds higher at 4 h after the CHX treatment than in the control group (Figure 2). Therefore, the present animal model was considered to have sustained mild liver damage.

The PET images with [^{18}F]FEDAC for the rats at 1 h, 2 h, 4 h, and 6 h after CHX treatment reflected the occurrence and progress of liver damage (Figure 3). Comparisons of liver images and $AUC_{0-30\ min}$ values between the control and CHX-treated groups indicated that the levels of radioactivity and radiotracer binding gradually elevated in the livers along with the severity of damage. At 4 h after CHX treatment, compared to that of the control group, the $AUC_{0-30\ min}$ value of [^{18}F]FEDAC increased to 1.8-fold.

The localization of TSPO in the liver was detected by immunohistochemical staining assay (Figures 4 and 5). In the controls, strong fluorescence representing TSPO expression was detected in parts of the Kupffer cells, intra-lobular bile duct, and hepatic arteriole of the portal triad, and with weak signals from the portal vein. TSPO level in hepatocytes was low regardless of CHX treatment. Our present results were consistent with the distribution patterns of TSPO immunoreactivity in human liver [26]. On the other hand, it has been reported that TSPO subcellular locations in rat liver are present not only in hepatocyte mitochondria but also in a non-mitochondrial fraction of the non-parenchymal cells with a possible biliary epithelial cell plasma membrane locations

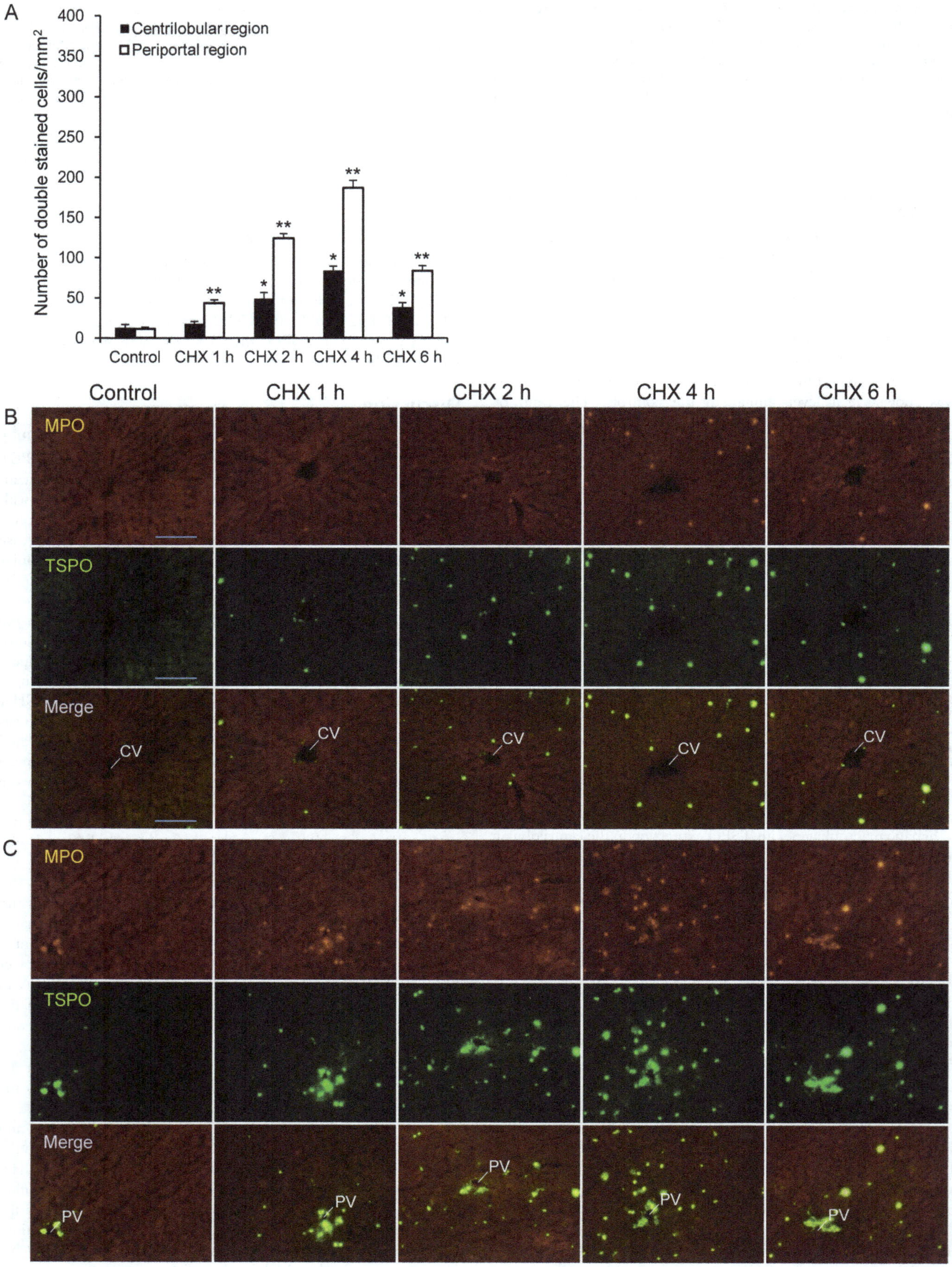
A
400
350
300
250
200
150
100
50
0
Number of double stained cells/mm2
Centrilobular region
Periportal region
Control
CHX 1 h
CHX 2 h
CHX 4 h
CHX 6 h
Control
CHX 1 h
CHX 2 h
CHX 4 h
CHX 6 h
B
MPO
TSPO
Merge
CV
C
MPO
TSPO
Merge
PV

Figure 5. Increased TSPO levels expressed in neutrophiles in liver tissues after CHX treatment. (A) The number of double immunofluorescence staining cells of MPO and TSPO in the centrilobular and periportal regions of the rat hepatic lobules. A significant difference ($p<0.05$) was seen for the following comparisons, *: centrilobular region, control versus CHX 2 h, 4 h, or 6 h; **: periportal region, control versus all CHX treatment groups. (B, C) Double immunofluorescence labeling of MPO (red) and TSPO (green) in the centrilobular region (B) and the periportal region (C). Neutrophils with TSPO expression increased after CHX treatment, and higher number of double stained cells was observed in the periportal region than in the centrilobular region CHX treatment. Abbreviations: central vein (CV), portal vein (PV). Scale bar: 100< μm.

[27], although TSPO was mainly localized in the cellular mitochondria of various tissues [18]. Our present finding supports the presence of TSPO in a non-mitochondrial fraction of biliary epithelial cells, although TSPO function in the bile duct is still unknown.

The present CHX treatment induced an increase in the number of cells containing TSPO, which were expressed in macrophages and neutrophils. The activated macrophages and neutrophils in both the periportal and centrilobular regions increased and were the highest at 4 h after the treatment. The hepatic TSPO mRNA expression also indicated similar changes in activated immune cell numbers over time (Figure 6). Because the TSPO mRNA levels in phagocytic cells, such as monocytes and polymorphonuclear cells were reported to be 7–8 fold higher than that in natural killer cells and B and T lymphocytes [20], the effect of lymphocytes on the TSPO level is considered to be much less than that of macrophages and neutrophils. It was indicated that the increase in TSPO in activated macrophages and neutrophils was mainly responsible for the increase in [^{18}F]FEDAC uptake in the CHX-treated livers.

Kupffer cells, the main residential macrophages in liver, are known to have a functional heterogeneity that is related to their position in the liver acinus. In the periportal region, Kupffer cells including large and heterogeneous lysosomes have high endocytic activity and high lysosomal enzyme activity. Previous studies showed that Kupffer cells are distributed over the periportal and centrilobular regions in a ratio of 1.5–2 in normal rat liver [28,29]. Our present results showed that TSPO expressed in macrophages in control livers was 1.7-fold higher in the periportal region than that in the centrilobular region. This ratio of TSPO expression in macrophages was close to that of the whole hepatic lobule of a normal rat. On the other hand, treatment with CHX induced an increase in TSPO expressed in macrophages in the periportal region more than that in the centrilobular region, and the ratio increased to 3 at 4 h after the treatment. It is known that blood from both the portal vein and hepatic artery contained in the portal tracts of the periportal region mixes together in the sinusoids and empties into the central vein of the centrilobular region [30]. In the sinusoids, Kupffer cells are perfectly situated to clear endotoxins from the passing blood and to phagocytose debris and microorganisms. In addition, Kupffer cells also pass through the space of Disse to make direct contact with hepatocytes and to phagocytose apoptotic hepatocytes [13]. Therefore, we assume that TSPO may play a role in the function of Kupffer cells.

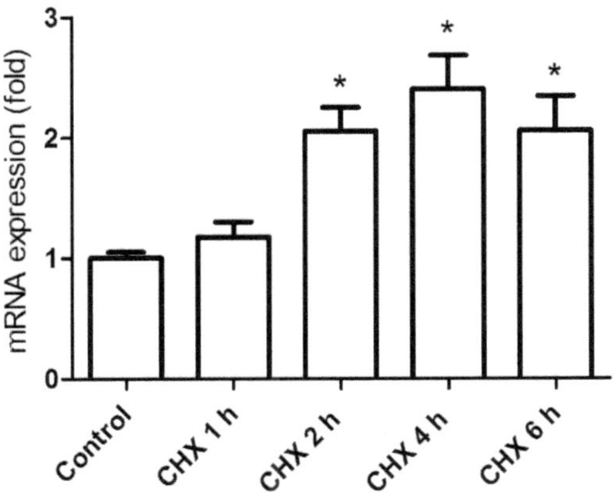

Figure 6. Effect of CHX treatment on the mRNA expression of TSPO. Hepatic TSPO mRNA expression was increased at 2 h (2.1 fold), 4 h (2.4 fold) and 6 h (2.1 fold) after CHX treatment compared with the control group. A significant difference ($p<0.05$) was seen in the following comparisons, *: control versus CHX 2 h, 4 h, or 6 h.

Acute liver injury from drug-induced liver damage, though uncommon, is of concern for both patients and medical doctors. In clinical practice, ultrasound assessment is a first line screening procedure for liver damage. However, inter-observer variability and poor reproducibility limit its usefulness. CT and MRI are more sensitive for liver damage than ultrasound. These modalities are shown in reformatted projections to fit the liver sonograms, but lack sensitivity and specificity for differentiating liver damage from other liver diseases and for assessing damage severity.

PET imaging with [^{18}F]FDG, the most commonly used radiotracer, has been used to detect and characterize malignant tumors and several liver diseases [6]. However, no significant uptake of [^{18}F]FDG was found in the present liver damage model and no observatory difference in liver uptake was observed between the control and CHX-treated groups (data not shown). In contrast with [^{18}F]FDG, PET with [^{18}F]FEDAC could noninvasively visualize liver damage by monitoring the increase in macrophages and neutrophils associated with early stages of liver damage, which could help elucidate the pathological mechanisms in liver damage induced by various drugs in the human liver. Early evaluation of liver damage is important for timely and accurate therapeutic interventions in patients suffering this disease. Therefore, using TSPO as a biomarker for PET imaging could eventually help establish a reliable and non-invasive method for monitoring liver damage. In combination with other modalities, such as serum assessment, ultrasound, CT and MRI, PET could give a reliable and accurate diagnosis of liver damage.

Conclusion

The present findings indicate the feasibility of PET-TSPO imaging. This PET study shows excellent sensitivity and imaging quality for the detection and quantification of TSPO expression associated with the occurrence and progression of liver damage. [^{18}F]FEDAC-PET appears to be a promising tool for studies involving the human liver.

Acknowledgments

We thank M. Higuchi (National Institute of Radiological Science) for providing us with antibody NP155 for mouse TSPO and for their technical support. We are grateful to the staff of our institute for their technical support and assistance with cyclotron operation, radionuclide production, and animal experiments.

Author Contributions

Conceived and designed the experiments: AH MRZ. Performed the experiments: AH JY LX TY HW K. Kawamura. Analyzed the data: AH JY. Contributed reagents/materials/analysis tools: K. Kumata MF MO NN. Wrote the paper: AH MRZ.

References

1. Lammert C, Bjornsson E, Niklasson A, Chalasani N (2010) Oral medications with significant hepatic metabolism at higher risk for hepatic adverse events. Hepatology 51: 615–620.
2. M'Kada H, Perazzo H, Munteanu M, Ngo Y, Ramanujam N, et al. (2012) Real time identification of drug-induced liver injury (DILI) through daily screening of ALT results: a prospective pilot cohort study. PLoS ONE 7: e42418.
3. Lewis JH (2012) The adaptive response (drug tolerance) helps to prevent drug-induced liver injury. Gastroenterol Hepatol 8: 333–336.
4. Marino G, Zimmerman HJ, Lewis JH (2001) Management of drug-induced liver disease. Curr Gastroenterol Rep 3: 38–48.
5. Boll DT, Merkle EM (2009) Diffuse liver disease: strategies for hepatic CT and MR imaging. Radiographics 29: 1591–1614.
6. Trojan J, Schroeder O, Raedle J, Baum RP, Herrmann G, et al. (1999) Fluorine-18 positron emission tomography for imaging of hepatocellular carcinoma. Am J Gastroenterol 94: 3314–3319.
7. Dhirapong A, Yang GX, Nadler S, Zhang W, Tsuneyama K, et al. (2013) Therapeutic effect of cytotoxic T lymphocyte antigen 4/immunoglobulin on a murine model of primary biliary cirrhosis. Hepatology 57: 708–715.
8. Proctor W R, Chakraborty M, Chea LS, Morrison JC, Berkson JD, et al. (2013) Eosinophils mediate the pathogenesis of halothane-induced liver injury in mice. Hepatology 57: 2026–2036.
9. Weber LW, Boll M, Stampfl A (2003) Hepatotoxicity and mechanism of action of haloalkanes: carbon tetrachloride as a toxicological model. Crit Rev Toxicol 33: 105–136.
10. Faa G, Ledda-Columbano GM, Ambu R, Congiu T, Coni P, et al. (1994) An electron microscopic study of apoptosis induced by cycloheximide in rat liver. Liver 14: 270–278.
11. Higami Y, Tanaka K, Tsuchiya T, Shimokawa I (2000) Intravenous injection of cycloheximide induces apoptosis and up-regulates p53 and Fas receptor expression in the rat liver in vivo. Mutat Res 457: 105–111.
12. Ito K, Kiyosawa N, Kumagai K, Manabe S, Matsunuma N, et al. (2006) Molecular mechanism investigation of cycloheximide-induced hepatocyte apoptosis in rat livers by morphological and microarray analysis. Toxicology 219: 175–186.
13. Racanelli V, Rehermann B (2006) The liver as an immunological organ. Hepatology 43: S54–62.
14. Canbay A, Feldstein AE, Higuchi H, Werneburg N, Grambihler A, et al. (2003) Kupffer cell engulfment of apoptotic bodies stimulates death ligand and cytokine expression. Hepatology 38: 1188–1198.
15. Dahle MK, Øverland G, Myhre AE, Stuestøl JF, Hartung T, et al. (2004) The phosphatidylinositol 3-kinase/protein kinase B signaling pathway is activated by lipoteichoic acid and plays a role in Kupffer cell production of interleukin-6 (IL-6) and IL-10. Infect Immun 72: 5704–5711.
16. Kurosaka K, Watanabe N, Kobayashi Y (2001) Production of proinflammatory cytokines by resident tissue macrophages after phagocytosis of apoptotic cells. Cell Immunol 211: 1–7.
17. Kumagai K, Ito K, Ando Y, Hakamata S, Teranishi M, et al. (2009) Neutralization of IL-10 exacerbates cycloheximide-induced hepatocellular apoptosis and necrosis. Toxicol Pathol 37: 536–546.
18. Papadopoulos V, Baraldi M, Guilarte TR, Knudsen TB, Lacapère JJ, et al. (2006) Translocator protein (18 kDa): new nomenclature for the peripheral-type benzodiazepine receptor based on its structure and molecular function. Trends Pharmacol Sci 27: 402–409.
19. Giatzakis C, Papadopoulos V (2004) Differential utilization of the promoter of peripheral-type benzodiazepine receptor by steroidogenic versus nonsteroidogenic cell lines and the role of Sp1 and Sp3 in the regulation of basal activity. Endocrinology 145: 1113–1123.
20. Canat X, Carayon P, Bouaboula M, Cahard D, Shire D, et al. (1993) Distribution profile and properties of peripheral-type benzodiazepine receptors on human hemopoietic cells. Life Sci 52: 107–118.
21. Scarf AM, Kassiou M (2011) The translocator protein. J Nucl Med 52: 677–680.
22. Yui J, Maeda J, Kumata K, Kawamura K, Yanamoto K, et al. (2010) ^{18}F-FEAC and ^{18}F-FEDAC: PET of the monkey brain and imaging of translocator protein (18 kDa) in the infarcted rat brain. J Nucl Med 51: 1301–1309.
23. Hatori A, Yui J, Yamasaki T, Xie L, Kumata K, et al. (2012) PET imaging of lung inflammation with [^{18}F]FEDAC, a radioligand for translocator protein (18 kDa). PLoS ONE 7: e45065.
24. Xie L, Yui J, Hatori A, Yamasaki T, Kumata K, et al. (2012) Translocator protein (18 kDa), a potential molecular imaging biomarker for non-invasively distinguishing non-alcoholic fatty liver disease. J Hepatol 57: 1076–1082.
25. Ji B, Maeda J, Sawada M, Ono M, Okauchi T, et al. (2008) Imaging of peripheral benzodiazepine receptor expression as biomarkers of detrimental versus beneficial glial responses in mouse models of Alzheimer's and other CNS pathologies. J Neurosci 28: 12255–12267.
26. Bribes E, Carrière D, Goubet C, Galiegue S, Casellas P, et al. (1996) Immunohistochemical assessment of the peripheral benzodiazepine receptor in human tissues. J Histochem Cytochem 52: 19–28.
27. Woods MJ, Zisterer DM, Williams DC (1996) Two cellular and subcellular locations for the peripheral-type benzodiazepine receptor in rat liver. Biochem Pharmacol 51: 1283–1292.
28. Bouwens L, Baekeland M, De Zanger R, Wisse E (1986) Quantitation, tissue distribution and proliferation kinetics of Kupffer cells in normal rat liver. Hepatology 6: 718–722.
29. Sleyster EC, Knook DL (1982) Relation between localization and function of rat liver Kupffer cells. Lab Invest 47: 484–490.
30. Yokoyama Y., Wawrzyniak A, Sarmadi AM, Baveja R, Gruber HE, et al. (2006) Hepatic arterial flow becomes the primary supply of sinusoids following partial portal vein ligation in rats. J Gastroenterol Hepatol 21: 1567–1574.

16

Quantitative Comparison of PET and Bremsstrahlung SPECT for Imaging the In Vivo Yttrium-90 Microsphere Distribution after Liver Radioembolization

Mattijs Elschot*, Bart J. Vermolen, Marnix G. E. H. Lam, Bart de Keizer, Maurice A. A. J. van den Bosch, Hugo W. A. M. de Jong

Department of Radiology and Nuclear Medicine, University Medical Center Utrecht, Utrecht, The Netherlands

Abstract

Background: After yttrium-90 (^{90}Y) microsphere radioembolization (RE), evaluation of extrahepatic activity and liver dosimetry is typically performed on ^{90}Y Bremsstrahlung SPECT images. Since these images demonstrate a low quantitative accuracy, ^{90}Y PET has been suggested as an alternative. The aim of this study is to quantitatively compare SPECT and state-of-the-art PET on the ability to detect small accumulations of ^{90}Y and on the accuracy of liver dosimetry.

Methodology/Principal Findings: SPECT/CT and PET/CT phantom data were acquired using several acquisition and reconstruction protocols, including resolution recovery and Time-Of-Flight (TOF) PET. Image contrast and noise were compared using a torso-shaped phantom containing six hot spheres of various sizes. The ability to detect extra- and intrahepatic accumulations of activity was tested by quantitative evaluation of the visibility and unique detectability of the phantom hot spheres. Image-based dose estimates of the phantom were compared to the true dose. For clinical illustration, the SPECT and PET-based estimated liver dose distributions of five RE patients were compared. At equal noise level, PET showed higher contrast recovery coefficients than SPECT. The highest contrast recovery coefficients were obtained with TOF PET reconstruction including resolution recovery. All six spheres were consistently visible on SPECT and PET images, but PET was able to uniquely detect smaller spheres than SPECT. TOF PET-based estimates of the dose in the phantom spheres were more accurate than SPECT-based dose estimates, with underestimations ranging from 45% (10-mm sphere) to 11% (37-mm sphere) for PET, and 75% to 58% for SPECT, respectively. The differences between TOF PET and SPECT dose-estimates were supported by the patient data.

Conclusions/Significance: In this study we quantitatively demonstrated that the image quality of state-of-the-art PET is superior over Bremsstrahlung SPECT for the assessment of the ^{90}Y microsphere distribution after radioembolization.

Editor: Erica Villa, University of Modena & Reggio Emilia, Italy

Funding: This work was funded by the University Medical Center Utrecht. The funders had no role in study design, data collection and analysis, decision to publish, or preparation of the manuscript.

Competing Interests: The authors have declared that no competing interests exist.

* E-mail: m.elschot@umcutrecht.nl

Introduction

Intra-arterial radioembolization (RE) using microspheres labeled with the high-energy beta-emitter yttrium-90 (^{90}Y), is used in clinical practice for treatment of unresectable liver tumours [1,2]. Prior to RE, prophylactic coil-embolization of arteries communicating with the gastrointestinal (GI) tract is performed, followed by administration of technetium-99m macroaggregated-albumin (^{99m}Tc-MAA) particles. Subsequent gamma camera imaging is used to assess any extrahepatic particle deposition, which is a contra-indication for RE. Also, the percentage of particles that shunts to the lungs is measured, which may lead to adjustment of the ^{90}Y dose [3]. After administration of the ^{90}Y microspheres, a post-therapy ^{90}Y Bremsstrahlung SPECT scan is performed for two reasons. First, ^{90}Y may unexpectedly be present outside the liver, despite a favorable distribution on the ^{99m}Tc-MAA scan. Accumulation of ^{90}Y microspheres in organs other than the liver will likely cause serious complications, like ulceration and bleedings in the GI tract [4,5]. Therefore, severe pain after treatment should be aggressively managed to prevent development of more serious complications [5], which may be facilitated by early detection of possible extrahepatic activity [6]. Second, the intrahepatic microsphere distribution over tumourous and non-tumourous liver tissue is expected to be an important predictor of treatment efficacy [7]. Post-therapy imaging facilitates estimation of the tumour and non-tumour absorbed radiation dose on the image-based microsphere distribution.

Unfortunately, the low photon yield and continuous nature of the Bremsstrahlung X-ray spectrum limit the quantitative accuracy of ^{90}Y Bremsstrahlung SPECT. Per MBq, approximately 23000 Bremsstrahlung photons with energy higher than 50 keV are produced by interaction of the beta particle with tissue [8], therefore acquisition in a wide energy window is required to maximize sensitivity. The absence of a photopeak prohibits the use of simple window-based scatter rejection, scatter correction, and attenuation correction techniques, and penetration of high-energy photons through the collimator septa leads to further loss of image contrast [9]. Recent efforts to optimize reconstruction algorithms, e.g. by compensation for scatter and collimator blurring with pre-calculated ^{90}Y point-spread functions (PSF) [8,10], have improved the quantitative accuracy of ^{90}Y Bremsstrahlung SPECT, but are not widely available in the clinic to date.

Yttrium-90 PET was recently shown to be feasible in phantoms and patients and may be an interesting alternative to Bremsstrahlung SPECT [11]. Per MBq, ^{90}Y emits 32 positrons per second with a maximum energy of 758 keV [12,13]. Consequently, annihilation photon pairs are produced approximately 700 times less often than Bremsstrahlung photons (E >50 keV). Nevertheless, ^{90}Y PET may allow for the detection of extrahepatic activity and accurate tumour and liver dose estimation, since the spatial resolution is expected to be comparable to that of ^{18}F PET, which has a maximum positron energy of 633 keV [14]. Additionally, advanced correction techniques for scatter, random, and attenuation effects that are clinically available for ^{18}F PET, can be directly applied to ^{90}Y PET [15]. Several groups have successfully assessed the post-therapy ^{90}Y microsphere distribution in RE patients [11,16–19].

To date, no systematic studies have quantitatively compared clinically available ^{90}Y PET with Bremsstrahlung SPECT. The potential for accurately assessing the intra- and extrahepatic microsphere distribution is determined by fundamental limitations of the imaging modality. The first objective of this study was to quantitatively evaluate and compare the contrast and noise characteristics of ^{90}Y PET and SPECT images, which are relevant parameters for activity detection and liver dosimetry in clinical practice. Image contrast depends on spatial resolution and on other effects that distort quantification of local ^{90}Y content, like photon attenuation, photon scatter, collimator penetration and random coincidences. Image noise is dependent on sensitivity and on the stochastic nature of attenuation, scatter and collimation. The second objective was to quantitatively compare ^{90}Y PET and SPECT on the ability to detect small accumulations of ^{90}Y inside and outside the liver, and on the accuracy of liver dose estimates, based on the recorded ^{90}Y distribution. All quantitative results were obtained in phantom experiments. Additionally, Bremsstrahlung SPECT and PET scans of five ^{90}Y RE patients were evaluated to support the results of the phantom study.

Materials and Methods

Ethics Statement

Dual post-treatment imaging using both SPECT/CT and PET/CT techniques was part of the quality control protocol for implementation of ^{90}Y-PET imaging as the standard post-radioembolization procedure. All data were retrospectively analyzed, written patient informed consent was therefore not sought nor documented. The institutional review board (IRB) of the University Medical Center Utrecht approves this type of retrospective study and waives the requirements for patient informed consent. The image data were handled anonymously, in accordance with the Declaration of Helsinki and the regulations of the IRB.

Scanners, Acquisition and Reconstruction

PET/CT data were acquired on a state-of-the-art Siemens mCT Time-Of-Flight (TOF) PET/CT scanner (Siemens Medical Solutions USA, Inc.). The mCT combines a whole body LSO PET scanner with a 40-slice CT scanner. The PET component is equipped with a large axial field-of-view (FOV) of 21.8 cm and wide acceptance angle of 13.2° to maximize sensitivity. In whole body mode, consecutive bed positions overlap approximately 43%. A detailed characterization of the physical and clinical performance of the mCT was performed by Jakoby *et al* [20]. PET data were acquired with a lower- and upper-level discriminator of 435 keV and 650 keV, respectively. Three reconstruction algorithms were compared, all including correction for random coincidences, scatter and attenuation [20]. The first algorithm was fully 3D iterative attenuation weighted ordinary Poisson ordered subset expectation maximization (OP-OSEM) reconstruction [21] ('iterative'), the second algorithm was iterative reconstruction extended with a PSF model of the detector response [22] ('iterative+PSF'), and the third was iterative reconstruction including PSF and TOF information ('iterative+PSF+TOF'). Images were reconstructed using 3 iterations with 24 or 21 (iterative+PSF+TOF) subsets and a 5 mm full-width at half-maximum (FWHM) Gaussian post-reconstruction filter. The reconstructed voxel size was $2\times2\times2$ mm^3.

SPECT/CT data were acquired on a Siemens Symbia T16 system (Siemens Medical Solutions USA, Inc.). The Symbia T16 combines a dual detector SPECT scanner with a 16-slice CT scanner. The SPECT detectors are equipped with 3/8 inch thick crystals. All our experiments were performed with the high-energy collimators mounted, which proved to be the best option for ^{90}Y imaging with maximum resolution and contrast [9,23]. SPECT data were acquired in a 105–195 keV energy window [8,24], using 120 projections over 360° and a 256×256 matrix with a pixel size of 2.4×2.4 mm^2. Images were reconstructed with two different reconstruction algorithms. The first algorithm was 2D OSEM reconstruction including correction for attenuation with an effective broad beam linear attenuation coefficient ('iterative'), and the second algorithm was iterative reconstruction including a Gaussian PSF model of the geometric collimator-detector response of the camera [25] ('iterative+PSF'). In both cases 8 iterations with 8 subsets were used without post-reconstruction filtering. The reconstructed voxel size was $2.4\times2.4\times2.4$ mm^3.

Phantom Set Up

The NEMA 2007/IEC 2008 PET Image Quality (IQ) Phantom, which is designed for evaluation of reconstructed image quality and activity recovery, was used for all phantom experiments to allow for direct comparison between the two modalities [26]. The phantom consists of a fillable torso-shaped compartment (volume = 9700 ml) containing six fillable coplanar spheres (inner diameter = 10, 13, 17, 22, 28, and 37 mm) and a cylindrical lung insert.

Table 1 lists the separately performed phantom experiments. PET data were acquired in one bed position centered on the spheres. Since the PET FOV covering a whole liver requires two bed positions (30 cm in axial direction) and for SPECT one FOV (40 cm) is sufficient, all PET scan times were set to half the SPECT scan times. The initial ^{90}Y activity concentration in the spheres ($[A]_{sph}$) and background compartment ($[A]_{bkg}$) was 2.40 and 0 MBq ml^{-1}, respectively. All six spheres were filled with activity, which slightly deviates from the NEMA recommendations. After performing experiments 1, ^{90}Y was added to the background for experiments 2–4, resulting in $[A]_{bkg} = 0.27$ MBq ml^{-1}. The total activity in the phantom was 119 and 2600 MBq, for experiments 1, and 2–4, respectively. Instead of adjusting the activity in the phantom, the scan times were prolonged ×2 and ×4 times in experiments 2–4 to obtain the simulated activity concentrations given in Table 1. This approach was deemed valid, because both the measured total activity and the maximum simulated total

Table 1. Phantom experiments.

Exp.	Ratio	Modality	Real scan time (min.)	$[A]_{sph}$ (MBq ml^{-1})	$[A]_{bkg}$ (MBq ml^{-1})
1P	1:0	PET	15	2.4 (real)	0 (real)
1S	1:0	SPECT	30	2.4 (real)	0 (real)
2P	9:1	PET	15	2.4 (real)	0.27 (real)
2S	9:1	SPECT	30	2.4 (real)	0.27 (real)
3P	9:1	PET	30	4.8 (simulated)	0.54 (simulated)
3S	9:1	SPECT	60	4.8 (simulated)	0.54 (simulated)
4P	9:1	PET	60	9.6 (simulated)	1.09 (simulated)
4S	9:1	SPECT	120	9.6 (simulated)	1.09 (simulated)

activity, which corresponded to approximately 2600 MBq for a 2000 ml liver, were within the linear range (i.e. no dead time effects) of ^{90}Y PET and Bremsstrahlung SPECT [9,11].

Image Contrast and Noise

Image contrast and noise measurements were obtained from phantom experiments 4 (Table 1), representing a clinically realistic liver background activity concentration of 1.09 MBq ml^{-1}. For comparison: using the body surface area (BSA) method (see 'Patients' section), the mean activity concentration in a 1.5 kg liver with 10% tumour involvement of an 'average' patient (1.70 m, 70 kg) would be 1.14 MBq ml^{-1}. Six circular hot sphere regions of interest (ROIs) were automatically delineated on the CT slice through the center of the spheres, covering the inner compartment voxels of each of the six phantom spheres. A background ROI was delineated on the same slice consisting of all voxels that fell within the physical phantom boundaries, excluding the voxels belonging to the hot sphere ROIs and the lung insert. For each reconstructed SPECT and PET volume, contrast recovery coefficients (Q_H) were calculated with equation 1.

$$Q_H = \frac{C_H/C_B - 1}{R-1} \times 100\% \tag{1}$$

Here, C_H is the mean intensity in the hot sphere ROIs, C_B is the mean intensity in the background ROI and R is the true sphere-to-background activity concentration ratio. As a measure of image noise, the coefficient of variation (CV) was calculated with equation 2.

$$CV = \frac{STDV_B}{C_B} \times 100\% \tag{2}$$

Here, STDVB is the standard deviation in the background ROI.

Detectability

The ability to detect small accumulations of activity (detectability) in a region without background activity is important for evaluation of extrahepatic microsphere deposition. Additionally, the detectability of activity in a region with background activity is important when intrahepatic tumour identification is based on the contrast in the SPECT and PET scans, e.g. using isocontours when the target volume cannot be derived from a CT or MRI scan.

A hot spot of activity can only be accurately identified, if it can be reliably distinguished from the background, i.e. if it is visible. The visibility (υ_H) of the six hot spheres was tested by quantitative evaluation of the hot sphere and background signal; for each hot sphere the effective contrast-to-noise ratio (CNR) was calculated according to equation 3.

$$v_H = \frac{C_H - C_B}{STDV_B} \times \sqrt{N_{voxels}} \tag{3}$$

with C_H, C_B, and $STDV_B$ as defined in the previous section and N_{voxels} the number of voxels in the hot sphere ROI. Subsequently, a hot sphere was scored 'visible' when υ_H was larger than 4, in accordance with the Rose criterion [27,28].

In addition to the visibility criterion, which is an established method for detection of false negatives, a new method is presented to evaluate the presence of false positive hot spots. Since accumulations of activity are not 'uniquely detectable' if false positives are present, we will refer to this criterion as 'unique detectability' in the remainder of this work. The unique detectability of the six hot spheres was evaluated in five consecutive background slices, placed five cm away from the slice through the center of the spheres. Circular ROIs to test for false positives ($ROI_{TEST-FP}$) with the same diameter as the hot sphere ROIs were centered on all phantom voxels in the five slices. The visibility ($\upsilon_{TEST-FP}$) of each $ROI_{TEST-FP}$ was calculated with equation 4.

$$v_{TEST-FP} = \frac{C_{TEST-FP} - C_B}{STDV_B} \times \sqrt{N_{voxels}} \tag{4}$$

Here, $C_{TEST-FP}$ is the mean intensity in $ROI_{TEST-FP}$, C_B the mean intensity in the background ROI of the same slice (consisting of all voxels falling within the phantom boundaries, excluding the lung insert), $STDV_B$ the standard deviation in the background ROI and N_{voxels} the number of voxels in $ROI_{TEST-FP}$. We investigated two different criteria to score a sphere 'uniquely detectable'. According to the first criterion, a visible hot sphere was scored 'uniquely detectable', if $\upsilon_{TEST-FP}$ was smaller than 4 for all $ROI_{TEST-FP}$ of the same size, i.e. if none of the corresponding $ROI_{TEST-FP}$ were visible according to the Rose criterion. Translated to clinical practice, this criterion measures whether any visible hot spot of a certain diameter can be reliably characterized as 'true positive'. According to the second criterion, a visible hot sphere was scored 'uniquely detectable' if $\upsilon_{TEST-FP}$ was smaller than υ_H for all $ROI_{TEST-FP}$ of the same size, i.e. if the hot sphere was better visible than all corresponding $ROI_{TEST-FP}$. This criterion is less strict and measures whether the visible hot spot with the highest CNR can be reliably characterized as 'true positive'.

When using CNR with the relaxation term $\sqrt{N_{voxels}}$ for evaluation of the visibility of hot spots, a uniform count density in the hot spot ROI is assumed. However, the mean intensities of the relatively small hot sphere and false positive ROIs are susceptible to outliers and may therefore not accurately represent human perception. Median values, on the other hand, are less sensitive to outliers and may be a better measure for this purpose. Consequently, equations 3 and 4 were also evaluated using median intensities for C_H and $C_{TEST\text{-}FP}$, respectively. The 'median-based' hot sphere visibility and unique detectability results were presented next to their 'mean-based' equivalents. Data from experiments 1 (Table 1) were used to analyze the extrahepatic detectability and experiments 2–4 were used to mimic the intrahepatic situation, for three different activity concentrations.

Patients

Radioembolization with ^{90}Y-labelled resin microspheres (SIR-Spheres, Sirtex Medical, Sydney, Australia) was performed in 5 consecutive patients (2 women, 3 men; mean age +/− SD, 56.8+/−13.0 y; age range 43–76 y) according to the international consensus report from the Radioembolization Brachytherapy Oncology Consortium [3]. The BSA method was used to calculate the activities (A) administered to the patients, according to the equation A (GBq) = BSA−0.2+ V_T/V_L, with BSA (m^2) = 0.20247 * height$^{0.725}$ * weight$^{0.725}$, and V_T and V_L the tumour and whole liver volume derived from CT or MRI, respectively. Dose adjustments were not required, since the percentage ^{99m}Tc-MAA lung shunting was below 10% for all patients. Four patients were diagnosed with liver metastases (2 colorectal carcinomas, 1 nasopharyngeal carcinoma, and 1 mammary carcinoma) and one patient was diagnosed with hepatocellular carcinoma. Four patients received whole liver treatment and one patient received left lobar treatment. PET data were acquired in two bed positions (total scan length 30 cm) centered on the liver, whereas the SPECT axial FOV was 40 cm. SPECT and PET data were both acquired in 30 minutes, which was considered the maximum desirable scan time for a RE patient. All patient and treatment characteristics are summarized in Table 2.

Absorbed Dose Estimation

Phantom. The iterative+PSF+TOF PET and iterative+PSF SPECT images of experiments 4 (Table 1) were used to evaluate the accuracy of dosimetry. Calibration factors to convert the PET and SPECT images into units of activity were determined by dividing the total reconstructed counts in the phantom by the known activity in the phantom. A digital phantom representing the 'true activity distribution' (TRUE) was constructed from a segmented high-resolution CT dataset (voxel size 0.6×0.6×0.6 mm^3). Activity concentrations of 1.09 MBq ml^{-1} and 9.6 MBq ml^{-1} were applied to the segmented 3D background ROI and 3D hot sphere ROIs, respectively. Dose maps were calculated from the PET, SPECT, and TRUE activity images by convolution with the appropriate ^{90}Y 3D dose-point kernel (DPK), in accordance with MIRD Pamphlet No. 17 [29]. For this purpose, DPKs with the same voxel sizes as the high-resolution CT, SPECT and PET images were calculated using the Monte Carlo engine MCNPX 2.5.0 [30].

Table 2. Patient and treatment characteristics.

Patient	Primary[a]	Lobes[b]	V_L[c]	V_T[d]	A_A[e]	A_S[f]	A_P[g]
1	CRC	W	2481	153	1714	1303	1602
2	CRC	W	1835	50	1852	1483	1499
3	NPC	W	1230	72	1199	922	1109
4	MC	L	383	20	281	216	270
5	HCC	W	3050	178	1177	916	927

[a]Primary disease: CRC = colorectal carcinoma; NPC = nasopharyngeal carcinoma; MC = mammary carcinoma; HCC = hepatocellular carcinoma.
[b]Lobes treated: W = whole liver treatment; L = left lobar treatment.
[c]V_L = treated liver volume (ml).
[d]V_T = volume of tumours in treated liver volume (ml).
[e]A_A = Activity administered to the patient, at time of administration (MBq).
[f]A_S = Activity at time of SPECT acquisition (MBq).
[g]A_P = Activity at time of PET acquisition (MBq).

Three-dimensional ROIs of the fillable spheres and a 2000 ml background region were delineated on the CT scans, altogether representing a liver with tumours. Cumulative dose-volume histograms (CDVH) and mean absorbed doses were calculated for all ROIs. Additionally, the mean absorbed doses in the hot sphere ROIs were corrected for incomplete activity recovery due to partial volume effects (PVE), by multiplication with the corresponding correction factors calculated as R * C_B/C_H. Errors in the uncorrected and corrected SPECT and PET-based dose estimates were calculated in comparison to the TRUE dose.

Patients. Patient data were reconstructed with the same settings as the phantom data. Three-dimensional liver ROIs were manually delineated on the CT scans. To be able to mutually compare the SPECT and PET-based dose distributions, the liver ROI of each patient was segmented into a low-dose ROI and a high-dose ROI. The high-dose ROI included all voxels that had on one or both modalities an activity concentration of at least two times the mean liver concentration. The low-dose ROI consisted of the other liver voxels, i.e. the liver ROI excluding the high-dose ROI. The resulting 'integrated' SPECT/PET ROIs allowed for an unbiased, direct comparison of the dose distribution between the modalities. Following conversion of PET and SPECT activity images into dose maps, CDVH and mean absorbed doses were calculated for all ROIs.

Results

Image Contrast and Noise

Figure 1 shows that iterative+PSF+TOF reconstruction resulted in PET images with the highest contrast recovery. Iterative+PSF reconstruction resulted in the highest contrast recovery for SPECT. PET contrast recovery coefficients were substantially higher than those of SPECT in all spheres. In comparison, both image contrast and image noise were higher in PET than in SPECT (Figure 2A), which is also evident from the transversal slices through the phantom in Figure 2B and 2C. The noise level in the PET images was substantially reduced when reconstructed with 1 iteration and a 15 mm FWHM post-reconstruction filter (equal noise (EQN) PET), approximately to the noise level of the SPECT images (approximately 18% CV, Figure 2A and 2D). This set-up allows for a fair comparison of image contrast. At equal noise level, all PET images still showed higher contrast than SPECT, although contrast was lost in comparison with PET images reconstructed with optimal settings.

Detectability

From Table 3 it can be appreciated that the 'mean-based' and 'median-based' visibility results were equal for all images but one. The unique detectability results differed between the 'mean-based'

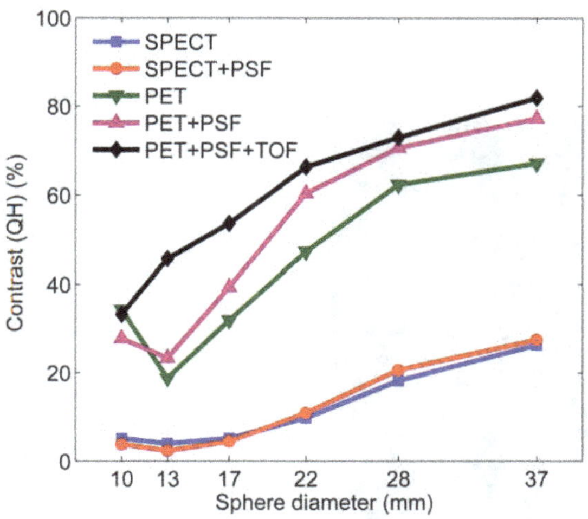

Figure 1. Contrast recovery as a function of sphere diameter for all reconstruction methods.

and 'median-based' approach, for both detectability criteria. From Figure 3 it is apparent the 'mean-based' approach detected more false positives than the 'median-based' approach. Being less affected by outliers, the 'median-based' approach only detected the more or less uniform false positives regions and was therefore considered the best approach for false positive detection. Consequently, in the remainder of this section the 'median-based' results are reported for hot sphere visibility and unique detectability. Table 3 and Figure 3 show that in the extrahepatic situation, all six spheres were visible on SPECT and PET images according to the Rose criterion. According to the criterion $\upsilon_{TEST\text{-}FP}<4$, none of the spheres were uniquely detectable with SPECT, whereas the smallest sphere uniquely detectable with PET was 28 mm in diameter. According to the criterion $\upsilon_{TEST\text{-}FP}<\upsilon_H$, all hot spheres in the cold background were uniquely detectable with PET, whereas the smallest sphere uniquely detectable with SPECT was 13 mm in diameter. For all three activity concentrations of the intrahepatic situation, all six spheres were visible with both SPECT and PET, but none of them was uniquely detectable according to the criterion $\upsilon_{TEST\text{-}FP}<4$. According to the criterion $\upsilon_{TEST\text{-}FP}<\upsilon_H$, the smallest sphere uniquely detectable with PET was 13 mm in diameter, whereas this was 22 mm for SPECT, for all activity concentrations.

Absorbed Dose Estimation

Phantom. The error of the uncorrected (in brackets: corrected for PVE) PET dose estimates ranged from −11% (+6%) for the largest sphere to −45% (+40%) for the smallest sphere (Table 4). For SPECT the errors were larger, ranging from −58% (+18%) to −75% (+69%). Figure 4 shows that the PET-based CDVH of the hot sphere ROI followed the true CDVH more closely than the SPECT-based CDVH. The higher image noise in TOF PET was reflected by the flattened slope of the CDVH curve.

Patients. For all patients, the difference between the estimated dose in the high-dose ROI and the low-dose ROI was larger for PET than for SPECT (Table 5). This effect is also illustrated by the CDVH and fused images of patient 2 in Figure 5. Images of patients 1, 3, 4, and 5 are provided as Figure S1, Figure S2, Figure S3 and Figure S4, respectively.

Discussion

In this study, we quantitatively compared the accuracy of ^{90}Y Bremsstrahlung SPECT and state-of-the-art PET for the assessment of the intra- and extrahepatic microsphere distribution after radioembolization, using the physical parameters image contrast and image noise, and the clinically relevant parameters detectability and dosimetry. We realize that image contrast and noise not only depend on the fundamental limitations of the imaging modalities, but also on acquisition and reconstruction settings; e.g., a well-known property of iterative reconstruction algorithms is that contrast can be maximized at the cost of noise amplification by varying the number of iterations [31]. Before defining the study setup as published, we evaluated image contrast and noise for various energy windows (wide: 50–250 keV [6,9,23,32–35];

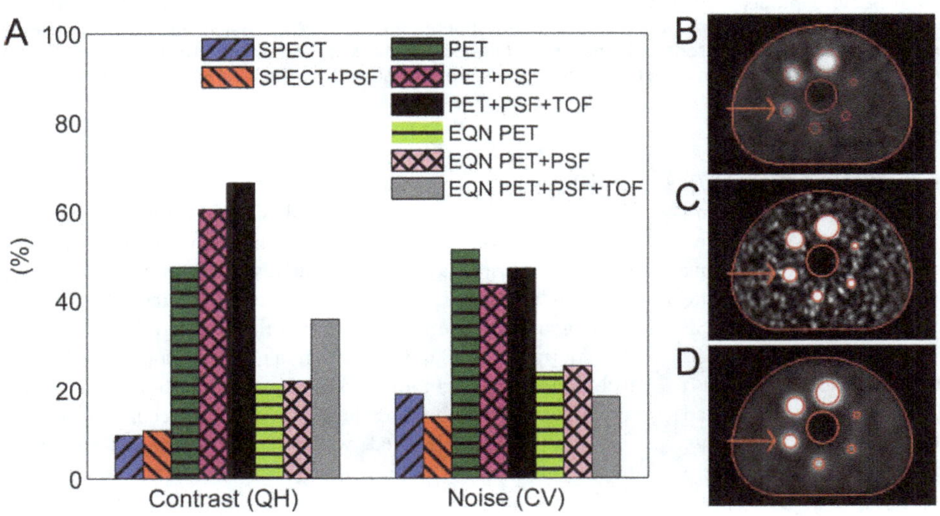

Figure 2. PET and SPECT contrast recovery and image noise. Contrast recovery and image noise in the 22-mm sphere for all reconstruction methods (A), the slice through the center of the SPECT volume (iterative+PSF) (B), the slice through the center of the PET volume (iterative+PSF+TOF) (C), and the slice through the center of the PET volume (iterative+PSF+TOF) reconstructed with SPECT-like noise level (D). All images were linearly window-leveled from 0 to 4 times the mean intensity in the background ROI. The boundaries of the central lung insert, the six hot sphere ROIs, and the background ROI are illustrated by the red lines and the 22-mm sphere is indicated by the arrow.

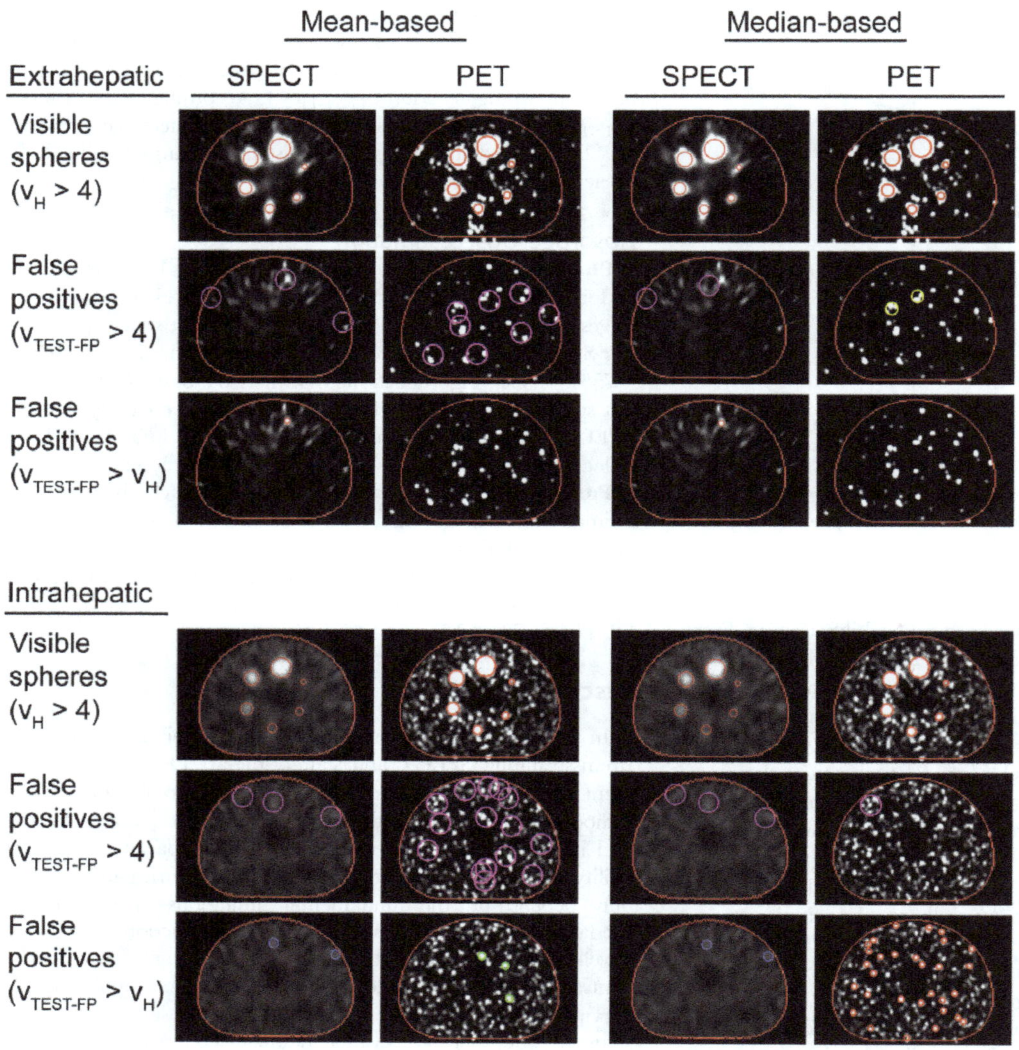

Figure 3. Visualization of the visibility and unique detectability results. The activity concentration in the hot spheres was 2.4 MBq ml^{-1} for both the images without (rows 1–3) and with background activity (rows 4–6). In the 1st and 4th row, the SPECT+PSF (1st and 3rd column) and PET+PSF+TOF (2nd and 4th column) slices are overlaid with the location of the visible phantom spheres (red). In rows 2, 3, 5 and 6 a background slice is overlaid with the location of false positive regions. For illustrative reasons, only the largest false positive ROIs are shown (red: 10 mm; green: 13 mm; blue: 17 mm; yellow: 22 mm; purple: 37 mm). Clustered ROIs with connecting center voxels are represented by the ROI with the highest $\upsilon_{TEST-FP}$ value.

medium-wide: 105–195 keV [8,24]; small: 76–105 keV [36,37], SPECT only), various numbers of iterations (1, 3, 5, and 8), and various post-reconstruction filters (0, 5, and 10 mm FWHM). The settings resulting in the highest image contrast were the starting point for this study. The results imply that ^{90}Y Bremsstrahlung SPECT and PET image contrast is improved by inclusion of a PSF model in the reconstruction process. The PET image contrast is further improved by inclusion of TOF information, which also resulted in slightly higher image noise. The latter can be attributed to faster convergence of TOF reconstruction [20]. At similar noise level, all PET algorithms demonstrated higher contrast recovery coefficients than optimal SPECT. Therefore, we conclude that the image quality of ^{90}Y state-of-the-art PET outperforms Bremsstrahlung SPECT.

In comparison with ^{18}F PET and ^{99m}Tc SPECT, the Q_H of ^{90}Y were consistently lower (e.g. 66% (^{90}Y) vs 71% (^{18}F) and 11% (^{90}Y) vs 57% (^{99m}Tc) for the 22-mm sphere, data not shown). The large difference in SPECT Q_H can probably be attributed to the low spatial resolution and the large amount of photon scatter and septal penetration with ^{90}Y [9], all of which increase the PVE. Recent work on ^{90}Y SPECT reconstruction demonstrated that image contrast may be substantially improved by including accurate models of the scattered and penetrated photons, but these algorithms are not available in the clinic to date [8,10]. To the contrary, PET reconstruction algorithms include advanced techniques to correct for random coincidences, photon scatter, and attenuation effects. Nevertheless, a slight difference in Q_H between ^{90}Y and ^{18}F was observed, which was probably not caused by resolution effects; the difference in spatial resolution was estimated to be within 1%, using the analytical resolution model of Lubberink and Herzog [38]. Instead, the intensity in the low-count background region may have been overestimated, possibly due to sparsity of the (smoothed) delayed coincidences sinogram that is used for random correction in the OP-OSEM algorithm [39]. This effect has also been observed in dynamic studies with

Table 3. Extra- and intrahepatic visibility and unique detectibility.

	Extrahepatic	Intrahepatic		
	$[A]_{sph}$ (MBq ml^{-1})	$[A]_{sph}$ (MBq ml^{-1})		
	2.4	9.6	4.8	2.4
Visible: υ_H >4				
SPECT	10 (10)	10 (10)	13 (13)	10 (10)
SPECT+PSF	10 (10)	10 (10)	10 (10)	10 (10)
PET	10 (10)	10 (10)	10 (10)	10 (13)
PET+PSF	10 (10)	10 (10)	10 (10)	10 (10)
PET+PSF+TOF	10 (10)	10 (10)	10 (10)	10 (10)
Uniquely detectable: $\upsilon_{TEST\text{-}FP}$<4				
SPECT	X (X)	X (X)	X (X)	X (X)
SPECT+PSF	X (X)	X (X)	X (X)	X (X)
PET	X (37)	X (X)	X (X)	X (X)
PET+PSF	X (X)	X (X)	X (X)	X (X)
PET+PSF+TOF	X (28)	X (X)	X (X)	X (X)
Uniquely detectable: $\upsilon_{TEST\text{-}FP}$< υ_H				
SPECT	17 (17)	22 (22)	22 (22)	22 (28)
SPECT+PSF	13 (13)	22 (22)	22 (22)	22 (22)
PET	13 (13)	17 (17)	17 (17)	13 (22)
PET+PSF	13 (13)	17 (17)	13 (17)	13 (22)
PET+PSF+TOF	10 (10)	10 (13)	13 (13)	17 (13)

The extra- and intrahepatic activity distribution is represented by hot spheres in a cold and warm background, respectively. For each image, the diameters (mm) of the first 'mean-based' visible and uniquely detectable spheres are given, followed by the diameters of the 'median-based' results in brackets. 'X' means that none of the spheres were uniquely detectable.

short frame rates [40]. Further research is required to fully understand the clinical impact of these effects.

Inadvertent extrahepatic deposition of activity may be detected directly post-treatment on ^{90}Y SPECT or PET images. Ahmadzadehfar *et al* showed that detection of extrahepatic activity on Bremsstrahlung SPECT/CT scans predicted GI ulcers with a sensitivity of 87% and a specificity of 100%, despite low image quality [6]. In this study, we investigated the detectability of accumulations of activity of different sizes with the well-known Rose criterion for detection of false negatives and with a new method for detection of false positives. The 'median-based' unique detectability approach was deemed better than its 'mean-based' equivalent, since the latter tended to erroneously classify non-uniform regions as 'false positive'. We demonstrated that the visibility of intra- and extrahepatic accumulations of activity was equal between SPECT and PET, for the investigated sphere sizes and activity concentration ratios. Unique detectability with the $\upsilon_{TEST\text{-}FP}< \upsilon_H$ criterion demonstrated larger differences between PET and SPECT than the $\upsilon_{TEST\text{-}FP}<4$ criterion, but will depend on the activity concentration in the hot spheres. Nevertheless, according to both criteria, PET was able to uniquely detect smaller accumulations of activity than SPECT, endorsing the use of (TOF) PET/CT instead of SPECT/CT. Given the relative simplicity of the detectability models used, we should emphasize that the results of our phantom study should not be interpreted as the lower limits of (lesion) detection performance by a human observer, but merely as a comparison between ^{90}Y SPECT and PET. The results are likely to be dependent on acquisition and reconstruction settings, which were optimized for image contrast in this study. Optimization of the imaging protocols for noise, e.g. by increasing the FWHM of the post-reconstruction filter, may improve the unique detectability of hot spots.

Accurate tumour and liver dosimetry can improve RE patient care, e.g. by facilitating (selective) re-treatment of tumourous tissue that did not receive a sufficient dose during the first treatment. The relationship between the ^{99m}Tc-MAA SPECT-based tumour absorbed dose and tumour response is reported in numerous publications investigating the possibilities of treatment optimization by individualized ^{99m}Tc-MAA SPECT-based dose planning (e.g. [7,33,41]). To the contrary, publications on the ^{90}Y SPECT or PET-based dose-response relation are relatively sparse [42,43]. The latter approach has the advantage of imaging the real ^{90}Y microsphere distribution, which avoids the question of accurate prediction of the microsphere distribution with ^{99m}Tc-MAA, but it is not used for individualized treatment planning. Using phantom experiments, we demonstrated that ^{90}Y TOF PET-based dose estimates were more accurate than Bremsstrahlung SPECT-based dose estimates. Based on the incomplete contrast recovery observed in the image quality phantom, dose underestimations with both PET and SPECT were to be expected. SPECT-based absorbed dose estimates in the high-dose regions of the phantom were lower than those of PET, which was supported by the results of our patient study. When correcting the hot sphere mean dose estimates for PVE, the absolute dose errors were reduced, but dose overestimations up to 69% were still observed. The use of PVE correction factors is restricted to correction of mean ROI values, and PVE correction was therefore applied to the mean absorbed dose values of the hot sphere ROIs. Due to the range of the beta-particles, however, the mean absorbed dose in the hot sphere ROIs not only depends on the locally absorbed energy as a result of activity in the ROIs itself, but also on the energy absorbed as a result of activity in adjacent background voxels. With hot spheres

Table 4. Phantom dosimetry.

	Phantom ROI						
	10	13	17	22	28	37	BKG
SPECT	76 (516)	69 (514)	78 (511)	102 (487)	143 (484)	181 (508)	61
PET	167 (431)	224 (432)	255 (433)	333 (475)	324 (426)	384 (457)	60
TRUE	306	341	372	395	412	432	52

The uncorrected mean dose (Gy) in the 6 hot sphere ROIs and the background ROI (BKG), followed by the mean dose corrected for PVE in brackets (spheres only). The TRUE dose represents the actual dose in the phantom.

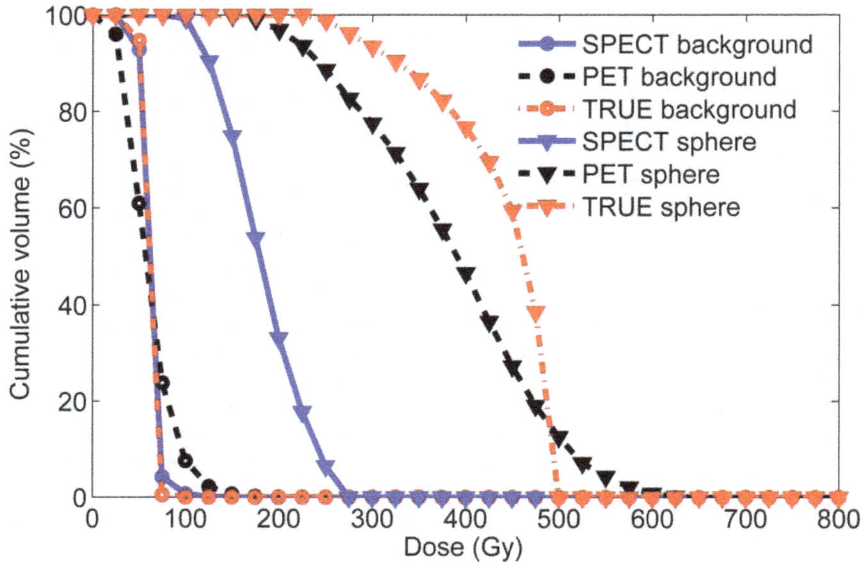

Figure 4. Phantom dosimetry. CDVH of the phantom background ROI and the ROI of the 37-mm diameter sphere. The presented doses were not corrected for PVE.

in a warm background, PVE result in an underestimation of the first contribution to the mean absorbed dose, whereas the latter contribution is overestimated. Consequently, application of the activity-based PVE correction factors leads to erroneous up-scaling of the adjacent background voxels' contribution to the mean absorbed dose in the hot sphere ROIs. This effect is stronger for smaller spheres, due to the relatively large amount of adjacent background voxels, and stronger for SPECT than for PET, due to the higher correction factors of the first. For dosimetry purposes, a better approach may be to determine correction factors on dose images, which not only include PVE but also DPK effects. However, these dose correction factors will strongly depend on the activity concentration ratio between ROIs and adjacent background voxels, which undesirably complicates PVE correction in clinical practice. For this reason, we chose not to correct the mean dose estimates in the patient study for PVE effects. The results of the patient study indicate that the use of high-resolution PET can potentially improve dose-response relationships on the level of the tumour for ^{90}Y RE. The evaluation of the estimated absorbed liver dose in low-dose and high-dose regions, which did not necessarily coincide with healthy liver and tumour regions, did not harm the conclusions presented in this study, since the primary aim was a quantitative comparison of the ^{90}Y SPECT and PET-based dose distribution, and not clinical liver dosimetry. Evaluation of the absorbed dose to tumourous and healthy liver tissue should be performed in a larger (prospective) patient study and is beyond the scope of this study.

Conclusion

This study demonstrates that the ^{90}Y image quality of state-of-the-art PET is superior over Bremsstrahlung SPECT for the assessment of the microsphere distribution after radioemboliza-

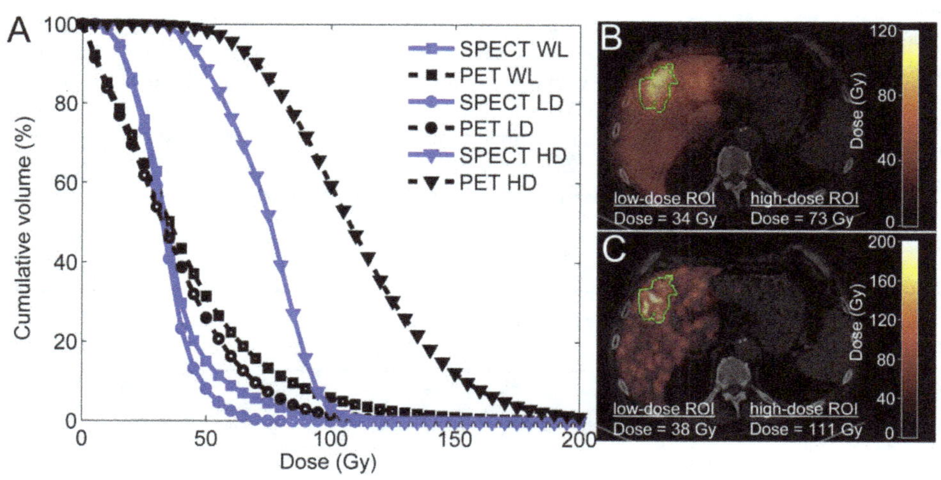

Figure 5. Patient 2 dosimetry. The CDVH of the whole liver (WL), low-dose (LD) and high-dose (HD) ROIs of patient 2 (A), a transversal slice through the SPECT-based dose map, fused with CT (B), and the same transversal slice through the PET-based dose map (C). The boundary of the high-dose ROI is depicted by the green line.

Table 5. Patient dosimetry.

	Patient ROI									
	1		2		3		4		5	
	LD	HD	LD	HD	LD	HD	LD	HD	LD	HD
SPECT	26	37	34	73	30	53	22	36	12	31
PET	29	85	38	111	33	80	26	58	11	47

The mean dose (Gy) in the low-dose ROI (LD) and the high-dose ROI (HD) are given for all patients.

tion. Intra- and extrahepatic hot spots of 10 mm in diameter or larger are visible on SPECT and PET images, but PET is able to uniquely detect smaller accumulations of activity than SPECT. Additionally, TOF PET-based dose estimates are more accurate than SPECT-based dose estimates, which give large underestimations in high-dose regions.

Supporting Information

Figure S1 Patient 1 dosimetry. The CDVH of the whole liver (WL), low-dose (LD) and high-dose (HD) ROIs of patient 1 (A), a transversal slice through the SPECT-based dose map, fused with CT (B), and the same transversal slice through the PET-based dose map (C). The boundary of the high-dose ROI is depicted by the green line.

Figure S2 Patient 3 dosimetry. The CDVH of the whole liver (WL), low-dose (LD) and high-dose (HD) ROIs of patient 3 (A), a transversal slice through the SPECT-based dose map, fused with CT (B), and the same transversal slice through the PET-based dose map (C). The boundary of the high-dose ROI is depicted by the green line.

Figure S3 Patient 4 dosimetry. The CDVH of the whole liver (WL), low-dose (LD) and high-dose (HD) ROIs of patient 4 (A), a transversal slice through the SPECT-based dose map, fused with CT (B), and the same transversal slice through the PET-based dose map (C). The boundary of the high-dose ROI is depicted by the green line.

Figure S4 Patient 5 dosimetry. The CDVH of the whole liver (WL), low-dose (LD) and high-dose (HD) ROIs of patient 5 (A), a transversal slice through the SPECT-based dose map, fused with CT (B), and the same transversal slice through the PET-based dose map (C). The boundary of the high-dose ROI is depicted by the green line.

Author Contributions

Conceived and designed the experiments: ME BJV MGEHL HJ. Performed the experiments: ME BJV BdK MAAJvdB. Analyzed the data: ME BJV HWAMdJ. Contributed reagents/materials/analysis tools: ME BJV. Wrote the paper: ME BJV MGEHL BdK MAAJvdB HWAMdJ.

References

1. Vente MA, Wondergem M, van der Tweel I, van den Bosch MA, Zonnenberg BA, et al. (2009) Yttrium-90 microsphere radioembolization for the treatment of liver malignancies: a structured meta-analysis. Eur Radiol 19: 951–959.
2. Kennedy AS, Salem R (2010) Radioembolization (yttrium-90 microspheres) for primary and metastatic hepatic malignancies. Cancer J 16: 163–175.
3. Kennedy AS, Nag S, Salem R, Murthy R, Mcewan AJ, et al. (2007) Recommendations for radioembolization of hepatic malignancies using yttrium-90 microsphere brachytherapy: A consensus panel report from the Radioembolization Brachytherapy Oncology Consortium. Int J Radiat Oncol Biol Phys 68: 13–23.
4. Murthy R, Brown DB, Salem R, Meranze SG, Coldwell DM, et al. (2007) Gastrointestinal complications associated with hepatic arterial yttrium-90 microsphere therapy. J Vasc Interv Radiol 18: 553–562.
5. Riaz A, Lewandowski RJ, Kulik LM, Mulcahy MF, Sato KT, et al. (2009) Complications Following Radioembolization with Yttrium-90 Microspheres: A Comprehensive Literature Review. J Vasc Interv Radiol 20: 1121–1130.
6. Ahmadzadehfar H, Muckle M, Sabet A, Kuhl C, Biermann K, et al. (2010) The significance of Bremsstrahlung SPECT-CT of the Abdomen after Yttrium 90 microsphere selective internal radiation treatment (SIRT) in the early Diagnosis of SIRT-Induced Extrahepatic Side Effects. Eur J Nucl Med Mol Imaging 37: S264–S264.
7. Chiesa C, Maccauro M, Romito R, Spreafico C, Pellizzari S, et al. (2011) Need, feasibility and convenience of dosimetric treatment planning in liver selective internal radiation therapy with Y-90 microspheres: the experience of the National Cancer Institute of Milan. Q J Nucl Med Mol Imag 55: 168–197.
8. Minarik D, Sjogreen GK, Ljungberg M (2008) Evaluation of quantitative (90)Y SPECT based on experimental phantom studies. Phys Med Biol 53: 5689–5703.
9. Elschot M, Nijsen JFW, Dam AJ, de Jong HWAM (2011) Quantitative Evaluation of Scintillation Camera Imaging Characteristics of Isotopes Used in Liver Radioembolization. PLoS ONE 6: e26174.
10. Rong X, Du Y, Ljungberg M, Rault E, Vandenberghe S, et al. (2012) Development and evaluation of an improved quantitative Y-90 bremsstrahlung SPECT method. Med Phys 39: 2346–2358.
11. Lhommel R, van Elmbt L, Goffette P, Van den Eynde M, Jamar F, et al. (2010) Feasibility of (90)Y TOF PET-based dosimetry in liver metastasis therapy using SIR-Spheres. Eur J Nucl Med Mol Imaging 37: 1654–1662.
12. Langhoff H, Hennies HH (1961) Zum Experimentellen Nachweis Von Zweiquantenzerfall Beim 0+-0+-Ubergang des Zr90. Z Phys A At Nucl 164: 166–173.
13. Nickles RJ, Roberts AD, Nye JA, Converse AK, Barnhart TE, et al. (2004) Assaying and PET imaging of yttrium-90: 1>34ppm>0. Conf Record of IEEE Nuclear Science Symp and Medical Imaging Conf. 3412–3414.
14. Bailey DL, Karp JS, Surti S (2003) Physics and instrumentation in PET. In: Valk PE, Bailey DL, Townsend DW, Maisey MN. Positron Emission Tomography: Basic Science and Clinical Practice. London: Springer-Verlag. 41–67.
15. van Elmbt L, Walrand S, Lhommel R, Jamar F, Pauwels S (2010) Quantitative comparison between LYSO and BGO PET-tomographs in 90Y imaging. Eur J Nucl Med Mol Imaging 37: S293–S293.
16. Lhommel R, Goffette P, Van den Eynde M, Jamar F, Pauwels S, et al. (2009) Yttrium-90 TOF PET scan demonstrates high-resolution biodistribution after liver SIRT. Eur J Nucl Med Mol Imaging 36: 1696–1696.
17. Werner MK, Brechtel K, Beyer T, Dittmann H, Pfannenberg C, et al. (2010) PET/CT for the assessment and quantification of Y-90 biodistribution after selective internal radiotherapy (SIRT) of liver metastases. Eur J Nucl Med Mol Imaging 37: 407–408.
18. Gates VL, Esmail AAH, Marshall K, Spies S, Salem R (2011) Internal Pair Production of (90)Y Permits Hepatic Localization of Microspheres Using Routine PET: Proof of Concept. J Nucl Med 52: 72–76.
19. D'Arienzo M, Chiaramida P, Chiacchiararelli L, Coniglio A, Cianni R, et al. (2012) Y-90 PET-based dosimetry after selective internal radiotherapy treatments. Nuc Med Comm 33: 633–640.
20. Jakoby BW, Bercier Y, Conti M, Casey ME, Bendriem B, et al. (2011) Physical and clinical performance of the mCT time-of-flight PET/CT scanner. Phys Med Biol 56: 2375–2389.
21. Comtat C, Kinahan PE, Defrise M, Michel C, Townsend DW (1998) Fast reconstruction of 3D PET data with accurate statistical modeling. IEEE Trans Nucl Sci 45: 1083–1089.

22. Panin VY, Kehren F, Michel C, Casey M (2006) Fully 3-D PET reconstruction with system matrix derived from point source measurements. IEEE Trans Med Imag 25: 907–921.
23. Shen S, DeNardo GL, Yuan A, DeNardo DA, DeNardo SJ (1994) Planar gamma camera imaging and quantitation of yttrium-90 bremsstrahlung. J Nucl Med 35: 1381–1389.
24. Minarik D, Ljungberg M, Segars P, Gleisner KS (2009) Evaluation of quantitative planar 90Y bremsstrahlung whole-body imaging. Phys Med Biol 54: 5873–5883.
25. Tsui BMW, Hu HB, Gilland DR, Gullberg GT (1988) Implementation of Simultaneous Attenuation and Detector Response Correction in Spect. IEEE Trans Nucl Sci 35: 778–783.
26. National Electrical Manufacturers Association (2007) NEMA Standards Publication NU 2-2007: Performance Measurements of Positron Emission Tomographs. Rosslyn, VA: National Electrical Manufacturers Association.
27. Cherry SR., Sorenson JA, Phelps ME (2003) Physics in Nuclear Medicine. Philadelphia: Saunders. 290.
28. Rose A (1948) The Sensitivity Performance of the Human Eye on An Absolute Scale. J Opt Soc Am 38: 196–208.
29. Bolch WE, Bouchet LG, Robertson JS, Wessels BW, Siegel JA, et al. (1999) MIRD pamphlet No. 17: the dosimetry of nonuniform activity distributions–radionuclide S values at the voxel level. Medical Internal Radiation Dose Committee. J Nucl Med 40: 11S–36S.
30. Hendricks JS, McKinney GW, Waters LS, Roberts TS, Egdorf HW et al (2005) MCNPX Extensions, Version 2.5.0. Los Alamos, CA: Los Alamos National Laboratory Report LA-UR-05-2675.
31. Hutton BF, Hudson HM, Beekman FJ (1997) A clinical perspective of accelerated statistical reconstruction. Eur J Nucl Med Mol Imaging 24: 797–808.
32. Clarke LP, Cullom SJ, Shaw R, Reece C, Penney BC, et al. (1992) Bremsstrahlung Imaging Using the Gamma-Camera - Factors Affecting Attenuation. J Nucl Med 33: 161–166.
33. Flamen P, Vanderlinden B, Delatte P, Ghanem G, Ameye L, et al. (2008) Multimodality imaging can predict the metabolic response of unresectable colorectal liver metastases to radioembolization therapy with Yttrium-90 labeled resin microspheres. Phys Med Biol 53: 6591–6603.
34. Fabbri C, Sarti G, Cremonesi M, Ferrari M, Di DA, et al. (2009) Quantitative analysis of 90Y Bremsstrahlung SPECT-CT images for application to 3D patient-specific dosimetry. Cancer Biother Radiopharm 24: 145–154.
35. Ito S, Kurosawa H, Kasahara H, Teraoka S, Ariga E, et al. (2009) (90)Y bremsstrahlung emission computed tomography using gamma cameras. Ann Nucl Med 23: 257–267.
36. Mansberg R, Sorensen N, Mansberg V, Van der Wall H (2007) Yttrium 90 Bremsstrahlung SPECT/CT scan demonstrating areas of tracer/tumour uptake. Eur J Nucl Med Mol Imaging 34: 1887.
37. Knesaurek K, Machac J, Muzinic M, DaCosta M, Zhang Z, et al. (2010) Quantitative comparison of yttrium-90 (90Y)-microspheres and technetium-99m (99mTc)-macroaggregated albumin SPECT images for planning 90Y therapy of liver cancer. Technol Cancer Res Treat 9: 253–262.
38. Lubberink M, Herzog H (2011) Quantitative imaging of (124)I and (86)Y with PET. Eur J Nucl Med Mol Imaging 38: 10–18.
39. Comtat C, Bataille F, Michel C, Jones JP, Sibomana M, et al. (2004) OSEM-3D reconstruction strategies for the ECAT HRRT. Conf Record of IEEE Nuclear Science Symp and Medical Imaging Conf. 3492–3496.
40. van Velden FHP, Kloet RW, van Berckel BNM, Wolfensberger SPA, Lammertsma AA et al. (2008) Comparison of 3D-OP-OSEM and 3D-FBP reconstruction algorithms for High-Resolution Research Tomograph studies: effects of randoms estimation methods. Phys Med Biol 53: 3217–3230.
41. Garin E, Lenoir L, Rolland Y, Edeline J, Mesbah H, et al. (2012) Dosimetry Based on Tc-99m-Macroaggregated Albumin SPECT/CT Accurately Predicts Tumor Response and Survival in Hepatocellular Carcinoma Patients Treated with Y-90-Loaded Glass Microspheres: Preliminary Results. J Nucl Med 53: 255–263.
42. Strigari L, Sciuto R, Rea S, Carpanese L, Pizzi G, et al. (2010) Efficacy and Toxicity Related to Treatment of Hepatocellular Carcinoma with Y-90-SIR Spheres: Radiobiologic Considerations. J Nucl Med 51: 1377–1385.
43. Walrand S, Lhommel R, Goffette P, Van den Eynde M, Pauwels S, et al. (2012) Hemoglobin level significantly impacts the tumor cell survival fraction in humans after internal radiotherapy. EJNMMI Research 2: 20.

Applying of Hierarchical Clustering to Analysis of Protein Patterns in the Human Cancer-Associated Liver

Natalia A. Petushkova[1]*, Mikhail A. Pyatnitskiy[1], Vladislav A. Rudenko[2], Olesya V. Larina[1], Oxana P. Trifonova[1], Julya S. Kisrieva[1], Natalia F. Samenkova[1], Galina P. Kuznetsova[1], Irina I. Karuzina[1], Andrey V. Lisitsa[1,2]

1 V. N. Orekhovich Institute of Biomedical Chemistry, Russian Academy of Medical Sciences, Moscow, Russia, **2** Postgen Tech LLC, Moscow, Russia

Abstract

Background: There are two ways that statistical methods can learn from biomedical data. One way is to learn classifiers to identify diseases and to predict outcomes using the training dataset with established diagnosis for each sample. When the training dataset is not available the task can be to mine for presence of meaningful groups (clusters) of samples and to explore underlying data structure (unsupervised learning).

Results: We investigated the proteomic profiles of the cytosolic fraction of human liver samples using two-dimensional electrophoresis (2DE). Samples were resected upon surgical treatment of hepatic metastases in colorectal cancer. Unsupervised hierarchical clustering of 2DE gel images (n = 18) revealed a pair of clusters, containing 11 and 7 samples. Previously we used the same specimens to measure biochemical profiles based on cytochrome P450-dependent enzymatic activities and also found that samples were clearly divided into two well-separated groups by cluster analysis. It turned out that groups by enzyme activity almost perfectly match to the groups identified from proteomic data. Of the 271 reproducible spots on our 2DE gels, we selected 15 to distinguish the human liver cytosolic clusters. Using MALDI-TOF peptide mass fingerprinting, we identified 12 proteins for the selected spots, including known cancer-associated species.

Conclusions/Significance: Our results highlight the importance of hierarchical cluster analysis of proteomic data, and showed concordance between results of biochemical and proteomic approaches. Grouping of the human liver samples and/or patients into differing clusters may provide insights into possible molecular mechanism of drug metabolism and creates a rationale for personalized treatment.

Editor: Silvia Mazzuca, Università della Calabria, Italy

Funding: The work was supported by the Ministry of Education and Science of the Russian Federation, State Contract No. 16.522.12.2002. The funders had no role in study design, data collection and analysis, decision to publish, or preparation of the manuscript.

Competing Interests: Two authors are employed also by a commercial company Postgen Tech LLC, but they did not receive payment or services from the company for any aspect of the submitted work (including but not limited to grants, data monitoring board, study design, manuscript preparation, statistical analysis, etc.).

* Email: natalia.petushkova@ibmc.msk.ru

Introduction

Hepatic metastases usually progressively damage liver function and are highly malignant and refractory to conventional therapies [1]. Understanding the molecular and biological mechanisms of colorectal cancer may allow for the development of further therapeutic strategies designed to prevent and treat liver metastases [2,3]. Furthermore, molecular-based therapies can extend time to liver recurrence after curative resection and may prolong patient survival. The development of more effective and less toxic anticancer strategies also will allow for the personalization of therapeutic regimens according to the molecular features of individual patients [4].

Proteomic studies of liver samples can help to identify specific protein markers for metastases [5]. One of the most frequently used procedures for characterization of the protein components of biological systems is two-dimensional polyacrylamide gel electrophoresis (2DE) in combination with mass spectrometry. Typically, 2DE is used to compare changes in protein level, modification, and degradation between treated and untreated samples [6]. Proteomic changes can be revealed by gel image analysis after visualization by staining and identification of protein species with altered expression or in post-translational states [7].

Most studies based on 2DE analysis of protein profiles in colorectal cancer are conducted on tissue lysate of colorectal adenocarcinoma, adjacent normal colon mucosa, and liver metastases [8–10]. Such a strategy is largely limited to abundant proteins (e.g., structural proteins, glycolytic enzymes, annexins, cathepsins, and heat shock proteins) that are overexpressed in several cancers [8]. However, these proteins may hamper the identification of low-abundance proteins, such as membrane proteins, which play a fundamental role in cell signaling, cell-cell interactions, communication, and transport mechanisms, and are drug targets [11]. Targeted approaches associated with the isolation from clinical material subproteomes, such as the secretome, proteasome, plasma-membrane fraction, nuclear matrix, etc., have emerged recently. Subcellular fractionation combined with mass spectrometry techniques is a powerful approach to uncover novel, low abundant, specific colorectal-associated proteins and candidate biomarkers [8]. For example, 1687 protein spots were observed on large format gels (24×33 cm) of a soluble protein fraction of cancerous and normal mucosa tissues and it was shown that the intensity of ≥96% protein spots was scattered within 2-fold differences and >90.5% within 1.5-fold differences [12]. For a human liver cytosolic fraction on 17×24 cm gels, 2-fold fewer protein spots (911 spots) were matched [13]. 2DE image analyses showed that the number of protein spots were significantly changed in primary cancer and hepatic metastatic lesions. Reportedly, the membrane fraction of primary cancer and hepatic metastases demonstrated loss of protein content (i.e., the number of matched protein spots on 2DE gels) compared to the membrane fraction of normal colorectal mucosa [10]. Muto et al. [12] generally reported that the proteome of normal tissue may be more homogeneous than that of tumor tissues.

Earlier, we described an approach to discriminate liver microsomal samples into certain classes based on biochemical profiles [14]. In this report, an experimental design to compare the biochemical and proteomic profiles is presented (Figure 1). In the first stage of this approach the biochemical profile was obtained. It included 12 parameters, namely activity of NADPH-cytochrome P450 reductase, cytochrome P450 content and 10 cytochrome P450-dependent monooxygenase activities with marker substrates. Purely from unsupervised statistical analysis of biochemical profiles of human liver microsomes we derived that patterns of the liver monooxygenase system formed two well-separated groups (Figure 1, **A**). It was shown that at least 6 variables were significantly different between two major clusters of human liver microsomal samples having p-value <0.05 with Bonferroni correction. In addition, it was found that changes in NADPH-cytochrome P450 reductase activity comprise the main factor, responsible for separation of biochemical profiles between two groups of patients [14].

To correlate the HLC protein profile, as defined by 2DE, with biochemical activities of the microsomal system we used previously collected morphologically normal liver specimens surrounding hepatic metastases of colon cancer. Ultracentrifugation protocol was employed to yield human liver cytosol and microsomal fractions from the same liver specimen. The current study was conducted to compare the sample clusters obtained according to microsomal biochemical activity (Figure 1, **A**) with the respective cytosolic proteomic profiles (Figure 1, **B**). Furthermore, we were interested in the identification of soluble proteins, which may be somehow related to the activity of membrane-bound cytochromes P450.

Materials and Methods

Ethical procedures

All samples from residual liver after histological analysis were approved by the Department of Pathological Anatomy of the National Research Center of Surgery, Russian Academy of Medical Sciences (Moscow, Russia). Informed consent was obtained from all patients. Individuals agreed to participate in the study according the local institution's ethical committee of the National Research Centre of Surgery. Samples have been described in previous publications [14,15].

Chemicals

2-[4-(2-hydroxyethyl)piperazin-1-yl]ethanesulfonic acid, phenylmethanesulfonylfluoride (PMSF), 2.5-dihydroxybenzoic acid, ethylenediaminetetraacetic acid (EDTA), nicotinamide adenine dinucleotide phosphate, sodium dithionite, trypsin, and sodium deoxycholate were purchased from Sigma-Aldrich (St. Louis, MO, USA); acetonitrile and trifluoroacetic acid were purchased from ICN Pharmaceuticals Inc. (Costa Mesa, CA, USA); Coomassie Brilliant Blue R-250 was purchased from Fluka (Seelze, Germany). Modified trypsin (catalog no. V511C) was obtained from Promega (Madison, WI, USA). Other chemicals were purchased from Reakhim-Penza, LLC (Penza, Russia).

2.3 Tissue samples and preparation

The human soluble liver protein fractions were prepared in our previous study (stored at −80°C prior to usage) from resected and discarded masses of surrounding liver tissues, which were taken from patients (n = 23) undergoing hepatic surgery [14]. Samples of morphologically normal liver (3–10 g,) were obtained from the distal edge of the resection, at least 5 cm off the tumor. Samples were diagnosed by histopathology.

As consisted with conditions of the experiment, we did not take into consideration any personalized information about patients or concerning patient treatment. However, collection of samples was performed according to the following instructions: (1) all patients were under severe cancer disease, which led to the surgery of liver maybe after a prior chemotherapy; (2) no radiotherapy was performed before surgery; (3) no evidence of endocrine or metabolic disease; (4) no severe infection was detected; (4) patients' dietary requirements were managed by the National Research Center of Surgery to a relatively uniform standard; as a result, exogenous dietary influence on metabolic profiling was limited to the lowest level. The resected samples were placed immediately on ice prior to obtaining the human liver microsomal fraction [14] and HLC. All preparation procedures were performed at 0–4°C. The liver samples were homogenized in two volumes of homogenization buffer, containing 1 mM EDTA, 1 mM dithiotreitol (DTT), 0.1 mM PMSF, and 150 mM KCl using a glass Potter Elvehjem homogenizer with a teflon pestle (Sartorius Stedim Biotech GmbH, Goettingen, Germany). The liver homogenate was successively centrifuged at 10,000×g for 20 min and 105,000×g for 70 min. The pellet (microsomal fraction) was analyzed as described in our previous study [14]. In the present study, the supernatant was used as the HLC fraction. The protein concentration of the HLC samples was estimated using the Bradford assay [16] with bovine serum albumin as a standard.

Prefractionation of HLC samples prior to two-dimensional polyacrylamide gel electrophoresis

Aliquot of HLC (200 μL, 13.2±5.6 mg of protein) was mixed with 1 mL of cold 10% trichloroacetic acid (TCA) in acetone (v/v), containing 0.07% mercaptoethanol. After a 3-h incubation at −18°C, the mixture was centrifuged at 20,000×g for 10 min (4°C). The supernatant was discarded and the pellet was dissolved in 5 mL of cold acetone, containing 0.07% mercaptoethanol, and centrifuged as described above. The supernatant was discarded and the resulting pellet was used for protein separation by 2DE.

Two-dimensional polyacrylamide gel electrophoresis (2DE)

2DE of HLC proteins was performed as described by the manufacturer (Bio-Rad, Hercules, CA, USA). For each HLC sample, the resulting pellet was dissolved in 200 μL of rehydration buffer (4 M urea, 2 M thiourea, 4% 3-[(3-cholamidopropyl)-dimethylammonio]-1-propane sulfonate, 50 mM DTT, and 0.5%

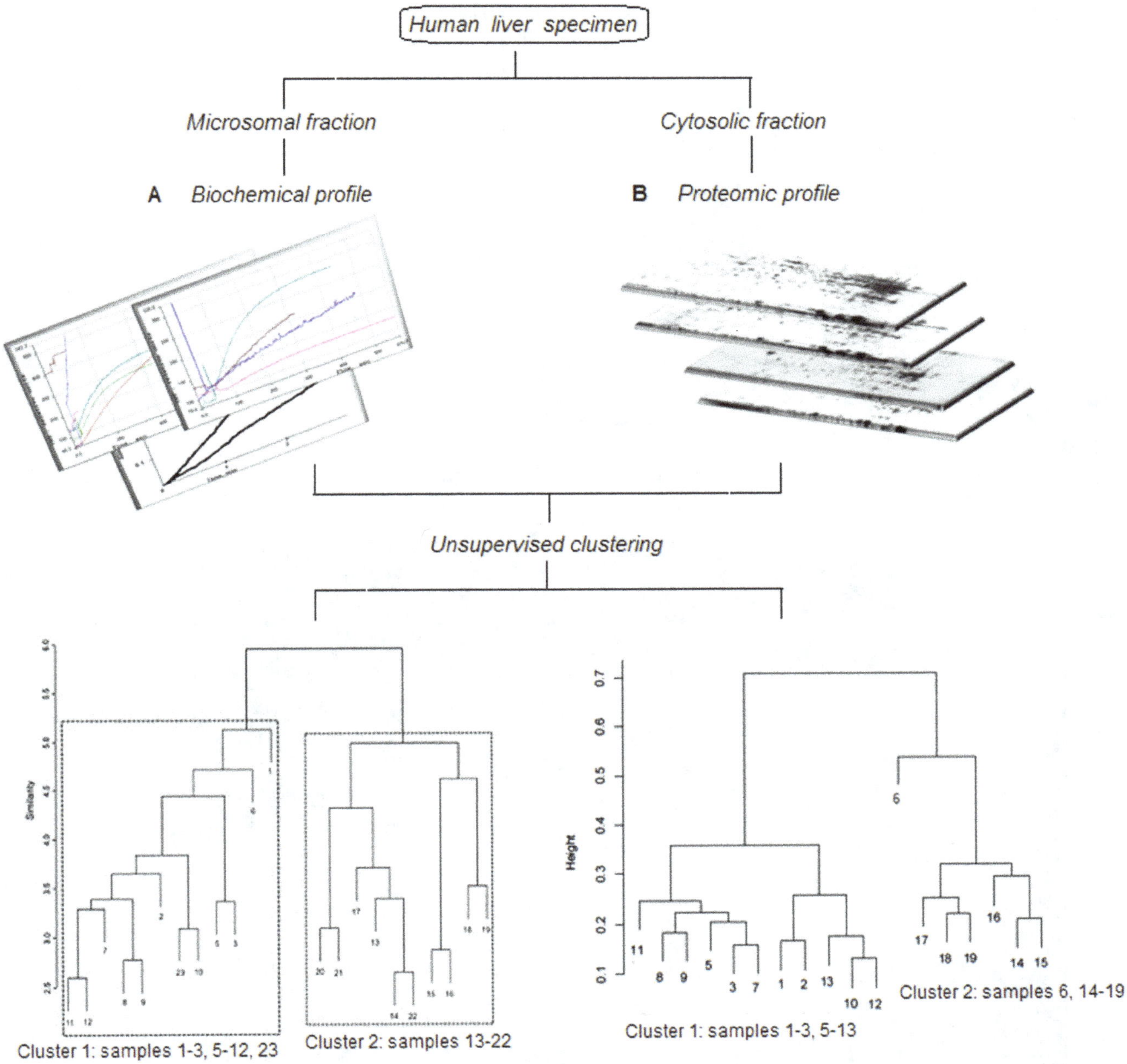

Figure 1. Schematic description of the comparative analysis of human liver biochemical (A) and proteomic (B) profiles. (**A**) The profile included 12 parameters, namely activity of NADPH-cytochrome P450 reductase, cytochrome P450 content and cytochrome P450-dependent monooxygenase activities with marker substrates (Petushkova et al., 2010). (**B**) The profile included 2DE images.

ampholine). Proteins were loaded by passive rehydration onto 11-cm, nonlinear, immobilized, pH gradient (IPG, pH 3–10) strips overnight (14 h) at 50 V and for a further 30 min at 250 V. Isoelectric focusing (IEF) was performed using the Protean IEF Cell (Bio-Rad) with an applied gradient 250–5500 V for a total of 35,000 V·h. All IEF steps were performed at 20°C. Following IEF, IPG gel strips were equilibrated in equilibration buffer (50 mM Tris-HCl, pH 6.8, 6 M urea, 2% sodium dodecyl sulphate (SDS), 20% glycerol) containing 1% DTT and shaken for 30 min at 50 rpm on an orbital shaker [17]. The IPG strips were then transferred to the equilibration solution, containing 2.5% acrylamide, and shaken for an additional 30 min before separation on a polyacrylamide gel (135×80×1.0 mm, 4% stocking gel, and 12% resolving gel). Separation in the second dimension was performed using the Mini-Protean Dodeca Cell (Bio-Rad) and Tris-glycine buffer (25 mM Tris base and 192 mM glycine), containing 0.1% SDS, at 150 V. Run time was approximately 60 min and upon the exit of bromophenol blue into the buffer, the electrophoretic separation was considered complete.

Protein visualization and image analysis

Gels were subjected to silver staining [18], gel images were acquired using a GS-800 Calibrated Densitometer (Bio-Rad) and uploaded into the proprietary digital image analysis software GelEditor. It is written in Java and supportsl tools for loading images, automated spot detection based on Laplacian of Gaussian Filter, manual spot detection, matching of protein profiles, and an

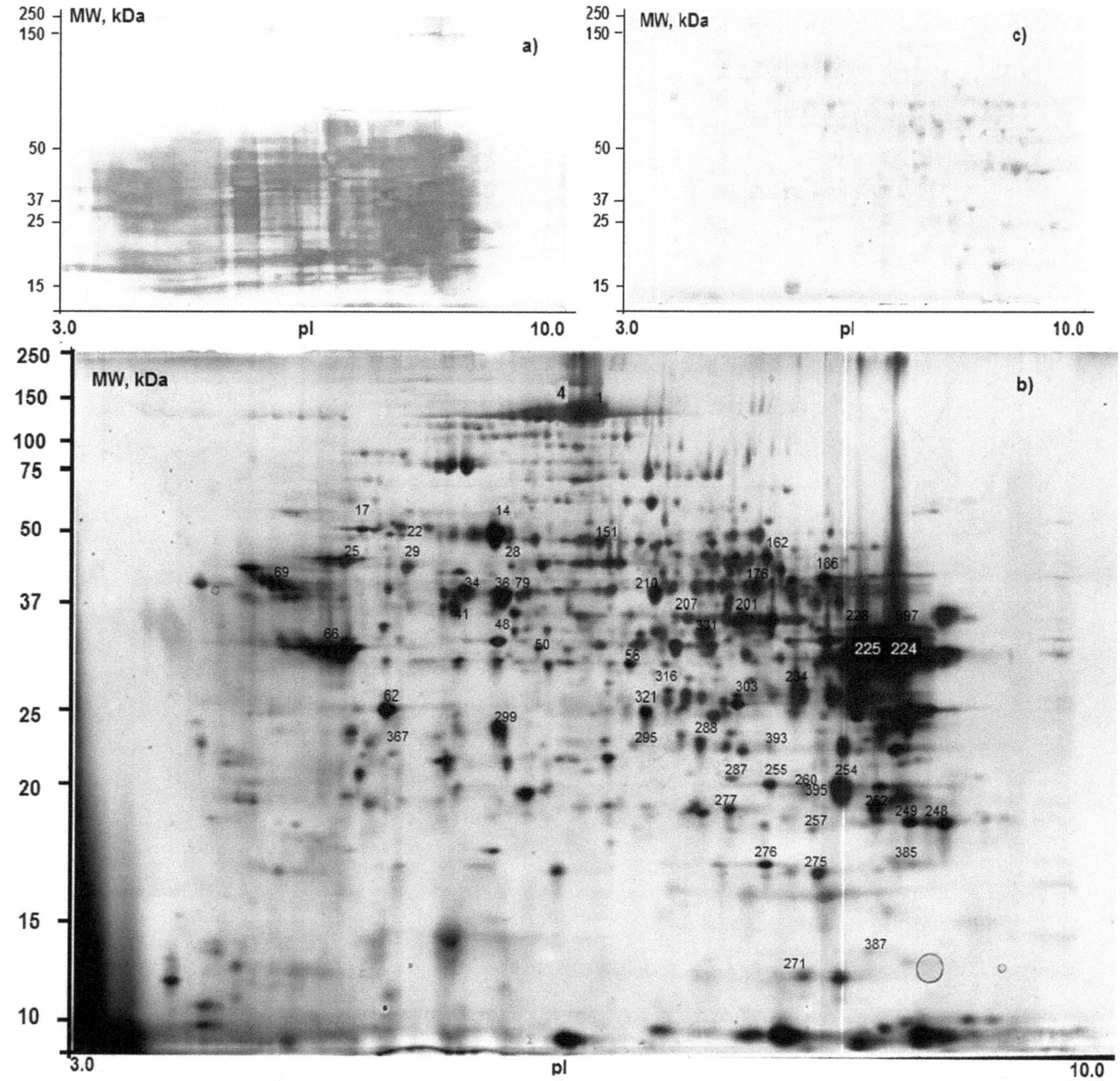

Figure 2. A Typical 2DE images of master gel no. 6, technical run 1. 30 μg of the human soluble liver protein fraction (HLC) was separated by 2DE and visualized by silver staining (*a* and *b*) or Coomassie Brilliant Blue staining (*c*): *a* – HLC before pretreatment with trichloroacetic acid in acetone; *b* and *c* – HLC after pretreatment. Using Coomassie staining nearly 100 protein spots could be revealed, but using silver staining labeling up to 687 protein spots were automatically detected. Spots nos. 14, 25, 34, 36, 48, 56, 62, 63, 66, 210, 214, 219, 247, 252, 275, 276, 279, 301, 321, 322, and 408 are common for all 2DE gels of 19 human liver cytosol samples.

option to save the reports (Figure S1). The spot intensity on the gel was calculated as the sum of the pixels in a manually detected spot. The GelEditor software can be freely downloaded from www.bioinformatics.ru/geleditor.zip.

In-gel digestion

The protein spots ($\sim$3 mm^3) were excised from the gel using modified 250-μL tips and destained with 50 μL of 100 mM $K_3[Fe(CN)_6]$ and 100 mM sodium thiosulfate in a ratio of 1:1 (v/v) per gel piece at room temperature for 30 min. Afterwards, the gel pieces were washed with water at room temperature and shaken for 15 min at 50 rpm on an orbital shaker. The procedure was repeated three times. Then, the gel pieces were washed twice with 150 μL of 50 mM NH_4HCO_3 in 50% acetonitrile at 37°C, shaken for 15 min at 50 rpm on an orbital shaker, and incubated for 15 min in dehydration solution (100% acetonitrile). After the acetonitrile was removed and the gel pieces dried, 8±2.0 μL of trypsin solution (25 ng/μL modified trypsin in 50 mM bicarbonate ammonium) was added and the mixture was incubated at 37°C overnight. Then, 15 μL of 0.7% trifluoroacetic acid were added to

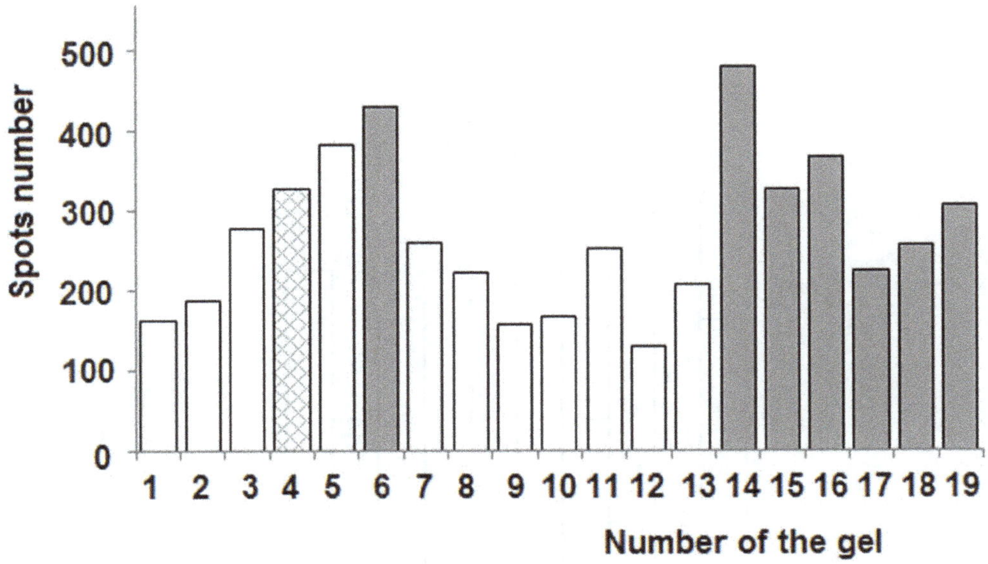

Figure 3. The number of protein spots after manual processing of 19 2DE gel images for the human liver cytosol using the proprietary GelEditor software. Gels belonging to cluster 1 are shown in white columns. Gels belonging to cluster 2 are shown in gray columns. Gel which removed from all subsequent data processing is shown in the shaded column.

each gel piece and the samples were incubated for 2 h at room temperature. The extracted tryptic peptides were used for mass spectrometric analysis.

Matrix-assisted laser desorption-ionization time-of-flight mass spectrometry (MALDI-TOF MS)

Each mixture of proteolytic peptides (1 µL) was spotted on a MALDI target (600/384 Anchor chip; Bruker Daltonik GmbH, Bremen, Germany) in three replicates and air-dried. For ionization, a solution of 2.5-dihydrobenzoic acid (3 mg/mL) in acetonitrile and 0.7% trifluoroacetic acid (1:1 v/v) was used. Mass spectra in the *m/z* range of 600–4000 were manually acquired using FlexControl software (Bruker Daltonik GmbH) in the reflection/delayed extraction mode with an accelerating voltage of 25 kV and a 135-ns delay using the Ultraflex II MALDI-TOF MS analyzer (Bruker Daltonik GmbH). All mass spectra represented signals averaging 100 laser shots from one location on a sample spot. From each sample spot, 4–6 mass spectra were acquired. Laser fluency was adjusted above the desorption threshold of the matrix to obtain the best resolution and the

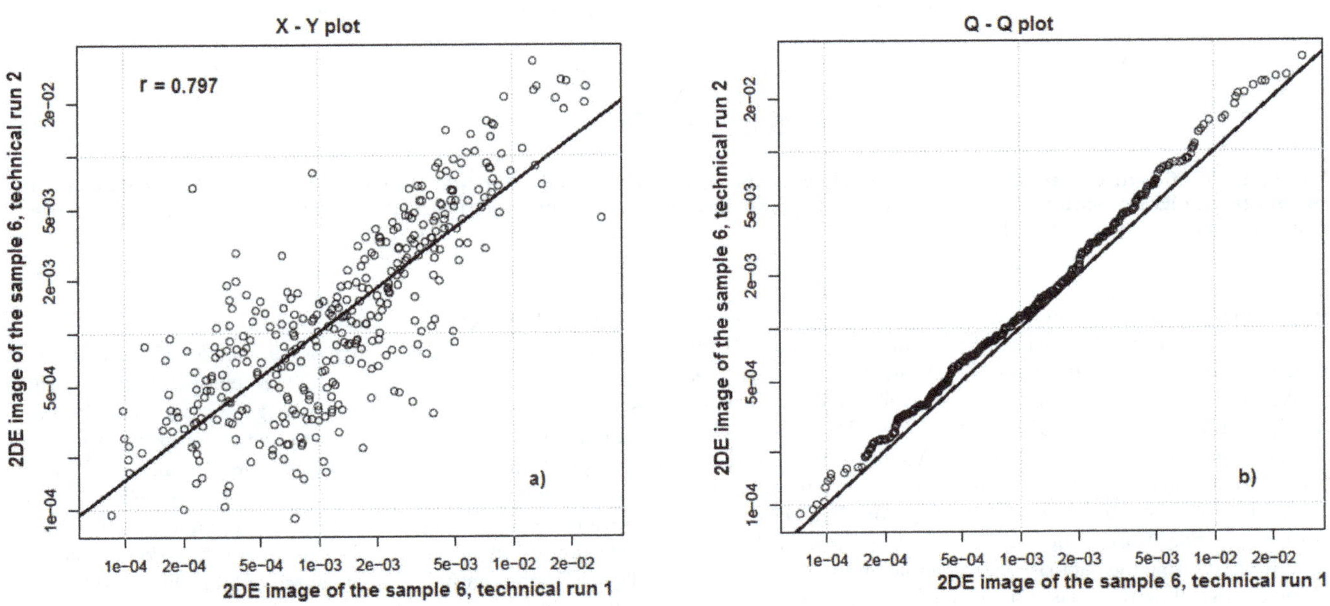

Figure 4. Reproducibility of quantitative data in 2DE images from human liver cytosolic fraction. Normalized spot intensities from two technical runs of the gel no. 6 illustrated by X – Y plot and quantile-quantile (Q – Q) plot. The X – Y plot shows strong correlation between spot intensities with a Pearson correlation coefficient r = 0.797 (**a**). Q – Q plot shows high similarity between spot intensities distribution (**b**). Intensity of each matched spot on the gel was normalized per overall intensity of matched spots within this gel.

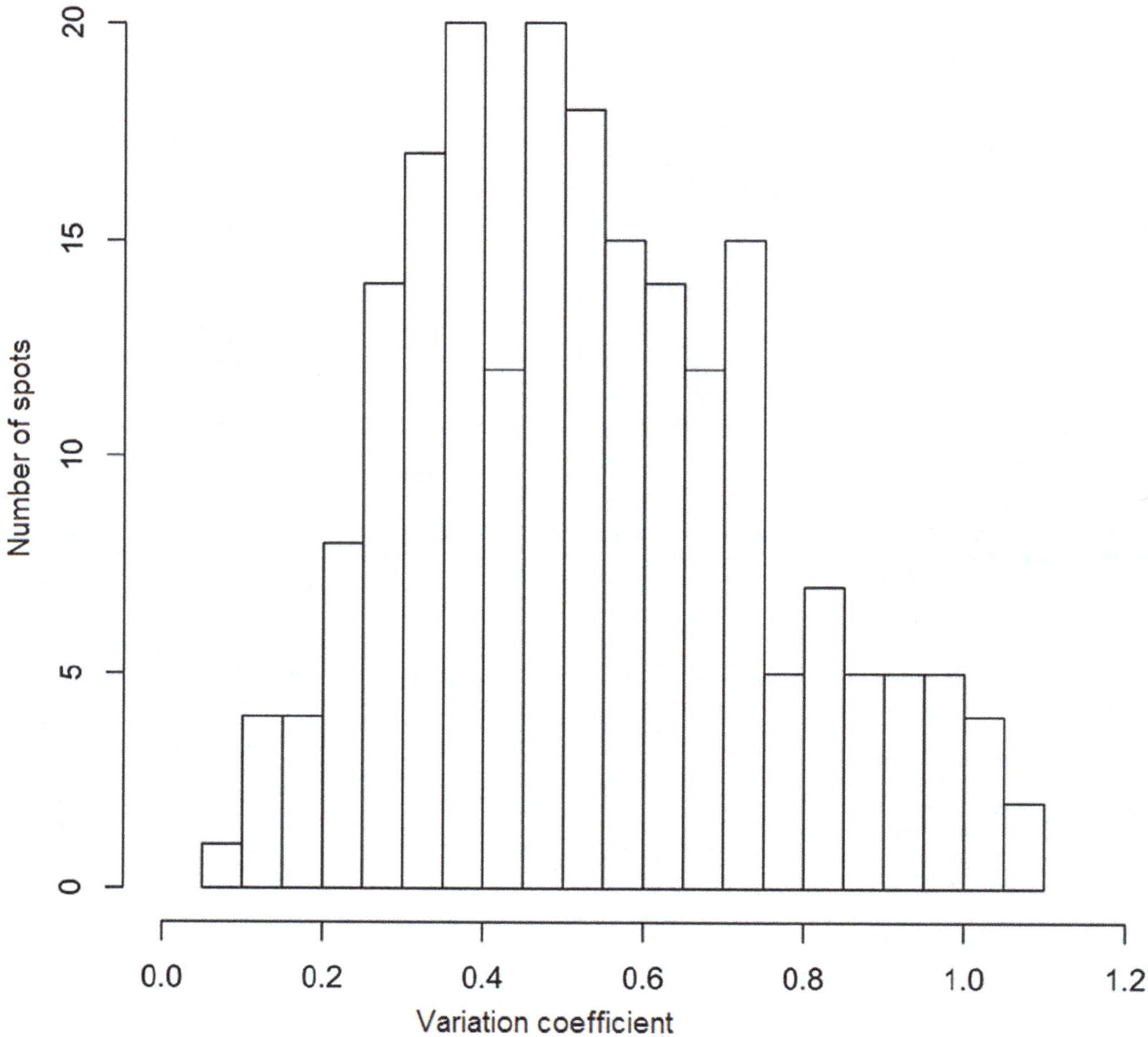

Figure 5. Coefficient of variation for 207 matched spots on the master-gel after manual matching of four 2DE gels using the proprietary GelEditor software for the human liver cytosol (sample 6). Intensity of each matched spot on the gel was normalized per overall intensity of matched spots within this gel.

highest mass measurement accuracy. Signals with an S/N ratio > 6 and a maximum of 100 peaks per spectrum were used to build peak lists with the SNAP algorithm (FlexAnalysis software ver. 2.0; Bruker Daltonik GmbH) and internally calibrated with trypsin autolysis products (*m/z* 842.5094 and 2211.1046 Da, respectively). Resulting peak lists were used to search against the UniProtKB/Swiss-Prot database (UniProt release 2012_09 - September 11, 2012). Identification by peptide mass fingerprinting (PMF) was performed using Mascot software (Matrix Science, Inc., Boston, MA, USA). During the database search, a maximum of one missed cleavage was allowed, a mass tolerance of 80 ppm was used, and variable modifications, such as methionine oxidation and cysteine modification with acrylamide, were taken into account. The appropriated m/z tolerance (80 ppm) was estimated as maximum mass deviation based on statistical distribution of mass errors in all spectra and its standard deviation.

Statistical analysis

The initial dataset consisted of 19 samples (2DE gels), each characterized on average by 271±99 protein spots/features (Table S1). Gel no. 6 was used as the master gel for the manual spot-to-spot alignment. Since we were interested in comparing the results with prior knowledge on biochemical profiles measured for the same samples [14], we also excluded gel no.4 because in our previous study it was considered as an outlier; so we had a collection of 18 gel images. To ensure study reproducibility and decrease noise sensitivity, we analyzed only qualitative differences between gels in terms of presence/absence of a certain protein spots. Each gel was replicated three times and the best replica was selected by visual inspection of separation quality. Final dataset was presented as a binary matrix **D** consisting of 18 rows (gels images) and 389 columns (spots) where $d_{ij} = 1$ if j-th spot was

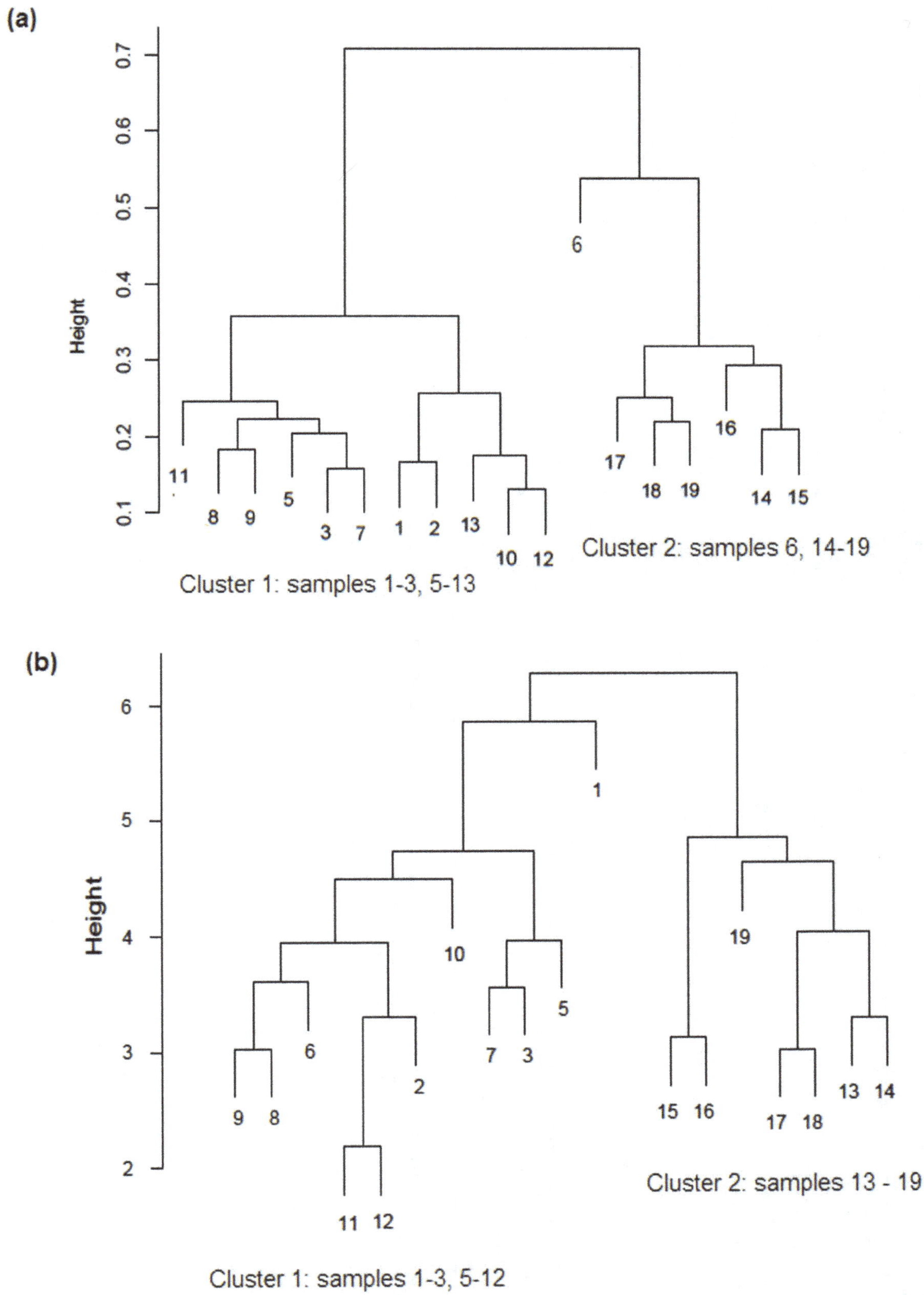

Figure 6. Hierarchical clustering applied to 2DE gel images of the human liver cytosol (a) and cytochrome P450 enzymes activities (mol/min/nmol P450) of the human liver microsomes (b). Two major clusters can be seen.

present on i-th gel, otherwise $d_{ij} = 0$. For gel clustering, we used Ward's method. Distance metric between two binary vectors was defined as number of bits where those vectors differ (also known as Hamming distance). All computations and graphics were per-

Table 1. Proteins differentially presented in cluster 1 vs cluster 2 of the human liver cytosol.

Spot ID	Protein name	Assession number[a]	Gene name	MW, Da	pI	Mascot score[b]	Seq.cov, %	Molecular class
1	*Carbamoyl-phosphate synthetase I	P31327	CPS1	164835	6.3	338	34	Enzyme: Ligase
4	*Pseudopodium-enriched atypical kinase 1	Q9H792	PEAK1	192986	6.46	60	15	Enzyme: Transferase
28	**Heat shock 70 kDa protein 1A/1B	P08107	HSPA1A	70009	5.48	118	35	Chaperone protein
28	**Bifunctional epoxide hydrolase 2	P34913	EPHX2	62575	5.91	80	23	Enzyme: Hydrolase
50	**Selenium binding protein 1	Q13228	SELENBP1	52358	5.93	261	61	Protein transport
248	**Glyceraldehyde-3-phosphate dehydrogenase	P04406	GAPDH	36030	8.57	103	59	Enzyme: Oxidoreductase
248	**Quinone oxidoreductase	Q08257	CRYZ	35185	8.56	68	49	Enzyme: Oxidoreductase
253	**Fructose-bisphosphate aldolase B	P05062	ALDOB	39448	8.01	171	59	Enzyme: Lyase
253	** Glyoxylate reductase/hydroxypyruvate reductase	Q9UBQ7	GRHPR	35646	7.01	59	42	Enzyme: Oxidoreductase
257	**Superoxide dismutase [Mn], mitochonderial	P04179	SOD2	24707	8.35	140	53	Enzyme: Oxidoreductase
260	**Carbonic anhydrase II	P00918	CA2	29228	6.87	64	30	Enzyme: Lyase
260	**Carbonic anhydrase I	P00915	CA1	28852	6.59	140	57	Enzyme: Lyase
295	**Phenazine biosynthesis-like domain-containing protein	P30039	PBLD	31765	6.06	256	81	Enzyme: Isomerase
367	**Nicotinamide N-methyltransferase	P40261	NNMT	29555	5.56	105	39	Enzyme:Methyltransferase
387	**L-xylulose reductase	Q7Z4W1	DCXR	25897	8.33	90	43	Enzyme: Oxidoreductase
395	**Triosephosphate isomerase isoform2	P60174	TPI1	30772	5.65	265	79	Enzyme: Isomerase

[a]Protein accession number as SwissProt at http://www.expasy.org/uniprot.
[b]MASCOT score from MASCOT protein database search at http://www.matrixscience.com, where the score >56 is statistically significant ($p<0.05$).
*The proteins that had been identified in the gels of cluster 1 and are absent in gels of cluster 2.
**The proteins that had been identified in the gels of cluster 2 and are absent in gels of cluster 1.

formed with R statistical language (www.r-project.org). The source code of the data analysis script can be found in Data Analysis Script S1. To measure the similarity between two data clusterings, we calculated the adjusted Rand index whose value is in the range between −1 and +1, where +1 corresponds to perfect agreement between partitions.

Results and Discussion

In our experiments all samples were taken from one category of patients: surgically treated for liver metastases arising from colon cancer (Figure 1). Therefore, our aim was not to find differences between norm and cancer, but rather to explore structure inside one-group dataset, describing human liver drug-metabolizing system and cytosol fraction (the present study). In previous study regarding drug metabolism [14] despite relatively modest sample size (n = 22) our results undoubtedly confirmed presence of two clusters in data. We computed silhouette width criteria for cluster validity, which showed that presence of two clusters is confirmed with very high confidence ($p<0.0001$). Therefore the revealed heterogeneity within one equally treated group of patients was a background for the currently reported proteomic investigation.

2DE analysis of HLC

Studies on human liver tissues have been conducted to identify if there are groups of samples distinctive in their proteomes. The HLC proteome was characterized by a representative collection of 19 samples separated by 2DE on middle format gels in three replicates, thus a total of 58 2DE images were examined. The best 2DE replicates were selected from the technical runs according to the separation quality (Figure S2). The selected representative images were converted to the spot lists and further clustered using the unsupervised method. Consistently with our previous work with liver microsomes here we used an unsupervised approach because the clinical information regarding the resected liver samples was unavailable.

We rejected some samples due to low quality 2DE separation because of peculiarities in sample preparation (Figure 2). The typical 2DE images of the Ag-stained gel of sample no. 6 before and after prefractionation with TCA in acetone (see Materials and Methods) are shown in Figure 2, ***a*** and ***b***. Without prefractionation, 2DE of cytosol fraction hampers separation of protein spots (Figure 2***a***). Figure 2***b*** is a representative master gel image showing separation of proteins from human liver tissue after TCA/acetone precipitation. This practice is often employed to remove contaminants because it minimizes protein degradation [19], but TCA/acetone precipitation was insufficient to obtain appropriate gel images of the HLC sample nos. 20–23, so we excluded these samples from further analyses. In total, 687 protein spots were resolved on a silver-stained 2DE gel from HLC sample no.6, technical run #1, using spot detection tool of GelEditor software. In addition to the silver staining based on protocol of Shevchenko et al. [18] Coomassie blue staining was also probed in this study and approximately only 100 protein spots were detected on the same gel no.6 (Figure 2***c***).

The obtained gel images were examined to characterize spot reproducibility and variability. We observed that 96% of the protein spots were at the lower boundary of detection limit of silver thiosulfate with a normalized intensity < 0.02 relative units. A medium intensity of 0.02–0.04 units was observed for 2% of spots, while 1% of spots was of high abundance with relative intensity of >0.1 unit.

Further, we selected the master gel as the best gel with the highest number of spots and minimal range of scattering of the average intensity of each spot. The master gel corresponded to sample no 6. To estimate the technical variation of our experimental setup, we conducted four independent replicative runs of HLC sample no. 6 at different times. At first step of analysis we used number of spots as a rough measure of gel reproducibility. A total of 449, 420, 444, and 406 protein spots were detected in these runs in the ranges of pI 3.5–10.0 and MW 10–250 kDa. The observed average number of spots was 430 ± 20, which was comparable to earlier data obtained from the cytoplasmic fraction of primary human hepatocytes in HepG2 and Hep2B cell lines [20]. The remaining gels contained sufficiently fewer spots, as shown in Figure 3 for 19 HLC samples. In the whole series, the average number of manually detected protein spots was 271 ± 99 (mean ± SD, n = 58). The spot quantities were three-fold lower compared to the earlier reported results of cytosolic fraction analysis of human liver tissue samples [13,21,22]. The difference in spot number was probably due to the 2DE setup, as we used 11-cm IPG strips instead of 17 cm, used by Wimmer et al. [13] and Kim et al. [23], and so the gradients for isoelectric focusing were shorter. Kim et al. [23] analyzed tumor and nontumor regions of resected liver cancer tissues by identification of cytosolic proteins using 2DE and MALDI-TOF-MS. They used silver staining for protein detection on the gels and observed up to 1060 spots and identified 127 proteins; they also reported that a problem with the variability of spot intensities was decided using normalized intensities.

To evaluate gel-to-gel variability, we compared the spots between four replicated gel images obtained from sample no. 6 by using the manual spot matching feature of the proprietary GelEditor software (Figure S1). Each replicate was manually aligned to the master image, which contained a maximum number of spots. We found that 102 spots were present in at least three replicates, 80 spots matched one-half of the gels, while 58 spots were present on the master gel only. Finally, 47% of the spots (209 spots) matched all four replicated 2DE images.

To determine the reproducibility of 2DE, we investigated technical runs of the HLC sample 6, analyzed the normalized intensities of each spot, and plotted those against each other on an X–Y and a quantile - quantile (Q–Q) plots [24]. The X–Y plots for the sample no.6, technical run #1 (master gel) compared with the same sample, technical run #2 show a Pearson correlation coefficient $r = 0.797$ (Figure 4***a***). We performed such analysis for all four technical runs of the gel 6 and determined the average Pearson's correlation coefficient which was equal 0.72 ± 0.06 (mean±95% confidence interval). The magnitude of the correlation coefficient $r>0.7$ suggests a strong correlation, while Q-Q plots were used as a graphical tool for comparing two distributions to each other. Two data sets would be considered identical if the points in the Q-Q plots lie close to a regression line $y = x$. As shown in Figure 4b this criterion is perfectly fulfilled for HLC proteins.

The highly reproducible spots (209) were used to estimate the spot intensity variation across four replicates for HLC sample no 6. In the coefficient of variation (CV) distribution histogram (see Figure 5), 65% of spots were characterized by a CV <0.6. This degree of variation between the replicated gels was comparable to the CV observed between normal tissue vs. various cancer stages [9,25]. For example, Shi et al. [9] observed an average CV of 62–69% in 1223 spot features from 18 2D-DIGE spot profiles amongst different sample groups (normal colon mucosa, primary colorectal cancer, and liver metastases). The authors found that both primary and secondary tumors displayed a significantly higher degree of spot volume variations than the normal colon.

Generally, the CV depends on the type of biological material, as well as sample preparation and spot detection approaches [26,27]. In silver staining, the matching spots prepared and run under identical conditions vary in intensities; therefore, it is difficult to achieve reproducibility even with parallel replicates [26]. Therefore, as our gels were poorly reproducible in the intensities of the matching spots, we did not use intensity values for further analysis, but converted the spots into binary format: either there is a spot, or not.

3.2 Unsupervised clustering of the gels and microsomal samples

We used cluster analysis to separate gels and elucidate groups in our collection of liver samples. Initially, spots on each 2DE gel were collated to the spots on the master gel (no. 6#1) using Perl script (Data Analysis Script S2). Our results were formatted into a table in which the rows indicated the protein spots and the columns represented HLC samples. If the protein spot was present on the HLC gel and master gel, the cell value was set at "1", otherwise if the spot was absent on the next HLC gel, it was set at "0". We performed hierarchical cluster analysis of the data matrix using Ward's method coupled with the Hamming distance metric. Clustering of 2DE gels of the HLC samples was visualized as a dendrogram (Figure 6***a***). Two major clusters were clearly distinguished: the first (cluster no. 1) was formed by gels nos. 1–3, 5, and 7–13, while the second (cluster no. 2) included gels nos. 6 technical run #3, and 14–19. So, Ward's method yielded two groups of liver samples. Interestingly, the histogram in Figure 3 preliminarily pointed to the existence of two clusters for the HLC samples. The average number of manually detected protein spots on gels from clusters nos. 1 and 2 were 219±72 and 342±91 (mean ± SD), respectively; however, the difference in the number of spots was statistically insignificant ($p>0.05$, n = 18).

According to our previous data, human liver microsomes also segregated into two groups [14]: the first contained samples nos. 1–3, 5–12, and 23, whereas the second contained samples nos. 13–22 (Figure 1**A**). Thus, there was a correlation between sample clustering emerged from the two absolutely different experimental approaches.

The Rand index was 0.58, indicating a significant match [27] between biochemical and proteomic data. A slight difference between group composition of the HLC samples and the human liver microsomal (drug-metabolizing) system was found. These changes were particular to HLC samples nos. 6 and 13, assigned to cluster nos. 2 and 1, contrary to their previous clustering by biochemical profiling. As can be seen from the dendrogram in Figure 6***a***, gel no. 6 (technical run 3 of the master gel) can be formally attributed to cluster no. 2, as it is located at a sufficient distance from the centroid of this cluster.

Due to problems with 2DE, the present study included 18 HLC samples vs. 22 microsomal fractions in our previous research [14]. We re-used biochemical data for hierarchical clustering with only 18 (instead of 22) corresponding microsomal samples and obtained consistent results. Again, two groups were observed: sample nos. 1–3 and 5–12 in cluster no. 1, and sample nos. 13–19 in cluster no. 2 (Figure 6***b***). As seen in the dendrograms (Figures 6 ***a*** and ***b***), the human liver samples and/or patients fell into the same subgroup within the same cluster. For example, samples nos. 3 and 7 were occupied neighboring leaf of cluster no. 1 both in biochemical and proteomic analyses, while samples nos. 8 and 9 were neighboring within cluster no. 1, and samples nos. 17 and 18– within cluster no. 2.

We attempted to elucidate the characteristic features for the clusters. The number of protein spots was not significantly different, so the number of the different protein species coincided in both groups. These results indicated, that even under changing biochemical conditions, the number of proteins is generally preserved in the liver cytosol.

Next, we analyzed changes in the intensity level of the spots, which contributed to the differentiations between clusters. Differences between the two HLC groups shown in Figure 6 ***a,*** were observed in 15 protein spots. In details, it appeared that in cluster no. 1, there were three spots (## 1, 4, and 8) that were absent in cluster no. 2.

Although there were no significant differences in the number of spots between clusters, it was observed that gels from cluster no. 1 generally contain less number of spots than gels from cluster no. 2. It was apparent already from the Figure 3, that clusters separate themselves in accordance with the number of spots. In a biochemical survey, we observed the higher activity of drug metabolizing enzymes for the samples of cluster no. 1, where the number of spots was lesser. Vice-a-versa for the gels with larger number of spots in cytosolic fraction the activity of microsomal enzymes diminished. It could be that there is no functional isolation between cytosolic and microsomal fraction. The deficiency of microsomal activity could be compensated by increased activity and/or content of cytosolic proteins.

We identified the particular forms of the proteins (2DE spots), which contributed to the differentiation between clusters of HLC samples. As mentioned already the differences between clusters shown in Figure 6***a*** and/or differences between two groups of HLC were observed in fifteen 2DE spots, three of which were specific for cluster no. 1 (## 1, 4 and 8 in Figure 2***c***). The rest twelve spots were present only in cluster no. 2 but not in cluster no. 1 (## 28, 50, 248, 253, 257, 260, 295, 367, 379, 381, 378 and 395).

The clustered gels were relatively similar in patterns of the differentially presented spots. Of 219 spots observed on the 2DE gel images from cluster no. 1, 13% of the spots were present on each gel, while those relating to cluster no. 2, practically the same portion (16%) of the spots were reproducible in all of the images in the group. From this observation we expect that the observed differences between clusters were not the consequence of individual variability between patients, but rather due to the variability between the cohorts specifically responding to chemotherapy exposure. On the other hand, the stratification of the cohorts can be explained by the different susceptibility to the chemotherapy or some patients may have lacked presurgical treatment.

Protein identification by MALDI-TOF mass spectrometry

Spots indicating differences between clusters were excised from some gels and identified by MALDI-TOF-MS. For each protein spot, we acquired 6–8 MALDI-TOF mass spectra from each of the two replicated positions on the MALDI target per protein spot. By averaging the *m/z* values in spectra the greatest MASCOT score for protein matching and the highest percentage of sequence coverage were selected (Figure S3). All of these spots were also analyzed using Mr and pI (Table I). Approximately 90% of the identified proteins had sequence coverage exceeding 25% (47±18%). In 44% of the cases, the identified proteins were the single candidate with significant score (173±85) leading to their unambiguous identification. Among 16 proteins presented in Table 1 four proteins, namely pseudopodium-enriched atypical kinase 1 (Q9H792, spot ID # 4), quinone oxidoreductase (P04406, #248), glyoxylate reductase/hydroxypyruvate reductase (Q9UBQ7, #253), and carbonic anhydrase II (P00918, #260) exhibited a score lower of 70. These identifications were confirmed as these proteins migrated within a range consistent with expected mass and pI values. Note, that three of these proteins were secondary residents in the spot identified at the background of the major protein species. For example, spot #253 contained two proteins: fructose-bisphosphate aldolase B (P05062) and glyoxylate reductase/hydroxypyruvate reductase (Q9UBQ7), which were identified with the score 171 and 59, respectively.

Table 1 presents the results of the identification performed by peptide mass fingerprinting (PMF). PMF spectra should be used cautiously, as identification results vary with tolerance value [28,29]; and peptide mass tolerance should receive a special attention regarding such parameters of PMF search engines as taxonomy, cleavage enzyme, the number of peptides matched, etc. Earlier we observed that human liver microsomal protein identification results show the dependency with a maximum at 0.15 Da (120 ppm) [15,30]. Herein applying the same method for HLC protein identification we obtained that peptide mass tolerance value achieved optimum at 60–90 ppm.

Among the proteins specific to the samples of cluster no. 1 carbamoyl phosphate synthetase I was normally found in hepatocytes. Cardona et al. [26] have shown that the development of small-intestinal adenocarcinoma is associated with colorectal cancer and loss of this protein may be of use to diagnose difficult cases. In the HLC samples belonging to group 2, following proteins were identified: carbonic anhydrase I (CA1, P00915), dicarbonyl/L-xylulose reductase (DCXR, Q7Z4W1), and selenium-binding protein 1 (SBP1, Q13228). CA isoforms have an important role in cancer development and altered CA1 protein levels can support the protective effects of changes in diet and vegetable consumption against colorectal cancer [31]. CA1 is down-regulated in cancerous vs. normal tissues and can be used as candidate prognostic biomarker to indicate good survival prediction for colorectal cancer patients [32]. DCXR has been proposed as a potential biomarker of human adenocarcinoma [33]. Differentially expressed SBP1 also demonstrated anti-cancer potential as its overexpression in HCT116 cells induced H_2O_2-mediated apoptosis, inhibited cell migration in vitro, and inhibited tumor growth in nude mice [34]. SBP1 suppression may contribute to the rapid progression of colorectal carcinoma, while higher SBP1 level is associated with differentiation of normal colonic epithelia and may be a positive prognostic factor for survival in stage III colorectal carcinoma [35,36].

2DE gels of all 18 HLC samples shared 21 common protein spots (see legend for Figure 2*b*), while identification by MALDI-TOF PMF was acquired only for 13 spots of sufficient intensity. Among them there were: malate dehydrogenase cytoplasmic (P40925), aldehyde dehydrogenase 1 (ALDH1, P00352), heat shock cognate (P11142), biliverdin reductase B (P30043), and aminoacylase-1 (Q03154). The amount of proteins listed above was higher in colorectal cancer cells vs. normal colorectal epithelial cells and may present a clinically useful prognostic biomarker of colorectal cancer [37–39]. For most of the detected spots no significant difference was observed between normalized intensities on 2DE gels belonging to clusters nos. 1 and 2. For example, the intensities of spot #48 (aminoacylase-1) were 0.0076 ± 0.037 and 0.0072 ± 0.0021, in clusters nos. 1 and 2, respectively. The same situation was also observed for spot #275 (biliverdin reductase B) -0.0128 ± 0.0149 (cluster no. 1) and 0.0098 ± 0.0040 (cluster no. 2). Nevertheless, the change in the staining intensity of one particular spot deserved attention: the intensity of spot #210 (ALDH1) was 0.0174 ± 0.0051 in cluster no. 1 and 0.0114 ± 0.0051 in cluster no. 2. The difference in spot intensities was statistically significant ($p<0.001$, $n=18$) and indicated that ALDH1 was 1.5-fold over-expressed in HLC samples of cluster no. 1 compared with its level in HLC samples of cluster no. 2. Lohberger et al. [40] demonstrated that cancer cells with high ALDH1 level were more resistant to commonly used chemotherapeutic agents, such as doxorubicin, epirubicin, and cisplatin, than cells with low ALDH1 amount.

The obtained data showed that the division of liver cytosolic fractions into two groups correlated with the segregation of liver microsomal fractions obtained earlier from the same samples. Characterization of the changes specific to the biochemical and proteomic profiles of human liver samples from patients with the same diagnostic category (i.e., colorectal cancer liver metastases, which may have led to hepatic surgery after prior chemotherapy) may suggest poor survival prediction in cluster no. 1 patients because of two reasons. First, human liver microsomes and/or the patients belonging to this cluster were characterized by a significant increase in activity of phase I metabolizing enzymes vs. activities of drug-metabolizing enzymes in microsomes from cluster no. 2 [14]. It was shown that higher enzymatic activities lead to lower treatment efficacy influenced (decreased) the survival time after chemotherapy [41,42]. Second, in HLC samples from group 1, the enzymes CA1, SBP1, and DCXR were absent. Down-regulation of these proteins serves as prognostic biomarkers for poor survival prediction in colorectal cancer patients [33,35,36].

Concluding remarks

This functional proteomic study integrated multi-parametric data from two sets of experiments. First, we performed biochemical analysis of liver microsomes, while another set was produced by 2DE analysis of cytosolic fractions. We observed that both sets of experiments were concordant, as samples were clustered in similar ways. Notably, the unsupervised method was used to unravel the clusters; therefore, results of the biochemical experiments did not affected sample segregation in proteome profiling.

Earlier, we observed significant changes in biochemical activities and explained them as different susceptibilities and/or expose patients to pre-operative chemotherapy. In the current follow-up study, the proteomic analysis confirmed two classes of samples and enabled the identification of proteins that were altered concordantly with changes in activity of phase I drug-metabolizing enzymes.

We introduced the application of unsupervised learning to compare the biochemical properties of hepatocytes and changes of the amount of particular forms of the proteins at the proteome level. The presented biochemical-to-proteome profiling approach is essentially different from the conventional proteomic studies, in which samples are attributed to the classes determined by clinical diagnoses.

Supporting Information

Figure S1 GelEditor software: Brief Description and application.

Figure S2 2DE images of human liver cytosolic fraction (19 samples). 30 µg of the human soluble liver protein fraction after pretreatment with trichloroacetic acid in acetone separated by 2D-PAGE were visualized by silver staining.

Figure S3 Mass spectrometric characterization of proteins differentially presented in cluster 1 vs cluster 2 of the human liver cytosol: a) Fructose-bisphosphate aldolase B; b) Carbamoyl-phosphate synthetase I; c) Glyceraldehyde-3-phosphate dehydrogenase; d) Glyoxylate reductase/hydroxypyruvate reductase; e) Selenium binding protein 1; and f) Superoxide dismutase [Mn], mitochondrial. (A) MALDI-TOF mass spectra of the tryptic digests of the spots on 2DE gels of human liver cytosolic fraction. Labeled peaks (*) correspond to the matched peptides of identified proteins. (B) The sequence coverage of identified protein. Matched peptides shown in bold red.

Table S1 Normalized intensities of the spots on 2DE gels of human liver cytosolic fraction.

Data Analysis Script S1 R script for statistical data analysis (process.r).

Data Analysis Script S2 Perl script for spot preprocessing (match_gels.pl).

Author Contributions

Conceived and designed the experiments: AVL NAP IIK. Performed the experiments: OVL OPT JSK NFS. Analyzed the data: NAP MAP VAR AVL. Contributed reagents/materials/analysis tools: GPK MAP. Wrote the paper: NAP AVL.

References

1. Mayer-Kuckuk P, Banerjee D, Kemeny N, Fong Y, Bertino JR (2002) Molecular therapies for colorectal cancer metastatic to the liver. Mol Ther 5: 492–500.
2. Ruan DT, Warren RS (2005) Liver-directed therapies in colorectal cancer. Semin Oncol 32(1): 85–94.
3. Wray CJ, Rilo HL, Ahmad SA (2004) Colon cancer angiogenesis and antiangiogenic therapy. Expert Opin Investig Drugs. Expert Opin Investig Drugs 13(6): 631–641.
4. Lise M, Mocellin S, Pilati P, Nitti D (2005) Colorectal liver metastasis: towards the integration of conventional and molecularly targeted therapeutic approaches. Frontiers in Bioscience 10: 3042–3057.
5. Macgregor PF, Squire JA (2002) Application of microarrays to the analysis of gene expression in cancer. Clin Chem 48: 1170–1177.
6. Celis J, Gromov P (1999) 2D protein electrophoresis: can it be perfected? Curr Opin Biotechnol 10: 16–21.
7. Karp NA, Lilley KS (2007) Design and analysis issues in quantitative proteomics studies. Practical Proteomics 1: 42–50.
8. Jimenez CR, Knol JC, Meijer GA, Fijneman RJ (2010) Proteomics of colorectal cancer: overview of discovery studies and identification of commonly identified cancer-associated proteins and candidate CRC serum markers. J Proteomics 73: 1873–1895.
9. Shi H, Hood KA, Hayes MT, Stubbs RS (2011) Proteomic analyses of advanced colorectal cancer by laser capture microdissection and two-dimensional difference gel electrophoresis. J Proteomics 75(2): 339–351.
10. Yu B, Li SY, An P, Zhang YN, Liang ZJ, et al. (2004) Comparative study of proteome between primary cancer and hepatic metastatic tumor in colorectal cancer. World J Gastroenterol 10(18): 2652–2656.
11. Alfonso P, Canamero M, Fernandez-Carbonie F, Nunez A, Casal JI (2008) Proteome analysis of membrane fractions in colorectal carcinomas by using 2D-DIGE saturation labeling. J Proteome Res 7: 4247–4255.
12. Muto T, Taniguchi H, Kushima R, Tsuda H, Yonemori H, et al. (2011) Global expression study in colorectal cancer on proteins with alkaline isoelectric point by two-dimensional difference gel electrophoresis. J Proteomics 74(6): 858–873.
13. Wimmer H, Gundacker NC, Griss J, Haudek VJ, Stättner S, et al. (2009) Introducing the CPL/MUW proteome database: interpretation of human liver and liver cancer proteome profiles by referring to isolated primary cells. Electrophoresis 30(12): 2076–2089.
14. Petushkova NA, Pyatnitskiy MA, Lisitsa AV, Larina OV, Kuznetsova GP, et al. (2010) Computational approach to characterization of human liver drug-metabolizing enzymes. Eur J Pharm Sci 41(2): 305–311.
15. Petushkova NA, Larina OV, Chernobrovkin AL, Trifonova OP, Kisrieva YS, et al. (2012) Optimization of the SDS-PAGE gel slicing approach for identification of human liver microsomal proteins via MALDI-TOF mass spectrometry. J Proteomics Bioinform 5: 40–49 Available: http://omicsonline.org/optimization-of-the-sds-page-gel-slicing-approach-for-identification-of-human-liver-microsomal-proteins-via-maldi-tof-mass-spectrometry-jpb.1000211.pdf.
16. Bradford MM (1976) A rapid and sensitive method for the quantitation of microgram quantities of protein utilizing the principle of protein-dye binding. Anal Biochem 72: 248–254.
17. Kulkarni YM, Suarez V, Klinke DJ2nd (2010) Inferring predominant pathways in cellular models of breast cancer using limited sample proteomic profiling. BMC Cancer 10: 291–302.
18. Shevchenko A, Wilm M, Vorm O, Mann M (1996) Mass spectrometric sequencing of proteins silver-stained polyacrylamide gels. Anal Chem 68(5): 850–858.
19. Slany A, Haudek VJ, Zwickl H, Gundacker NC, Grusch M, et al. (2010) Cell characterization by proteome profiling applied to primary hepatocytes and hepatocyte cell lines Hep-G2 and Hep-3B. J Proteome Res 9: 6–21.
20. Corona G, De Lorenzo E, Elia C, Simula MP, Avellini C, et al. (2010) Differential proteomic analysis of hepatocellular carcinoma. Int J Oncol 36(1): 93–99.
21. Choe LH, Lee KH (2003) Quantitative and qualitative measure of intralaboratory two-dimensional protein gel reproducibility and the effects of sample preparation, sample load, and image analysis. Electrophoresis 24: 3500–3507.
22. Kwong KY, Bloom GC, Yang I, Boulware D, Coppola D, et al. (2005) Synchronous global assessment of gene and protein expression in colorectal cancer progression. Genomics 86: 142–158.
23. Kim J, Kim SH, Lee SU, Ha GH, Kang DG, et al. (2002) Proteome analysis of human liver tumor tissue by two-dimensional gel electrophoresis and matrix assisted laser desorption/ionization-mass spectrometry for identification of disease-related proteins. Electrophoresis 23(24): 4142–4156.
24. Techritz S, Lützkendorf S, Bazant E, Becker S, Klose J, et al. (2013) Quantitative and qualitative 2D electrophoretic analysis of differentially expressed mitochondrial proteins from five mouse organs. Proteomics 13(1): 179–195.
25. Voss T, Haberl P (2000) Observations on the reproducibility and matching efficiency of two-dimensional electrophoresis gels: consequences for comprehensive data analysis. Electrophoresis 21(16): 3345–3350.
26. Cardona DM, Zhang X, Liu C (2009) Loss of carbamoyl phosphate synthetase I in small-intestinal adenocarcinoma. Am J Clin Pathol 132(6): 877–882.
27. Rand W (1971) Objective criteria for the evaluation of clustering methods. J American Statistical association 66(336): 846–850.
28. Ossipova E, Fenyö D, Eriksson J (2006) Optimizing search conditions for the mass fingerprint-based identification of proteins. Proteomics 6: 2079–2085.
29. Jain R, Wagner M (2010) Kolmogorov-Smirnov scores and intrinsic mass tolerances for peptide mass fingerprinting. J Proteome Res 9: 737–742.
30. Chernobrovkin AL, Trifonova OP, Petushkova NA, Ponomarenko EA, Lisitsa AV (2011) Selection of the peptide mass tolerance value for the protein identification with peptide mass fingerprinting. Bioorg Khim 37: 132–136.
31. Breikers G, van Breda SG, Bouwman FG, van Herwijnen MH, Renes J, et al. (2006) Potential protein markers for nutritional health effects on colorectal cancer in the mouse as revealed by proteomics analysis. Proteomics 6: 2844–2852.
32. Peng Y, Li X, Wu M, Yang J, Liu M, et al. (2012) New prognosis biomarkers identified by dynamic proteomic analysis of colorectal cancer. Mol Biosyst 8(11): 3077–8308.
33. Cho-Vega JH, Tsavachidis S, Do KA, Nakagawa J, Medeiros LJ, et al. (2007) Dicarbonyl/L-xylulose reductase: a potential biomarker identified by laser-capture microdissection-micro serial analysis of gene expression of human prostate adenocarcinoma. Cancer Epidemiol Biomarkers Prev 16(12): 2615–2622.
34. Pohl NM, Tong C, Fang W, Bi X, Li T, et al. (2009) Transcriptional regulation and biological functions of selenium-binding protein 1 in colorectal cancer in vitro and in nude mouse xenografts. PLoS One 4(11): 1–6.
35. Kim H, Kang HJ, You KT, Kim SH, Lee KY, et al. (2006) Suppression of human selenium-binding protein 1 is a late event in colorectal carcinogenesis and is associated with poor survival. Proteomics 6: 3466–3476.
36. Li T, Yang W, Li M, Byun DS, Tong C, et al. (2008) Expression of selenium-binding protein 1 characterizes intestinal cell maturation and predicts survival for patients with colorectal cancer. Mol Nutr.Food Res 52: 1289–1299.
37. Shi H, Hayes MT, Kirana C, Miller RJ, Keating JP, et al. (2013) Overexpression of aminoacylase 1 is associated with colorectal cancer progression. Hum Pathol 44(6): 1089–1097.
38. Melle C, Ernst G, Scheibner O, Kaufmann R, Schimmel B, et al. (2007) Identification of specific protein markers in microdissected hepatocellular carcinoma. J Proteome Res 6: 306–315.
39. Albrethsen J, Bøgebo R, Gammeltoft S, Olsen J, Winther B, et al. (2005) Upregulated expression of human neutrophil peptides 1, 2 and 3 (HNP 1–3) in colon cancer serum and tumors: a biomarker study. BMC Cancer 5: 8.
40. Lohberger B, Rinner B, Stuendl N, Absenger M, Liegl-Atzwanger B, et al. (2012) Aldehyde dehydrogenase 1, a potential marker for cancer stem cells in human sarcoma. PLoS One 7(8): e43664.
41. Lentz F, Tran A, Rey E, Pons G, Tréluyer JM (2005) Pharmacogenomics of fluorouracil, irinotecan, and oxaliplatin in hepatic metastases of colorectal cancer: clinical implications. Am J Pharmacogenomics 5(1): 21–33.
42. Rochat B (2005) Role of cytochrome P450 activity in the fate of anticancer agents and in drug resistance: focus on tamoxifen, paclitaxel and imatinib metabolism. Clin Pharmacokinet 44(4): 349–366.

Is 3-Tesla Gd-EOB-DTPA-Enhanced MRI with Diffusion-Weighted Imaging Superior to 64-Slice Contrast-Enhanced CT for the Diagnosis of Hepatocellular Carcinoma?

Bettina Maiwald*, Donald Lobsien, Thomas Kahn, Patrick Stumpp

Department of Diagnostic and Interventional Radiology, University of Leipzig, Leipzig, Germany

Abstract

Objectives: To compare 64-slice contrast-enhanced computed tomography (CT) with 3-Tesla magnetic resonance imaging (MRI) using Gd-EOB-DTPA for the diagnosis of hepatocellular carcinoma (HCC) and evaluate the utility of diffusion-weighted imaging (DWI) in this setting.

Methods: 3-phase-liver-CT was performed in fifty patients (42 male, 8 female) with suspected or proven HCC. The patients were subjected to a 3-Tesla-MRI-examination with Gd-EOB-DTPA and diffusion weighted imaging (DWI) at b-values of 0, 50 and 400 s/mm^2. The apparent diffusion coefficient (ADC)-value was determined for each lesion detected in DWI. The histopathological report after resection or biopsy of a lesion served as the gold standard, and a surrogate of follow-up or complementary imaging techniques in combination with clinical and paraclinical parameters was used in unresected lesions. Diagnostic accuracy, sensitivity, specificity, and positive and negative predictive values were evaluated for each technique.

Results: MRI detected slightly more lesions that were considered suspicious for HCC per patient compared to CT (2.7 versus 2.3, respectively). ADC-measurements in HCC showed notably heterogeneous values with a median of $1.2\pm0.5\times10^{-3}$ mm^2/s (range from 0.07 ± 0.1 to $3.0\pm0.1\times10^{-3}$ mm^2/s). MRI showed similar diagnostic accuracy, sensitivity, and positive and negative predictive values compared to CT (AUC 0.837, sensitivity 92%, PPV 80% and NPV 90% for MRI vs. AUC 0.798, sensitivity 85%, PPV 79% and NPV 82% for CT; not significant). Specificity was 75% for both techniques.

Conclusions: Our study did not show a statistically significant difference in detection in detection of HCC between MRI and CT. Gd-EOB-DTPA-enhanced MRI tended to detect more lesions per patient compared to contrast-enhanced CT; therefore, we would recommend this modality as the first-choice imaging method for the detection of HCC and therapeutic decisions. However, contrast-enhanced CT was not inferior in our study, so that it can be a useful image modality for follow-up examinations.

Editor: Andreas-Claudius Hoffmann, West German Cancer Center, Germany

Funding: This work was supported by a research grant from Bayer Vital, Leverkusen, Germany. This was used to buy contrast media for the MRI-examination. The funders had no role in study design, data collection and analysis, decision to publish, or preparation of the manuscript. None of the author received specific funding for this work. www.bayerpharma.com.

Competing Interests: The study was supported by a research grant from Bayer Vital, Leverkusen, Germany but this did not modify the authors' results and conclusion in any way. It was used to buy contrast media (Gd-EOB-DTPA (Primovist®)) for the MRI-examination of the patients. This contrast medium is a specific tool in imaging liver lesions since it is metabolized by the hepatocytes. It is officially approved by the European Medicines Agency (EMA) as well as by the Food and Drug Administration (FDA) in the USA and the authors currently use it daily in clinical routine. The funders had no role in study design, data collection and analysis, decision to publish or preparation of the manuscript. The authors' employments were not paid by the research grant. None of the authors received personal funding for this work and therefore no personal competing interests exist.

* Email: bettina.maiwald@medizin.uni-leipzig.de

Introduction

Hepatocellular carcinoma (HCC) is one of the most common malignancies worldwide. Liver cirrhosis is a precancerous condition associated with the development of HCC. Other important risk factors include chronic hepatitis B and C, as well as alcohol abuse. The sequential carcinogenesis from regenerative nodules to overt HCC has been described previously, and the *de novo* development of HCC without prior liver cirrhosis has also been delineated [1–5].

HCC can be diagnosed by various imaging modalities, including ultrasound, multidetector computed tomography (CT) and magnetic resonance imaging (MRI). Despite these versatile imaging modalities, correct characterization of HCC versus other liver lesions remains a challenging task, and a definite diagnosis often cannot be made based on imaging alone [6]. However, in cancer patients, a precise diagnosis is important for optimal treatment planning [2,7].

Concerning advanced magnetic resonance techniques, diffusion weighted imaging (DWI) has the ability to differentiate between malignant and benign liver lesions [8–12]. A recently developed liver-specific contrast medium, Gd-EOB-DTPA (Gadolinium-ethoxybenzyl-diethylene-triamine-pentaacetic-acid), is a paramagnetic contrast agent with properties of extracellular and hepatobiliary contrast media for use in MR imaging of the liver. This reagent allows for dynamic perfusion imaging and the evaluation of liver function. Gd-EOB-DTPA is taken up in hepatocytes to approximately 50% via OATP-1 (organic anion transporter protein-1), increasing the signal intensity of the liver parenchyma approximately 20 min after injection [13–16]. Several studies have demonstrated that this reagent improved the detection and characterization of focal liver lesions [17–19].

High field-strength MRI at 3.0 Tesla provides better tissue contrast compared to 1.5 Tesla due to a greater signal-to-noise ratio, improved image quality, higher resolution imaging and faster scanning times [20].

The aim of this study was to compare the diagnostic power of CT with 3 Tesla MRI using Gd-EOB-DTPA for the diagnosis of HCC and to evaluate the diagnostic impact of DWI with apparent diffusion coefficient (ADC) quantification in this setting.

Material and Methods

Patient Selection

Fifty patients (mean age 60.6 years, range 29–84 years, mean body weight 79,8 kg, range 45–120 kg, 42 male, 8 female, Table 1) with suspected or proven HCC were included in this prospective single-centre study to evaluate the diagnostic performance of contrast-enhanced CT and Gd-EOB-DTPA-enhanced MRI in terms of lesion detection. Inclusion criteria were suspicious findings in the US or/and increased laboratory parameters (e.g., alpha-fetoprotein). Exclusion criteria were renal failure, allergy to contrast agents, hyperthyreoidism, pregnancy and, especially for the MRI-examination, pacemaker or other non-compatible implants and claustrophobia. The aetiology of liver cirrhosis in the patient cohort was as follows: 26 patients with alcohol induced liver cirrhosis, 2 with Hepatitis B- and 3 with Hepatitis C-related chronic liver disease, 3 patients with hemochromatosis, one with Budd-Chiari-Syndrome and one with non-alcoholic steatohepatitis. 14 patients had cryptogenic liver cirrhosis. Based on the Child-Pugh-Classification, the severity of liver cirrhosis was classified as class A in 27 patients, class B in 16 patients and class C in 7 patients [Table 1].

The histopathological report after resection or biopsy of a lesion served as the gold standard for diagnosis, whereas a surrogate of follow-up (after 6 months) or complementary imaging technique (ultrasound, digital subtraction angiography) in combination with clinical (loss of weight, general state) and paraclinical parameters (especially alpha-fetoprotein) was used in unresected lesions.

This study was approved by the ethics committee of the medical faculty of the University of Leipzig, and all patients provided written informed consent.

Imaging technique

Multiphase-CT was performed using two different scanners (Brilliance 64/iCT; Philips Healthcare, Eindhoven, Netherlands) with identical parameters to prevent bias within the CT: collimation of 0.625 mm, rotation time of 0.75 s, tube voltage of 120 kV, tube current 200 mAs and adjusted with automatic dose modulation, reconstructed slice thickness of 3 mm, matrix 512*512). The contrast agent (Iopromide Ultravist 370, Bayer Vital GmbH, Leverkusen, Germany) was applied at a constant volume of 100 ml at a rate of 3 ml/s (Power injector mississippi, Ulrich Medical, Ulm, Germany). The unenhanced phase, early arterial phase 10 s after bolustracking (positioning the respective region of interest in the abdominal aorta just above the coeliac trunk, threshold 150 HU) and portal venous phase 60 s after reaching the threshold were acquired.

Subsequent MRI (median time: 2.2 days, range 0–30d) was performed in all subjects using a 3.0 Tesla scanner (TrioTim, Siemens Medical Solutions, Erlangen, Germany). The study protocol consisted of the following sequences:

(1) T2w-HASTE (half-fourier acquisition single-shot turbo spin echo) coronal and axial
(2) T1w-VIBE (volume-interpolated breath-hold examination) coronal unenhanced, axial unenhanced and dynamic after contrast medium was applied (Gd-EOB-DTPA (Primovist), Bayer Vital GmbH, Leverkusen, Germany) at 0.1 ml/kg bodyweight at a rate of 2 ml/s using a power injector (Spectris solaris EP, Medrad, Dusseldorf, Germany), followed by a 30 ml saline flush. Scanning times were as follows: arterial phase, 2 s; portalvenous phase, 30–40, equilibrium phase, 2–3 min; and hepatobiliary phase, 20 min after the contrast bolus reached the abdominal aorta.
(3) Diffusion-weighted sequence coronal and axial (b-value 0, 50 and 400 s/mm^2)
(4) T2w TSE (turbo spin echo) with fat saturation coronal
(5) T1w in phase and opposed phase axial

See Table 2 for more details concerning the sequences.

Imaging analysis

Image analysis focused on the number, size and detectability of liver lesions, as well as image quality. A radiologist with 10 years of experience in abdominal imaging performed the analysis using a picture archiving and communication system workstation (Magic-View 1000, Siemens Medical Solutions, Erlangen, Germany). The observer was aware of the patients being at risk of HCC, but otherwise blinded to all patient data. Diagnosis of HCC was based on hypervascularization in the arterial phase and washout in the portal venous phase or delayed phase, as suggested by the European Association for the Study of the Liver and the American Association for the Study of Liver Disease for MRI and CT [1]. In addition, focal areas with a suspicious hypointense signal in the hepatobiliary phase were used to detect HCC [21] (Figure 1). The radiologist recorded the presence and anatomical location of lesions, as well as diagnostic confidence using the following 5-point scale: 1 = definitely not HCC, 2 = probably not HCC, 3 = equivocal, 4 = probably HCC, 5 = definitely HCC.

Lesion detectability and image quality were evaluated using a 5-point rating-scale (1 = excellent, 2 = good, 3 = fair, 4 = poor, 5 = unacceptable). The average largest tumour diameter was determined using a measuring tool integrated in the workstation software.

ADC-values were measured for each clearly demarcated lesion in ADC-map by drawing a circular region of interest into the tumour that encompassed as much of the lesion as possible while excluding vascular structures and necrotic tissue.

Imaging analysis was accomplished according to the following settings:

Table 1. Demographics, aetiology of liver cirrhosis and patients clinical condition.

Gender	
Male	42
Female	8
Mean age (years)	60.6 (range 29–84)
Mean weight (kg)	79.8 (range 45–120)
Aetiology of liver cirrhosis	
Alcoholic disease	26
Hepatitis B	2
Hepatitis C	3
Haemochromatosis	3
Budd-Chiari-Syndrome	1
Non-alcoholic steatohepatosis	1
Cryptogenic	14
Child Pugh Status	
A (5–6)	27
B (7–9)	16
C (10–15)	7

1) In general, CT-scans were compared with

2) complete MRI-examinations (including conventional dynamic MRI with hepatobiliary phase and DWI).

To estimate the impact of the hepatobiliary phase and diffusion-weighted imaging, MRI-data were subdivided into three sets:

3) conventional dynamic MRI without the hepatobiliary phase and DWI

4) dynamic MRI including the hepatobiliary phase

5) MRI including diffusion-weighted sequences.

In addition, the observer evaluated the reading time.

Statistical analysis

Statistical analysis was performed using SPSS 20.0 for Windows (statistical package for social sciences 20.0, Chicago, IL, USA) and Microsoft Excel (Microsoft, Redmond, WA, USA). The diagnostic performance of each technique was assessed by measuring the area under the curve (AUC) of the free-response receiver operating characteristic analysis (ROC-curve) on a lesion-per-patient-basis.

Sensitivity, specificity, and positive and negative predictive values were calculated for patients assigned a diagnostic confidence level of 4 and 5 (probably and definitely HCC). In addition, we included patients with a confidence level of 3, because in clinical routine, a suspicious lesion must be clarified (e.g., by further imaging or biopsy). The differences in the ROC-curves, sensitivities, specificities, positive predictive value (PPV) and negative predictive value (NPV) were statistically analysed using a binomial test. Student's t-test was used to calculate significant differences for image quality, detectability and reading time between the image modalities, P-values <0.05 were considered significantly different.

Table 2. MR Imaging Parameters.

Parameter	T2-weighted (HASTE)	T1-weighted (VIBE)	DWI	T2-weighted TSE	T1-weighted in and out of phase
Imaging plane	Coronal and axial	Coronal and axial unenhanced, axial enhanced	Coronal and axial	Coronal	Axial
Fat saturation	No	Yes	Yes	Yes	No
Respiratory triggering	Breath-hold (12 s)	Breath-hold (16 s)	Respiratory-triggered	Respiratory-triggered	Breath-hold (18 s)
Repetition time (TR)	800 ms	2.92 ms	2000 ms	2000 ms	212 ms
Echo time (TE)	83 s	0.86 ms	60 ms	81 ms	2.32 ms
Flip angle	160°	10°	-	120°	65°
Bandwidth	781 Hz/Px	540 Hz/Px	1736 Hz/Px	260 Hz/Px	930 Hz/Px
Field of view (FOV)	450 mm	400 mm	380 mm	400 mm	380 mm
Slice thickness	5 mm	3 mm	5 mm	5 mm	5 mm
Matrix	320*256	256*200	192*154	320*224	256*200

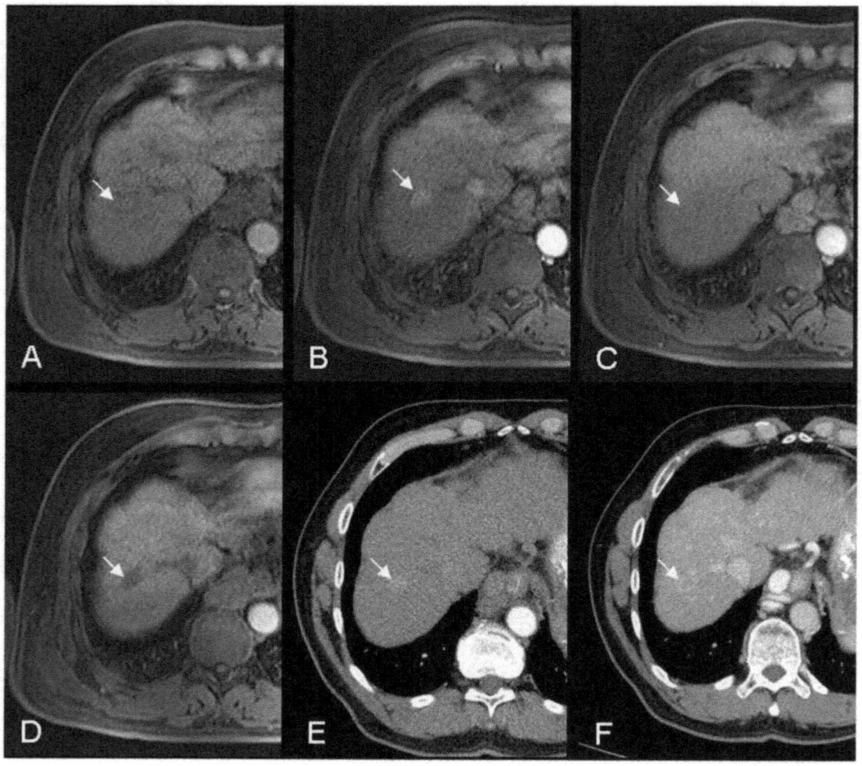

Figure 1. A 59-year-old male patient with liver cirrhosis (Child A) and HCC (arrow) in segment 7. Axial images: A) lesion is barely visible using unenhanced T1w-VIBE, B) marked arterial enhancement in T1w-VIBE following i.v. administration of contrast medium, C) typical washout of the lesion in the equilibrium phase (T1w-VIBE), and D) a clear hypointense lesion in the hepatobiliary phase (20 min after contrast agent injection, T1w-VIBE). Similar behaviour was observed with typical contrast medium enhancement in CT: E) early arterial phase after bolus tracking and F) washout in the portal venous phase with pseudocapsule.

Results

In 35 of 50 patients, the histopathological report after resection or biopsy of a lesion served as the gold standard for diagnosis, and in 24 of these 35 patients, the diagnosis of HCC was proven histopathologically. In 2 additional cases, HCC was diagnosed at follow-up (after 6 months) via clinical and paraclinical parameters.

In our study, 26 of 50 patients were positive for HCC (MRI-related: 9 patients with one lesion, 4 patients with 2 lesions, 3 patients with 3 lesions and 10 patients with 4 or more lesions).

ROC-curves for MRI displayed similar AUCs as observed for CT (0.837 vs. 0.798, $p=0.48$). Sensitivity and positive and negative predictive values were measured for both methods (sensitivity 92%, PPV 80% and NPV 90% for MRI vs. sensitivity 85%, PPV 79% and NPV 82% for CT). Specificity was 75% for both techniques (see Table 3 and Figure 2). False positives resulted from numerous metastases of a neuroendocrine carcinoma, one adenoma and regenerative nodules. Because we calculated sensitivity, specificity, and positive and negative predictive values on a per-patient-basis, our subset analyses revealed no differences.

On a *liver-lesion-per-patient basis*, we detected slightly more lesions that were suspicious for HCC using MRI compared to CT, but this value did not reach statistical significance (mean, 2.7 for MRI versus 2.3 for CT, $p=0.256$, Figure 3). One additional HCC was identified with aid of the hepatobiliary phase compared to conventional dynamic MRI; this lesion measured 8 mm in diameter (Figure 4). Compared to Gadolinium-EOB-DTPA-enhanced MRI-images evaluated with the hepatobiliary phase, no additional lesions were detected by DWI. However, DWI identified one additional malignant lesion compared to conventional dynamic MRI-scan. This was the same 8 mm diameter lesion that was observed with the hepatobiliary phase, and this finding impacted patient treatment (Figure 4).

Lesion size was similar using both methods, with an average greatest diameter of 33 mm for CT and 32 mm for MRI (measured in the arterial phase T1w VIBE; $p=0.195$). Twenty malignant neoplasms were >3 cm, 16 lesions were 2–3 cm and 35 lesions were <2 cm, as determined by MRI-scans.

ADC-measurements in 32 lesions showed extremely heterogeneous values, with a mean of $1.2\pm0.5\times10^{-3}$ mm^2/s (range, 0.07 ± 0.1 to $3.0\pm0.1\times10^{-3}$ mm^2/s; Figure 5).

The radiologist reported that the *detectability* of lesions was similar using both methods using a 5-point rating scale (2.6 for CT and 2.7 for MRI, $p=0.807$; range from 2.6 to 4.0 between sequences, 1 = excellent, 5 = unacceptable). The ability of MRI to detect lesions was significantly better using the hepatobilary phase (2.2, range from 1 to 4) compared to conventional dynamic MRI (2.9, $p=0.005$), but the difference was not significantly different compared to DWI (2.6, $p=0.125$).

Image quality (2.2 for CT vs. 2.3 for MRI, $p=0.249$, 2 = good, 3 = fair) was more scattered within MR sequences (1.8 in T1w HASTE and 2.9 in T2w TSE). Image quality was rated better for the hepatobiliary phase and conventional dynamic MRI than for DWI (2.0 for hepatobiliary phase, 2.1 for dynamic MRI without hepatobiliary phase and 2.7 for DWI, $p<0.001$). No significant disparity was noted between conventional dynamic MRI and the hepatobiliary phase ($p=0.342$).

Table 3. Diagnostic accuracy, sensitivity, specificity, PPV and NPV for MRI and CT (binomial test, $p<0.05=$ significant).

	MRI	CT	P-value
Diagnostic accuracy (AUC)	0.837	0.798	0.4795
Sensitivity	0.92	0.85	0.4795
Specificity	0.75	0.75	1.000
PPV	0.80	0.79	0.500
NPV	0.90	0.82	1.000

The average *reading time* for MR-images was16.9 min and significantly longer than the reading time for CT-scans, which averaged 4.5 min. ($p<0.001$).

Discussion

Accuracy

In our study, MRI showed similar diagnostic accuracy for the detection of HCC compared to CT. Reports by Akai et al. and Lee et al. demonstrated similar results with a tendency to higher diagnostic accuracy for MRI, but also without statistically significant differences [22,23]. One explanation for this discrepancy might be the high number of suspicious lesions with a diameter greater than 3 cm in our study population. Haradome et al. also showed no difference in diagnostic accuracy between conventional dynamic MRI and CT. However, using the hepatobiliary phase, MRI displayed significantly higher accuracy than CT, especially for lesions smaller than 1.5 cm [24]. Kim demonstrated that MRI has better sensitivity for the detection of HCCs due to an increased delineation of hypointensity of HCC at a three-minute late phase and a hepatocyte phase [25], supporting previous reports [26–28]. While these studies report that CT is inferior to MRI, the use of different contrast agents, older scanner technology and different scanning parameters of the CTs must be taken into account. Similar to our study parameters, several groups used an early arterial phase [25,27]. For example, Chan et al. described better conspicuity for hepatocellular carcinomas using a bolus tracking delay of 6s for achieving the arterial phase [29]. Other studies state that the late arterial phase (e.g., approximately 14–30 s from 100 HU-threshold) is the optimal scan window for the detection of HCC [30]. Moreover, differences in histopathological subtypes of HCC might also yield different enhancement patterns [31], making it difficult to clearly specify standard examination protocols.

Detectability and number of lesions

Although the reader rated the subjective detectability of liver lesions similarly for MRI and CT, slightly more liver lesions per patient were detected using 3T MRI. Although this did not reach statistical significance, it is important for therapeutic decisions because liver transplantation can achieve excellent results in patients with HCC according to the benchmark defined by the Milan criteria (solitary HCC of less than 5 cm or with up to three nodules of less than 3 cm) [32–34]. Furthermore, decision to surgically resect tumours or use minimally invasive therapies (i.e., radiofrequency ablation (RFA), laser-induced interstitial thermotherapy (LITT), microwave ablation (MWA), cryoablation and transarterial chemoembolisation (TACE), etc.) depends on number and size of hepatocellular carcinomas, as visualised using CT or MRI [35,36].

In our study, the detectability of lesions using MRI with the hepatobiliary phase 20 min after i.v. injection of Gd-EOB-DTPA was significantly better than conventional dynamic MRI. In one patient a suspicious lesion with a diameter of 8 mm was only observed with the hepatobiliary phase and DWI, but not with conventional dynamic MRI (Figure 4). This lesion changed the therapeutic management of the patient because it was the 4th HCC suspicious lesion in his liver, which excluded him from the liver transplantation list according to the Milan criteria [32]. These data support several studies reporting that Gd-EOB-DTPA enhanced MRI is superior to conventional dynamic MRI [17,21,24].

Gd-EOB-DTPA is a gadolinium-based, liver specific MRI contrast medium that allows diagnosis derived from haemodynamics during the extracellular phase and measures hepatocellular function during the hepatobiliary phase. Information regarding the degree of cellular differentiation might also be possible [18]. Concerning the timing of hepatobiliary phase imaging, Motosugi

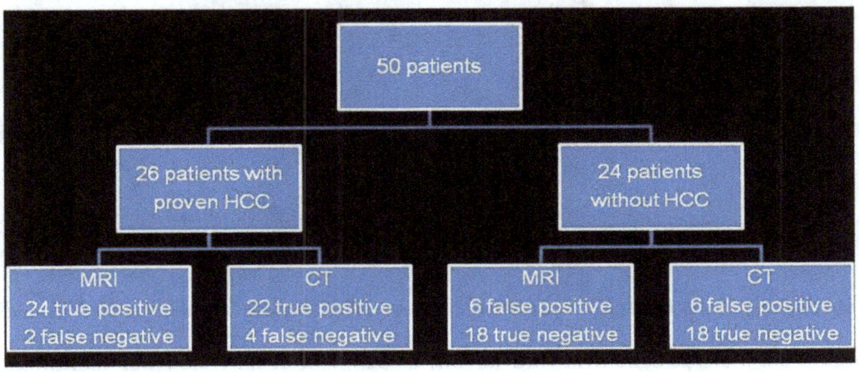

Figure 2. Flow chart for identification of patients with HCC in MRI and CT.

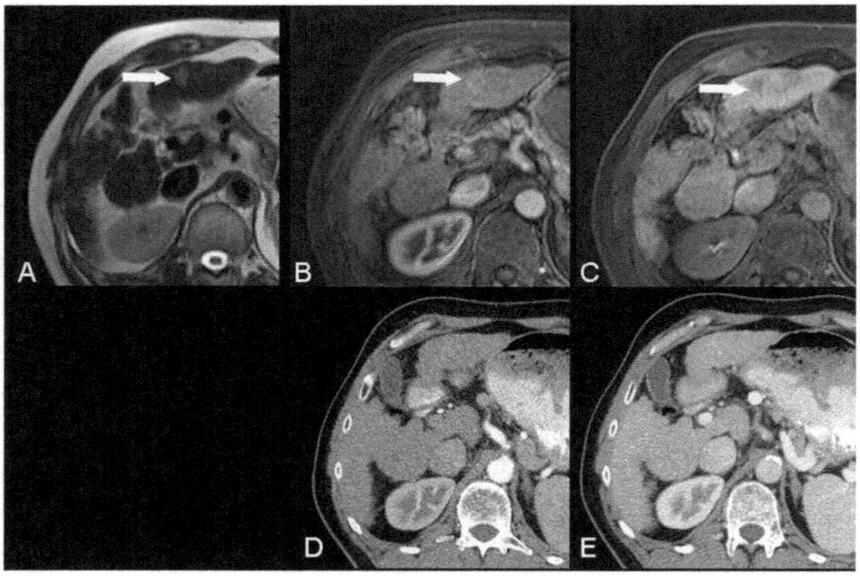

Figure 3. A 59-year-old male patient with liver cirrhosis and HCC (arrow) in S3 was only observed using MRI: *A*) markedly hyperintense HCC in T2w-HASTE axial, *B*) typical arterial enhancement in T1w-VIBE, and *C*) hypointense lesion in the hepatobiliary phase. No lesion was detected using CT: *D*) early arterial phase and *E*) portal venous phase.

et al. described that if the liver parenchyma is sufficiently enhanced 10 min after injection, no further imaging is necessary to detect focal liver lesions. However, the visual liver to spleen contrast scores 20 min after injection were frequently higher than 10 min images in patients with chronic liver diseases. These data indicate that a longer delay of 20 min might be more useful for patients with chronic liver diseases [37]. Because all of our patients suffered from chronic liver disease, we acquired hepatobiliary phase images 20 min after contrast application.

DWI

DWI is commonly used in liver imaging to assess various focal lesions. In particular, DWI has a higher detection rate and diagnostic performance for small, malignant liver lesions com-

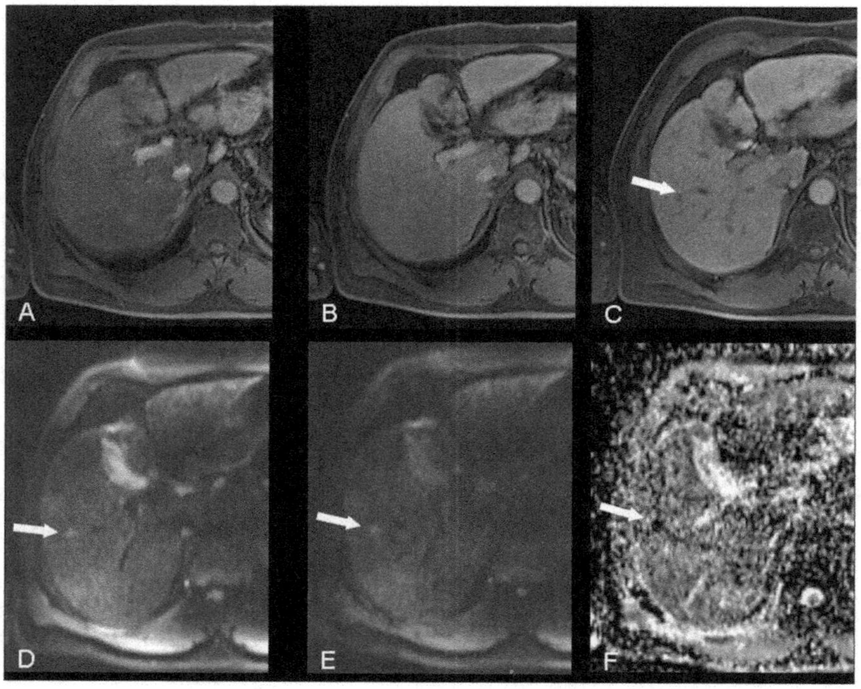

Figure 4. MRI of a 53-years-old male patient with HCC (arrow) in Segment 5: no lesion was identified in the arterial (A) and equilibrium phases (B), a small hypointense lesion was only observed in the hepatobiliary phase (C) and in DWI, where it is seen as a hyperintense lesion in b 50- (D) and b 400-images (E) and hypointense in the ADC-map (F).

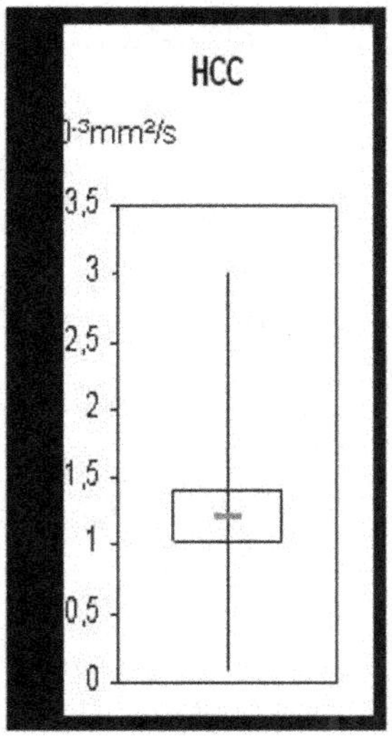

Figure 5. Range of ADC-values (10^{-3} mm²/s) in lesions suspicious for HCC.

pared to conventional dynamic MRI with different contrast agents; however, these results are not always significant [38–40]. A recent study by Holzapfel et al. reported no significant difference in diagnostic accuracy and sensitivity between diffusion weighted imaging, Gd-EOB-DTPA-enhanced imaging and combined imaging for the detection of focal liver lesions. However, for lesions smaller than 10 mm, a combination of DWI and Gd-EOB-DTPA significantly increased the overall detection rate. Similar to our findings regarding HCC-related diagnostic accuracy, Gadolinium-enhanced MRI and the combination of DWI and Gd-EOB-DTPA enhanced MRI demonstrated equal results [41]. In our 50 patients, just one additional HCC suspicious lesion was detected with DWI compared to conventional dynamic MRI, an 8 mm lesion that was also detected with hepatobiliary phase imaging. Therefore, DWI did not improve the detection of HCC compared to imaging with Gd-EOB-DTPA in our study.

Park et al. also demonstrated that DWI was outperformed by contrast enhanced T1-weighted imaging for the detection of HCC, but it represents a reasonable alternative [42]. However, if Gd-EOB-DTPA is used in the hepatic imaging, a time gap occurs between the equilibrium phase and the hepatobiliary phase, and because there is no significant impact of contrast media on achieving diffusion-weighted imaging and ADC-maps [43–45]. This gap can easily be filled with respiratory-triggered, diffusion-weighted imaging, which can provide additional information for the characterization of focal liver lesions. An important advantage of DWI is that no contrast agent is necessary, a property that is especially valuable for patients with poor renal function [39]. In our department, diffusion-weighted MR imaging is part of the routine liver protocol for all patients.

The potential to differentiate between benign and malignant liver lesions using ADC-quantification was previously reported in the literature [8–12]. Several thresholds have been proposed to accomplish this task, but there is still considerable overlap between benign and malignant liver lesions [9]. Vandecavaeye confirmed that there is no significant difference in ADC between malignant and benign lesions in patients with cirrhotic liver disease [46]. In our study, the mean ADC-value of HCC lesions was $1.2\pm0.5\times10^{-3}$ mm^2/s, which is similar to values reported in the literature. For example, Naoto measured an ADC-value of $1.31\pm0.28\times10^{-3}$ mm^2/s [12], and Holzapfel reported an ADC-value of $1.12\pm0.28\times10^{-3}$ mm^2/s for a small number of HCC samples [9]. These variances are likely due to differential cellularity of the tumours [47]. Another influential factor are the b-values chosen for DWI. In our study, we used relatively low b-values (b = 0, 50 and 400 s/mm^2), which have the disadvantage of being influenced by perfusion effects. Measured ADC-values tend to decrease as the b-value increases [48]. However, the use of low (perfusion-sensitive) b-values has several advantages: it provides a higher signal-to-noise ratio and more anatomical information of the liver, it is less sensitive to eddy current-induced distortions and it suppresses signals from the hepatic vasculature, which improves the detectability of perivascular lesions [49–51]. Further investigations are needed to determine the best b-values for liver imaging.

Our study has some limitations. First, there was a bias in patient recruitment because we included patients with proven or suspected HCC. This stipulation might result in an overestimation of specificity. Second, we could not achieve a histological proof for every detected lesion due to ethical reasons, so we had to use follow-up examinations and surrogates of clinical and paraclinical findings to confirm the presence of lesions. For this reason, we calculated sensitivity, specificity, and positive and negative predictive values on a patient basis. Third, our study group was relatively small, and further studies with more patients might yield statistically significant results. Fourth, we used a first generation MR-scanner with 3 Tesla, which can suffer from B0 artefacts within the liver parenchyma. Newer MR-Scanners with different coil and RF impulse designs (i.e., the TrueForm and Multi-Transmit) reduce these artefacts and can increase the diagnostic ability for liver imaging. Finally, we only determined ADC-values for suspicious lesions that were clearly visible in the ADC-map. However, our ADC-values were comparable to the values given in literature.

Conclusions

Our study did not show a statistically significant difference in detection of HCC between 3-Tesla Gd-EOB-DTPA-enhanced MRI with diffusion-weighted imaging and 64-slice contrast-enhanced CT.

As we detected slightly more lesions per patient using MRI, we recommend this imaging modality as the first-choice imaging method for the detection of HCC and individual therapeutic decisions. However, contrast-enhanced CT was not inferior in our study, indicating that it represents a useful image modality when MRI is not available or for follow-up examinations.

Author Contributions

Conceived and designed the experiments: BM PS. Performed the experiments: BM. Analyzed the data: PS DL BM. Contributed reagents/materials/analysis tools: BM PS TK. Wrote the paper: BM DL TK PS.

References

1. Bruix J, Sherman M (2005) Management of hepatocellular carcinoma. Hepatology 42: 1208–36
2. Kudo M (2010) The 2008 Okuda lecture: Management of hepatocellular carcinoma: from surveillance to molecular targeted therapy. J Gastroenterol Hepatol 25: 439–52

3. El-Serag HB (2007) Epidemiology of hepatocellular carcinoma in USA. Hepatol Res 37: S88–94
4. Tannapfel A, Wittekind C (2003) Pathology of hepatocellular carcinoma. Chir Gastroenterol 19: 225–230.
5. Tanimoto A, Lee JM, Murakami T, Huppertz A, Kudo M, et al. (2009) Consensus report of the 2nd International Forum for Liver MRI. Eur Radiol 19: S975–89
6. Zech CJ, Reiser MF, Herrmann KA (2009) Imaging of hepatocellular carcinoma by computed tomography and magnetic resonance imaging: state of art. Dig Dis 27: 114–24
7. Rempp H, Boss A, Helmberger T, Pereira P (2011) The current role of minimally invasive therapies in the management of liver tumors. Abdom Imaging 36: 635–47
8. Bruegel M, Holzapfel K, Gaa J, Woertler K, Waldt S, et al. (2008) Characterization of focal liver lesions by ADC measurements using a respiratory triggered diffusion-weighted single-shot echo-planar MR imaging technique. Eur Radiol 18: 477–85
9. Holzapfel K, Bruegel M, Eiber M, Ganter C, Schuster T, et al. (2010) Characterization of small (≤10 mm) focal liver lesions: value of respiratory-triggered echo-planar diffusion-weighted MR imaging. Eur J Radiol 76: 89–95
10. Moteki T, Ishizaka H, Horikoshi H, Matsumoto M (1995) Differentiation between hemangiomas and hepatocellular carcinomas with the apparent diffusion coefficient calculated from turboFLASH MR images. J Magn Reson Imaging 5: 187–91
11. Kim T, Murakami T, Takahashi S, Hori M, Tsuda K, et al. (1995) Diffusion-weighted single-shot echoplanar MR imaging for liver disease. AJR Am J - Roentgenol 173: 393–8
12. Koike N, Cho A, Nasu K, Seto K, Nagaya S, et al. (2009) Role of diffusion-weighted magnetic resonance imaging in the differential diagnosis of focal hepatic lesions. World J Gastroenterol 14; 15: 5805–12
13. Hamm B, Staks T, Mühler A, Bollow M, Taupitz M, et al. (1995) Phase I clinical evaluation of Gd-EOB-DTPA as a hepatobiliary MR contrast agent: safety, pharmacokinetics, and MR imaging. Radiology 195: 785–92
14. Clément O, Mühler A, Vexler V, Berthezène Y, Brasch RC (1992) Gadolinium-ethoxybenzyl-DTPA, a new liver-specific magnetic resonance contrast agent. Kinetic and enhancement patterns in normal and cholestatic rats. Invest Radiol 27: 612–9
15. Schuhmann-Giampieri G, Schmitt-Willich H, Press WR, Negishi C, Weinmann HJ, et al. (1992) Preclinical evaluation of Gd-EOB-DTPA as a contrast agent in MR imaging of the hepatobiliary system. Radiology 183: 59–64
16. Weinmann HJ, Schuhmann-Giampieri G, Schmitt-Willich H, Vogler H, Frenzel T, et al. (1991) A new lipophilic gadolinium chelate as a tissue-specific contrast medium for MRI. Magn Reson Med 22: 233–7
17. Huppertz A, Balzer T, Blakeborough A, Breuer J, Giovagnoni A, et al. (2004) Improved detection of focal liver lesions at MR imaging: multicenter comparison of gadoxetic acid-enhanced MR images with intraoperative findings. Radiology 230: 266–75
18. Huppertz A, Haraida S, Kraus A, Zech CJ, Scheidler J, et al. (2005) Enhancement of focal liver lesions at gadoxetic acid-enhanced MR imaging: correlation with histopathologic findings and spiral CT—initial observations. Radiology 234: 468–78
19. Reimer P, Rummeny EJ, Shamsi K, Balzer T, Daldrup HE, et al. (1996) Phase II clinical evaluation of Gd-EOB-DTPA: dose, safety aspects, and pulse sequence. Radiology 199: 177–83
20. Low RN (2007) Abdominal MRI advances in the detection of liver tumours and characterisation. Lancet Oncol 8: 525–35
21. Ahn SS, Kim MJ, Lim JS, Hong HS, Chung YE, et al. (2010) Added value of gadoxeticacid-enhanced hepatobiliary phase MR imaging in the diagnosis of hepatocellular carcinoma. Radiology 255: 459–66
22. Akai H, Kiryu S, Matsuda I, Satou J, Takao H, et al. (2011) Detection of hepatocellular carcinoma by Gd-EOB-DTPA-enhanced liver MRI: Comparison with triple phase 64 detector row helical CT. Eur J Radiol 80: 310–5
23. Lee CH, Kim KA, Lee J, Park YS, Choi JW, et al. (2012) Using low tube voltage (80kVp) quadruple phase liver CT for the detection of hepatocellular carcinoma: Two-year experience and comparison with Gd-EOB-DTPA enhanced liver MRI. Eur J Radiol 81: e605–11
24. Haradome H, Grazioli L, Tinti R, Morone M, Motosugi U, et al. (2011) Additional value of gadoxetic acid-DTPA-enhanced hepatobiliary phase MR imaging in the diagnosis of early-stage hepatocellular carcinoma: comparison with dynamic triple-phase multidetector CT imaging. J Magn Reson Imaging 34: 69–78
25. Kim YK, Kim CS, Han YM, Kwak HS, Jin GY, et al. (2009) Detection of hepatocellular carcinoma: gadoxetic acid-enhanced 3-dimensional magnetic resonance imaging versus multi-detector row computed tomography. J Comput Assist Tomogr 33: 844–50
26. Di Martino M, Marin D, Guerrisi A, Baski M, Galati F, et al. (2010) Intraindividual comparison of gadoxetate disodium-enhanced MR imaging and 64-section multidetector CT in the Detection of hepatocellular carcinoma in patients with cirrhosis. Radiology 256: 806–16
27. Pitton MB, Kloeckner R, Herber S, Otto G, Kreitner KF, et al. (2009) MRI versus 64-row MDCT for diagnosis of hepatocellular carcinoma. World J Gastroenterol 15: 6044–51
28. Sano K, Ichikawa T, Motosugi U, Sou H, Muhi AM, et al. (2011) Imaging study of early hepatocellular carcinoma: usefulness of gadoxetic acid-enhanced MR imaging. Radiology 261: 834–44
29. Chan R, Kumar G, Abdullah B, Ng Kh, Vijayananthan A, et al. (2011) Optimising the scan delay for arterial phase imaging of the liver using the bolus tracking technique. Biomed Imaging Interv J 7: e12
30. Kim MJ, Choi JY, Lim JS, Kim JY, Kim JH, et al. (2006) Optimal scan window for detection of hypervascular hepatocellular carcinomas during MDCT examination. AJR Am J Roentgenol 187: 198–206
31. Lee JH, Lee JM, Kim SJ, Baek JH, Yun SH, et al. (2012) Enhancement patterns of hepatocellular carcinomas on multiphasicmultidetector row CT: comparison with pathological differentiation. Br J Radiol 85: e573–83
32. Mazzaferro V, Bhoori S, Sposito C, Bongini M, Langer M, et al. (2011) Milan criteria in liver transplantation for hepatocellular carcinoma: an evidence-based analysis of 15 years of experience. Liver Transpl 17: S44–57
33. Cauchy F, Fuks D, Belghiti J (2012) HCC: current surgical treatment concepts. Langenbecks Arch Surg 397: 681–95
34. Mazzaferro V, Regalia E, Doci R, Andreola S, Pulvirenti A, et al. (1996) Liver transplantation for the treatment of small hepatocellular carcinomas in patients with cirrhosis. N Engl J Med 334: 693–699
35. Llovet JM (2005) Updated treatment approach to hepatocellular carcinoma. J Gastroenterol 40: 225–35
36. Kudo M, Okanoue T (2007) Japan Society of Hepatology. Management of hepatocellular carcinoma in Japan: consensus-based clinical practice manual proposed by the Japan Society of Hepatology. Oncology 72: S2–15
37. Motosugi U, Ichikawa T, Tominaga L, Sou H, Sano K, et al. (2009) Delay before the hepatocyte phase of Gd-EOB-DTPA-enhanced MR imaging: is it possible to shorten the examination time? Eur Radiol 19: 2623–9
38. Kim YK, Lee MW, Lee WJ, Kim SH, Rhim H, et al. (2012) Diagnostic accuracy and sensitivity of diffusion-weighted and of gdoxetic acid-enhanced 3-T MR Imaging alone or in combination in the detection of small liver metastasis (≤ 1.5 cm in diameter). Invest Radiol 47: 159–66
39. Yu JS, Chung JJ, Kim JH, Cho ES, Kim DJ, et al. (2011) Detection of small intrahepatic metastases of hepatocellular carcinomas using diffusion-weighted imaging: comparison with conventional dynamic MRI. Magn Reson Imaging 29: 985–92
40. Chung J, Yu JS, Kim DJ, Chung JJ, Kim JH, et al. (2011) Hypervascular hepatocellular carcinoma in the cirrhotic liver: diffusion-weighted imaging versus superparamagnetic iron oxide-enhanced MRI. Magn Reson Imaging 29: 1235–43
41. Holzapfel K, Eiber MJ, Fingerie AA, Bruegel M, Rummeny EJ, et al. (2012) Detection, classification, and characterization of focal liver lesions: value of diffusion-weighted MR imaging, gadoxetic acid-enhanced MR imaging and the combination of both methods. Abdom Imaging 37: 74–82
42. Park MS, Kim S, Patel J, Hajdu CH, Do RK, et al. (2012) Hepatocellular carcinoma: Detection with diffusion-weighted vs. contrast-enhanced MRI in pre-transplant patients. Hepatology 56: 140–8
43. Kinner S, Umutlu L, Blex S, Maderwald S, Antoch G, et al. (2012) Diffusion weighted MR imaging in patients with HCC and liver cirrhosis after administration of different gadolinium contrast agents: Is it still reliable? Eur J Radiol 81: 625–8
44. Choi JS, Kim MJ, Choi JY, Park MS, Lim JS, et al. (2010) Diffusion-weighted MR imaging of liver on 3.0-Tesla system: effect of intravenous administration of gadoxetic acid disodium. Eur Radiol 20: 1052–60
45. Chiu FY, Jao JC, Chen CY, Liu GC, Jaw TS, et al. (2005) Effect of intravenous gadolinium-DTPA on diffusion-weighted magnetic resonance images for evaluation of focal hepatic lesions. J Comput Assist Tomogr 29: 176–80
46. Vandecaveye V, De Keyzer F, Verslype C, Op de Beeck K, Komuta M, et al. (2009) Diffusion-weighted MRI provides additional value to conventional dynamic contrast-enhanced MRI for detection of hepatocellular carcinoma. Eur Radiol 19: 2456–66
47. Koike N, Cho A, Nasu K, Seto K, Nagaya S, et al. (2009) Role of diffusion-weighted magnetic resonance imaging in the differential diagnosis of focal hepatic lesions. World J Gastroenterol 15: 5805–12
48. Hollingsworth KG, Lomas DJ (2006) Influence of perfusion on hepatic MR diffusion measurement. NMR Biomed 19: 231–5
49. Nasu K, Kuroki Y, Nawano S, Kuroki S, Tsukamoto T, et al. (2006) Hepatic metastases: diffusion-weighted sensitivity-encoding versus SPIO-enhanced MR imaging. Radiology 239: 122–30
50. Goshima S, Kanematsu M, Kondo H, Yokoyama R, Kajita K, et al. (2008) Diffusion-weighted imaging of the liver: optimizing b value for the detection and characterization of benign and malignant hepatic lesions. J Magn Reson Imaging 28: 691–7
51. Takahara T, Kwee TC (2012) Low b-value diffusion-weighted imaging: Emerging applications in the body. J Magn Reson Imaging 35: 1266–73

19

Design and Development of a Robotized System Coupled to µCT Imaging for Intratumoral Drug Evaluation in a HCC Mouse Model

Gaétan Bour[1]*, Fernand Martel[2], Laurent Goffin[3], Bernard Bayle[3], Jacques Gangloff[3], Marc Aprahamian[1], Jacques Marescaux[1], Jean-Marc Egly[1,2]*

1 Institut de Recherche contre les Cancers de l'Appareil Digestif (IRCAD), Strasbourg, France, **2** IGBMC, Department of Functional Genomics and Cancer, CNRS/INSERM/ Université de Strasbourg, BP 163, Illkirch, C. U. Strasbourg, Strasbourg, France, **3** ICube laboratory UMR, CNRS 7357, University of Strasbourg, Strasbourg, France

Abstract

Hepatocellular carcinoma (HCC) is one of the most common cancer related deaths worldwide. One of the main challenges in cancer treatment is drug delivery to target cancer cells specifically. Preclinical evaluation of intratumoral drugs in orthotopic liver cancer mouse models is difficult, as percutaneous injection hardly can be precisely performed manually. In the present study we have characterized a hepatoma model developing a single tumor nodule by implantation of Hep55.1C cells in the liver of syngeneic C57BL/6J mice. Tumor evolution was followed up by µCT imaging, and at the histological and molecular levels. This orthotopic, poorly differentiated mouse HCC model expressing fibrosis, inflammation and cancer markers was used to assess the efficacy of drugs. We took advantage of the high precision of a previously developed robotized system for automated, image-guided intratumoral needle insertion, to administer every week in the tumor of the Hep55.1C mouse model. A significant tumor growth inhibition was observed using our robotized system, whereas manual intraperitoneal administration had no effect, by comparison to untreated control mice.

Editor: Kalpana Ghoshal, The Ohio State University, United States of America

Funding: The work was supported by the following: European Research Council Advanced Scientists grants (JME, http://erc.europa.eu/advanced-grants); Institut National du Cancer (INCA-2008-041, http://www.e-cancer.fr/); and Association de la Recherche contre le Cancer (ARC-N°3153, http://www.recherche-cancer.net/) (MA JME). The funders had no role in study design, data collection and analysis, decision to publish, or preparation of the manuscript.

Competing Interests: The authors have declared that no competing interests exist.

* Email: bour.gaetan@gmail.com (GB); egly@igbmc.fr (JME)

Introduction

Hepatocellular carcinoma (HCC) represents 80–85% of the primary malignant liver tumors and is the 3rd most common cancer related death worldwide, with a high increase in developed countries [1]. One of the main challenges in cancer treatment is the targeting of the drug to the tumor to increase the local concentration of the therapeutic agent and avoid major side effects on healthy tissues [2]. This is addressed by using either specifically formulated drug vehicles [2] or targeted therapies delivered by intravenous administration. Some cancers like early HCC can also be treated by radiofrequency, thermal ablation or percutaneous ethanol or acetic acid injection in the tumor [3]. Moreover, among the recent developments in cancer treatment, viral based gene therapy often requires an intratumoral administration [4–7]. Intratumoral injection is also frequently performed in the preclinical steps on animal models to develop and assess the efficacy of new therapies [8–13].

For many decades, carcinogenesis studies as well as assays in drug therapy utilized tumor rodent models. The recent development of medical imaging especially micro CT scanner (µCT), allows to follow the evolution of the disease and/or the therapy at high resolution, on the same model animal; it also make it possible to perform preclinical drug evaluation in a non-invasive manner on orthotopic rodent cancer models [14,15]. Additionally such experimental procedures might avoid the intense use of animal models.

Several types of cancer animal models are reported to study hepatocellular carcinoma [16]: (i) genetically engineered mice developing spontaneous tumors; (ii) chemical induction using carcinogens; (iii) xenograft models, in which HCC cells or tumors from human origin are injected subcutaneously or orthotopically into the liver of immunocompromised mice; (iv) syngeneic graft of rodent HCC cells or tumors; (iv) viral hepatocarcinogenesis. Graft of HCC cell lines is the fastest model as it allows tumor growth within days after implantation [14,15].

In the present study, we characterized a hepatoma model in immunocompetent mice, obtained by implantation of Hep55.1C cells [17] in the liver of syngeneic C57BL/6J mice. We demonstrated that this mouse model can be used to assess the efficacy of drugs taking advantage of a robotized system developed for automated, image-guided intratumoral administration [18].

Results

Development of a restrainer bed system for *in vivo* imaging

Since most μCT scanners do not allow to perform robotized procedures under CT guidance in real-time, we designed a robotized-cell and a process to use pre-operative scan data to precisely target the affected organ. However, the use of μCT scanner analysis for further robotized investigations has to be performed in well-defined conditions. First of all, the animal has to be maintained anesthetized during the whole procedure. We then modeled a dedicated bed for 4–8 week-old mice by Computer Assisted Design (Figure 1A). This bed is composed of three different parts: (i) the support frame of the bed that can be placed inside the μCT scanner, lipped on the existing carbon bed for imaging, as well as in the robotized cell for the image-guided robotized intratumoral administration of the drug. The mouse is maintained under gaseous anesthesia during the entire procedure; (ii) the hemi-cylindrical mouse restrainer that is plugged and screwed in the support frame, firmly restraining the animal in a comfortable position on its back (Figure 1B) to expose the abdomen of the mouse. A sterile operative field stuck on the shaved abdomen ensures that the mouse does not slide during the transfer from the scanner to the robotized cell. In addition, tensing the skin and compressing the abdomen facilitates the penetration of the needle during the robotized insertion step; (iii) the removable registration cover [18,19] screwed on the support frame, overlaps the mouse on the restrainer part (Figure 1C) during the imaging recording after which it will be removed prior to the needle insertion. A needle insertion system was developed [18], keeping into account the size of the animal, the skin elasticity and the internal organ displacement. A particular attention was paid to the choice of the needle, which length, diameter, and bevel must be compatible with either drug injection or biopsy. Except for the final injection, all the steps are automated, from the positioning outside the animal, to the insertion in the animal.

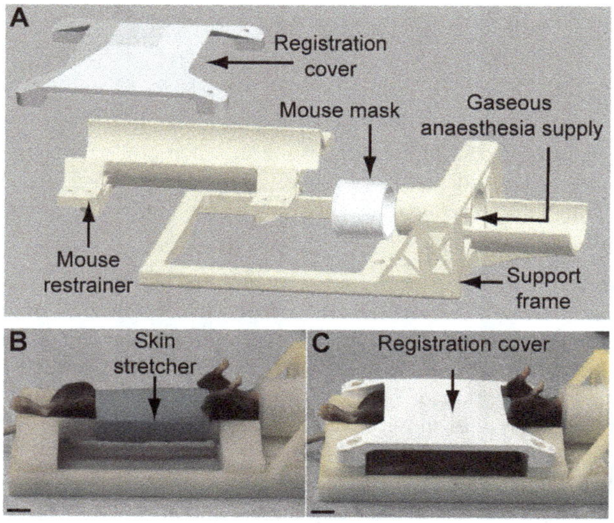

Figure 1. Mouse restrainer and robotized needle injector for intratumoral drug administration. **(A)** Description of the mouse restrainer bed. **(B)** View of a mouse restrained under gaseous anesthesia. The animal is tightly fixed on a hemicylindrical shell by a sterile operative field stuck on the abdomen. A sensor placed on the back of the mouse monitors respiration. **(C)** A dedicated registration cover is screwed on the bed frame during μCT scan imaging and registration by structured light projection.

Hepp55.1C cells induce fast growing orthotopic HCC

In parallel, to develop a HCC tumor model that would be accepted by immune competent mice, Hep55.1C and Hepa1.6 rodent HCC cell lines [17,20] were screened for their sensitivity to human standard therapeutic drugs for HCC and their tumorigenicity. We observed that Hep55.1C cells were more sensitive to Doxorubicin and Sorafenib than Hepa1.6 cells: IC50 values for Doxorubicin being around 0.10 μg/ml for Hep55.1C and 0.20 μg/ml for Hepa1.6, and in the range 6.6–10 μg/ml and 10–12.5 μg/ml respectively for Sorafenib (Figure 2A and 2B). Interestingly, Hep55.1C cells were found to be much more tumorigenic than Hepa1.6 cells, as all mice injected subcutaneously with Hep55.1C cells developed tumors, whereas Hepa1.6 tumors were observed in only 15% of the mice (Figure 2C).

We next followed HCC evolution in the Hep55.1C syngeneic orthotopic graft mouse model by recurrent μCT imaging and histological evaluation (Figure 3). An intrahepatic HCC was initiated by injection of 2×10^6 Hep55.1C cells either directly into the liver left lateral lobe or indirectly via the spleen. Macroscopically, Hep55.1C tumors appeared either as a white large nodule or as multiple small white nodules under liver capsule (Figure S1A and S1B). By micro CT imaging, contrast enhancement of the liver allowed a clear identification of the tumor nodules (TN) that remained hypo dense by comparison to normal contrast-enhanced liver (Figure S1C and S1D).

We focused on the intrahepatic graft model that developed single, well localized tumor nodules identified by μCT imaging, and more adapted to evaluate drug. The small nodule (initiated by the Hep55.1C cells) visualized at 2 weeks (in green on Figure 3A), expended progressively in the lobe (Figure 3B). The 3D reconstructions highlight the rapid increase in tumor volume from 5 to 9 weeks, rising from 2% to 40% (Figure 3B–C). Indeed, at 9 weeks, a large nodule invaded the left lateral liver lobe as well as the peritoneal cavity. We observed that the median survival was around 8 weeks, concurrently with the strong increase of tumor size (Figure S2). Similar results were also obtained by grafting Hep55.1C cells in male mice [21].

The progression of the tumor was also followed by histological examination. At 2 weeks after graft, Hep55.1C tumors presented small sized cells with an increasing nuclear/cytoplasm ratio and empty vesicles (right panel black arrows in Figure 3D) that could correspond to vesicular steatosis, in line with positive oil red O staining of tumor frozen section (Figure S3A). At that stage, Hep55.1C tumor cells were highly proliferative, as depicted by a Ki67 index of 40 (fraction of green positive nuclei in figure S3B), comparable to the Ki67 score observed in human HCC [22]. At 5 weeks the tumor exhibited a pseudo glandular aspect similar to a cholangiocarcinoma (Figure 3E, closed white arrows) and presented some features of non-alcoholic steatohepatitis (NASH) with vesicular steatosis (black arrow). At 9 weeks after graft, Hep55.1C tumors corresponded to a poorly differentiated human HCC (Grade III/IV) with a very dense fibrotic structure, and tumor cells with an almost invisible cytoplasm. Some glandular structures and vessels (indicated respectively by open and closed white arrows, Figure 3F) were observed at the periphery of the tumors. The presence of tumor neo-angiogenesis was assessed by immunofluorescence microscopy; we observed a labeling of vessels by the specific endothelial cell marker PECAM-1/CD31 (green staining in figure S3C). In addition, a very strong fibrosis appeared in early and advanced Hep55-1C tumors (Figure 3E–F) as visualized by silver and Sirius red staining for reticulin and collagen respectively

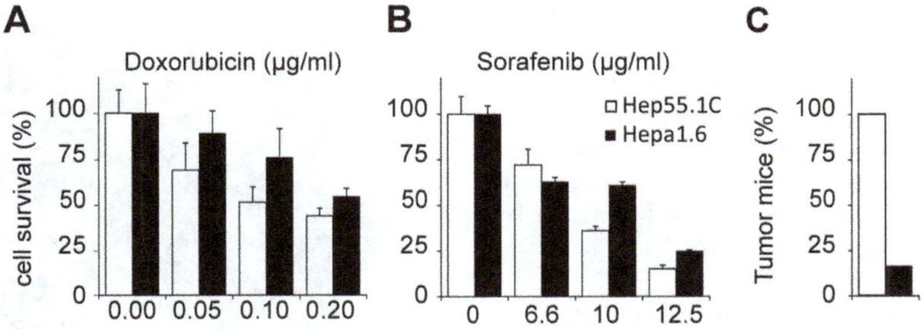

Figure 2. Screening of mouse hepatoma cell lines for chemical sensitivity and tumorigenicity. Hepa1.6 and Hep55.1C cells were exposed to Doxorubicin (**A**) and Sorafenib (**B**) for 3 days and assessed for toxicity using a cell proliferation assay. Results are shown as the mean +/− SD of triplicates. (**C**) Percentage of C57BL6J mice (n = 6) with palpable tumor two weeks after subcutaneous injection of either 10^6 Hepa1.6 or Hep55.1C in the back mice.

(Figure S3D and data not shown). Fibers of collagen and reticulin were scattered throughout the tumor, invading the anarchic Tumor cells and surrounding the pseudo glandular structures (white arrow in figure S3D. The presence of reticulin and collagen fibers inside the tumor is independent of animal sex, fibrosis deposition being observed following orthotopic graft of Hep55.1C cells in both male and female mice (data not shown).

We further investigated for the presence of fibrotic genes by RT-qPCR on Hep55.1C tumor extract (Figure 4). We observed a strong expression of type 1 collagen (COLA1), a major extracellular matrix component by comparison to surrounding normal liver cell extract. As collagen is mainly deposited by during fibrosis, the overexpression of both alpha smooth muscle actin (ASMA), and matrix metalloproteinase 3 (MMP3) genes, two activated stellate cells (HSC) markers was noted in tumor cells extract compared to wild type cells. Moreover, an increase in the mRNA level of signaling molecules associated with inflammation and hepatic stellate cell activation like interleukin-6 (IL-6), platelet derived growth factor beta (PDGFB); transforming growth factor beta (TGFB) was also marked by comparison to the surrounding liver cells (Figure 4). However, no expression of fibronectin 1 (FN-1), another extracellular matrix protein and fibrosis marker, was observed. Interestingly, we found that Hep55.1C tumor do not express albumin, a liver specific gene, in line with its poorly differentiated state. On the contrary, cyclin D1 (CCND1), implicated in cell cycle regulation and often dysregulated in cancers, and osteopontin (SPP1) a HCC marker [23–25], were highly expressed. The HCC specific marker alpha fetoprotein (AFP) was also overexpressed in the tumor extract (Figure 4), but also in the adjacent liver presumably as a consequence of liver

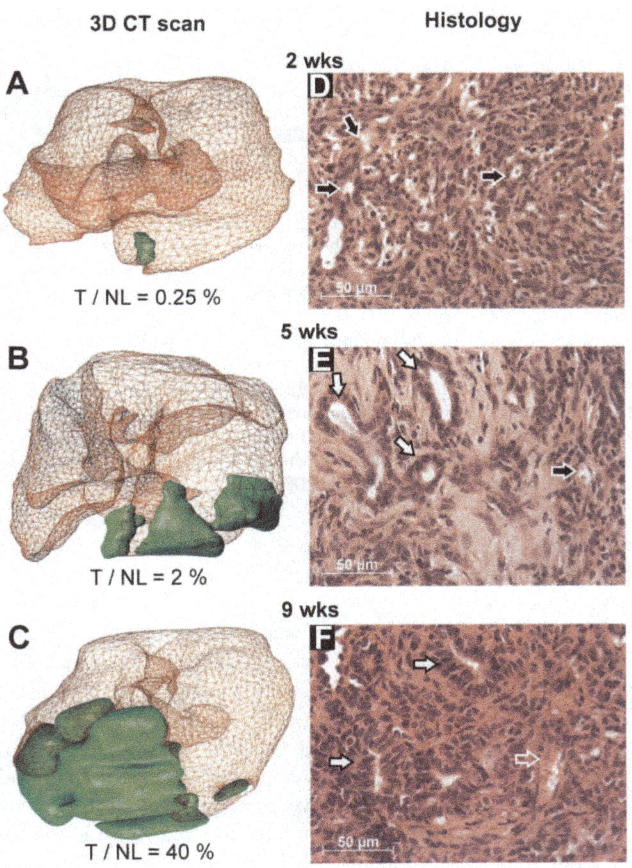

Figure 3. Evolution of tumor after intra liver injection of Hep55.1C cells. Evolution of liver tumor was followed by μCT scan imaging and histology two (**A, D**), five (**B, E**) and nine (**C, F**) weeks after Hep55.1C cells grafted in the liver of C57BL6/J mice. (**A–C**) 3D reconstructions from representative μCT scan showing the normal liver (red) and the tumor (green). Tumor/normal liver volume ratio (T/NL) computed from 3D reconstruction is indicated. (**D–F**) H&E staining of formalin fixed paraffin embedded tumors (black arrow: vesicle, closed white arrow: glandular structure; open white arrow: red blood cells).

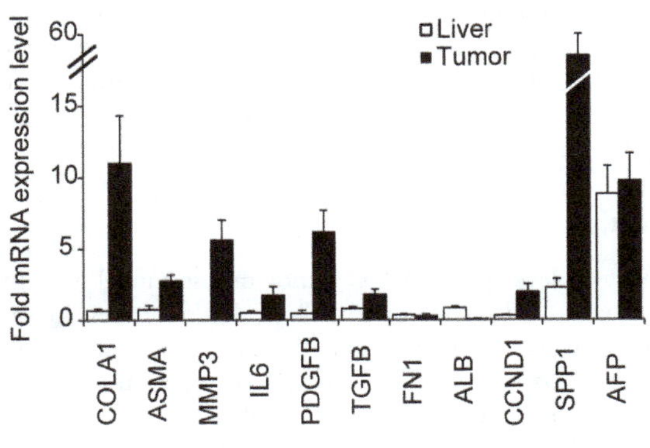

Figure 4. Hep55.1C tumors markers. Expression of COLA1, ASMA, MMP3, FN1 fibrosis markers, IL6, PDGFB, TGFB inflammation markers and ALB, CCND1, SPP1, AFP cancer markers was assessed by RTqPCR from Hep55.1C tumor and corresponding surrounding normal liver. Relative mRNA level of each gene was normalized to the level of the housekeeping gene 36B4. Results are expressed as the mean +/− SEM for at least 3 animals.

injury and regeneration consecutive to the graft and tumor growth [26].

The graft of Hep55.1C cells in the syngeneic mice liver allows the fast growth of a highly differentiated tumor, expressing fibrotic and cancer marker genes. Pretreatment of the mice with diethylnitrosamine for 4 weeks to induce liver fibrosis prior to Hep55.1C cell graft did not modify tumor growth and marker gene expression (Figure S4 and data not shown).

Robotized intratumoral injection inhibits Hep55.1C tumor growth

Having set up and followed the evolution of HCC tumor in mice, we evaluated the potency of intratumoral drug administration, using our system for image-guided robotized needle positioning [18]. μCT scan imaging helps to precisely position the needle of a disposable syringe filed with a test drug at the center of the tumor; the needle is positioned by a robot with a deviation lower than 0.3 mm (Figure S5 and [18]). We compared the growth of hepatic tumors in untreated mice to mice either treated intratumorally (IT) with Doxorubicin using our automated positioning system, or injected intraperitoneally (IP). For intratumoral injection, a 29G needle was used to facilitate the insertion while limiting damaging effects on tumors. In addition, it has been demonstrated in previous studies that the sole intratumoral injection of inactive compounds in rodent models of human cancers did not inhibit tumor growth [27,28]. Thus we postulated that a reduced tumor growth in the IT group could be attributed to the antineoplastic effect of Doxorubicin on tumor cells.

Treatment started two weeks after Hep55.1C cell inoculation in a liver lobe, once tumor was detected by μCT scan. In the IT group, each of the 3 mice was subjected to robotized administration of 10 μl of Doxorubicin, at the center of the tumor. In the IP group, the same amount of drug was injected manually in the peritoneum at the vicinity of the tumor. Tumor volume was determined for each mouse at each time point by 3D reconstruction from the μCT scan data (Figure 5A). Tumors resected at the end of the experiment after 3 weeks of treatment were smaller in the IT group than in the IP and control group. μCT scan follow up demonstrated that IT injection of Doxorubicin decreased tumor growing rate by comparison to untreated mice, as tumor volume in the IT group was significantly smaller than in the control group after 2 weeks (Figure 5B). However, no statistical difference was observed after manual IP injection of Doxorubicin, tumor growth being only slightly affected by drug administration (Figure 5B). In addition, a statistical increase in apoptosis was evidenced by TUNEL assay in the tumor injected intratumorally with Doxorubicin by comparison to the non-treated control group (Figure S6).

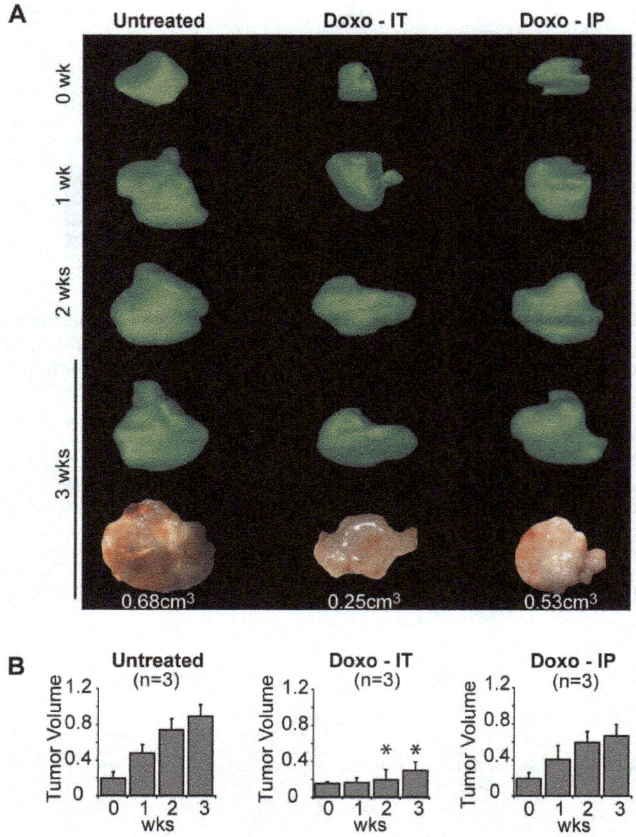

Figure 5. Treatment of Hep55.1C mouse HCC model by Doxorubicin. Mice bearing orthotopic HCC tumors were treated by recurrent automated robotized intratumoral injection (IT, n = 3) or manual intraperitoneal (IP, n = 3) of Doxorubicin; untreated mice (n = 3) were used as control of tumor growth. (**A**) Representative 3-weeks follow-up by μCT scan imaging and 3D reconstruction of tumor development. Volumes of the tumors resected at the end of the experiment were measured. (**B**) Tumor volume was computed at each time point from the 3D reconstructions of the tumors in untreated (left), IT (middle) or IP (right) injected mice (mean +/− SEM, star (*) indicates a difference with untreated control at the same time point with $p<0.05$).
doi:10.1371/journal.pone.0106675.g005

Discussion

Here we have developed a HCC tumor mouse model and an automated image-guided system to follow the tumor evolution overtime and evaluate the potency of anti-cancer drugs. Among all HCC animal models, tumor cell graft is most appropriate for rapid development of a single tumor nodule. One of the main limitations of the tumor graft model in immune-competent animals is tumor rejection. The Hepa1.6 cells [20] are rejected in the majority of C57BL/6J mice [29–36], probably due to differences between cell line and host haplotypes. On the contrary, we observed that the Hep55.1C cell line, deriving from a C57BL/6J tumor [17], is tumorigenic after subcutaneous, intra hepatic or intra splenic injection, in 100% of both male and female mice. This model, based on the Hep55.1C cells harboring a mutation in the β-catenin pathway [17,37] represents a reproducible HCC model in the C57BL/6J mouse strain, which has a low susceptibility to spontaneous cancers.

At the histological level, these tumor cells resemble a poorly differentiated human HCC, with small sized cell, a high proliferation index, and duct like structures. A high level of fibrosis was also evidenced in the tumor as reported for other syngeneic or xenogeneic liver tumor models in mouse [38,39]. At the molecular level, an increased expression of inflammatory and pro-fibrotic genes has been observed, in line with hepatic stellate cell activation. Recent studies demonstrated that hepatic stellate cells not only play a major role in fibrosis, but also in liver development, regeneration, and cancer, notably by promoting HCC cell growth [40–42]. The Hep55.1C tumors being vascularized, expressing some human cancer and HCC markers like osteopontin, cyclin D1 and AFP, the model seemed suitable to analyze the effect of anti-cancer or anti-fibrotic drugs.

Several therapies in preclinical development or evaluated in clinical trials require intratumoral administration [4–6,43–45] that helps to reduce toxicity on normal tissue and improve treatment efficacy as concentration is locally increased. In rodents, one of the main constraints is the small size of the tumor necessitating to perform a laparotomy [35] for direct injection in orthotopic tumors. We here have designed a dedicated animal restrainer bed allowing both reproducible positioning of the animal in the µCT scan for longitudinal follow-up, and firm animal restrainment for accurate percutaneous needle insertion. Our image guided system for percutaneous drug administration did not damage surrounding tissues (see also [18,19]).

By combining µCT imaging and 3D reconstructions [15,21], we localized and computed the volume of liver tumors after intrahepatic or intrasplenic graft of Hep55.1C cells. As an example, we demonstrated that the robotized intratumoral injection of low amount of Doxorubicin, a drug used notably for transarterial chemoembolization of HCC [46], significantly reduced tumor growth by around 60% after 3 weeks, whereas manual intraperitoneal administration of the same amount of drug has no significant effect on tumor evolution.

The high accuracy of the system would also allow to perform recurrent tumor micro biopsy to analyze on the same animal at the molecular level, the evolution of specific markers, notably in response to drug administration. Due to the high level of fibrosis in the tumor, this model could also be used to test anti fibrotic drugs. Further developments will include the reduction of the duration of the robotized procedure for routine use on larger groups of animal, and also the development of a microbiopsy needle to retrieve biological samples from recurrent robotized biopsies.

Materials and Methods

Ethics statement

The project was approved by the local ethics committee (ICOMETH), under the permit number 38.2011.01.011. All experiments were performed under gaseous anesthesia, and animals were euthanized by overdosage of anesthesia followed by cervical dislocation.

Cell lines

Hep-55.1C derived from DENA induced HCC in C57BL/6J mouse [17] was obtained from Cell Lines Service (Eppelheim, Germany) and maintained in Dulbecco's modified Eagle's medium supplemented with 4.5 g/L glucose and 10% fetal bovine serum in a 5% CO2 humidified chamber. The Hepa1.6 cell line derived from an HCC tumor in a C57L/J mouse [20] was obtained from ATCC and maintained in Dulbecco's modified Eagle's medium supplemented with 1 g/L glucose and 10% fetal bovine serum in a 5% CO2 humidified chamber.

Cytotoxicity assay

24 h before treatment, 1.5 10^3 Hep55.1C or Hepa1.6 cells were seeded in 96 well plates. 50–70% confluent cells were treated with Sorafenib (Nexavar, Bayer), Doxorubicin (Adriamycin, Pfizer) or DMSO for 72 h and MTT (Sigma-Aldrich) dissolved in DMEM was added to the cells for 4 h. MTT formazan crystals were then dissolved in isopropanol: HCl (10:1) containing 0.01% NP-40. Background absorbance at 690 nm was subtracted from the measurement at 570 nm.

Mouse Hepatoma tumor model

C57BL/6J mice (Janvier Labs, France) experiments were realized under anesthesia, following FELASA recommendations and local ethics committee approval. For subcutaneous tumor, 10^6 cells resuspended in PBS (Sigma-Aldrich) where injected subcutaneously in the back of anaesthetized mice. For orthotopic tumor graft, 2×10^6 Hep55.1C cells were injected in the left liver lateral lobe of anaesthetized 8 week-old mice after midline laparotomy as described in [21]. Diffuse HCC was induced after injection of 2×10^6 Hep55.1C cells in PBS into the spleen of C57BL/6J mice following subcostal incision under gaseous anesthesia.

Mouse Scanning procedure

MicroCT images were obtained on a micro CAT II scanner (Imtek Inc, Siemens) at 80 kVp X-ray voltage and 500 µA anode current under general gaseous anesthesia with isoflurane (Abbott). Respiratory-gated images were acquired with a voxel size of 119×119×119 µm, corresponding to a scanned volume of 6.1×6.1×6.1 cm to encompass the whole registration cover.

Four hours before imaging, animals were injected intraperitoneally with 6 µl/g Fenestra LC (ART, Canada) liver contrast agent. This polyiodinated contrast agent is taken-up specifically by normal hepatocytes via the ApoE cell surface receptors [47,48]. Five min before µCT scan the mouse was anaesthetized, the abdomen was shaved and disinfected. The mouse was then positioned on the restrainer bed and fastened with a sterile sticky operative field. A pressure pad placed on the back of the mouse and connected to a pressure transducer served to gate µCT imaging and needle insertion on animal respiration.

µCT images exported by the AMIRA software were processed with VR-Render (available at http://www.ircad.fr/softwares) for visualization and planning or with 3DVPM for tumor segmentation, 3D reconstruction and to compute tumor volume [49,50].

Histology

Excised tumors and normal liver were fixed in 10% formalin and embedded in paraffin after dehydration in ethanol and xylene substitute. 5 µm thick sections were stained with Eosin and Haematoxylin for morphometric analyses. Reticulin was stained with silver according to Gordon and Sweet [51], collagen was stained with Sirius Red (Euromedex, France). For immunofluorescence, tissue was frozen in OCT embedding medium above liquid nitrogen. After permeabilization/fixation in 4% PFA, 0.1% Triton X-100 in PBS, 5 µm thick cryosection were saturated with PBS-5% BSA, and incubated with primary anti-PECAM-1 or anti-Ki-67 (Santa Cruz Biotech) and secondary AlexaFluor 488 anti-Rabbit antibodies. Lipid vesicles were stained using Oil Red O (Sigma-Aldrich, France) on frozen section. For apoptosis detection, TUNEL assay was performed on paraffin sections using the Apoptag Red in situ detection kit (Merck Millipore, France), according to the manufacturer recommendations. Images were acquired with an Axiophot microscope equipped with a CDD camera (Axiocam, Carl Zeiss) and processed with Photoshop CS4.

RT-PCR

Tumor and normal liver samples were homogenized in a Fastprep apparatus (MP Biomedical) in Lysis Matrix B tubes (MP Biomedical) containing lysis buffer (Sigma). RNAs were purified with the mammalian Genelute kit from Sigma, according to the manufacturer recommendations. 3 µg of RNA were used as template for reverse transcription with random hexamer in the presence of 200 units of Superscript II reverse transcriptase (Invitrogen). cDNA were analyzed by real time quantitative PCR on a Chromo4 (Biorad), using Quantitect mastermix (Qiagen). Primer sequences for the PCR were as follows: 36B4: 5′-GAGGTCACTGTGCCAGCTCA-3′ and 5′-GAAGGTGTACTCAGTCTCCA-3′; AFP: 5′-GGCAAAGCCC-TACAGACCA-3′ and 5′-TAAACGCCCAAAGCATCAC-3′; ALB: 5′-CCCTGTTGCTGAGACTTGCT-3′ and 5′-CTGAGGTGC-TTTCTGGGTGT-3′; ASMA: 5′-GGCTGTGCTGTCCCTCT-ATG-3′ and 5′-TCTCACGCTCGGCAGTAGTC-3′; CCND1:

5′-AACTACCTGGACCGCTTCCT-3′ and 5′-GCTTGTTCT-CATCCGCCTCT-3′; COLA1: 5′-TTTGGAGAGAGCATGAC-CGA-3′ and 5′-AAGTTCCGGTGTGACTCGTG-3′; IL-6: 5′-AGGATACCACTCCCAACAGAC-3′ and 5′-AGTGCATCATC-GTTGTTCATAC-3′; FN1: 5′-CCACCTCGAGCCCGTTATAG-3′ and 5′-GCAGAGGCTGCAGGGTAGTA-3′; MMP3: 5′-CAC-GAGGAGCTAGCAGGTTA-3′ and 5′-TCCAACTGCGAAGA-TCCACT-3′; PDGFB: 5′-CCGGTCCAGGTGAGAAAGAT-3′ and 5′-AATAACCCTGCCCACACTCT-3′; SPP1: 5′-GCTTG-GCTTATGGACTGAGG-3′ and 5′-CTCTCCTGGCTCTCT-TTGGA-3′; TGFB: 5′-ATTCAGCGCTCACTGCTCTT-3′ and 5′-ACTTCCAACCCAGGTCCTTC-3′.

Robotic System Design

The robotized procedure for image-guided percutaneous injection has been described [18]. Briefly, a specific mouse restrainer bed (Figure 1A–C) was developed and prototyped by stereolithography (Initial, France) in ABS-like epoxy resin (Protogen 18420) to maintain the animal during the different steps of the procedure. Animal respiration is monitored via a custom developed software using a pressure pad placed on the back of the animal and connected to a Unik5000 pressure transducer (GE, France) linked to a USB multifunction I/O NI 6800 (National Instruments, France). Following mouse imaging in the μCT scan, the needle insertion is performed in a robotized cell according to the trajectory defined in the μCT scan images, from the skin entry point to the center of the tumor. The robotized system is composed of a 6-degree of freedom (DOF) robotic arm RV-1A (Mitsubishi), holding a needle injector and able to reproduce the motion of a human arm with high accuracy and excellent repeatability (+/−0.02 mm). Two stereoscopic cameras (AVT Marlin, Stemmer Imaging, France) are fixed on a tripod to observe the mouse bed with an angle of about 55°. A grid projector fixed on the top of the robotized cell projects structured light on the bed as detailed in [18]. The needle injector is composed of a high speed linear motorized stage M-663 (PI France S.A.S) driven by a C-867 controller (PI France S.A.S). A disposable 29G Myjector syringe (Terumo/Thermo Fisher, France) filed with the drug is fixed on the needle injector prior to the calibration of the system.

Non-invasive follow-up of HCC evolution and intratumoral robotized drug administration

Nine mice bearing an orthotopic Hep55.1C hepatoma tumor were randomly assigned to 3 groups. IP mice received every week 10 μl of a solution of Doxorubicin at 2 mg/ml intraperitoneally under anesthesia; robotized intratumoral injection of Doxorubicin was applied to IT mice, and untreated mice were used as control. Tumor volume was determined every week by μCT imaging and 3D reconstruction of the tumors using 3DVPM [49]. Mean tumor volumes and standard deviations were determined for each group at each time point. When tumor volume reached 5% of total body weight, as determined by μCT imaging, (assuming 1 cm^3 of tumor weights 1 g) in one mouse, the experiments was stopped, all mice were sacrificed, and the tumors dissected.

Supporting Information

Figure S1 Orthotopic HCC development after inoculation of hepatoma cells in the liver or in the spleen. Hep55.1C cells were surgically injected either in the liver left lateral lobe (**A, C**) or in the spleen (**B, D**) of C57BL/6J mice. (**A**) Macroscopic appearance of a unique tumor nodule (TN) 6 weeks after Hep55.1C cell inoculation in the liver (L). (**B**) Macroscopic appearance of multiple sub capsular tumor nodules (TN) 6 weeks after Hep55.1C cells injection in the spleen. (**C, D**) Contrast enhanced μCT imaging was performed 6 weeks after Hep55.1C cell inoculation. Hypodense tumor nodules (TN) in normal liver lobes (L) and in the spleen (S) are delineated by dotted lines (scale bar: 3 mm).

Figure S2 Mice survival after intrahepatic Hep55.1C cell injection correlates with increased tumor volume determined by μCT-scan. The evolution Hep55.1C orthotopically grafted mice (n = 20) was followed over 18 weeks (black line). Tumor volume (dashed line) was measured on a subset of animals (n = 6) by contrast enhanced μCT scan. For ethical reasons, animal were sacrificed when tumor size exceeded the maximal ethical volume or when humane endpoints were reached.

Figure S3 Histological characterization of Hep55.1C tumors. (**A**) Oil red O staining of lipid vesicles in Hep55.1c tumor 2 weeks after graft. (**B**) Proliferative tumor cells evidenced by immunofluorescent staining of the nuclear Ki-67 cell proliferation marker (green). Nuclei were counterstained with DAPI (blue). (**C**) Tumor vascularization evidenced by PECAM-1 endothelial cell marker immunofluorescent staining (green) 5 weeks after graft. (**D**) Silver staining of reticulin fibers in Hep55.1C tumors demonstrating the presence of fibrosis (black arrow) surrounding duct like structures (white arrow) 9 weeks after graft.

Figure S4 Fibrosis induction by diethylnitrosamine. Fibrosis was induced in the liver of C57BL6/J mice prior to Hep55.1C cell graft by weekly DENA injection. (**A**) Liver fibrosis evidenced by increased Sirius red staining of the collagen fibers (black arrow). (**B**) Western Blot demonstrates the increased expression of ASMA following activation of Hepatic Stellate Cells by DENA.

Figure S5 In vitro evaluation of image guided robotized needle positioning. (**A**) Volume Rendering view from μCT scan of the mouse restrainer bed filed with an 80%parafin: 20%solvent phantom. 22 virtual targets were defined in this phantom (yellow sphere, only 7 targets (T1 to T7) are represented). (**B**) Axial view of the needle track observed on a post-operative μCT scan of the phantom after robotized positioning. The distance between the targeted position (T1) and the needle tip stop was measured to calculate the precision of the procedure. (**C**) Box plot representing the positioning precision in the three dimensions for from 3 independent experiments on 22 targets (mean: white dash; 1st and 3rd percentile: white rectangle; min/max values: black dashes).

Figure S6 Intratumoral injection of Doxorubicin increases apoptosis. Apoptosis was evidenced in tumors from the non-treated control group (**A, B**) and from the intratumorally injected group (**C, D**) by indirect TUNEL assay. Nuclei were counterstained with DAPI. (**E**) Mean positive nuclei observed per microscope field of view at magnification 40x.

Acknowledgments

We thank Francine Gosse for excellent technical expertise. Thanks are also due to Emmanuel Compe and Luc Soler for fruitful discussion.

Author Contributions

Conceived and designed the experiments: GB FM LG BB JG MA JM JME. Performed the experiments: GB FM LG. Analyzed the data: GB FM LG BB JG MA JM JME. Contributed reagents/materials/analysis tools: GBM FM LG. Contributed to the writing of the manuscript: GB FM LG BB JG MA JM JME.

References

1. Llovet JM, Burroughs A and Bruix J (2003) Hepatocellular carcinoma. Lancet 362: 1907–1917.
2. Arias JL (2011) Drug delivery strategies in targeting cancer: current concepts and future developments. Curr Drug Targets 12: 1094–1095.
3. Shiina S, Teratani T, Obi S, Sato S, Tateishi R, et al. (2005) A Randomized Controlled Trial of Radiofrequency Ablation With Ethanol Injection for Small Hepatocellular Carcinoma. Gastroenterology 129: 122–130.
4. Harrington KJ, Hingorani M, Tanay MA, Hickey J, Bhide SA, et al. (2010) Phase I/II study of oncolytic HSV GM-CSF in combination with radiotherapy and cisplatin in untreated stage III/IV squamous cell cancer of the head and neck. Clin Cancer Res 16: 4005–4015.
5. Harrington KJ, Karapanagiotou EM, Roulstone V, Twigger KR, White CL, et al. (2010) Two-stage phase I dose-escalation study of intratumoral reovirus type 3 dearing and palliative radiotherapy in patients with advanced cancers. Clin Cancer Res 16: 3067–3077.
6. Park BH, Hwang T, Liu TC, Sze DY, Kim JS, et al. (2008) Use of a targeted oncolytic poxvirus, JX-594, in patients with refractory primary or metastatic liver cancer: a phase I trial. Lancet Oncol 9: 533–542.
7. Sung MW, Yeh HC, Thung SN, Schwartz ME, Mandeli JP, et al. (2001) Intratumoral adenovirus-mediated suicide gene transfer for hepatic metastases from colorectal adenocarcinoma: results of a phase I clinical trial. Mol Ther 4: 182–191.
8. Borovjagin AV, McNally LR, Wang M, Curiel DT, MacDougall MJ, et al. (2010) Noninvasive monitoring of mRFP1- and mCherry-labeled oncolytic adenoviruses in an orthotopic breast cancer model by spectral imaging. Mol Imaging 9: 59–75.
9. Fernandes MS, Gomes EM, Butcher LD, Hernandez-Alcoceba R, Chang D, et al. (2009) Growth inhibition of human multiple myeloma cells by an oncolytic adenovirus carrying the CD40 ligand transgene. Clin Cancer Res 15: 4847–4856.
10. Kolodkin-Gal D, Zamir G, Edden Y, Pikarsky E, Pikarsky A, et al. (2008) Herpes simplex virus type 1 preferentially targets human colon carcinoma: role of extracellular matrix. J Virol 82: 999–1010.
11. Lun X, Chan J, Zhou H, Sun B, Kelly JJ, et al. (2010) Efficacy and safety/toxicity study of recombinant vaccinia virus JX-594 in two immunocompetent animal models of glioma. Mol Ther 18: 1927–1936.
12. Penheiter AR, Wegman TR, Classic KL, Dingli D, Bender CE, et al. (2010) Sodium iodide symporter (NIS)-mediated radiovirotherapy for pancreatic cancer. AJR Am J Roentgenol 195: 341–349.
13. Suggitt M and Bibby MC (2005) 50 years of preclinical anticancer drug screening: empirical to target-driven approaches. Clin Cancer Res 11: 971–981.
14. Akladios CY, Bour G, Balboni G, Mutter D, Marescaux J, et al. (2011) [Contribution of microCT structural imaging to preclinical evaluation of hepatocellular carcinoma chemotherapeutics on orthotopic graft in ACI rats]. Bull Cancer 98: 120–132.
15. Aprahamian M, Bour G, Akladios CY, Fylaktakidou K, Greferath R, et al. (2011) Myo-InositolTrisPyroPhosphate treatment leads to HIF-1alpha suppression and eradication of early hepatoma tumors in rats. Chembiochem 12: 777–783.
16. Leenders MW, Nijkamp MW and Borel Rinkes IH (2008) Mouse models in liver cancer research: a review of current literature. World J Gastroenterol 14: 6915–6923.
17. Kress S, Konig J, Schweizer J, Lohrke H, Bauer-Hofmann R, et al. (1992) p53 mutations are absent from carcinogen-induced mouse liver tumors but occur in cell lines established from these tumors. Mol Carcinog 6: 148–158.
18. Goffin L, Bour G, Martel F, Nicolau S, Gangloff J, et al. (2013) Design and In Vivo Evaluation of a Robotized Needle Insertion System for Small Animals. Biomedical Engineering, IEEE Transactions on 60: 2193–2204.
19. Ayadi A, Bour G, Aprahamian M, Bayle B, Graebling P, et al. (2007) Fully automated image-guided needle insertion: application to small animal biopsies. Conf Proc IEEE Eng Med Biol Soc 2007: 194–197.
20. Darlington GJ, Bernhard HP, Miller RA and Ruddle FH (1980) Expression of liver phenotypes in cultured mouse hepatoma cells. J Natl Cancer Inst 64: 809–819.
21. Bousserouel S, Bour G, Kauntz H, Gosse F, Marescaux J, et al. (2012) Silibinin inhibits tumor growth in a murine orthotopic hepatocarcinoma model and activates the TRAIL apoptotic signaling pathway. Anticancer Res 32: 2455–2462.
22. Grigioni WF, D'Errico A, Bacci F, Gaudio M, Mazziotti A, et al. (1989) Primary liver neoplasms: evaluation of proliferative index using MoAb Ki67. J Pathol 158: 23–29.
23. Luo JH, Ren B, Keryanov S, Tseng GC, Rao UN, et al. (2006) Transcriptomic and genomic analysis of human hepatocellular carcinomas and hepatoblastomas. Hepatology 44: 1012–1024.
24. Gotoh M, Sakamoto M, Kanetaka K, Chuuma M and Hirohashi S (2002) Overexpression of osteopontin in hepatocellular carcinoma. Pathol Int 52: 19–24.
25. Wu JC, Sun BS, Ren N, Ye QH and Qin LX (2010) Genomic aberrations in hepatocellular carcinoma related to osteopontin expression detected by array-CGH. J Cancer Res Clin Oncol 136: 595–601.
26. Bisgaard HC, Nagy Ton PPT, Hu Z and Thorgeirsson SS (1994) Modulation of keratin 14 and α-fetoprotein expression during hepatic oval cell proliferation and liver regeneration. Journal of Cellular Physiology 159: 475–484.
27. Angelova AL, Aprahamian M, Balboni G, Delecluse HJ, Feederle R, et al. (2009) Oncolytic rat parvovirus H-1PV, a candidate for the treatment of human lymphoma: In vitro and in vivo studies. Mol Ther 17: 1164–1172.
28. Li J, Bonifati S, Hristov G, Marttila T, Valmary-Degano S, et al. (2013) Synergistic combination of valproic acid and oncolytic parvovirus H-1PV as a potential therapy against cervical and pancreatic carcinomas. EMBO molecular medicine 5: 1537–1555.
29. Nakatsuka K, Sugiyama H, Nakagawa Y and Takahashi H (1999) Purification of antigenic peptide from murine hepatoma cells recognized by Class-I major histocompatibility complex molecule-restricted cytotoxic T-lymphocytes induced with B7-1-gene-transfected hepatoma cells. J Hepatol 30: 1119–1129.
30. Zhang BN, Watanabe S, Kohyama M, Saijo K, Kusakabe M, et al. (2000) Tumor formation suppressed in gammadeltaT knock-out mice. Cancer Lett 153: 63–66.
31. Dan Q, Sanchez R, Delgado C, Wepsic HT, Morgan K, et al. (2001) Non-immunogenic murine hepatocellular carcinoma Hepa1-6 cells expressing the membrane form of macrophage colony stimulating factor are rejected in vivo and lead to CD8+ T-cell immunity against the parental tumor. Mol Ther 4: 427–437.
32. Ohira M, Ohdan H, Mitsuta H, Ishiyama K, Tanaka Y, et al. (2006) Adoptive transfer of TRAIL-expressing natural killer cells prevents recurrence of hepatocellular carcinoma after partial hepatectomy. Transplantation 82: 1712–1719.
33. Si S, Sun Y, Li Z, Ge W, Zhang X, et al. (2006) Gene therapy by membrane-expressed superantigen for alpha-fetoprotein-producing hepatocellular carcinoma. Gene Ther 13: 1603–1610.
34. Nie F, Xu HX, Lu MD, Wang Y and Tang Q (2008) Anti-angiogenic gene therapy for hepatocellular carcinoma mediated by microbubble-enhanced ultrasound exposure: an in vivo experimental study. J Drug Target 16: 389–395.
35. Wang G, Dong X, Tian W, Lu Y, Hu J, et al. (2013) Evaluation of miR-122-regulated suicide gene therapy for hepatocellular carcinoma in an orthotopic mouse model. Chin J Cancer Res 25: 646–655.
36. Tamaki S, Homma S, Enomoto Y, Komita H, Zeniya M, et al. (2005) Autoimmune hepatic inflammation by vaccination of mice with dendritic cells loaded with well-differentiated hepatocellular carcinoma cells and administration of interleukin-12. Clin Immunol 117: 280–293.
37. Schwarz M, Wanke I, Wulbrand U, Moennikes O and Buchmann A (2003) Role of connexin32 and beta-catenin in tumor promotion in mouse liver. Toxicol Pathol 31: 99–102.
38. Shouval D, Schuger L, Levij IS, Reid LM, Neeman Z, et al. (1988) Comparative morphology and tumourigenicity of human hepatocellular carcinoma cell lines in athymic rats and mice. Virchows Arch A Pathol Anat Histopathol 412: 595–606.
39. Higashi N, Ishii H, Fujiwara T, Morimoto-Tomita M and Irimura T (2002) Redistribution of fibroblasts and macrophages as micrometastases develop into established liver metastases. Clin Exp Metastasis 19: 631–638.
40. Amann T, Bataille F, Spruss T, Muhlbauer M, Gabele E, et al. (2009) Activated hepatic stellate cells promote tumorigenicity of hepatocellular carcinoma. Cancer Sci 100: 646–653.
41. Yin C, Evason KJ, Asahina K and Stainier DYR (2013) Hepatic stellate cells in liver development, regeneration, and cancer. The Journal of Clinical Investigation 123: 1902–1910.
42. Coulouarn C, Corlu A, Glaise D, Guenon I, Thorgeirsson SS, et al. (2012) Hepatocyte-stellate cell cross-talk in the liver engenders a permissive inflammatory microenvironment that drives progression in hepatocellular carcinoma. Cancer Res 72: 2533–2542.
43. Carpentier A, Metellus P, Ursu R, Zohar S, Lafitte F, et al. (2010) Intracerebral administration of CpG oligonucleotide for patients with recurrent glioblastoma: a phase II study. Neuro Oncol 12: 401–408.
44. Kang YM, Kim GH, Kim JI, Kim DY, Lee BN, et al. (2011) In vivo efficacy of an intratumorally injected in situ-forming doxorubicin/poly(ethylene glycol)-b-polycaprolactone diblock copolymer. Biomaterials 32: 4556–4564.
45. Santamaria E, Mora MI, Carro-Roldan E, Molina M, Fernandez-Irigoyen J, et al. (2009) Identification of replication-competent HSV-1 Cgal+ strain targets in a mouse model of human hepatocarcinoma xenograft. J Proteomics 73: 153–160.

46. Huang K, Zhou Q, Wang R, Cheng D and Ma Y (2013) Doxorubicin-eluting Bead versus Conventional Transarterial Chemoembolization for the Treatment of HCC: a Meta-Analysis. J Gastroenterol Hepatol.
47. Weber SM, Peterson KA, Durkee B, Qi C, Longino M, et al. (2004) Imaging of murine liver tumor using microCT with a hepatocyte-selective contrast agent: accuracy is dependent on adequate contrast enhancement. J Surg Res 119: 41–45.
48. Weichert JP, Lee FT, Jr., Chosy SG, Longino MA, Kuhlman JE, et al. (2000) Combined hepatocyte-selective and blood-pool contrast agents for the CT detection of experimental liver tumors in rabbits. Radiology 216: 865–871.
49. Fasquel JB, Agnus V, Moreau J, Soler L and Marescaux J (2006) An interactive medical image segmentation system based on the optimal management of regions of interest using topological medical knowledge. Comput Methods Programs Biomed 82: 216–230.
50. Soler L, Nicolau S, Pessaux P, Mutter D and Marescaux J (2014) Real-time 3D image reconstruction guidance in liver resection surgery. Hepatobiliary surgery and nutrition 3: 73–81.
51. Gordon H and Sweet HH (1936) A simple method for the silver impregnation of reticulin. American Journal of Pathology 12: 545.

Associated Factors of Atrophic Gastritis Diagnosed by Double-Contrast Upper Gastrointestinal Barium X-Ray Radiography

Nobutake Yamamichi[1]*, Chigaya Hirano[2], Takeshi Shimamoto[1,2], Chihiro Minatsuki[1], Yu Takahashi[1], Chiemi Nakayama[1], Rie Matsuda[1], Mitsuhiro Fujishiro[1], Maki Konno-Shimizu[1], Jun Kato[3], Shinya Kodashima[1], Satoshi Ono[1], Keiko Niimi[1], Satoshi Mochizuki[1], Yosuke Tsuji[1], Yoshiki Sakaguchi[1], Itsuko Asada-Hirayama[1], Chihiro Takeuchi[1], Seiichi Yakabi[1], Hikaru Kakimoto[1], Ryoichi Wada[2], Toru Mitsushima[2], Masao Ichinose[3], Kazuhiko Koike[1]

1 Department of Gastroenterology, Graduate School of Medicine, The University of Tokyo, Tokyo, Japan, **2** Department of Gastroenterology, Kameda Medical Center Makuhari, Chiba, Japan, **3** Second Department of Internal Medicine, Wakayama Medical University, Wakayama, Japan

Abstract

Background: Double-contrast upper gastrointestinal barium X-ray radiography (UGI-XR) is one of the most widely conducted gastric cancer screening methods. It has been executed to find gastric cancer, but has not been usually executed to detect premalignant atrophic mucosa of stomach. To understand the meaning of UGI-XR-based atrophic gastritis, we analyzed its association with several causative factors including *Helicobacter pylori* (HP) infection.

Methods: We evaluated 6,901 healthy adults in Japan. UGI-XR-based atrophic gastritis was diagnosed based on the irregular shape of areae gastricae and its expansion in the stomach.

Results: Of the 6,433 subjects with no history of HP eradication and free from gastric acid suppressants, 1,936 were diagnosed as UGI-XR-based atrophic gastritis (mild: 234, moderate: 822, severe: 880). These were univariately associated with serum HP IgG and serum pepsinogen I/II ratio with statistical significance. The multiple logistic analysis calculating standardized coefficients (β) and odds ratio (OR) demonstrated that serum HP IgG ($\beta = 1.499$, OR = 4.48), current smoking ($\beta = 0.526$, OR = 1.69), age ($\beta = 0.401$, OR = 1.49), low serum pepsinogen I/II ratio ($\beta = 0.339$, OR = 1.40), and male gender ($\beta = 0.306$, OR = 1.36) showed significant positive association with UGI-XR-based atrophic gastritis whereas drinking and body mass index did not. Among the age/sex/smoking/drinking-matched 227 pairs derived from chronically HP-infected and successfully HP-eradicated subjects, UGI-XR-based atrophic gastritis was detected in 99.1% of the former but in only 59.5% of the latter subjects ($p < 0.0001$). Contrastively, UGI-XR-based atrophic gastritis was detected in 13 of 14 HP-positive proton pump inhibitor users (92.9%) and 33 of 34 HP-positive histamine H_2-receptor antagonist users (97.1%), which are not significantly different from gastric acid suppressant-free subjects.

Conclusions: The presence of UGI-XR-based atrophic gastritis is positively associated with *Helicobacter pylori* infection, current smoking, age, decreased serum pepsinogen I/II ratio, and male gender. Eradication of *Helicobacter pylori* seems to superficially improve UGI-XR-based atrophic gastritis whereas intake of gastric acid suppressants does not.

Editor: Mitsunobu R. Kano, Okayama University, Japan

Funding: This work was supported in part by a research grant from Takeda Science Foundation, in part by a research grant from the Daiwa Security Health Foundation, and also in part by Grant-in-Aid for Scientific Research (C) from the Japan Society for the Promotion of Science. All the funders had no role in study design, data collection and analysis, decision to publish, or preparation of manuscript.

Competing Interests: The authors have declared that no competing interests exist.

* Email: nyamamic-tky@umin.ac.jp

Introduction

The incidence and mortality of gastric cancer has gradually fallen in the recent several decades, but it is still the second leading cause of cancer death worldwide [1,2]. Many gastric cancer screening methods have been developed and executed especially in East Asia, where a high incidence of gastric cancer is observed [3]. Among them, the double-contrast upper gastrointestinal barium X-ray radiography (UGI-XR) is one of the most widely used screening methods for gastric cancer. It has been conducted in

Japan since 1960's as the nationwide mass screening for stomach cancer [3,4,5]. Many previous studies suggested that regularly-scheduled UGI-XR may lead to a reduced risk of mortality from gastric cancer [4,6,7,8]. Therefore, UGI-XR is at present the only one method of gastric cancer screening officially authenticated in Japan [9], though other screening methods with endoscopy or serum pepsinogens are gradually spreading [10,11].

Nowadays, an issue to be solved for UGI-XR-based gastric cancer screening is coming about. UGI-XR has been mainly performed to find gastric cancer and other lesions such as erosion, ulcer, polyp, and so on. But regrettably, atrophic gastritis detected by UGI-XR has not been usually assessed. One of the reasons for that is probably the time when UGI-XR-based gastric cancer screening began: around 1960's in Japan, the prevalence of *Helicobacter pylori* (*H. pylori*)-induced gastritis was extremely high [3,5]. In the past several decades, however, the infection rate of *H. pylori* has been decreased worldwide [12,13,14,15]: consequently, clinical significance of evaluating UGI-XR-based atrophic gastritis become relatively higher today. Another more important reason is inadequate validation of the meaning of "atrophic gastritis" diagnosed by UGI-XR. At present, it is well established that chronic *H. pylori* infection mostly causes pathological gastritis with mucosal atrophy and precancerous intestinal metaplasia [16,17,18,19,20]. However, there is no clear evidence that "UGI-XR-based" atrophic gastritis coincides with *H. pylori*-induced "pathological" gastritis or "endoscopy-based" atrophic gastritis.

Based on these backgrounds, the purpose of this study is evaluating associations of "UGI-XR-based" atrophic gastritis with several causative factors including chronic *H. pylori* infection. Through the large-scale analysis of healthy adults in Japan, we have challenged the unsolved but important problem: the meaning of "atrophic gastritis" diagnosed by UGI-XR. We further expect that our results will improve the efficacy of gastric cancer screening via establishing precise evaluation of premalignant UGI-XR-based atrophic gastritis. Prediction of future cancer risk based on UGI-XR-based atrophic gastritis should increase the value of gastric cancer screening with barium X-ray.

Materials and Methods

Study Subjects

The study population was 20,773 subjects who received medical checkup at Kameda Medical Center Makuhari (Chiba-shi, Chiba, Japan) in 2010 and agreed with participating in our study. In cases where health checkup was performed twice in 2010, the former data was used. Criteria for exclusion were insufficient data for analysis or history of gastrectomy. This study was approved by the ethics committee of the University of Tokyo, and written informed consents were obtained from all the study participants according to the Declaration of Helsinki.

Double-contrast Upper Gastrointestinal Barium X-ray Radiography (UGI-XR)

Five minutes after intramuscular injection of spasmolytic agent (10 mg of scopolamine butylbromide), the subject drank 150 ml of barium (220 w/v %) in one gulp. X-ray images were then taken as follows; 1) double-contrast right anterior oblique view of the upper and lower esophagus in the near-supine standing position, 2) single-contrast frontal view of the stomach in the supine standing position, 3) double-contrast frontal image of the stomach in the supine position, 4) double-contrast right anterior oblique view of the stomach in the near-supine position, 5) double-contrast left anterior oblique view of the stomach in the near-supine position, 6) double-contrast right lateral view of the stomach in the horizontal position, 7) single-contrast frontal view of the stomach in the prone position, 8) double-contrast frontal view of the stomach in the prone position with the head down, 9) double-contrast frontal view of the stomach in the prone standing position, 10) double-contrast left anterior oblique view of the stomach in the prone position with the head down, 11) double-contrast left lateral view of the stomach in the horizontal position, 12) double-contrast left anterior oblique view of the stomach in the near-supine half-standing position (Schatzki's position), 13) double-contrast left anterior oblique view of the stomach in the near-supine position ("Barium divided" image), and 14) double-contrast right anterior oblique view of the stomach in the near-supine half-standing position.

Definition of Atrophic Gastritis Based on the Double-contrast Barium X-ray Radiography (UGI-XR-based atrophic gastritis)

The characteristics of gastritis in the double-contrast barium X-ray images have been described by a few reports [21,22]. By referring to them, in our previous report [23], we diagnosed gastritis based on the enlarged areae gastricae and/or hypertrophic gastritis with thickened folds on the greater curvature. It is also well known that atrophic gastritis usually extends from the antrum to body and fornix [19]. Taken these into consideration, we classified the double-contrast barium X-ray images of stomach into four types, on the basis of the irregular shapes of areae gastricae and their expansion as follows;

(A: normal) No atrophic change can be observed in stomach. The areae gastricae cannot be detected or can be recognized as small, round, and regular shapes in all the mucosal surface of stomach (Figure 1a).

(B: mild) The mucosal atrophy is mostly limited to gastric antrum. The enlarged areae gastricae with slight angularity and irregularity are observed in the restricted mucosal surface of stomach (Figure 1b).

(C: moderate) The mucosal atrophy extends from gastric antrum to body (corpus) and/or fornix. The obviously enlarged areae gastricae with considerable angularity and irregularity are observed in most or all mucosal surface of stomach (Figure 1c).

(D: severe) The severe atrophic change entirely covers the mucosal surface of stomach. The small or even absent areae gastricae diffusely extend in stomach, accompanied with irregularly rugged mucosal surface (Figure 1D).

Disgnosis of Atrophic Gastritis by Endoscopy

Atrophic patterns of gastric mucosa by endoscopy were classified into seven classes according to the Kimura-Takemoto classification [24,25]: no atrophic change (C0), three closed type atrophy patterns (C1, C2, C3), and three open type atrophy patterns (O1, O2, O3).

Evaluation of Serum anti-*Helicobacter pylori* IgG, Serum Pepsinogens (PGs), Alcohol Intake, and Smoking

Serum anti-*H. pylori* IgG, pepsinogen I, and pepsinogen II were measured using commercial kits (E-plate "EIKEN" Helicobacter pylori antibody and E-Plate "EIKEN" Pepsinogen I and II, Eiken Chemical Co LTD., Tokyo, Japan) as we had previously reported [26,27,28]. According to the manufacture's instruction, titer of *H. pylori* IgG $\geq$10 U/ml was considered as *H. pylori*-positive. Recently, it has been suggested that titer of *H. pylori* IgG $<$ 10 U/ml should be reconsidered from the standpoint of mucosal

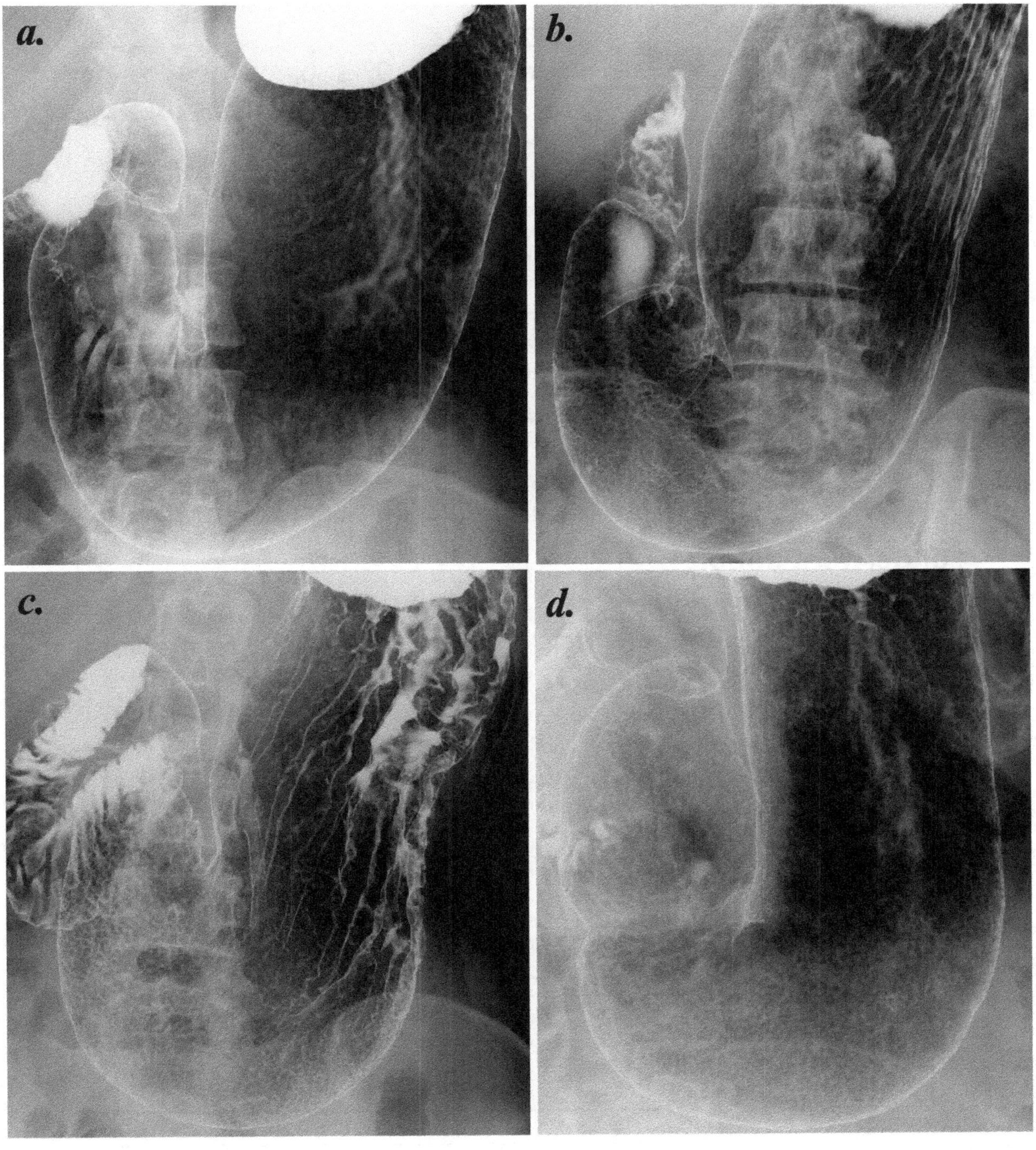

Figure 1. Typical four images of stomach by double-contrast upper gastrointestinal barium X-ray radiography (UGI-XR). (a) Normal stomach with no atrophic change of gastric mucosa. (b) Mild gastritis in which atrophic change mostly exists in gastric antrum and angle, accompanied with slightly enlarged irregular areae gastricae. (c) Moderate gastritis in which atrophic change extends from gastric antrum to body and/or fornix, accompanied with obviously enlarged irregular areae gastricae. (d) Severe gastritis in which atrophic change covers the entire stomach, accompanied with obscured small or even absent areae gastricae.

atrophic change or gastric cancer risk [29,30]. Therefore, we further divided "*H. pylori*-negative" subjects into "≥3 and < 10 U/ml (gray-zone titer of *H. pylori* IgG)" and "<3 U/ml (absolutely negative for *H. pylori* IgG)". In accordance with previous reports [28,31,32], ratios of serum pepsinogen I and II (pepsinogen I [ng/ml]/pepsinogen II [ng/ml]) were classified into ">3", ">2 and ≤3", and "≤2".

For alcohol intake, the study subjects were scored according to the 5-grade scale (never, seldom, sometimes, often, and always), and further categorized into "rarely drinking" group (never or seldom) and "usually drinking" group (sometimes, often, or always). For smoking, the subjects were classified into three groups: "current smoker" group, "past habitual smoker" group, and "lifelong nonsmoker" group.

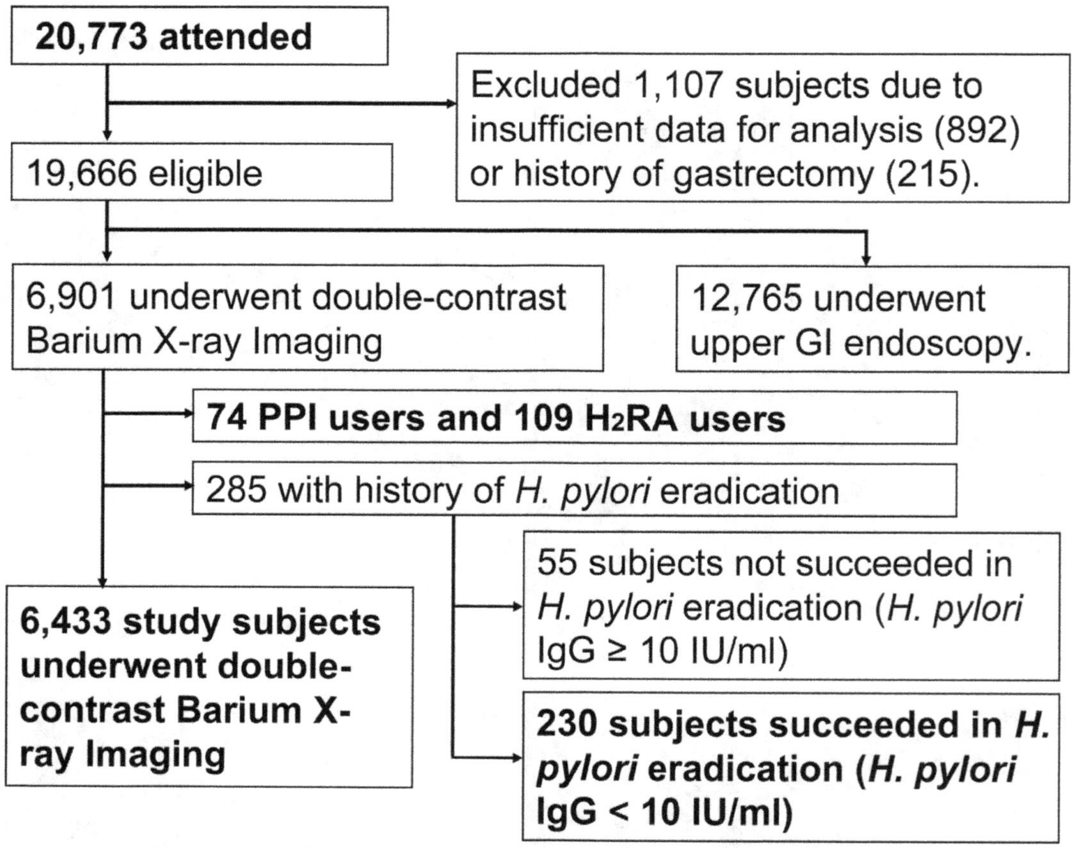

Figure 2. Study flowchart of the present study.

Endoscopy-based atrophic gastritis (Kimura-Takemoto classification of mucosal atrophic change in stomach)			UGI-XR-based atrophic gastritis: -	UGI-XR-based atrophic gastritis: +			
			Normal	Mild	Moderate	Severe	Total
	-	C0	84	1	3	0	88
	+	C1	6	0	1	1	8
	+	C2	4	2	5	4	15
	+	C3	1	0	3	1	5
	+	O1	0	0	9	7	16
	+	O2	0	0	3	11	14
	+	O3	0	0	0	4	4
		Total	95	3	24	28	150

(Polychoric correlation coefficient: r=0.9330)

Figure 3. Relationship between the four grades of UGI-XR-based atrophic gastritis and the extent of endoscopy-based atrophic gastritis classified into seven categories according to the Kimura-Takemoto classification (C0 with no atrophic change and C1-O3 with various degrees of endoscopy-based atrophic change of gastric mucosa).

a.

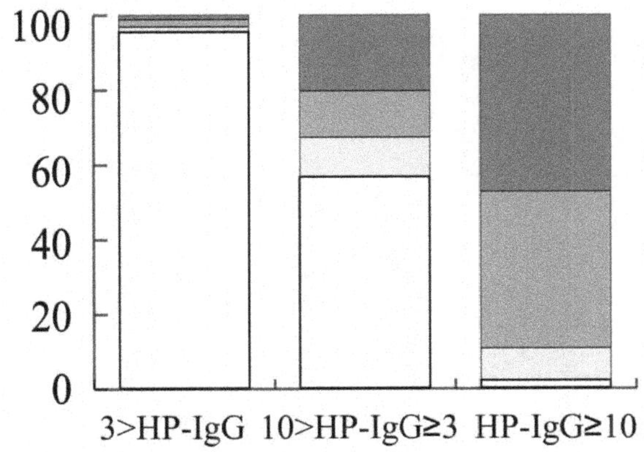

UGI-XR-based Gastritis	A	B	C	D	Total
3 > HP-IgG	4337 (95.5%)	66 (1.5%)	90 (2.0%)	48 (1.1%)	4541
10 > HP-IgG ≥ 3	124 (56.9%)	23 (10.6%)	27 (12.4%)	44 (20.2%)	218
HP-IgG ≥ 10	36 (2.2%)	145 (8.7%)	705 (42.1%)	788 (47.1%)	1674
Total	4497 (69.9%)	234 (3.6%)	822 (12.8%)	880 (13.7%)	6433

(p value<0.0001 by Cochran-Mantel-Haenszel trend test)

b.

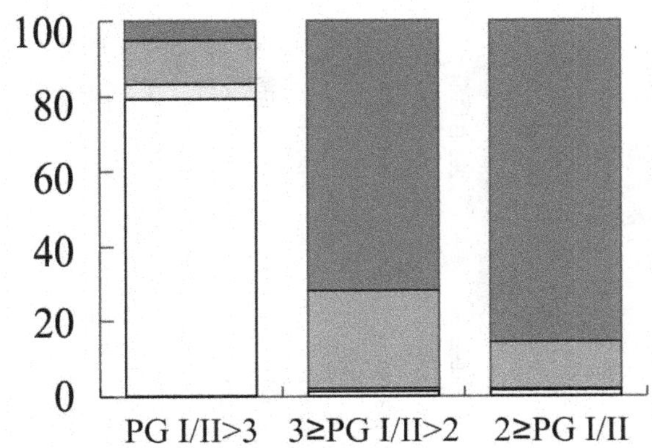

UGI-XR-based Gastritis	A	B	C	D	Total
PG I/II > 3	4486 (79.2%)	229 (4.0%)	656 (11.6%)	293 (5.2%)	5664
3 ≥ PG I/II > 2	7 (1.4%)	4 (0.8%)	135 (26.2%)	369 (71.7%)	515
2 ≥ PG I/II	4 (1.6%)	1 (0.4%)	31 (12.2%)	218 (85.8%)	254
Total	4497 (69.9%)	234 (3.6%)	822 (12.8%)	880 (13.7%)	6433

(p value<0.0001 by Cochran-Mantel-Haenszel trend test)

Figure 4. Distribution of our proposed four types of atrophic gastritis by double-contrast upper gastrointestinal barium X-ray radiography (A: normal, B: mild, C: moderate, D: severe) with titer of serum *Helicobacter pylori* IgG (a) or serum pepsinogen I/II ratio (b).

Statistical Analyses

We used JMP 10 software or SAS 9.1.3 (SAS Institute Inc. Cray, NC, USA) for statistical analyses and matching process. In the univariate analysis, associations between the presence of UGI-XR-based atrophic gastritis and seven variables were compared using the χ^2 test and Cochran-Mantel-Haenszel trend test. In the multivariate analysis, standardized coefficient and odds ratio of each variable were calculated using multiple logistic regression analysis. In the both analyses, p values <0.05 were considered as statistically significant.

To estimate the association between UGI-XR-based atrophic gastritis (normal, mild, moderate, and severe) and endoscopy-based atrophic gastritis (C0, C1, C2, C3, O1, O2, and O3 according to Kimura-Takemoto classification) [24,25], the polychoric correlation coefficient was calculated.

To evaluate the effect of *H. pylori* eradication on UGI-XR-based atrophic gastritis, the matching was performed to control age (±2 years), sex, smoking (current, past habitual, or lifelong non-smoking), and drinking ("rarely" or "usually") between the successfully *H. pylori*-eradicated subjects (negative for serum *H. pylori* IgG with history of eradication therapy) and the chronically *H. pylori*-infected subjects (positive for serum *H. pylori* IgG with no history of eradication therapy). Using the matched pairs of subjects, we applied Cochran-Mantel-Haenszel trend test, in which p value <0.05 was considered as statistically significant.

To evaluate the influence of gastric acid suppressants (proton pump inhibitors (PPI) and histamine H_2-receptor antagonist (H_2RA)) upon UGI-XR-based atrophic gastritis, we used Fisher's exact test in which p value <0.05 was considered as statistically significant.

Results and Discussion

Characteristics of the Study Subjects

Of the 20,773 subjects who participated in the study (Figure 2), we excluded 1,107 subjects with insufficient data or history of gastrectomy, and also excluded 12,765 subjects who underwent upper gastrointestinal (GI) endoscopy. Of the residual 6,901 subjects, we further excluded 74 PPI users, 109 H_2RA users, and 285 subjects who had underwent eradication therapy for *H. pylori*. The eligible 6,433 subjects comprised of 3,405 men and 3,028 women (a mean age of 47.4±8.8 years; range 20–83 years) were mainly analyzed in our present study (Figure 2).

Among the 6,433 main subjects for this study, only 1,674 (26.0%) were positive for *H. pylori*, which is consistent with the rapid decrease in prevalence of *H. pylori* infection in Japan [12,33]. Actually, for the data of healthy adults in our institutes located at Chiba prefecture in Japan, the seropositivity of *H. pylori* infection has markedly reduced from 47.0% (2,695 of 5,732

Table 1. Characteristics of the study subjects from the standpoint of atrophic gastritis diagnosed by double-contrast upper gastrointestinal barium X-ray radiography (UGI-XR-based atrophic gastritis).

Factor	Total 6,433 study subjects	1,936 subjects with UGI-XR-based atrophic gastritis	234 subjects with mild UGI-XR-based atrophic gastritis	822 subjects with moderate UGI-XR-based atrophic gastritis	880 subjects with severe UGI-XR-based atrophic gastritis	Residual 4,497 subjects without UGI-XR-based atrophic gastritis (normal)	*p* value
Age	47.7±8.8 y.o.	51.1±8.9 y.o.	48.4±8.4 y.o.	49.8±8.8 y.o.	53.0±8.7 y.o.	45.8±8.3 y.o.	<.0001*
<30	53 (0.8%)	5 (0.3%)	0 (0.0%)	3 (0.4%)	2 (0.2%)	48 (1.1%)	
≥30 and <40	1,274 (19.8%)	212 (11.0%)	40 (17.1%)	107 (13.0%)	65 (7.4%)	1,062 (23.6%)	
≥40 and <50	2,579 (40.1%)	600 (31.0%)	94 (40.2%)	286 (34.8%)	220 (25.0%)	1,979 (44.0%)	
≥50 and <60	1,909 (29.7%)	774 (40.0%)	76 (32.5%)	304 (37.0%)	394 (44.8%)	1,135 (25.2%)	
≥60 and <70	558 (8.7%)	308 (15.9%)	22 (9.4%)	111 (13.5%)	175 (19.9%)	250 (5.6%)	
≥70	60 (0.9%)	37 (1.9%)	2 (0.9%)	11 (1.3%)	24 (2.3%)	23 (0.5%)	
Sex							<.0001*
female	3,028 (47.1%)	828 (42.8%)	77 (32.9%)	366 (44.5%)	385 (43.8%)	2,200 (48.9%)	
male	3,405 (52.9%)	1,108 (57.2%)	157 (67.1%)	456 (55.5%)	495 (56.3%)	2,297 (51.1%)	
BMI	22.8±3.4	23.0±3.3	23.3±3.4	22.9±3.3	22.8±3.4	22.8±3.4	0.0079*
<18.5	451 (7.0%)	120 (6.2%)	17 (7.3%)	42 (5.1%)	61 (6.9%)	331 (7.4%)	
≥18.5 and <25	4,508 (70.1%)	1,337 (69.1%)	147 (62.8%)	587 (71.4%)	603 (68.5%)	3,171 (70.5%)	
≥25	1,474 (22.9%)	479 (24.7%)	70 (29.9%)	193 (23.5%)	216 (24.5%)	995 (22.1%)	
H. pylori IgG							<.0001*
<3	4,541 (70.6%)	204 (10.5%)	66 (28.2%)	90 (10.9%)	48 (5.5%)	4,337 (96.4%)	
<10 and ≥3	218 (3.4%)	94 (4.9%)	23 (9.8%)	27 (3.3%)	44 (5.0%)	124 (2.8%)	
≥10	1,674 (26.0%)	1,638 (84.6%)	145 (62.0%)	705 (85.8%)	788 (89.5%)	36 (0.8%)	
PG I/II ratio							<.0001*
>3	5,664 (88.0%)	1,178 (60.9%)	229 (97.9%)	656 (79.8%)	293 (33.3%)	4,486 (99.8%)	
≤3 and >2	515 (8.0%)	508 (26.2%)	4 (1.7%)	135 (16.4%)	369 (41.9%)	7 (0.2%)	
≤2	254 (3.9%)	250 (12.9%)	1 (0.4%)	31 (3.8%)	218 (24.8%)	4 (0.1%)	
Smoking							<.0001*
non smoker	3,511 (54.6%)	950 (49.1%)	92 (39.3%)	422 (51.3%)	436 (49.5%)	2,561 (57.0%)	
former smoker	1,622 (25.2%)	548 (28.3%)	73 (31.2%)	197 (24.0%)	278 (31.6%)	1,074 (23.9%)	
current smoker	1,300 (20.2%)	438 (22.6%)	69 (29.5%)	203 (24.7%)	166 (18.9%)	862 (19.2%)	
Alcohol							0.8881
rarely drinking	2,567 (39.9%)	770 (39.8%)	75 (32.1%)	319 (38.8%)	376 (42.7%)	1,797 (40.0%)	
usually drinking	3,866 (60.1%)	1,166 (60.2%)	159 (67.9%)	503 (61.2%)	504 (57.3%)	2,700 (60.0%)	

BMI, body mass index; *H. pylori*, *Helicobacter pylori*; PG, pepsinogen. The levels of significance (*p* value) for analyzing associations between UGI-XR-based atrophic gastritis and the seven causative factors were set at <0.05 (*), which were calculated by χ^2 test or Cochran-Mantel-Haenszel trend test.

Table 2. Multivariate analysis of the 6,433 study subjects evaluating associations of the seven background factors with UGI-XR-based atrophic gastritis (atrophic gastritis diagnosed by double-contrast upper gastrointestinal barium X-ray radiography).

Factor	Standardized coefficients	Odds ratio (95% C.I.)	*p* value
Age	0.401	1.49 (1.31–1.70)	<.0001*
Sex			
female	reference	reference	reference
male	0.306	1.36 (1.16–1.59)	0.0002*
BMI	−0.100	0.90 (0.80–1.03)	0.124
H. pylori IgG			
<3	reference	reference	reference
<10 and ≥3	0.479	1.61 (1.52–1.72)	<.0001*
≥10	1.499	4.48 (4.12–4.91)	<.0001*
PG I/II ratio			
>3	reference	reference	reference
≤3 and >2	0.270	1.31 (1.18–1.48)	<.0001*
≤2	0.339	1.40 (1.26–1.59)	<.0001*
Smoking			
non smoker	reference	reference	reference
former smoker	0.137	1.15 (0.98–1.33)	0.0773
current smoker	0.526	1.69 (1.49–1.93)	<.0001*
Alcohol			
rarely drinking	reference	reference	reference
usually drinking	0.051	1.05 (0.92–1.20)	0.449

BMI, body mass index; *H. pylori*, *Helicobacter pylori*; PG, pepsinogen. The level of significance in each factor was set at $p<0.05$ (*).

subjects in 1996–1997 [34]) to 26.0% (1,674 of 6,433 subjects in the present study) in only 14 short years.

The 285 subjects after *H. pylori* eradication therapy comprised of 230 subjects with serum *H. pylori* IgG <10 U/ml (certainly succeeded in *H. pylori* eradication) and 55 subjects with serum *H. pylori* IgG ≥10 U/ml (probably not succeeded in *H. pylori* eradication or on the way of negative conversion of serum *H. pylori* IgG). Aside from the main 6,433 study subjects, we additionally analyzed the above-mentioned 74 PPI users, 109 H_2RA users, and 230 "successfully *H. pylori*-eradicated" subjects (Figure 2).

Validation of our defined "UGI-XR-based" Atrophic Gastritis by comparing "Endoscopy-based" Atrophic Gastritis

In our previous work [23], 29 (97%) of 30 subjects positive for serum anti-*H. pylori* IgG were diagnosed as gastritis by UGI-XR, which convinced us the sufficient detection of *H. pylori*-induced chronic gastritis by barium X-ray. In the present study, we classified the UGI-XR-based atrophic gastritis into four types as above-mentioned (Figure 1). To validate this classification, the extent of endoscopy-based atrophic gastritis were simultaneously evaluated among the 150 subjects randomly selected (Figure 3).

Table 3. Comparison between the matched pairs of 227 subjects with chronic infection of *H. pylori* and after successful eradication of *H. pylori*, focusing on the presence of UGI-XR-based atrophic gastritis (atrophic gastritis diagnosed by double-contrast upper gastrointestinal barium X-ray radiography).

	Presence of UGI-XR-based atrophic gastritis (mild, moderate, severe)	Absence of UGI-XR-based atrophic gastritis (normal)	Total
The 227 matched subjects after successful eradication of *H. pylori*	135 (59.5%)	92 (40.5%)	227 (100%)
The 227 matched subjects with chronic *H. pylori* infection	225 (99.1%)	2 (0.9%)	227 (100%)

($p<0.0001$ by Cochran-Mantel-Haenszel test).

Table 4. Comparison between the *H. pylori*-positive gastric acid suppressant (PPI or H_2RA) users and *H. pylori*-positive gastric acid suppressant-free subjects, focusing on the presence of UGI-XR-based gastritis (gastritis diagnosed by double-contrast upper gastrointestinal barium X-ray radiography).

	Presence of UGI-XR-based atrophic gastritis (mild, moderate, severe)	Absence of UGI-XR-based atrophic gastritis (normal)	Total	*p* value
H. pylori-positive and gastric acid suppressant-free subjects among the 6,433 main study subjects	1,638 (97.8%)	36 (2.1%)	1,674 (100%)	reference
H. pylori-positive subjects among the 74 PPI users	13 (92.9%)	1 (7.1%)	14 (100%)	0.2677
H. pylori-positive subjects among the 109 H_2RA users	33 (97.1%)	1 (2.9%)	34 (100%)	0.5286

For the PPI and H_2RA users each, the level of significance was set at $p<0.05$ (*) by Fisher's exact test.

On the basis of endoscopy-based atrophic gastritis, sensitivity and specificity of UGI-XR-based atrophic gastritis were 82.3% (51/62) and 95.5% (84/88) respectively. In addition, the four-grade categories of UGI-XR-based atrophic gastritis showed significant association with seven-grade classes of endoscopy-based atrophic gastritis (polychoric correlation coefficient: r = 0.9330). Actually, all the subjects (34/34) with severe endoscopy-based atrophic gastritis (namely, open type (O1–O3) atrophy according to Kimura-Takemoto classification [24,25]) were diagnosed as UGI-XR-based atrophic gastritis (Figure 3). Based on these results, we concluded that UGI-XR-based diagnosis used in this study can certainly reflect the atrophic mucosa of stomach.

The Four-grade Types of UGI-XR-based Atrophic Gastritis are Significantly Associated with the Titer of Serum *H. pylori* IgG and the Ratio of Serum Pepsinogen I and II

Based on the UGI-XR-based mucosal atrophy of stomach, the total 6,433 subjects with no history of *H. pylori* eradication and free from gastric acid suppressants were classified into four classes (Figure 4): 234 subjects with mild gastritis, 822 subjects with moderate gastritis, 880 subjects with severe gastritis, and residual 4,497 subjects without atrophic gastritis (normal).

We first evaluated associations of the four-grade UGI-XR-based atrophic gastritis with two serum markers: the titer of *H. pylori* IgG and the ratio of pepsinogen I and II reflecting the mucosal atrophy of stomach [32,35]. As shown in Figure 4a, UGI-XR-based atrophic gastritis significantly extends in proportion to rise in serum *H. pylori* IgG titer ($p<0.0001$). And as also shown in Figure 4b, the grade of UGI-XR-based atrophic gastritis meaningfully advances accompanied with decline in pepsinogen I/II ratio ($p<0.0001$). Though the effects of other causative factors should not be groundlessly underestimated, these results suggest that the four-grade categorization of UGI-XR-based atrophic gastritis strongly reflects chronic *H. pylori* infection and consequent mucosal atrophy of stomach.

Associated Background Factors of UGI-XR-based Atrophic Gastritis

The detailed characteristics of the 6,433 study subjects focusing on UGI-XR-based atrophic gastritis and the seven putative background factors are shown in Table 1. The results of univariate analyses concerning the seven factors are also denoted. It is clear that old age, male gender, a high titer of serum *H. pylori* IgG, low ratio of serum pepsinogen I/II, and a habit of smoking show strongly positive association with the presence of UGI-XR-based atrophic gastritis.

We next executed multivariate analyses with these seven causative factors (Table 2). As was expected, a high titer of serum *H. pylori* IgG is the strongest associated factor for UGI-XR-based atrophic gastritis. Current smoking, old age, low ratio of serum pepsinogen I/II, and male gender also show significant association. In contrast, drinking as well as BMI (body mass index) has no meaningful association with UGI-XR-based atrophic gastritis: this unexpected but clear difference between drinking and smoking should be noted when considering the establishment of atrophic gastritis.

Eradication of *Helicobacter pylori* Seems to Superficially Improve UGI-XR-based Atrophic Gastritis

We next tried to evaluate the effect of *H. pylori* eradication upon UGI-XR-based atrophic gastritis. For this purpose, the matching was performed to control age (within±2 years), sex, smoking, and drinking between the 230 subjects succeeded in *H. pylori* eradication (negative for serum *H. pylori* IgG with history of eradication therapy) and the 1,674 subjects with chronic *H. pylori* infection (positive for serum *H. pylori* IgG with no history of eradication therapy).

Between the 227 matched pairs of subjects, prevalences of UGI-XR-based atrophic gastritis were markedly different with statistical significance (Table 3): it was detected in only 59.5% of the *H. pylori*-eradicated subjects but was detected in 99.1% of the chronically *H. pylori*-infected subjects ($p<0.0001$). These suggest that eradication of *H. pylori* diminishes the typical images of UGI-XR-based atrophic gastritis. In other words, chronic infection of *H. pylori* in the past cannot be efficiently detected by UGI-XR, after eradication therapy has been completed.

It has been reported that eradication of *H. pylori* can improve gastritis both pathologically [20,36,37] and endoscopically [38]. The result of our present study suggests that eradication of *H. pylori* can also relieve UGI-XR-based atrophic gastritis, which is defined by the irregular shapes of areae gastricae and their expansion in the stomach. However, this is not always a preferable result, since the superficial improvement of chronic gastritis does not considerably reduce the risk of gastric tumorigenesis [39,40,41,42]. It can be otherwise considered that UGI-XR cannot adequately distinguish the lifelong *H. pylori*-negative stomach (having a very low risk of gastric cancer [17,30,43]) from the *H. pylori*-eradicated stomach keeping a considerable risk for gastric canceration [40]. We are apprehensive that the difficulty in detecting *H. pylori*-eradicated stomach will be a formidable problem for UGI-XR-based gastric cancer screening.

Intakes of PPI and H_2RA Mostly do not Affect UGI-XR-based Atrophic Gastritis

We further evaluated the influence of gastric acid suppressants upon UGI-XR-based atrophic gastritis. Among the gastric acid suppressant users positive for serum *H. pylori* IgG (Table 4), UGI-XR-based atrophic gastritis was detected in 13 of 14 PPI users (92.9%) and 33 of 34 H_2RA users (97.1%). Though the statistical evaluation cannot be accurately calculated due to the small number of subjects, there seems to be no obvious differences compared to the *H. pylori*-positive 1,674 subjects free from gastric acid suppressants. To say the least, our results indicate that intakes of PPI and H_2RA mostly do not deteriorate the diagnostic quality of UGI-XR-based atrophic gastritis.

Conclusions

The presence of atrophic gastritis diagnosed by double-contrast upper gastrointestinal barium X-ray radiography (UGI-XR-based atrophic gastritis) is positively associated with *Helicobacter pylori* infection, current smoking, old age, decreased pepsinogen I/II ratio, and male gender. Eradication of *Helicobacter pylori* seems to superficially improve UGI-XR-based gastritis whereas intake of proton pump inhibitors or histamine H_2-receptor antagonist does not.

Acknowledgments

We are grateful to Mr. Minoru Okada, Mr. Masanori Fujiwara, and Mr. Masami Muraoka (Kameda Medical Center Makuhari, Chiba-shi, Chiba, Japan) for assistance with establishment and maintenance of the study database.

Author Contributions

Conceived and designed the experiments: NY CH TS TM MI. Performed the experiments: NY CH CM Y. Takahashi CN RM MKS. Analyzed the data: NY TS SK SO KN SM Y. Tsuji YS IAH CT SY HK RW. Contributed reagents/materials/analysis tools: NY CH TM. Contributed to the writing of the manuscript: NY CH TS MF JK MI KK.

References

1. Crew KD, Neugut AI (2006) Epidemiology of gastric cancer. World J Gastroenterol 12: 354–362.
2. Yamamichi N, Inada K, Ichinose M, Yamamichi-Nishina M, Mizutani T, et al. (2007) Frequent loss of Brm expression in gastric cancer correlates with histologic features and differentiation state. Cancer Res 67: 10727–10735.
3. Leung WK, Wu MS, Kakugawa Y, Kim JJ, Yeoh KG, et al. (2008) Screening for gastric cancer in Asia: current evidence and practice. Lancet Oncol 9: 279–287.
4. Lee KJ, Inoue M, Otani T, Iwasaki M, Sasazuki S, et al. (2006) Gastric cancer screening and subsequent risk of gastric cancer: a large-scale population-based cohort study, with a 13-year follow-up in Japan. Int J Cancer 118: 2315–2321.
5. Tsubono Y, Hisamichi S (2000) Screening for gastric cancer in Japan. Gastric Cancer 3: 9–18.
6. Oshima A, Hirata N, Ubukata T, Umeda K, Fujimoto I (1986) Evaluation of a mass screening program for stomach cancer with a case-control study design. Int J Cancer 38: 829–833.
7. Hisamichi S, Sugawara N (1984) Mass screening for gastric cancer by X-ray examination. Jpn J Clin Oncol 14: 211–223.
8. Mizoue T, Yoshimura T, Tokui N, Hoshiyama Y, Yatsuya H, et al. (2003) Prospective study of screening for stomach cancer in Japan. Int J Cancer 106: 103–107.
9. Hamashima C, Shibuya D, Yamazaki H, Inoue K, Fukao A, et al. (2008) The Japanese guidelines for gastric cancer screening. Jpn J Clin Oncol 38: 259–267.
10. Hosokawa O, Miyanaga T, Kaizaki Y, Hattori M, Dohden K, et al. (2008) Decreased death from gastric cancer by endoscopic screening: association with a population-based cancer registry. Scand J Gastroenterol 43: 1112–1115.
11. Miki K, Morita M, Sasajima M, Hoshina R, Kanda E, et al. (2003) Usefulness of gastric cancer screening using the serum pepsinogen test method. Am J Gastroenterol 98: 735–739.
12. Nakajima S, Nishiyama Y, Yamaoka M, Yasuoka T, Cho E (2010) Changes in the prevalence of Helicobacter pylori infection and gastrointestinal diseases in the past 17 years. J Gastroenterol Hepatol 25 Suppl 1: S99–S110.
13. Lee SY, Park HS, Yu SK, Sung IK, Jin CJ, et al. (2007) Decreasing prevalence of Helicobacter pylori infection: a 9-year observational study. Hepatogastroenterology 54: 630–633.
14. Brown LM (2000) Helicobacter pylori: epidemiology and routes of transmission. Epidemiol Rev 22: 283–297.
15. Bures J, Kopacova M, Koupil I, Seifert B, Skodova Fendrichova M, et al. (2012) Significant decrease in prevalence of Helicobacter pylori in the Czech Republic. World J Gastroenterol 18: 4412–4418.
16. Dixon MF, Genta RM, Yardley JH, Correa P (1996) Classification and grading of gastritis. The updated Sydney System. International Workshop on the Histopathology of Gastritis, Houston 1994. Am J Surg Pathol 20: 1161–1181.
17. Uemura N, Okamoto S, Yamamoto S, Matsumura N, Yamaguchi S, et al. (2001) Helicobacter pylori infection and the development of gastric cancer. N Engl J Med 345: 784–789.
18. Polk DB, Peek RM Jr (2010) Helicobacter pylori: gastric cancer and beyond. Nat Rev Cancer 10: 403–414.
19. Satoh K, Kimura K, Taniguchi Y, Yoshida Y, Kihira K, et al. (1996) Distribution of inflammation and atrophy in the stomach of Helicobacter pylori-positive and -negative patients with chronic gastritis. Am J Gastroenterol 91: 963–969.
20. Ohkusa T, Fujiki K, Takashimizu I, Kumagai J, Tanizawa T, et al. (2001) Improvement in atrophic gastritis and intestinal metaplasia in patients in whom Helicobacter pylori was eradicated. Ann Intern Med 134: 380–386.
21. Dheer S, Levine MS, Redfern RO, Metz DC, Rubesin SE, et al. (2002) Radiographically diagnosed antral gastritis: findings in patients with and without Helicobacter pylori infection. Br J Radiol 75: 805–811.
22. Rubesin SE, Levine MS, Laufer I (2008) Double-contrast upper gastrointestinal radiography: a pattern approach for diseases of the stomach. Radiology 246: 33–48.
23. Yamamichi N, Shimamoto T, Minatsuki C, Yoshida Y, Fujishiro M, et al. (2011) Postprandial fullness correlates with rapid inflow of gastric content into duodenum but not with chronic gastritis. BMC Gastroenterol 11: 140.
24. Kimura K (1972) Chronological transition of the fundic-pyloric border determined by stepwise biopsy of the lesser and greater curvatures of the stomach. Gastroenterology 63: 584–592.
25. Kimura K, Takemoto T (1969) An Endoscopic Recognition of the Atrophic Border and its Significance in Chronic Gastritis. Endoscopy 3: 87–97.
26. Takahashi Y, Yamamichi N, Shimamoto T, Mochizuki S, Fujishiro M, et al. (2013) Helicobacter pylori infection is positively associated with gallstones: a large-scale cross-sectional study in Japan. J Gastroenterol.
27. Minatsuki C, Yamamichi N, Shimamoto T, Kakimoto H, Takahashi Y, et al. (2013) Background factors of reflux esophagitis and non-erosive reflux disease: a cross-sectional study of 10,837 subjects in Japan. PLoS One 8: e69891.
28. Shimamoto T, Yamamichi N, Kodashima S, Takahashi Y, Fujishiro M, et al. (2013) No association of coffee consumption with gastric ulcer, duodenal ulcer, reflux esophagitis, and non-erosive reflux disease: a cross-sectional study of 8,013 healthy subjects in Japan. PLoS One 8: e65996.
29. Tatemichi M, Sasazuki S, Inoue M, Tsugane S (2009) Clinical significance of IgG antibody titer against Helicobacter pylori. Helicobacter 14: 231–236.
30. Ohata H, Kitauchi S, Yoshimura N, Mugitani K, Iwane M, et al. (2004) Progression of chronic atrophic gastritis associated with Helicobacter pylori infection increases risk of gastric cancer. Int J Cancer 109: 138–143.
31. Oishi Y, Kiyohara Y, Kubo M, Tanaka K, Tanizaki Y, et al. (2006) The serum pepsinogen test as a predictor of gastric cancer: the Hisayama study. Am J Epidemiol 163: 629–637.
32. Watabe H, Mitsushima T, Yamaji Y, Okamoto M, Wada R, et al. (2005) Predicting the development of gastric cancer from combining Helicobacter pylori antibodies and serum pepsinogen status: a prospective endoscopic cohort study. Gut 54: 764–768.
33. Shiota S, Murakami K, Fujioka T, Yamaoka Y (2010) Population-based strategies for Helicobacter pylori-associated disease management: a Japanese perspective. Expert Rev Gastroenterol Hepatol 4: 149–156.
34. Yamaji Y, Mitsushima T, Ikuma H, Okamoto M, Yoshida H, et al. (2001) Inverse background of Helicobacter pylori antibody and pepsinogen in reflux oesophagitis compared with gastric cancer: analysis of 5732 Japanese subjects. Gut 49: 335–340.
35. Miki K (2006) Gastric cancer screening using the serum pepsinogen test method. Gastric Cancer 9: 245–253.

36. Sung JJ, Lin SR, Ching JY, Zhou LY, To KF, et al. (2000) Atrophy and intestinal metaplasia one year after cure of H. pylori infection: a prospective, randomized study. Gastroenterology 119: 7–14.
37. Ito M, Haruma K, Kamada T, Mihara M, Kim S, et al. (2002) Helicobacter pylori eradication therapy improves atrophic gastritis and intestinal metaplasia: a 5-year prospective study of patients with atrophic gastritis. Aliment Pharmacol Ther 16: 1449–1456.
38. Kato M, Terao S, Adachi K, Nakajima S, Ando T, et al. (2013) Changes in endoscopic findings of gastritis after cure of H. pylori infection: multicenter prospective trial. Dig Endosc 25: 264–273.
39. Correa P, Fontham ET, Bravo JC, Bravo LE, Ruiz B, et al. (2000) Chemoprevention of gastric dysplasia: randomized trial of antioxidant supplements and anti-helicobacter pylori therapy. J Natl Cancer Inst 92: 1881–1888.
40. Fuccio L, Zagari RM, Eusebi LH, Laterza L, Cennamo V, et al. (2009) Meta-analysis: can Helicobacter pylori eradication treatment reduce the risk for gastric cancer? Ann Intern Med 151: 121–128.
41. Wong BC, Lam SK, Wong WM, Chen JS, Zheng TT, et al. (2004) Helicobacter pylori eradication to prevent gastric cancer in a high-risk region of China: a randomized controlled trial. JAMA 291: 187–194.
42. Leung WK, Lin SR, Ching JY, To KF, Ng EK, et al. (2004) Factors predicting progression of gastric intestinal metaplasia: results of a randomised trial on Helicobacter pylori eradication. Gut 53: 1244–1249.
43. Correa P, Houghton J (2007) Carcinogenesis of Helicobacter pylori. Gastroenterology 133: 659–672.

21

Liver Stiffness Measurement among Patients with Chronic Hepatitis B and C: Results from a 5-Year Prospective Study

Karen M. Christiansen, Belinda K. Mössner, Janne F. Hansen, Erik F. Jarnbjer, Court Pedersen, Peer B. Christensen*

Department of Infectious Diseases, Odense University Hospital, Odense, Denmark

Abstract

Liver stiffness measurement (LSM) is widely used to evaluate liver fibrosis, but longitudinal studies are rare. The current study was aimed to monitor LSM during follow-up, and to evaluate the association of LSM data with mortality and liver-related outcomes. We included all patients with chronic viral hepatitis and valid LSM using Fibroscan. Information about liver biopsy, antiviral treatment, and clinical outcome was obtained from medical records and national registers. The study included 845 patients: 597 (71%) with hepatitis C virus (HCV), 235 (28%) with hepatitis B virus (HBV) and 13 (2%) with dual infection. The initial LSM distribution (<7/7–9.9/10–16.9/≥17 kPa) was 58%/16%/14%/12%. Among patients with initial LSM values of 7–9.9 kPa, 60% of HCV patients and 83% of HBV patients showed LSM values of <7 kPa at the latest follow-up. Progression rates (defined as >20% and >2 kPa increase, with one measure >7 kPa) were 3.4/100 person years (PY) for HCV and 1.5/100 PY for HBV infected patients. Patients with LSM values of ≥17 kPa had the same liver-related complication incidence as patients with biopsy-proven cirrhosis (11.1 versus 12.1/100 PY). Thirteen liver-related deaths occurred among HCV patients (0.6/100 PY), but none among HBV patients. Among patients who died of liver-related causes, all but one had baseline LSM values of ≥17 kPa. Overall, patients with LSM values <17 kPa were not associated with adverse outcomes. In contrast, LSM values ≥17 kPa were associated with significant risk of liver-related problems. The results of the current study suggest that clinical decisions should not be taken based on a single LSM measurement.

Editor: Joseph George, Kanazawa Medical University, Japan

Funding: The authors have no support or funding to report.

Competing Interests: The authors have declared that no competing interests exist.

* Email: peer.christensen@dadlnet.dk

Introduction

In patients with viral hepatitis, morbidity and mortality are closely related to fibrosis development, which can lead to cirrhosis and end-stage liver disease. Liver biopsy is considered the gold standard method for fibrosis diagnosis; however, this procedure carries rare but serious complications and substantial problems with sampling variability and observer agreement [1]. Thus, alternative non-invasive methods have been eagerly pursued for decades [2,3].

Liver stiffness measurement (LSM) using the Fibroscan device from Echosens was originally introduced in clinical practice in 2003 [4]. This technique performs well in classifying patients at the extremes of no significant fibrosis (Metavir F0–F1) and cirrhosis (F4), but is less accurate for detecting significant fibrosis (F2–F3) [3]. Measurement can also be difficult in patients with narrow intercostal space and/or obesity, with invalid results reported in up to 20% of patients. Furthermore, several factors—including liver inflammation, right-sided heart failure, and measurement in the post-prandial state—may increase the LSM, thus overestimating the fibrosis present [5–8].

To date, there is no universal consensus regarding a normal LSM value, or how to define cut-offs for significant fibrosis and cirrhosis. LSM may vary with the etiology of liver fibrosis, as patients with hepatitis B virus (HBV) reportedly have lower LSM values than patients with hepatitis C virus (HCV) at the same stage of fibrosis [9]. Among blood donors with no signs of liver disease and in health care center-based screenings, median/95th percentile values have been reported to be 4.4/6.7 kiloPascal(kPa) and 5.3/8.0 kPa [10–12]. Two large meta-analyses determined cut-off values of 7.2/7.7 kPa for F2 and of 13.0/14.5 kPa for cirrhosis among patients with liver disease [13,14]. However, a large French multicenter study identified 17 kPa as a reliable cut-off for cirrhosis. Current Danish national guidelines for patients with viral hepatitis recommend 17 kPa as the cut-off for cirrhosis and 7 kPa as the upper limit of normal [15,16]. Liver-related morbidity and mortality is primarily seen in patients with cirrhosis, and LSM is significantly correlated with hepatic vein portal gradient (HVPG) [17,18]. To better discriminate between patients with and without substantial fibrosis (F2), algorithms have been developed to combine LSM with serological markers, but no individual test or algorithm has yet attained universal acceptance [3,19]. However,

LSM is currently used in clinical practice in Europe and was approved for use in the US in 2013.

The present study aimed to evaluate LSM over time in a well-defined population of patients with chronic viral hepatitis B or C. The hypothesis was that high or increasing LSM values would be predictive of liver-related morbidity and mortality.

Patients and Methods

This study included all patients whose first LSM was performed between May 1, 2007 (the date that our department began to implement LSM) and April 30, 2012. LSM examinations were performed using the Fibroscan 402 and M probe (Echosens, Paris, France) according to the manufacturer's guidelines. All examiners were certified by Echosens. In 2010, we introduced the use of the XL probe for obese patients, which was employed in 8% of all examinations. All measurements were automatically stored on the Fibroscan hard disk, with back-up on a central server. For the present study, personal ID (civil registration number) and LSM measurements were obtained from a file from the Fibroscan device. Vital status was obtained from the civil register at the end of observation (July 31, 2012), and causes of death were obtained from the register of death certificates. For 2012, information from the death certificate register was not yet available, and therefore causes of death were obtained from individual death certificates and hospital clinical records. Information about morbidity and antiviral treatment was obtained from hospital records.

This study was approved by the Local Committee on Biomedical Research Ethics (VF 20050089) and the Danish Data Protection Agency (2006-41-7196 and 2012-41-0079). Participants gave written informed consent.

Routine LSM was performed with no food restrictions. Patients with LSM above normal were offered a fasting LSM within 1–3 months. A valid LSM examination included 10 valid measurements, a success rate of 60%, and an interquartile range of measurements (IQR) below 30% of the median value. We considered an LSM of <7 kPa to be normal and an LSM of >17 kPa to indicate cirrhosis. Lacking previous guidelines to define a significant change in LSM over time, we applied the following definition: a 20% change in LSM value was regarded as significant if the observed change was ≥2 kPa and if at least one of the measurements was >7 kPa. The requirement of one absolute value above 7 kPa was included to avoid classifying trivial changes within the normal range as significant changes. This also compensated for the intra-individual stochastic variation observed by repeated measurements over short periods of time and for the precision of measurement (0.5 kPa). LSM was offered at least once yearly, and more frequently if deemed necessary. Patients with repeated LSM values in the range of 7–9 kPa were usually closely monitored, while patients with values of above 9 kPa were recommended to undergo biopsy or start treatment based on an overall evaluation. After 2010, patients with a confirmed LSM of >17 kPa were started on cirrhosis surveillance and treatment without biopsy.

Prior to 2007, cirrhosis was diagnosed based on liver biopsy, development of clinical decompensation (ascites, presence of esophageal varices with or without bleeding, encephalopathy, spontaneous bacterial peritonitis, or hepatorenal syndrome), or detection of hepatocellular carcinoma (HCC). Following the introduction of LSM, patients with LSM of >17 kPa were also classified as having cirrhosis. For incidence calculation, we excluded a lead-in phase of 6 months after the first LSM, in order to exclude the prevalent decompensation detected during the initial workup of an elevated first LSM.

The LSM natural history follow-up cohort included patients infected with HBV or HCV in whom two or more LSM were performed at least 3 months apart. We excluded patients with dual infection with HBV, HCV, and/or human immunodeficiency virus (HIV), and patients who were treated between January 1, 2006 and start of the inclusion period. Patients whose treatment started during follow-up (as part of the LSM natural history cohort) were censored at the date of last LSM before treatment initiation.

Statistical analysis was performed using Stata version 12. Nonparametric statistical tests (Fisher's exact test, chi-square test, and Wilcoxon rank-sum test, as appropriate) were employed, and results were reported with 95% confidence intervals (95% CI). A two-sided p value of <0.05 was considered significant.

Results

The study included a total of 845 patients with chronic viral hepatitis and a valid LSM examination. Of these patients, 71% (597) had hepatitis C, 28% (235) hepatitis B, and 2% (13) had both infections (Figure 1). Hepatitis B and C patients significantly differed in many aspects, with hepatitis C patients more commonly showing fibrosis-associated factors, such as older age, male gender, alcohol consumption, etc. Median LSM was 1.8 kPa higher in hepatitis C patients than hepatitis B patients (p<0.001; Table 1). Several liver test results were also significantly higher among hepatitis C patients (Table 2).

At first examination, the distribution of the predefined LSM categories was 57.8% <7 kPa, 16.1% 7.0–9.9 kPa, 14.1% 10–16.9 kPa, and 12.1% ≥17 kPa. The median number of LSMs performed was 3 (IQR, 2–4; range, 1–17). In the LSM natural history cohort, 315 patients were excluded (Figure 1). Among the remaining 530 patients, 93.6% (496) were treatment naïve and 6.4% (34) had been treated without success more than one year prior to inclusion. In this cohort, we performed 1926 valid scans during a median follow-up of 36 months, corresponding to a total of 1519 person years (PY) of observation (Table 1). Median LSM values were 6.6 kPa at the first examination, and 6.4 kPa at the last examination (p<0.001). Although we observed no clinically relevant change in the overall median LSM over time, a high proportion of individual patients changed LSM category during follow-up, including 30% (40/134) of hepatitis B patients and 36.9% (146/396) of hepatitis C patients (Table 3, Figures 2 and 3). Change in LSM category was most common for patients with an initial LSM value of between 7 and 10 kPa, among whom 83% (20/24) of HBV patients and 60% (45/75) of HCV patients had values below 7 kPa at the end of untreated follow-up (Figures 2 and 3).

Among patients with normal initial LSM values (≤7 kPa), 76% of HCV patients and 88% of HBV patients also had normal values at the end of follow-up. However, among the HCV patients whose first and last examination values were both in the normal range, 16% (25/155) had one or more LSM value of >7 kPa during the follow-up period, and 3% (4/155) had one or more LSM value of >10 kPa (none presented an LSM value of >17 kPa). Among the HBV patients with normal first and last LSM examination results, 9% (8/88) had one or more LSM values of >7 kPa, but none were above 10 kPa. Among untreated HCV patients, 10% (41/396) showed a persistent and significant increase in LSM values, corresponding to an incidence rate of 3.4/100 PY (95% CI, 2.5–4.7). Among untreated HBV patients, 4% (6/134) showed a persistent and significant increase in LSM, corresponding to an incidence rate of 1.5 (95% CI, 0.6–3.3)/100 PY.

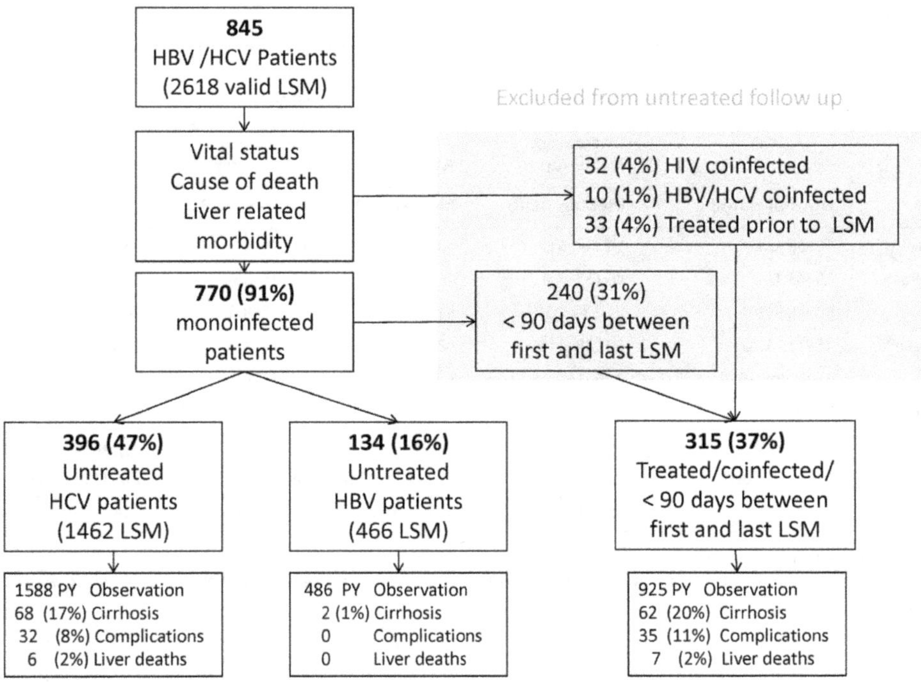

Figure 1. Flow chart of patients showing follow-up liver stiffness measurements.

During the study period, 105 biopsies were performed among the 845 patients, corresponding to 12% of the population (16% of HCV patients and 8% of HBV patients). These biopsies revealed significant fibrosis (≥F2) in 53%, and cirrhosis in 23% of biopsied patients. Among the 54 untreated patients subjected to biopsy, a cut-off of 17 kPa correctly classified 96% as having cirrhosis (sensitivity, 0.92; specificity, 0.95; likelyhood ratio of a positive test (LR+), 19; likelyhood ratio of a negative test (LR−), 0.1).

Cirrhosis

Among the 845 patients, 132 (16%) were classified as having cirrhosis—of whom 51 (39%) were diagnosed prior to the first

Table 1. Demographics of study populations.

	HCV		HBV		HCV/HBV, all
	Untreated follow-up	All	Untreated follow-up	All	p value
Male gender, n (%)	246 (62)	381 (64)	61 (46)	111 (47)	<0.001
Age at first scan (years), median (IQR)	45 (36–52)	45 (36–52)	34 (29–43)	36 (29–47)	<0.001
Injecting drug use (ever), n(%)	248 (63)	374 (63)	1 (1)	3 (1)	<0.001
Self reporet alcohol overuse (ever), n(%)	187 (47)	248 (42)	12 (9)	20 (9)	<0.001
Baseline liver stiffness, median(IQR)	6.9 (5.6–10.5)	6.9 (5.4–11.8)	5.2 (4.2–7)	5.2 (4.3–6.8)	<0.001
Baseline liver stiffness ≥17 kPa, n (%)	46 (12)	94 (16)	1 (1)	7 (3)	<0.001
Liver biopsy Metavir score*					
Fibrosis, median (IQR)	1.5 (1–3)	1.5 (1–3)	1 (0.5–1)	1 (0–1)	0.041
Activity, median (IQR)	0.5 (0–2)	1 (0–2)	0 (0–1.5)	0 (0–2)	0.224
Liver Biopsy with cirrhosis, n (%)	29 (7)	47 (8)	0 (0)	2 (1%)	<0.001
Observed clical decompentsations, n (%)	32 (8)	61 (10)	0 (0)	4 (2)	<0.001
Observed total deaths, n (%)	27 (7)	50 (8)	0 (0)	5 (2)	<0.001
Liver related deaths, n (%)**	5 (1)	12 (2)	0 (0)	0 (0)	0.030
Sum of follow up in person years	1133	2198	0 (0)	744	
Total, n (%)	396 (100)	597 (100)	134	234 (100)	

These data exclude 13 patients co-infected with HBV and HCV, and include 29 patients co-infected with HIV.
* Liver biopsy data for 68 patients with biopsy within one year of liver stiffness measurement.
**Excluding 1 hepatitis C patient with an unconfirmed liver-related cause of death.

Table 2. Laboratory tests at first liver stiffness measurement.

		HCV		HBV		HCV/HBV
		Untreated follow-up	All	Untreated follow-up	All	All
	Normal range	**Median (IQR)**	**Median (IQR)**	**Median (IQR)**	**Median (IQR)**	**p value**
Alanine aminotransferase	10-50 U/L	54 (34–91)	54 (34–95)	32 (23–47)	33 (23–49)	<0.001
Asparatate aminotransferase	15–45 U/L	46 (33–75)	46 (33–76)	30 (25–36)	30 (25–36)	<0.001
Alkaline phosphatase	80–285 U/L	81(63–103)	81 (64–105)	71 (57–84)	74 (60–89)	<0.001
Gamma-glutamyltranferase	15–115 U/L	60 (28–119)	58 (28–117)	21 (14–32)	21 (15–38)	<0.001
Bilirubin	5–25 μmol/L	8 (6–11)	8 (6–12)	8 (6–12)	8 (6–12)	0.983
International normalized ratio	0.9–1.2	1.0 (0.9–1.1)	1.0 (0.9–1.1)	1.0 (1.0–1.1)	1.0 (1.0–1.1)	0.003
Albumin	36–48 g/L	44 (42–46)	44(41–46)	45 (43–47)	44 (42–46)	0.319
Platelets	145–350 109/L	224 (175–278)	222 (170–272)	228 (194–282)	226 (193–226)	0.203
Total, n (%)*		396 (100)	597 (100)	134 (100)	234 (100)	

Excluding 13 patients co-infected with HBV and HCV.
All tests were performed within three months of the first liver stiffness measurement, except for aspartate aminotransferase, which was first introduced in 2011.
* Not all patients were tested for all analyses.

LSM, 56 (42%) within 6 months of the first LSM, and 25 (19%) during follow-up. Prior to the introduction of LSM, 67% of cirrhosis diagnoses were made based on biopsy and 33% based on clinical signs of decompensation. After the introduction of LSM, 61 patients (75%) were diagnosed with cirrhosis based on an LSM value of ≥17 kPa, 5 (6%) based on clinical signs, and 15 (19%) by biopsy. In all cases where cirrhosis was diagnosed by clinical signs alone, this diagnosis occurred during the initial workup (the 6-month lead-in phase). During the subsequent follow-up, no patient was diagnosed with cirrhosis based on clinical signs. Excluding the 6-month lead-in phase after the first LSM, the incidence of cirrhosis was 1.0/100 PY (95% CI, 0.6–1.4).

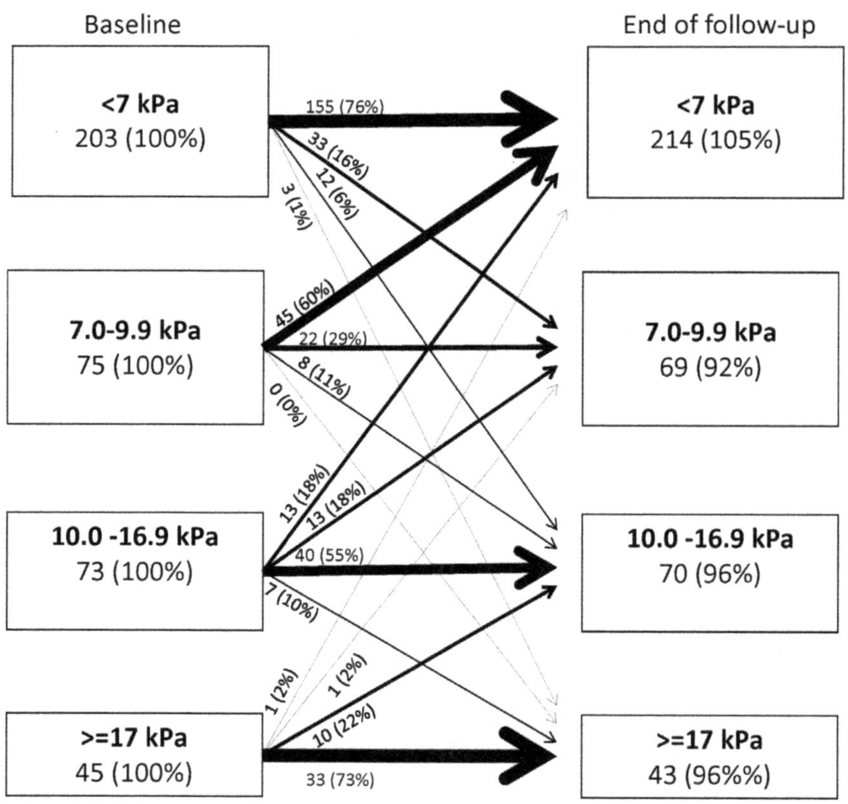

Figure 2. Changes in liver stiffness measurements over time among 396 untreated hepatitis C patients. Percentage values indicate percent of baseline group.

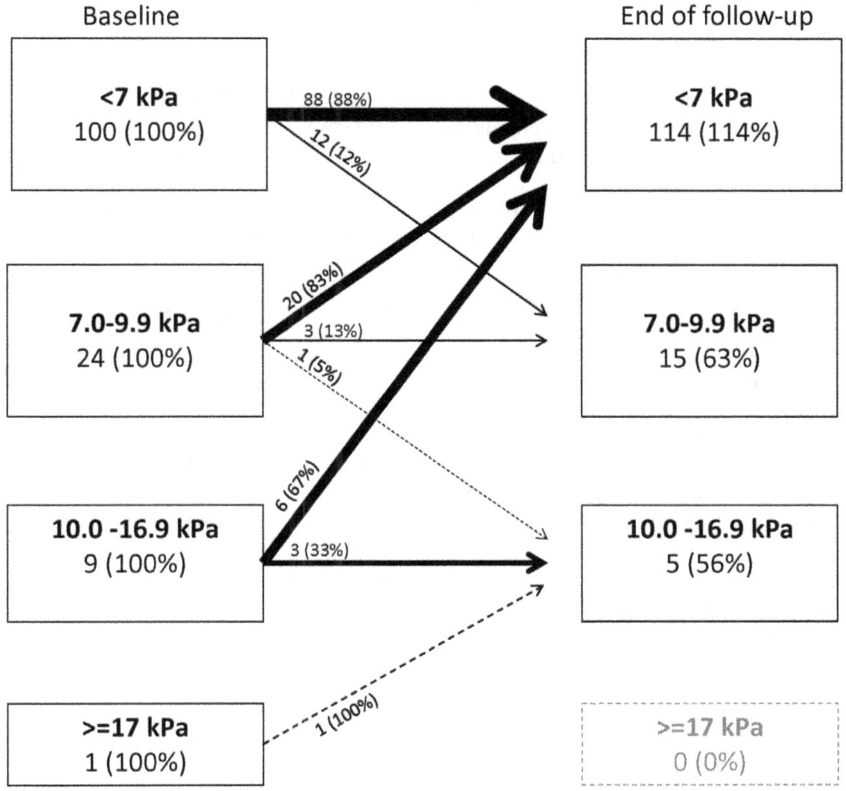

Figure 3. Changes in liver stiffness measurements over time among 134 untreated hepatitis B patients. Percentage values indicate percent of baseline group.

Decompensated liver disease

Overall, 103 liver-related complications occurred in 67 of 132 patients with cirrhosis (51%). Of these complications, 58 (56%) were observed among 32 patients (24%) during follow-up, corresponding to an 11.5/100 PY incidence of complications among patients with cirrhosis. During follow-up, liver-related complications occurred only among patients with a previous diagnosis of cirrhosis and who were infected with HCV (including one patient co-infected with HBV and HIV). Patients diagnosed with cirrhosis based on an LSM value of ≥17 kPa without biopsy had the same risk of complications during follow-up (incidence of

Table 3. Change between first and last liver stiffness measurements among 530 untreated patients who were monoinfected with viral hepatitis B or C and followed for >3 months.

	No change	Increase	Decrease	Total
First LSM (kPa)	**n (%)**	**n (%)**	**n (%)**	**n (%)**
Hepatitis C				
2.0–6.9	170 (83.7)	33 (16.3)	-	203 (100)
7.0–9.9	41 (54.7)	7 (9.3)	27 (36.0)	75 (100)
10.0–16.9	29 (39.7)	15 (20.5)	29 (39.7)	73 (100)
17.0–75.0	13 (28.9)	10 (29.4)	22 (48.9)	45 (100)
Total	253 (63.9)	15.9)	78 (19.7)	396 (100)
Hepatitis B				
2.0–6.9	93 (93.0)	7 (7.0)	-	100 (100)
7.0–9.9	6 (25.0)	1 (4.2)	17 (70.8)	24 (100)
10.0–16.9	1 (11.1)	2 (22.2)	6 (66.7)	9 (100)
17.0–75.0	1 (100.0)	0 (0.0)	0 (0.0)	1 (100)
Total	101 (74.4)	10 (13.3)	23 (12.2)	134 (100)

Change defined as: a difference of >20% of the primary measurement and of >2 kPa, with one measurement >7 kPa.

11.1/100 PY) as patients with biopsy-proven cirrhosis (12.1/100 PY; incidence rate ratio (IRR), 0.92; 95% CI, 0.4–2.0; p = 0.8).

Mortality

Among the 845 patients, 56 deaths occurred, corresponding to 1.9/100 PY of observation (95% CI, 1.4–2.4). Fifty of these deaths occurred among the 586 hepatitis C monoinfected patients, one of whom received a liver transplant, corresponding to 2.4/100 PY (95% CI, 1.7–3.1). The liver-related mortality was 0.65/100 PY (0.35–1.08) (13 deaths and one liver transplant) and death by drug-related causes was 0.51/100 PY (0.25–0.91) (11 deaths) (Table 3). Of the 13 liver-related events, 11 occurred among HCV patients with an initial LSM value of ≥17 kPa. The remaining two patients registered as death from liver-related causes had initial LSM values of <7 kPa. However, one was probably a registration error, as the repeat LSM value was 65 kPa and the patient had biopsy-proven cirrhosis prior to the first examination. The other patient had F1 fibrosis in a liver biopsy performed in 2004, 3 LSM values of <5.5 kPa during 2007–2010, and no clinical or biochemical signs of liver disease at last follow-up. The patient died 11 months later with no history of preceding illness. No autopsy was performed, and the death certificate was filled out by a private practitioner who stated liver coma to be the immediate cause of death, and cirrhosis due to hepatitis C as the underlying cause of death. We consider this cause of death unlikely. Excluding this patient, the liver-related mortality was 0.60/100 PY (12 deaths and one transplant) overall, and 2.5/100 PY for patients with cirrhosis.

Among the 217 monoinfected hepatitis B patients, 5 died, corresponding to 0.73/100 PY (0.23–1.69). No liver-related deaths were observed (97.5% CI, 0–0.43). Nine patients (4%) had an initial LSM value of >17 kPa, compatible with cirrhosis. Of these 9 patients, 7 started treatment, of whom 4 had LSM values of <17 kPa at end of follow-up (two with values in the normal range).

We found a high predictive value of initial LSM for liver-related deaths among the 845 patients in our cohort. The overall area under the receiver operating characteristics curve (AUROC) was 0.86, and the AUROC calculated excluding the two patients that we believe were not correctly classified was 0.96. No liver-related deaths occurred in patients with an initial LSM value of <17 kPa. In contrast, the prediction of overall mortality based on LSM was low (AUROC of 0.64) reflecting that only 23% (13/56) of the deaths observed in our cohort were considered to be liver related.

Discussion

The present single-center study evaluated the use of LSM to monitor liver fibrosis in a routine clinical setting over a five-year period with complete mortality follow-up. We found a significant spontaneous decrease in LSM values during untreated follow-up among patients with an initial LSM of <10 kPa. In contrast, patients with LSM values of ≥17 kPa had a clinically significant incidence of liver-related complications regardless of whether cirrhosis had also been diagnosed by biopsy.

Using our present definition of significant and persistent fibrosis progression (20% increase of a minimum of 2 kPa, with one value above 7 kPa, and all elevated values documented at least twice), such progression was observed in 3% of the untreated hepatitis C patients and 2% of the hepatitis B patients per year. Previous studies have reported similar rates of progression in HCV-infected drug users (median 3% progression during 1.8 years of follow-up) and among hemophiliacs (4.1/100 PY), although these studies did not use the same definition of fibrosis progression as our study [20,21]. The incidence of cirrhosis in our study was 1/100 PY during follow-up, which is in accordance with results from prior cohort studies of hepatitis C patients [22].

A striking finding of our present study was that many patients showed a decline in LSM values, or had fluctuating values during follow-up (Table 3). This confirms the results from our previous screening study showing that 30% (6/20) of drug users with an initial LSM value of >12 kPa had regressed to a median value of 8.4 kPa after three months. These data are also in agreement with the results reported by Mehta et al., demonstrating that 48% of patients with initial LSM values of between 8–12 kPa had one or more measurement of <8 kPa during follow-up [20,23]. A study of hemophiliacs showed that 32% exhibited more than 2 kPa of regression during 3.7 years of follow-up [21]. Among hepatitis B patients, Castera et al. [24] reported that 81% (9/11) with an initial LSM value of >7.2 kPa regressed to normal values during 22 months of follow-up, and Kim et al. [25] reported that 30% (34/114) of patients with F3+ in biopsy regressed more than 30% during 13 months. For comparison, studies using repeated biopsy have reported that up to 24% exhibited decreasing fibrosis during 3–4 years of untreated follow-up [24–26]. Our present study did not address the causes of the observed variations; however, our findings suggest that clinical decisions, such as treatment initiation, or prediction of prognosis for long-term liver-related complications should not be based on a single LSM measurement.

One major change that occurred at our clinic after LSM introduction was that we no longer observed patients who developed liver decompensation without a previous diagnosis of cirrhosis. Prior to LSM, one-third of our patients with cirrhosis were diagnosed based on decompensation [27]. Among these patients, cirrhosis had not been suspected or the patients had refused to undergo liver biopsy. Our present rates of complications (12.7/100 PY) and liver-related deaths (0.6/100 PY) were comparable to those previously reported in both LSM-based and biopsy-based studies, in which decompensation has been reported as 5–12/100 PY and liver-related mortality as 1/100 PY [18,28–31]. We observed few liver-related complications among hepatitis B patients; however, due to the low number of events, the incidence was not statistically different from that among hepatitis C patients. This is in contrast to Asian studies that have reported a similar or higher prevalence of cirrhosis and liver-related events among HBV patients compared to HCV patients [32–34]. Compared to the HCV patients in our study, the HBV patients showed fewer risk factors associated with cirrhosis; only 9 HBV patients had cirrhosis and 20% of all HBV patients received continuous nucleoside treatment during follow-up.

All of the above cited studies, as well as studies in hepatitis B patients, are in agreement with our finding that LSM was a strong predictor for liver-related events, with optimal cut-offs of 13–20 kPa for predicting events, and very low risk associated with values below 10 kPa [35]. This association was confirmed in a recent meta-analysis of LSM as a predictor of complications, showing a 22% increase in mortality per kPa increase in baseline LSM [36]. However, they did not report a lower threshold for complications.

Our study has several weaknesses. We focused on LSM examinations and did not include clinical or laboratory tests in the evaluation. These parameters would have improved patient characterization and probably would have increased the precision of our estimates, for instance hepatitis C patients had significantly higher liver enzymes than hepatitis B (Table 2). Several studies have found ALT to be an independent predictor of LSM value regression, and it has been suggested that LSM be combined with serological markers of fibrosis in order to increase diagnostic accuracy [3,37–39]. However the addition of laboratory data would have also limited the interpretation of LSM performance alone. The regression towards normal among patients with initial LSM values in the 7–10 kPa range could have partly been due to the fact that repeat scans were performed in the fasting state. However, after detection of an elevated LSM value, the patient was followed in the fasting state, as has been our standard practice since 2008. Additionally, the XL probe has been shown to produce values up to 1 kPa lower when compared to the median probe [40]. However, we used the XL probe in cases where the M probe did not give valid results, and thus very few patients had an initial valid scan with the M probe and a scan with the XL probe at the end of follow-up.

Conclusions

Over the past years, LSM has been widely introduced as a screening tool for fibrosis, with patients showing an LSM value above the normal range potentially being considered candidates for antiviral treatment. Our present study showed that the LSM values of many of these patients returned to within the normal range during untreated follow-up. Furthermore, no cases of liver-related death or morbidity were observed in patients with moderately and intermittently elevated LSM values. Our findings suggested that clinical decisions should not be based on a single elevated LSM measurement. Furthermore, our present results indicated that patients with LSM values of ≥17 kPa should enter surveillance for complications of cirrhosis.

Author Contributions

Conceived and designed the experiments: KC CP PBC. Performed the experiments: KC BKM JFH EFJ PBC. Analyzed the data: KC BKM JFH EFJ CP PBC. Wrote the paper: KC BKM JFH EFJ CP PBC.

References

1. Rockey DC, Caldwell SH, Goodman ZD, Nelson RC, Smith AD (2009) Liver biopsy. Hepatology 49: 1017–1044. 10.1002/hep.22742 [doi].
2. Manning DS, Afdhal NH (2008) Diagnosis and quantitation of fibrosis. Gastroenterology 134: 1670–1681. S0016-5085(08)00425-3 [pii];10.1053/j.gastro.2008.03.001 [doi].
3. Castera L (2012) Noninvasive methods to assess liver disease in patients with hepatitis B or C. Gastroenterology 142: 1293–1302. S0016-5085(12)00230-2 [pii];10.1053/j.gastro.2012.02.017 [doi].
4. Sandrin L, Fourquet B, Hasquenoph JM, Yon S, Fournier C, et al. (2003) Transient elastography: a new noninvasive method for assessment of hepatic fibrosis. Ultrasound Med Biol 29: 1705–1713.
5. Berzigotti A, De GA, Vukotic R, Siramolpiwat S, Abraldes JG, et al. (2013) Effect of meal ingestion on liver stiffness in patients with cirrhosis and portal hypertension. PLoS One 8: e58742. 10.1371/journal.pone.0058742 [doi]; PONE-D-12-38729 [pii].
6. Coco B, Oliveri F, Maina AM, Ciccorossi P, Sacco R, et al. (2007) Transient elastography: a new surrogate marker of liver fibrosis influenced by major changes of transaminases. J Viral Hepat 14: 360–369.
7. Arena U, Lupsor PM, Stasi C, Moscarella S, Assarat A, et al. (2013) Liver stiffness is influenced by a standardized meal in patients with chronic hepatitis C virus at different stages of fibrotic evolution. Hepatology 58: 65–72. 10.1002/hep.26343 [doi].
8. Millonig G, Friedrich S, Adolf S, Fonouni H, Golriz M, et al. (2010) Liver stiffness is directly influenced by central venous pressure. J Hepatol 52: 206–210. S0168-8278(09)00794-6 [pii];10.1016/j.jhep.2009.11.018 [doi].
9. Ganne-Carrie N, Ziol M, de Lédinghen V, Douvin C, Marcellin P, et al. (2006) Accuracy of liver stiffness measurement for the diagnosis of cirrhosis in patients with chronic liver diseases. Hepatology 44: 1511–1517.
10. Colombo S, Belloli L, Zaccanelli M, Badia E, Jamoletti C, et al. (2011) Normal liver stiffness and its determinants in healthy blood donors. Dig Liver Dis 43: 231–236. S1590-8658(10)00259-8 [pii];10.1016/j.dld.2010.07.008 [doi].
11. Roulot D, Czernichow S, Le CH, Costes JL, Vergnaud AC, et al. (2008) Liver stiffness values in apparently healthy subjects: Influence of gender and metabolic syndrome. J Hepatol 48: 606–613.
12. Roulot D, Costes JL, Buyck JF, Warzocha U, Gambier N, et al. (2011) Transient elastography as a screening tool for liver fibrosis and cirrhosis in a community-based population aged over 45 years. Gut 60: 977–984. gut.2010.221382 [pii];10.1136/gut.2010.221382 [doi].
13. Friedrich-Rust M, Ong MF, Martens S, Sarrazin C, Bojunga J, et al. (2008) Performance of transient elastography for the staging of liver fibrosis: a meta-analysis. Gastroenterology 134: 960–974. S0016-5085(08)00108-X [pii];10.1053/j.gastro.2008.01.034 [doi].
14. Tsochatzis EA, Gurusamy KS, Ntaoula S, Cholongitas E, Davidson BR, et al. (2011) Elastography for the diagnosis of severity of fibrosis in chronic liver disease: a meta-analysis of diagnostic accuracy. J Hepatol 54: 650–659. S0168-8278(10)00825-1 [pii];10.1016/j.jhep.2010.07.033 [doi].
15. Degos F, Perez P, Roche B, Mahmoudi A, Asselineau J, et al. (2010) Diagnostic accuracy of FibroScan and comparison to liver fibrosis biomarkers in chronic viral hepatitis: a multicenter prospective study (the FIBROSTIC study). J Hepatol 53: 1013–1021. S0168-8278(10)00692-6 [pii];10.1016/j.jhep.2010.05.035 [doi].
16. Christensen PB, Clausen MR, Krarup H, Laursen AL, Schlichting P, et al. (2012) Treatment for hepatitis B virus (HBV) and hepatitis C virus (HCV) infection - Danish national guidelines 2011. Dan Med J 59: C4465. C4465 [pii].
17. Castera L, Pinzani M, Bosch J (2012) Non invasive evaluation of portal hypertension using transient elastography. J Hepatol 56: 696–703. S0168-8278(11)00553-8 [pii];10.1016/j.jhep.2011.07.005 [doi].
18. Schuppan D, Afdhal NH (2008) Liver cirrhosis. Lancet 371: 838–851. S0140-6736(08)60383-9 [pii];10.1016/S0140-6736(08)60383-9 [doi].
19. Ydreborg M, Lisovskaja V, Lagging M, Christensen PB, Langeland N, et al. (2014) A Novel Fibrosis Index Comprising a Non-Cholesterol Sterol Accurately Predicts HCV-Related Liver Cirrhosis. PLoS One 9 e93601. doi: 10.1371/journal.pone.0093601.
20. Mehta SH, Kirk GD, Astemborski J, Sulkowski MS, Afdhal NH, et al. (2012) Stability of liver fibrosis among HCV-infected injection drug users. Antivir Ther 17: 813–821. 10.3851/IMP2085 [doi].
21. Fransen van de Putte DE, Fischer K, de Knegt RJ, Posthouwer D, van Erpecum KJ, et al. (2011) Liver stiffness measurements to assess progression of fibrosis in HCV-infected patients with inherited bleeding disorders. Haemophilia 17: e975–e980. 10.1111/j.1365-2516.2011.02542.x [doi].
22. Seeff LB (2009) The history of the "natural history" of hepatitis C (1968–2009). Liver Int 29 Suppl 1: 89–99. LIV1927 [pii];10.1111/j.1478-3231.2008.01927.x [doi].
23. Moessner BK, Jorgensen TR, Skamling M, Vyberg M, Junker P, et al. (2011) Outreach screening of drug users for cirrhosis with transient elastography. Addiction 106: 970–976. 10.1111/j.1360-0443.2010.03246.x [doi].
24. Ghany MG, Kleiner DE, Alter H, Doo E, Khokar F, et al. (2003) Progression of fibrosis in chronic hepatitis C. Gastroenterology 124: 97–104.
25. Marcellin P, Asselah T, Boyer N (2002) Fibrosis and disease progression in hepatitis C. Hepatology 36: S47–S56.
26. McHutchison J, Goodman Z, Patel K, Makhlouf H, Rodriguez-Torres M, et al. (2010) Farglitazar lacks antifibrotic activity in patients with chronic hepatitis C infection. Gastroenterology 138: 1365–73, 1373. S0016-5085(09)02111-8 [pii];10.1053/j.gastro.2009.12.003 [doi].
27. Dam FA, Schaffalitzky de Muckadell OB, Touborg LA (2012) Incidence, etiology and mortality of cirrhosis: a population-based cohort study. Scand J Gastroenterol 47: 702–709. 10.3109/00365521.2012.661759 [doi].
28. Klibansky DA, Mehta SH, Curry M, Nasser I, Challies T, et al. (2012) Transient elastography for predicting clinical outcomes in patients with chronic liver disease. J Viral Hepat 19: e184–e193. 10.1111/j.1365-2893.2011.01493.x [doi].
29. Missiha SB, Ostrowski M, Heathcote EJ (2008) Disease progression in chronic hepatitis C: modifiable and nonmodifiable factors. Gastroenterology 134: 1699–1714. S0016-5085(08)00348-X [pii];10.1053/j.gastro.2008.02.069 [doi].
30. Asrani SK, Kamath PS (2013) Natural history of cirrhosis. Curr Gastroenterol Rep 15: 308. 10.1007/s11894-012-0308-y [doi].
31. Vergniol J, Foucher J, Terrebonne E, Bernard PH, Le BB, et al. (2011) Noninvasive tests for fibrosis and liver stiffness predict 5-year outcomes of patients with chronic hepatitis C. Gastroenterology 140: 1970–9, 1979. S0016-5085(11)00270-8 [pii];10.1053/j.gastro.2011.02.058 [doi].
32. Cardoso AC, Carvalho-Filho RJ, Stern C, Dipumpo A, Giuily N, et al. (2012) Direct comparison of diagnostic performance of transient elastography in patients with chronic hepatitis B and chronic hepatitis C. Liver Int 32: 612–621. 10.1111/j.1478-3231.2011.02660.x [doi].
33. Jung KS, Kim SU, Ahn SH, Park YN, Kim DY, et al. (2011) Risk assessment of hepatitis B virus-related hepatocellular carcinoma development using liver stiffness measurement (FibroScan). Hepatology 53: 885–894. 10.1002/hep.24121 [doi].
34. Kim SU, Lee JH, Kim DY, Ahn SH, Jung KS, et al. (2012) Prediction of liver-related events using fibroscan in chronic hepatitis B patients showing advanced liver fibrosis. PLoS One 7: e36676. 10.1371/journal.pone.0036676 [doi]; PONE-D-12-00848 [pii].
35. de Lédinghen V, Vergniol J, Barthe C, Foucher J, Chermak F, et al. (2013) Non-invasive tests for fibrosis and liver stiffness predict 5-year survival of patients chronically infected with hepatitis B virus. Aliment Pharmacol Ther 37: 979–988. 10.1111/apt.12307 [doi].
36. Singh S, Fujii LL, Murad MH, Wang Z, Asrani SK, et al. (2013) Liver stiffness is associated with risk of decompensation, liver cancer, and death in patients with chronic liver diseases: a systematic review and meta-analysis. Clin Gastroenterol

Hepatol 11: 1573–1584. S1542-3565(13)01167-1 [pii];10.1016/j.cgh.2013.07.034 [doi].

37. Fung J, Lai CL, Wong DK, Seto WK, Hung I, et al. (2011) Significant changes in liver stiffness measurements in patients with chronic hepatitis B: 3-year follow-up study. J Viral Hepat 18: e200–e205. 10.1111/j.1365-2893.2010.01428.x [doi].
38. Poynard T, Vergniol J, Ngo Y, Foucher J, Munteanu M, et al. (2014) Staging chronic hepatitis C in seven categories using fibrosis biomarker (FibroTest) and transient elastography (FibroScan(R)). J Hepatol 60: 706–714. S0168-8278(13)00817-9 [pii];10.1016/j.jhep.2013.11.016 [doi].
39. Lannerstedt H, Konopski Z, Sandvik L, Haaland T, Loberg EM, et al. (2013) Combining transient elastography with FIB4 enhances sensitivity in detecting advanced fibrosis of the liver. Scand J Gastroenterol 48: 93–100. 10.3109/00365521.2012.746389 [doi].
40. de Lédinghen V, Wong VW, Vergniol J, Wong GL, Foucher J, et al. (2012) Diagnosis of liver fibrosis and cirrhosis using liver stiffness measurement: comparison between M and XL probe of FibroScan(R). J Hepatol 56: 833–839. S0168-8278(11)00855-5 [pii];10.1016/j.jhep.2011.10.017 [doi].

22

Phosphatidylcholine Alteration Identified using MALDI Imaging MS in HBV-Infected Mouse Livers and Virus-Mediated Regeneration Defects

Eun-Sook Park[1,2], Jeong Hwa Lee[4], Ji Hye Hong[4], Yong Kwang Park[1], Joon Won Lee[4], Won-Jae Lee[1], Jae Won Lee[4], Kwang Pyo Kim[4]*, Kyun-Hwan Kim[1,2,3]*

1 Department of Pharmacology and Center for Cancer Research and Diagnostic Medicine, IBST, School of Medicine, Konkuk University, Seoul, Korea, **2** KU Open Innovation Center, Konkuk University, Seoul, Korea, **3** Research Institute of Medical Sciences, Konkuk University, Seoul, Korea, **4** Department of Applied Chemistry, Kyung Hee University, Yongin, Gyeonggi, Korea

Abstract

In this study, we investigated whether hepatitis B virus (HBV) causes the alteration of lipid metabolism and composition during acute infection and liver regeneration in a mouse model. The liver controls lipid biogenesis and bile acid homeostasis. Infection of HBV causes various liver diseases and impairs liver regeneration. As there are very few reports available in the literature on lipid alterations by HBV infection or HBV-mediated liver injury, we have analyzed phospholipids that have important roles in liver regeneration by using matrix-assisted laser desorption/ionization (MALDI)-imaging mass spectrometry (IMS) in the livers of HBV model mice. As a result, we identified different phosphatidylcholines (PCs) showing significant changes in their composition as well as cationized ion adduct formation in HBV-infected mouse livers which are associated with virus-mediated regeneration defects. To find the factor of altered PCs, the expression kinetics of enzymes was also examined that regulate PC biosynthesis during liver regeneration. It is noteworthy that the expression of choline-phosphate cytidylyltransferase A (PCYT1A) was significantly delayed in wild type HBV-expressing livers. Moreover, the amount of hepatic total PC was also significantly decreased in wt HBV-expressing mice. These results suggest that infection of HBV alters the composition of PCs which may involve in HBV-mediated regeneration defects and liver disease.

Editor: Tony Wang, SRI International, United States of America

Funding: This work was supported by Proteogenomic Research Program, the Bio- and Medical Technology Development Program (Project No. 2012M3A9B6055305), and Basic Science Research Program (NRF-2013R1A1A3008681) through the National Research Foundation of the Ministry of Science, ICT & Future Planning. The funders had no role in study design, data collection and analysis, decision to publish, or preparation of the manuscript.

Competing Interests: The authors have declared that no competing interests exist.

* Email: kimkp@khu.ac.kr (KPK); khkim10@kku.ac.kr (KHK)

Introduction

Lipid metabolism is one of the essential liver functions and the aberrant metabolism of liver has been reported to cause liver diseases such as inflammation and fibrosis [1]. Infection of hepatitis B virus (HBV), which was estimated to affect 400 million people worldwide, also causes a variety of liver diseases including acute or chronic inflammation, cirrhosis, and hepatocellular carcinoma (HCC) [2–4]. It is well known that HBV infection provokes disturbance of lipid metabolism; however, little is known about virus-mediated lipid changes.

The liver has a unique ability to be regenerated after injury or partial hepatectomy through relatively well-defined and dynamic processes [5,6]. Such regenerative potential is essential for survival after acute or chronic liver injury. The hepatic regeneration is a highly complex process that involves variety of growth factors such as hepatocyte growth factor (HGF), interleukin (IL)-6, tumor necrosis factor (TNF)-α, and transforming growth factor (TGF)-β [5–10]. Multiple factors can influence regeneration processes by providing stimulatory or inhibitory signals for hepatocyte proliferation.

Liver regeneration after liver damages caused by hepatotoxins such as diet toxins and pathogen infections and surgical resection is critical for liver homeostasis. Since phospholipids are major components of the cell membrane, they have important roles during liver regeneration and lipid metabolism. In this regard, the aberrant accumulation of lipid and triglycerides were observed during liver regeneration after partial hepatectomy [11–13]. Lipids that accumulate during liver regeneration are thought to play some transient roles for the liver remnant by supplying the energy and membrane components needed for cell division [11,12]. Moreover, fatty acid composition is altered in liver after partial hepatectomy [14] and especially, the hepatic content of phospholipids is increased [15]. These observations suggest that phospholipid metabolism may be critically associated with the liver regeneration. Recently, we and other groups have reported that HBV infection can impair the liver regeneration through the HBV X protein (HBx) [16–20], suggesting that the altered biogenesis of phospholipids, is involved in the regeneration process after the liver injury caused by HBV infection. However, there have been no studies examining the effect of HBV infection on the alterations of phospholipids during infection or liver regeneration.

Currently, matrix-assisted laser desorption ionization (MALDI)-imaging mass spectrometry (IMS) is an established approach for detecting and localizing a large variety of endogenous molecules including drugs and their metabolites, proteins, peptides and phospholipids. In our previous studies, MALDI-IMS was applied to visualize the differential distributions of phospholipids in diseased lesions and adjacent normal regions of surgical tissues including the breast, lung, ovarian, and intrahepatic cholangiocarcinoma cancers as well as focal cerebral ischemia [21–25]. In this study, we applied MALDI-IMS to examine the distributions and alterations of phospholipids in livers with HBV infection and HBV-mediated regeneration defects. We showed that the composition of several phosphatidylcholines (PCs) and expression level of an enzyme for PC biosynthesis were significantly altered in livers with HBV infection and HBV-mediated regeneration defects.

Materials and Methods

Mouse model for HBV infection

A mouse model for acute HBV infection was used as previously described [19,26]. Briefly, six- to seven-week-old male BALB/c mice (n = 3 per group) were hydrodynamically injected with 25 ug of plasmid DNA (pGEM-4z, pHBV1.2 (wt), pHBV1.2 (HBx-)) into the tail vein in a volume of phosphate-buffered saline (PBS) equivalent to 10% of the mouse body weight. The total volume of DNA was delivered into the vein with high pressure within 4–6 seconds (hydrodynamic *in vivo* transfection). All procedures involving experimental animals were approved by the Animal Care Committee in Konkuk University.

Partial hepatectomy

To induce physiological liver regeneration in mice, a model of 70% partial hepatectomy was used as previously described [19,27]. Briefly, 4 days after hydrodynamic injection with DNA, approximately 70% of the total liver mass was resected after intraperitoneal administration of xylazine (10 ug/kg body weight) and zoletil 50 (10 mg/kg body weight). After anesthetization, the left lobe and a part of the median lobe of each mouse liver were removed through a mid-abdominal incision. After suturing the abdominal wall, the animals were returned to their cages and permitted to feed *ad libitum*. Liver regeneration was evaluated by the ratio of body weight and the liver weight 8 days after partial hepatectomy.

HBV antigen analysis and histological examination of mouse tissue

Surface antigen analysis was performed with mouse serum using the HBsAg detection enzyme-linked immunosorbent assay (ELISA) kit (Enzygnost HBsAg 5.0, Siemens, Erlangen, Germany). Liver tissues were fixed in 4% formaldehyde, embedded in paraffin and sectioned using a microtome. Paraffin sections were stained with hematoxylin and eosin (H&E) and examined using a microscope.

Proliferation assay of mouse hepatocytes

To evaluate the proliferation status of mouse hepatocytes after partial hepatectomy, the Ki67-labeling index was monitored as a proliferation marker. Ki67-stained hepatocytes were identified on 4-um tissue sections of paraffin-embedded liver samples according to the manufacturer's instructions (Cell Proliferation Kit, Amersham Life Science, Amersham, UK).

Tissue processing for MALDI analysis

Liver tissues (n = 2) extracted from mouse specimens were flash-frozen in liquid nitrogen and then stored at −80°C until use. The 10-um-thick tissue sections were cut in a temperature ranging from −20°C to −25°C using cryostat (Leica CM-1850, Leica Microsystems Inc., Solms, Germany). For MALDI-IMS experiments, tissue sections were thaw-mounted on indium-tin-oxide (ITO)-coated glass slides (HST Global, Inc., Hampton, VA, USA). The tissues were then frozen; incubated at 4°C, and at room temperature. Finally, the tissues were dried in a desiccator. For MALDI-MS profiling experiments, a binary matrix solution was prepared by dissolving 3.5 mg each of DHB and CHCA into 1 ml of 70% methanol containing 0.1% TFA as described previously [28], and for the imaging experiments the same matrix was added using ImagePrep (Bruker Daltonics, Billerica, MA, USA). Biological replicates per group were generated from two randomly selected mice.

MALDI imaging mass spectrometry analysis

Mass spectrometry experiments were performed using an Autoflex III mass spectrometer equipped with smart beam laser technology (Nd:YAG, 355 nm; Bruker Daltonics Inc.). Imaging experiments were performed in both positive and negative ion modes from single tissue section and all ions in the mass-to-charge (*m/z*) ratio range of 500–1,200 at a laser frequency of 200 Hz (3,000 consecutive laser shots) were detected in reflectron mode. For imaging experiments, the data acquisition was under the control of Flex software suite (FlexControl 3.0, FlexImaging 2.1, FlexAnalysis 3.3, Bruker Daltonics) and using a spatial resolution of 150 μm with 500 consecutive laser shots per pixel (50 laser shots per position of a random walk within each pixel). Before each data acquisition, an external calibration was conducted using phospholipid-mixed calibration standards with a mass range of 674–834 Da (positive ion mode) and 564–906 Da (negative ion mode). MALDI LIFT (MS/MS) analysis was directly performed on the tissue after MALDI MS. Different phospholipid species were identified by using LIFT data and lipid database (www.lipidmaps.org).

Clinpro Tools (version 2.2, Bruker Daltonics) and flexImaging software was used for MALDI imaging data processing, and all spectral intensities were divided by the obtained total ion count values. Ion intensities were evaluated by comparing ion pairs from liver sections of different experimental groups after normalization. The Top Hat baseline with a 10% minimal baseline width was used for baseline subtraction. Data reduction was performed at a factor of four.

Real-time-PCR (RT-PCR)

Whole mouse liver tissues were lysed using Trizol reagent (Invitrogen/Gibco BRL, Carlsbad, CA, USA) according to the manufacturer's instructions, and total RNAs were isolated. Reverse transcription reactions were performed using 2 ug of total RNA and M-MLV reverse transcriptase (iNtRON, Seoul, Korea) in a final reaction volume of 20 ul. The resulting cDNA was PCR-amplified under the following conditions: initial denaturation at 94°C for 5 min, followed by 25–30 cycles of 94°C (30 s), 58°C (30 s), and 72°C (30 s), with a final extension of 5 min at 72°C. The primer sequences used for amplifications were as follows: phosphate cytidylyltransferase 1, choline, alpha isoform (Pcyt1a), forward, 5′-AGGCTACTGTGACCGAGGTA-3′, reverse, 5′-AGTCACCCTGACATAGGGCT-3′; phosphatidylethanolamine N-methyltransferase (Pemt), forward, 5′-GAGAACTCGGAAGCTGAGCA-3′, reverse, 5′-CAGCACAAACACGAATCCCC-3′. Quantitative real-time PCR was performed using a

SYBR Green PCR Master Mix (Applied Biosystems, Foster City, CA, USA), and PCR amplification was conducted using the Applied Biosystems (ABI7500) real-time PCR machine. Relative quantification analysis was performed by the comparative ΔΔCt method. The results were presented as an n-fold difference relative to calibrator ($RQ = 2^{-\Delta\Delta C_t}$).

Western blot analysis

Each liver tissue was homogenized in RIPA buffer. Fifty μg of protein was separated by 10–12% SDS-PAGE gel and subjected to Western blot analysis. The primary antibodies used were anti-Pcyt1a (N-20, Santa Cruz Biotechnology, CA, USA) and anti-b-actin (Sigma Aldrich). As secondary antibody, appropriate peroxidase-conjugated secondary antibodies (Santa Cruz Biotechnology, CA, USA) were used. Chemiluminecent detection was done with the ECL Detection Reagent (GE Healthcare, Buckinghamshire, UK) and visualized with a LAS-4000 Luminescent Image analyzer (LAS-4000, Fuji, Tokyo, Japan).

Quantification of total PC amount

Mice were sacrificed after partial hepatectomy at indicated time points. The amount of total PC was measured by using phosphatidylcholine assay kit (Cell biolabs Inc, San Diego, CA) according to the manufacturer's instruction. At least three mice are used for the analysis of each group.

Data analysis

Data were obtained by at least 3 independent experiments and the values are presented as the mean ± standard deviation (SD). For MALDI-IMS analysis, two liver tissue samples per groups were independently analyzed. Differences between groups were tested for statistical significance using Student's *t*-test or analysis of variance. The statistical significance was set at $p < 0.05$.

Results

Characterization of mouse model of HBV infection and virus-induced inhibition of liver regeneration

To investigate whether HBV infection can alter the distribution or composition of phospholipids when regenerating liver using MALDI-IMS, we established a mouse model of HBV infection by hydrodynamically injecting the HBV genome [19,26]. The overall experimental scheme used in this study is depicted in Figure 1A. To validate whether the HBV mouse could express viral proteins, viral surface protein (HBsAg) was analyzed by ELISA using mice sera at 3 days after hydrodynamic injection. As shown in Figure 1B, both the replication-competent wt HBV (HBV1.2 (wt)) and the HBx-null HBV (HBV1.2 (HBx-)) can express a similar level of HBsAg protein in the serum of HBV infection (Fig. 1B).

More recently, we reported that HBV infection inhibits liver regeneration by epigenetic regulation of urokinase plasminogen activator through HBx [19]. In this study, to correlate the alterations in phospholipid metabolism with HBV-induced liver regeneration defects, we performed phospholipid profiling and imaging with MALDI-MS and MALDI-IMS using an experimental model of the partial hepatectomy after the hydrodynamic injection of wt HBV and HBx-negative HBV. Consistent with the results of our previous study [19], significant inhibition of liver regeneration at 8 days after partial hepatectomy was observed only in wt HBV infection (Fig. 1C and D). We also examined hepatocyte proliferation by counting the Ki67-positive cells (marker of cell proliferation) by immunohistochemical staining. Proliferation of hepatocytes was also markedly reduced in the liver tissues of wt HBV-expressing mice compared to control or HBx-null liver tissues (Fig. 1E). These results collectively suggest that our model is well established for further analysis of phospholipid imaging using MALDI-IMS.

MS spectra analyses from IMS by PCA and comparison of phospholipid imaging between control and HBV mice in regenerating livers

It was previously reported that the content of hepatic phospholipids which are the major components of cell membrane was altered after the partial hepatectomy [15]. Thus, we investigated whether HBV infection could alter the distribution of phospholipids in the regenerating liver using MALDI-IMS. Liver samples (n = 2 per group) extracted from mice of liver regeneration after partial hepatectomy were subjected to MALDI-IMS analysis in both positive and negative modes. Figure 2A shows the averaged MS spectra acquired from whole mouse liver tissue sections in positive ion mode. The spectra show more than 80 peaks (S/N>6) having specific *m/z* values with different relative intensities from different liver tissues under different experimental conditions (Mock, HBV1.2 (HBx-), and HBV1.2 (wt)) (Fig. 2A). The distribution of obtained MS data was also analyzed statistically by principal component analysis (PCA) and classification methods. PCA for total MS spectra was performed from each group using ClinProTools v2.2 (Bruker Daltonics). As a result, PCA provided a visual distinction on the basis of the detected ions according to three different experimental groups as shown in Figure 2B. Interestingly, PCA analysis for averaged MS spectra acquired in negative ion mode showed no significant changes, although more than 55 peaks (S/N>6) were detected (Figure S1).

Of a number of imaging data obtained using MALDI-IMS, we selected 17 ion images acquired in positive ion mode showing significant changes in their abundance in ion images of liver tissue sections from three different groups as shown in Figure 2C and 2D. Ion images from the biological replicates were listed in Figure S2. No significant alterations were observed in ion images in the negative ion mode (data not shown).

To identify the selected 17 ions in Figure 2C and 2D, we performed MS/MS analysis (Figure S3). From the spectra, these ions were identified as seven PCs with three different adducts (H^+, Na^+ and K^+), two sphingomyelins (SMs) and two lyso-phosphatidylcholines (LPCs) as listed in Table 1. Due to the low intensity of m/z 776.6 ion, the structure was not elucidated in these experiments. The phospholipids shown as 17 ion images were classified into 5 groups according to their patterns of level changes. Phospholipids belonging to A, B, and C groups generally showed decreased relative abundances in HBV1.2 (HBx-) and HBV1.2 (wt) compared to the mock, while ion intensities for phospholipids belonging to the D and E groups showed increased relative abundances in HBV1.2 (HBx-) and HBV1.2 (wt) compared to the mock. Phospholipids belonging to group A, SM (42:2) $[M+K]^+$ (m/z 851.8), SM (42:1) $[M+K]^+$ (m/z 853.6), PC (34:2) $[M+K]^+$ (m/z 796.6), PC (34:1) $[M+K]^+$ (m/z 798.6), and PC (36:2) $[M+K]^+$ (m/z 824.7), showed decreased ion intensities in HBV1.2 (HBx-) and HBV1.2 (wt) compared with the mock. Ion intensities of phospholipids belonging to group B, PC (32:4) $[M+Na]^+$ (m/z 748.5), PC (32:3) $[M+Na]^+$ (m/z 750.5) and m/z 776.6 (structure not identified), decreased gradually in the order of the mock, HBV1.2 (HBx-), and HBV1.2 (wt). However, phospholipids of group D, LPC (22:2) $[M+K]^+$ (m/z 614.2) and LPC (22:2) $[M+K]^+$ (m/z 616.2), showed higher ion intensities in HBV1.2 (HBx-) and HBV1.2 (wt) compared with the mock. Ion intensities of phospholipids of group E, PC (34:2) $[M+H]^+$ (m/z 758.7), PC (34:1) $[M+H]^+$ (m/z 760.6), PC (36:2) $[M+H]^+$ (m/z 786.7), and PC (38:6) $[M+H]^+$ (m/z 806.6), increased

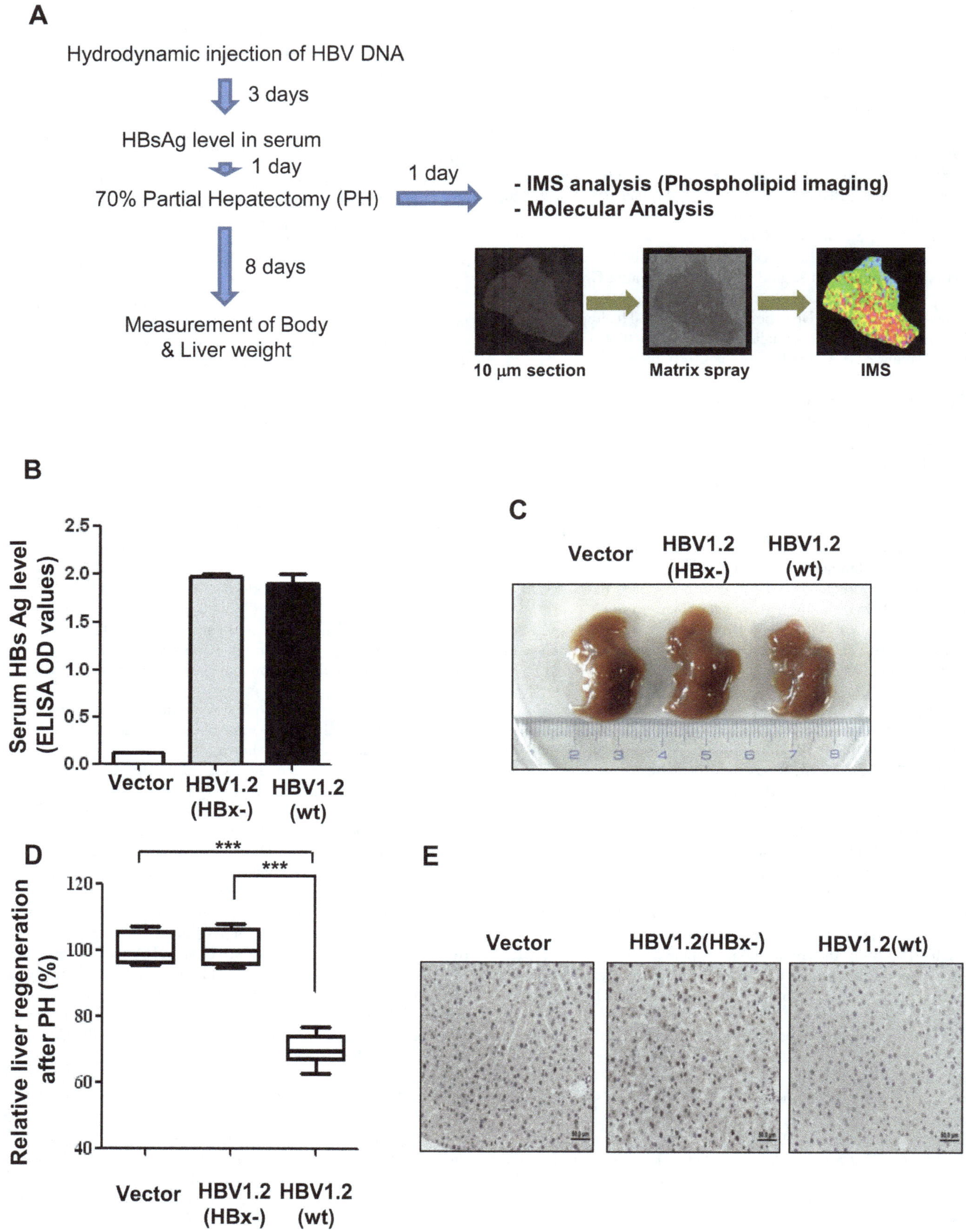

Figure 1. Characterization of HBV mouse model and virus-mediated inhibition of liver regeneration. (A) Overall scheme of experimental procedures. B–E. Validation and characterization of the mouse model of HBV infection used in this study. (B) The HBsAg level in mouse serum at 3 days after hydrodynamic injection. (C) Inhibition of liver regeneration by HBx in HBV mouse model. Macroscopic evaluation of regenerated livers of

HBV or HBx mouse model at 8 days after partial hepatectomy. (D) Box plots of liver weight/body weight at 8 days after partial hepatectomy. (E) Ki 67 (marker of cell proliferation) expression in formalin-fixed liver tissues obtained at 48 h after partial hepatectomy. Data are depicted as mean ±S.D. and are representative of three independent experiments. ***, P<0.001 compared with mock vector and HBV1.2 (HBx-) (n = 5~6 mice per each group).

gradually in the order of the mock, HBV1.2 (HBx-), and HBV1.2 (wt). Interestingly, phospholipids of group C, PC (32:0) $[M+K]^+$ (m/z 772.7) and PC (34:2) $[M+Na]^+$ (m/z 780.6), showed similar ion intensities between the mock and HBV1.2 (HBx-) and the significantly lower ion intensities in HBV1.2 (wt) compared with the mock and HBV1.2 (HBx-).

There was no significant difference in liver histology analyzed by H&E staining within the 3 groups (Fig. 2E). IMS data was applied to confirm not only lipid alteration but also the distribution of each ion in the tissue.

Analysis of potassium cationized adduct formation for selected phospholipids by IMS in regenerating livers

Interestingly, we observed distinct adduct formation for the most abundant PC species, PC (34:2), PC (34:1), and PC (36:2). Adduct formation of these PCs is different according to the mock and HBV infection with or without HBx expression (Fig. 3). The potassium cationized adducts of these PCs showed higher ion intensities than those protonated forms in the livers of control in which the regeneration is more active than in those of HBV infection. However, in the liver samples of HBV1.2 (HBx-) and HBV1.2 (wt), there was no significant difference in adduct formation. In the case of HBV1.2 (HBx-), the potassium cationized forms of PC (34:2) (m/z 796.6) and PC (36:2) (m/z 824.7) showed slightly higher intensities than those protonated forms. In particular, potassium cationized form of PC (34:1) (m/z 798.6) showed lower intensity than its protonated form in the liver of HBV1.2 (wt) (Fig. 3A). The MS/MS analysis was also applied to assign the formation of protonated form and potassium cationized form of PC (34:2), PC (34:1), and PC (36:2) (Fig. 3B). In the MS/MS data of PCs, the *m/z* 184 ion was mainly detected in its protonated form, whereas the ions at *m/z* 86, *m/z* 163 and *m/z* 184 were detected in their potassium cationized form. From the spectra it is observed that the protonated and potassium cationized PC forms of precursor ions ($[M+H]^+$ and $[M+K]^+$ ions) and fragment ions mainly show the neutral loss of $C_3H_{10}N$ (59 Da) (Fig. 3B).

It was previously reported that ($Na^+ + K^+$)-stimulated ATPase activity was increased in the hepatic plasma membranes of partially hepatectomized rat [29,30]. In this study, the high level of potassium cationized form in PCs was observed in the active liver regeneration after partial hepatectomy. However, in the HBV-infected liver, the level of potassium cationized form in PCs was reversed in the liver regeneration.

Kinetic analysis of major genes involved in PC synthesis in regenerating liver

The above results demonstrated that PCs are primarily differentially regulated by HBV infection during liver regeneration. Therefore, we investigated whether the expression of genes known to be involved in PC biosynthesis are altered by HBV infection. PC biosynthesis is generally known as being regulated by 2 pathways: the CDP-choline and phosphatidylethanolamine N-methyltransferase (PEMT) pathways [31]. The major enzymes that regulate these 2 pathways include choline-phosphate cytidylyltransferase A (PCYT1A) and PEMT, respectively (Fig. 4A).

To investigate the kinetic changes in these genes in regenerating liver, we determined the mRNA expression level of Pcyt1a and Pemt at several time points after partial hepatectomy. As shown in Figure 4B and 4C, the expression of Pcyt1a was strongly induced at 6 h after partial hepatectomy in the liver of control and HBx-negative HBV mice. However, in the liver of wt HBV infection, the expression level of Pcyt1a was significantly repressed. Interestingly, the expression was induced rather late after partial hepatectomy (24 h). The expression level of Pcyt1a protein was also delayed in the regenerating livers with wt HBV infection (Fig. 4D). To examine the consequence of altered expression of Pcyt1a enzyme, we measured the total amount of hepatic PCs at both early and late time points after partial hepatectomy. As shown in Figure 4E, the level of total PCs was significantly decreased only in the liver of wt HBV infected mice at 48 h after partial hepatectomy. These data demonstrated that the PC biosynthesis was disturbed by wt HBV infection during liver regeneration, suggesting that the regulation of Pcyt1a expression by HBx is involved in the mouse livers with HBV infection and virus-mediated regeneration defects.

Discussion

In this study, we analyzed the distribution and composition of differentially regulated phospholipids in regenerating livers with HBV infection using MALDI-IMS. Although we could not find significant alterations in phospholipid distribution across the liver tissue, we identified that several PCs altered in the regenerating livers of HBV-infected mice. Moreover, the kinetic changes in genes involved in PC biosynthesis were found in regenerating livers. It was demonstrated that PC biosynthesis is deregulated in the liver of HBV-infected mouse with the virus-mediated regeneration defects through a mechanism mediating the action of HBx protein. Reversely, in livers with HBX-null HBV infection, the recovery of liver regeneration was shown.

Recently, it was reported that the aberrant lipid metabolism mediates liver inflammation and fibrosis [1]. However, it is unclear whether the altered PCs observed in this study resulted from the aberrant lipid metabolism of liver. The chronic infection of HBV undoubtedly induces liver inflammation and fibrosis, indicating that the altered PCs are associated with HBV-related liver diseases.

We identified 17 phospholipids showing significant changes in regenerating liver tissues as shown in Figure 2C and 2D. Phospholipids in A and B groups were altered during HBV infection regardless of HBx expression (Fig. 2C). On the other hand, phospholipids in C, D and E groups showed prominent alterations only in the wt HBV-expressed regenerating liver (Fig. 2D). Phospholipids altered only by wt HBV infection were identified as several PCs. These results suggest that several phospholipids can be altered by HBV infection and it is expected that especially altered PCs (groups C, D, and E) may involve in inhibiting liver regeneration by HBx.

Of phospholipids, several PC represents significant alterations in the HBV 1.2 (wt) compared to the mock and HBV1.2 (HBx-). Thus, we investigated whether the infection of HBV affects PC biosynthesis known to be regulated by 2 pathways: the CDP-choline and phosphatidylethanolamine N-methyltransferase

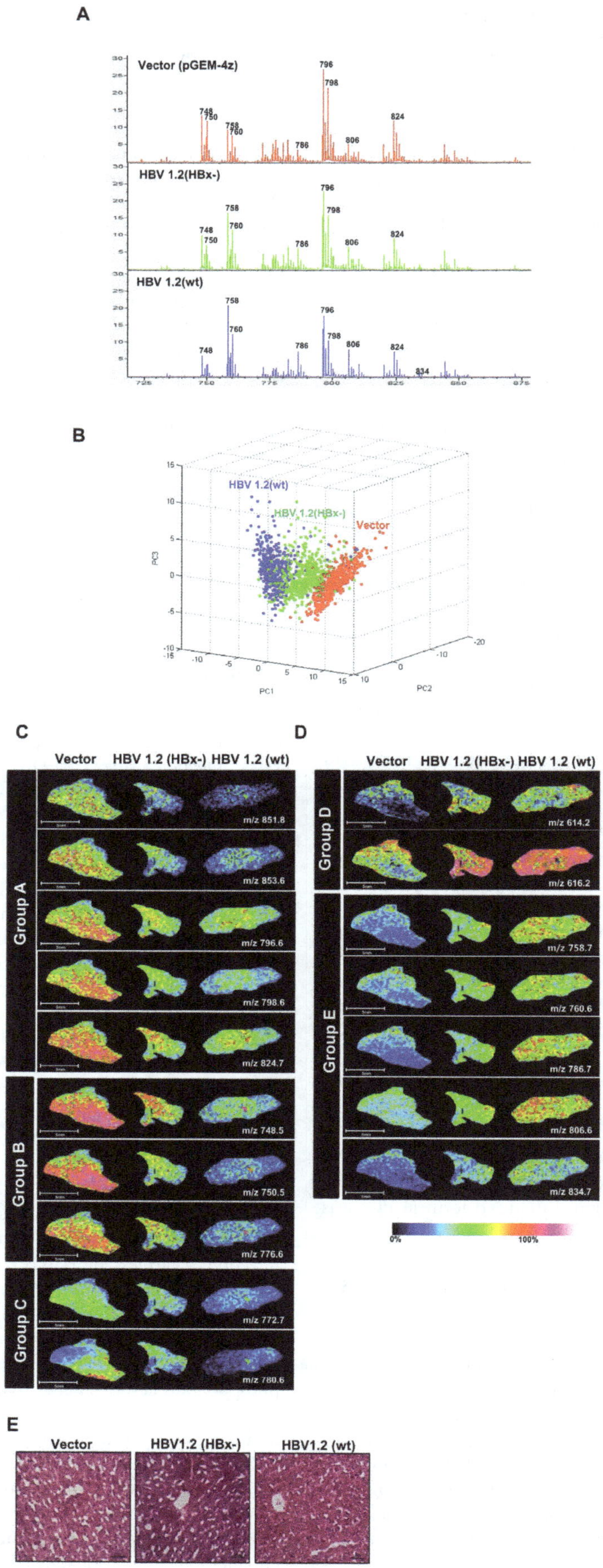
A
Vector (pGEM-4z)
HBV 1.2(HBx-)
HBV 1.2(wt)
748
750
758
760
786
796
798
806
824
834
B
HBV 1.2(wt)
HBV 1.2(HBx-)
Vector
PC1
PC2
PC3
C
D
Vector HBV 1.2 (HBx-) HBV 1.2 (wt)
Group A
Group B
Group C
Group D
Group E
m/z 851.8
m/z 853.6
m/z 796.6
m/z 798.6
m/z 824.7
m/z 748.5
m/z 750.5
m/z 776.6
m/z 772.7
m/z 780.6
m/z 614.2
m/z 616.2
m/z 758.7
m/z 760.6
m/z 786.7
m/z 806.6
m/z 834.7
0%
100%
E
Vector
HBV1.2 (HBx-)
HBV1.2 (wt)

Figure 2. PCA analysis of the averaged MS spectra of phosopholipids from liver tissue sections obtained from 3 different conditions in positive ionization mode and comparison of MALDI images of phospholipids in regenerating liver tissues after partial hepatectomy. (A) Typical MS spectra of liver tissue sections in 3 different conditions obtained from imaging mass spectrometry. (B) PCA analysis of the IMS data acquired in positive-ionization mode. (C, D) Representative MALDI images of molecular ions showing alterations in their levels according to HBV infection with or without HBx expression. (E) H&E-stained liver tissues 24 h after partial hepatectomy.

(PEMT) pathways. Several studies have demonstrated that 70% of PC synthesized in the liver is mediated through the CDP-choline pathway, while the remaining 30% is produced by the PEMT pathway [31]. Induction of PC biosynthesis has been shown to be an essential step in cell proliferation in various cells [32–34]. Martin *et al.* demonstrated that the amount of PC is increased in regenerating livers and the activity of an enzyme, PCYT1A which involves in PC biosynthesis is significantly enhanced after partial hepatectomy [35]. In this study, we examined the kinetic changes in PC synthesis-related genes in regenerating livers and found that the expression of PCYT1A is clearly elevated at 6 h after partial hepatectomy in control and HBx-negative HBV mice. However, PCYT1A expression was strongly suppressed in wt HBV 1.2 mice early after partial hepatectomy. These data indicate that HBV infection can disturb the expression kinetics of PCs and Pcyt1a through HBx protein.

Several studies have reported that altered liver plasma-membrane fluidity was observed between 15 and 24 h after partial hepatectomy which is associated with the altered composition of phospholipids and functional changes in liver plasma-membrane-bound enzymes [36,37]. The Na^+/K^+-ATPase (Na^+/K^+ pump) is located in the plasma membrane of all animal cells and responsible for up to two-third of energy expenditure in a cell. Cells maintain a low concentration of sodium ions and high levels of potassium ions within the cell in order to maintain the cell membrane potential. The (Na^+/K^+)-stimulated ATPase activity has shown to be increased in hepatic plasma membranes of partially hepatectomized rat [29,30]. In this study, the potassium cationized adduct forms of PC (34:2), PC (34:1) and PC (36:2) showed significantly higher intensities than their protonated forms in the livers of control as shown in Figure 3A. However, this pattern was not shown in the liver of HBx-null and wt HBV 1.2 mice. The phospholipid species PC (34:2) and PC (36:2) were also found in intact potassium cationized forms in the liver of HBV1.2 (HBx-), whereas PC (34:1) was mainly found in intact protonated forms in the liver of HBV1.2 (wt). Although the adduct formation is related to ionization in MS which is not related to biological phenomena but it showed significant differences indifferent liver tissues (Mock, HBV1.2 (HBx-), and HBV1.2 (wt)).

We previously demonstrated that the decrease of potassium cationized adduct formation in the focal ischemic region is due to energy failure by a decrease in Na^+/K^+-ATPase activity in this region [25]. Additionally, decreased Na^+/K^+ pump activity was observed due to lower potassium ion concentration in a necrotic region [38]. The low potassium ion concentration may cause the relatively lower intensity of potassium cationized forms of PCs in the liver of HBV1.2 (wt). Although further comprehensive studies are necessary to delineate whether HBV infection regulates ATPase activity, our results suggest that the activity of (Na^+/K^+)-stimulated ATPase is associated with regulating physiological liver regeneration during HBV infection.

Recently, Singh *et al.* have reported that autophagy regulates the lipid metabolism and metabolic syndrome in the liver [39]. Interestingly, HBx was reported to induce autophagy, which is required for HBV replication [40,41]. Thus, lipid alterations observed in our study may be associated with autophagy induced

Table 1. Phospholipids showing the alteration in regenerating liver tissues.

Group	*m/z*	Phospholipid Class	FA (Cn: Un)	Adduct
A	851.8	SM	42:2	K
	853.6	SM	42:1	K
	796.6	PC	34:2	K
	798.6	PC	34:1	K
	824.7	PC	36:2	K
B	748.5	PC	32:4	Na
	750.5	PC	32:3	Na
	776.6	-	-	-
C	772.7	PC	32:0	K
	780.6	PC	34:2	Na
D	614.2	LPC	22:2	K
	616.2	LPC	22:1	K
E	758.7	PC	34:2	H
	760.6	PC	34:1	H
	786.7	PC	36:2	H
	806.6	PC	38:6	H
	834.7	PC	40:6	H

Cn, total chain length; Un, total degree of unsaturation; SM, sphingomyelin; PC, phosphatidylcholine; LPC, lyso-phosphatidylcholine.

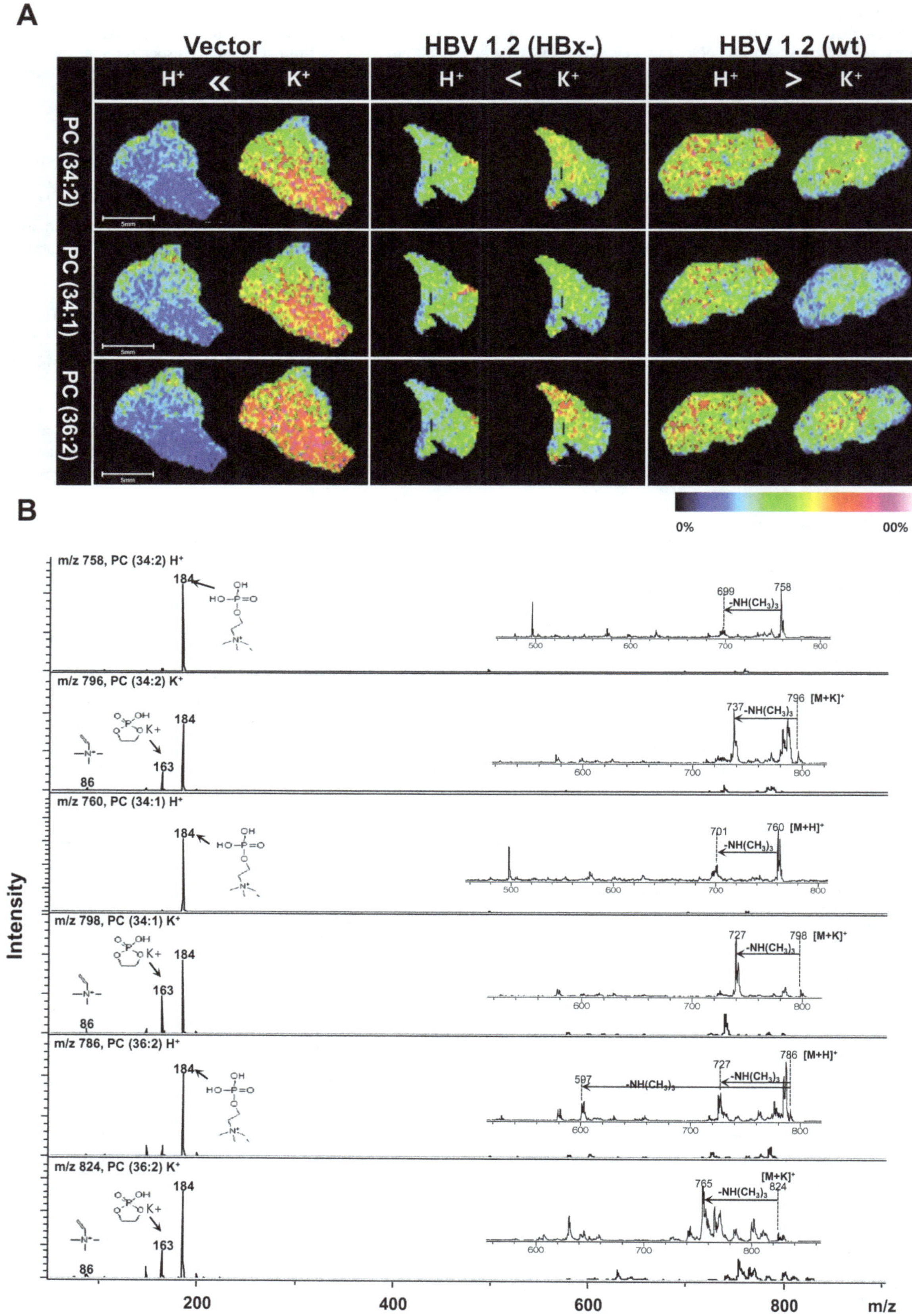

Figure 3. Analysis of selected phospholipids by IMS and MS/MS in regenerating liver tissues. (A) Comparison of the images of H^+ and K^+ adduct form of 3 PCs in regenerating liver tissues. (B) Validation of selected PCs $[M+H]^+$ and $[M+K]^+$ ions by MS/MS analysis.

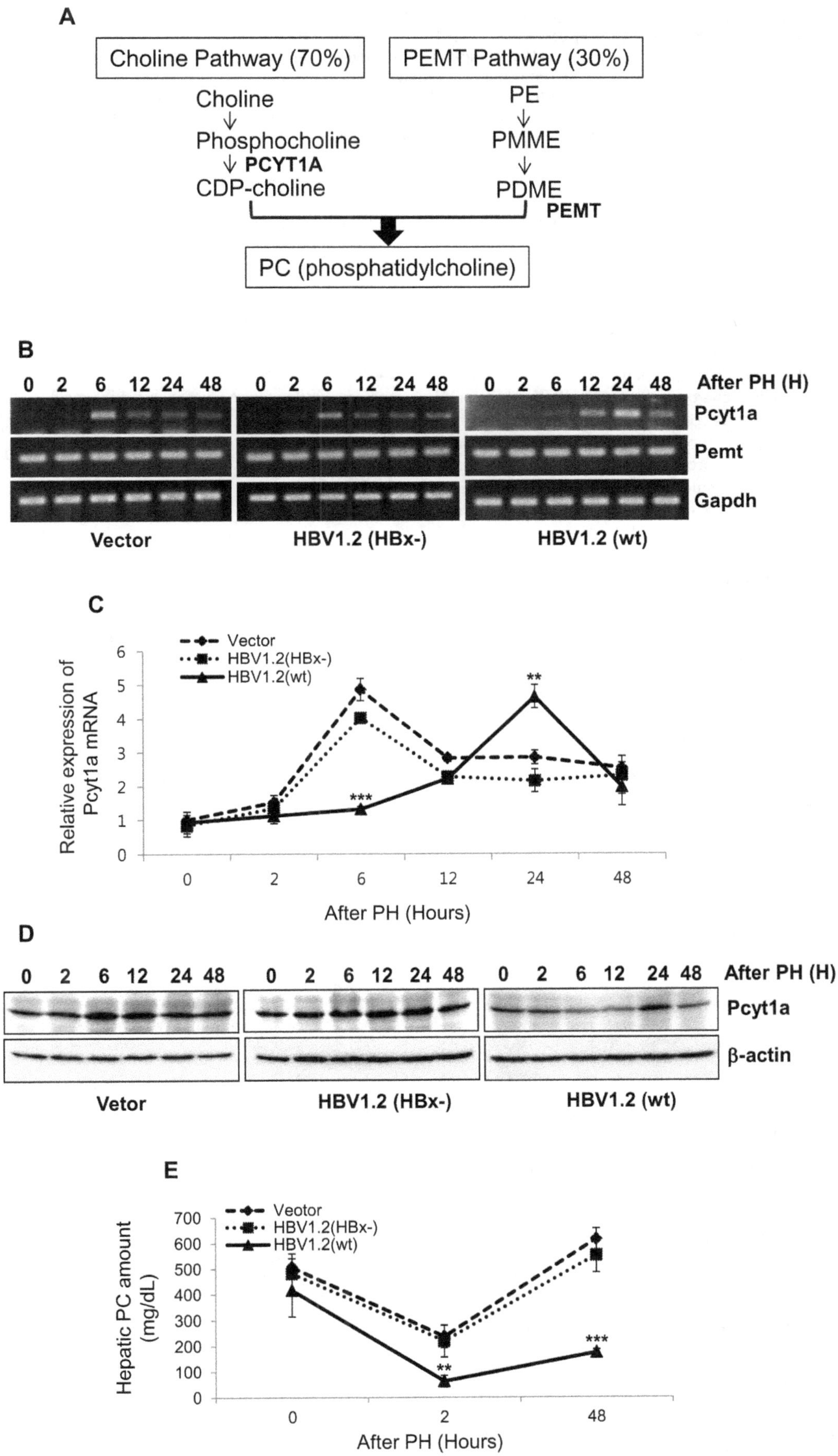
A
Choline Pathway (70%)
PEMT Pathway (30%)
Choline
Phosphocholine
PCYT1A
CDP-choline
PE
PMME
PDME
PEMT
PC (phosphatidylcholine)
B
0 2 6 12 24 48
After PH (H)
Pcyt1a
Pemt
Gapdh
Vector
HBV1.2 (HBx-)
HBV1.2 (wt)
C
Vector
HBV1.2(HBx-)
HBV1.2(wt)
Relative expression of Pcyt1a mRNA
After PH (Hours)
D
After PH (H)
Pcyt1a
β-actin
Vetor
HBV1.2 (HBx-)
HBV1.2 (wt)
E
Veotor
HBV1.2(HBx-)
HBV1.2(wt)
Hepatic PC amount (mg/dL)
After PH (Hours)

Figure 4. Kinetic analysis of phosphatidylcholines (PCs) synthesis-related genes and measurement of total PCs level in regenerating liver tissues after partial hepatectomy. (A) The schematic pathway of PC biosynthesis. PCYT1A, choline-phosphate cytidylyltransferase A; PE, phosphatidylethanolamine; PMME, triolein-phosphatidyl-N-monomethyl ethanolamine; PDME, triolein-phosphatidyl-N,N-dimethyl ethanolamine; PEMT, phosphatidylethanolamine N-methyltransferase. (B–C) Kinetic analysis of Pcyt1a and Pemt expression in liver tissues after partial hepatectomy. At indicated time intervals after partial hepatectomy, the mRNA expression of indicated genes was analyzed using semi-quantitative RT-PCR (B) and real-time PCR (C), and Western blot analysis (D). (E) Quantification of hepatic PCs level after partial hepatectomy. Data represent the mean ±S.D. and are representative of three independent experiments. **, P<0.01; ***, P<0.001 compared with mock vector and HBV1.2 (HBx-) (n = 3~4 mice per each group).

by HBx. Further studies on this issue will result in a better understanding of HBV-mediated liver diseases.

Conclusions

In conclusion, we analyzed the altered phospholipids using MALDI-IMS in regenerating livers of HBV mouse models. In this study, we identified several PCs and related enzymes that showed significant expression changes in the livers of HBV infection and HBV-mediated regeneration defects. These results suggest that HBV infection particularly through the HBx protein which induces alterations in PC expression and these are potentially involved in HBV-mediated regeneration defects and liver diseases. Further studies are needed to define the specific role of these altered PCs on HBV-mediated liver pathogenesis.

Supporting Information

Figure S1 PCA analysis of the averaged MS spectra of phospholipids from liver tissue sections obtained from 3 different conditions in negative ionization mode. (A) Typical MS spectra of liver tissue sections in 3 different conditions obtained from imaging mass spectrometry. (B) PCA analysis of the IMS data acquired in positive-ionization mode.

Figure S2 MALDI images of phospholipids from the biological replicate in regenerating liver tissues after partial hepatectomy. Alterations of phospholipid distribution showed similar tendency between biological replicates.

Figure S3 MS/MS data of 17 phospholipid ions listed in Table 1.

Author Contributions

Conceived and designed the experiments: ESP KHK KPK. Performed the experiments: ESP JHL JHH YKP Joon Won Lee WJL Jae Won Lee. Analyzed the data: ESP JHL Jae Won Lee. Contributed reagents/materials/analysis tools: ESP JHL JHH Jae Won Lee. Contributed to the writing of the manuscript: ESP KHK KPK.

References

1. Moustafa T, Fickert P, Magnes C, Guelly C, Thueringer A, et al. (2012) Alterations in Lipid Metabolism Mediate Inflammation, Fibrosis, and Proliferation in a Mouse Model of Chronic Cholestatic Liver Injury. Gastroenterology 142: 140–151.
2. Feitelson MA (1999) Hepatitis B virus in hepatocarcinogenesis. Journal of Cellular Physiology 181: 188–202.
3. Bréchot C, Gozuacik D, Murakami Y, Paterlini-Bréchot P (2000) Molecular bases for the development of hepatitis B virus (HBV)-related hepatocellular carcinoma (HCC). Seminars in Cancer Biology 10: 211–231.
4. Seeger C, Mason WS (2000) Hepatitis B virus biology. Microbiology and Molecular Biology Reviews 264: 51–68.
5. Taub R (2004) Liver regeneration: from myth to mechanism. Nature Reviews Molecular Cell Biology 5: 836–847.
6. Michalopoulos GK (2007) Liver regeneration. Journal of Cellular Physiology 213: 286–300.
7. Michalopoulos GK, DeFrances MC (1997) Liver regeneration. Science 276: 60–66.
8. Fausto N, Campbell JS, Riehle KJ (2006) Liver regeneration. Hepatology 43: S45–S53.
9. Michalopoulos GK (1990) Liver regeneration: molecular mechanisms of growth control. The FASEB Journal 4: 176–187.
10. Fausto N, Campbell JS, Riehle KJ (2012) Liver regeneration. Journal of Hepatology 57: 692–694.
11. Murray AB, Strecker W, Silz S (1981) Ultrastructural changes in rat hepatocytes after partial hepatectomy, and comparison with biochemical results. Journal of Cell Science 50: 433–448.
12. Delahunt TJ, Rubinste D (1970) Accumulation and release of triglycerides by rat liver following partial hepatectomy. Journal of Lipid Research 11: 536–543.
13. Miyamura N, Nakamura T, Goto-Inoue N, Zaima N, Hayasaka T, et al. (2011) Imaging mass spectrometry reveals characteristic changes in triglyceride and phospholipid species in regenerating mouse liver. Biochemical and Biophysical Research Communications 408: 120–125.
14. Glende EA, Morgan WS (1968) Alteration in liver lipid and lipid fatty acid composition after partial hepatectomy in rat. Experimental and Molecular Pathology 8: 190–200.
15. Fex G (1970) Phospholipid metabolism during regeneration of rat liver. Biochemical Journal 119: 743–747.
16. Tralhao JG, Roudier J, Morosan S, Giannini C, Tu H, et al. (2002) Paracrine in vivo inhibitory effects of hepatitis B virus X protein (HBx) on liver cell proliferation: an alternative mechanism of HBx-related pathogenesis. Proceedings of the National Academy Sciences 99: 6991–6996.
17. Wu BK, Li CC, Chen HJ, Chang JL, Jeng KS, et al. (2006) Blocking of G1/S transition and cell death in the regenerating liver of Hepatitis B virus X protein transgenic mice. Biochemical and Biophysical Research Communications 340: 916–928.
18. Hodgson AJ, Keasler VV, Slagle BL (2008) Premature cell cycle entry induced by hepatitis B virus regulatory HBx protein during compensatory liver regeneration. Cancer Research 68: 10341–10348.
19. Park ES, Park YK, Shin CY, Park SH, Ahn SH, et al. (2013) Hepatitis B virus inhibits liver regeneration via epigenetic regulation of urokinase-type plasminogen activator. Hepatology 58: 762–776.
20. Quétier I, Brezillon N, Duriez M, Massinet H, Giang E, et al. (2013) Hepatitis B virus HBx protein impairs liver regeneration through enhanced expression of IL-6 in transgenic mice. Journal of Hepatology 59: 285–291.
21. Kang S, Lee A, Park YS, Lee SC, Park SY, et al. (2011) Alteration in lipid and protein profiles of ovarian cancer: similarity to breast cancer. Inernational Journal of Gynecological Cancer 21: 1566–1572.
22. Lee GK, Lee HS, Park YS, Lee JH, Lee SC, et al. (2012) Lipid MALDI profile classifies non-small cell lung cancers according to the histologic type. Lung Cancer 76: 197–203.
23. Kang HS, Lee SC, Park YS, Jeon YE, Lee JH, et al. (2011) Protein and lipid MALDI profiles classify breast cancers according to the intrinsic subtype. BMC Cancer 11: 747–752.
24. Park YS, Yoo CW, Lee SC, Park SJ, Oh JH, et al (2011) Lipid profiles for intrahepatic cholangiocarcinoma identified using matrix-assisted laser desorption/ionization mass spectrometry. Clinica Chimica Acta 412: 1978–1982.
25. Shanta SR, Choi CS, Lee JH, Shin CY, Kim YJ, et al. (2012) Global changes in phospholipids identified by MALDI MS in rats with focal cerebral ischemia. Jounal of Lipid Research 53: 1823–1831.
26. Yang PL, Althage A, Chung J, Chisari FV (2002) Hydrodynamic injection of viral DNA: a mouse model of acute hepatitis B virus infection. Proceedings of the National Academy Sciences 99: 13825–13830.
27. Mitchell C, Willenbring H (2008) A reproducible and well-tolerated method for 2/3 partial hepatectomy in mice. Nature Protocols 3: 1167–1170.
28. Shanta SR, Zhou LH, Park YS, Kim YH, Kim Y, et al. (2011) Binary matrix for MALDI imaging mass spectrometry of phospholipids in both ion modes. Analytical Chemistry 83: 1252–1259.
29. Wright GH (1977) Changes in plasma membrane enzyme activities during liver regeneration in the rat. Biochimca et Biophysica Acta 470: 368–381.
30. Deliconstantinos G, Ramantanis G (1983) Alterations in the activities of hepatic plasma-membrane and microsomal enzymes during liver regeneration. Biochem Journal 212: 445–452.

31. Vance DE, Vance JE (2008) Phospholipid biosynthesis in eukaryotes. In Biochemistry of Lipids, Lipoproteins and Membranes. Edited by D.E. Vance and J.E. Vance. 5th ed. Elsevier, New York, N.Y. pp. 213–244.
32. Cornell R, Grove GL, Rothblat GH, Horwitz AF (1977) Lipid requirement for cell cycling: The effect of selective inhibition of lipid synthesis. Experimental Cell Research 109: 299–307.
33. Tercé F, Brun H, Vance DE (1994) Requirement of phosphatidylcholine for normal progression through the cell cycle in C3H/10T1/2 fibroblasts. Journal of Lipid Research 35: 2130–2142.
34. Cui Z, Houweling M, Chen MH, Record M, Chap H, et al. (1996) A genetic defect in phosphatidylcholine biosynthesis triggers apoptosis in Chinese hamster ovary cells. Journal of Biological Chemistry 271: 14668–14671.
35. Houwelling M, Tijburg LB, Jamil H, Vance DE, Nyathi CB, et al. (1991) Phosphatidylcholine metabolism in rat liver after partial hepatectomy. Evidence for increased activity and amount of CTP:phosphocholine cytidylyltransferase. Biochemical Journal 278: 347–351.
36. Van Hoeven RP, van Blitterswijk WJ, Emmelot P (1979) Fluorescence polarization measurements on normal and tumor cells and their corresponding plasma membrane. Biochimica et Biophysica Acta 551: 44–54.
37. Bruscalupi G, Curatola G, Lenaz G, Leoni S, Mangiantini MT, et al. (1980) Plasma membrane changes associated with rat liver regeneration. Biochimica et Biophysica Acta 597: 263–273.
38. Summers RM, Joseph PM, Kundel HL (1991) Sodium nuclear magnetic resonance imaging of neuroblastoma in the nude mouse. Investigative Radiology 26: 233–241.
39. Singh R, Kaushik S, Wang Y, Xiang Y, Novak I, et al. (2009) Autophagy regulates lipid metabolism. Nature 458: 1131–1135.
40. Sir D, Tian Y, Chen WL, Ann DK, Yen TS, et al. (2010) The early autophagic pathway is activated by hepatitis B virus and required for viral DNA replication. Proceedings of the National Academy Sciences USA 107: 4383–4388.
41. Tang H, Da L, Mao Y, Li Y, Li D, et al. (2010) Hepatitis B virus X protein sensitizes cells to starvation-induced autophagy via upregulation of beclin 1 expression. Hepatology 49: 60–71.

Permissions

All chapters in this book were first published in PLOS ONE, by The Public Library of Science; hereby published with permission under the Creative Commons Attribution License or equivalent. Every chapter published in this book has been scrutinized by our experts. Their significance has been extensively debated. The topics covered herein carry significant findings which will fuel the growth of the discipline. They may even be implemented as practical applications or may be referred to as a beginning point for another development.

The contributors of this book come from diverse backgrounds, making this book a truly international effort. This book will bring forth new frontiers with its revolutionizing research information and detailed analysis of the nascent developments around the world.

We would like to thank all the contributing authors for lending their expertise to make the book truly unique. They have played a crucial role in the development of this book. Without their invaluable contributions this book wouldn't have been possible. They have made vital efforts to compile up to date information on the varied aspects of this subject to make this book a valuable addition to the collection of many professionals and students.

This book was conceptualized with the vision of imparting up-to-date information and advanced data in this field. To ensure the same, a matchless editorial board was set up. Every individual on the board went through rigorous rounds of assessment to prove their worth. After which they invested a large part of their time researching and compiling the most relevant data for our readers.

The editorial board has been involved in producing this book since its inception. They have spent rigorous hours researching and exploring the diverse topics which have resulted in the successful publishing of this book. They have passed on their knowledge of decades through this book. To expedite this challenging task, the publisher supported the team at every step. A small team of assistant editors was also appointed to further simplify the editing procedure and attain best results for the readers.

Apart from the editorial board, the designing team has also invested a significant amount of their time in understanding the subject and creating the most relevant covers. They scrutinized every image to scout for the most suitable representation of the subject and create an appropriate cover for the book.

The publishing team has been an ardent support to the editorial, designing and production team. Their endless efforts to recruit the best for this project, has resulted in the accomplishment of this book. They are a veteran in the field of academics and their pool of knowledge is as vast as their experience in printing. Their expertise and guidance has proved useful at every step. Their uncompromising quality standards have made this book an exceptional effort. Their encouragement from time to time has been an inspiration for everyone.

The publisher and the editorial board hope that this book will prove to be a valuable piece of knowledge for researchers, students, practitioners and scholars across the globe.

List of Contributors

Michael Forsting and Thomas C. Lauenstein
Department of Diagnostic and Interventional Radiology and Neuroradiology, University Hospital Essen, Essen, Germany

Anja Fischer, Karsten Beiderwellen and Lale Umutlu
Department of Diagnostic and Interventional Radiology and Neuroradiology, University Hospital Essen, Essen, Germany
Erwin L. Hahn Institute for Magnetic Resonance Imaging, University Duisburg-Essen, Essen, Germany

Mark E. Ladd
Department of Diagnostic and Interventional Radiology and Neuroradiology, University Hospital Essen, Essen, Germany
Erwin L. Hahn Institute for Magnetic Resonance Imaging, University Duisburg-Essen, Essen, Germany
German Cancer Research Center (DKFZ), Heidelberg, Germany

Oliver Kraff and Stefan Maderwald
Erwin L.Hahn Institute for Magnetic Resonance Imaging, University Duisburg-Essen, Essen, Germany

Dou-dou Hu, Xin-min Li, Bao-en Wang and Xin-yan Zhao
Liver Research Center, Beijing Friendship Hospital, Capital Medical University, Beijing, China

Yu Chen
Institute of High Energy Physics, Chinese Academy of Sciences, Beijing, China

Ali Bihi
International School of Capital Medical University. Beijing, China

Tai-ling Wang
Department of Pathology, China-Japan Friendship Hospital, Beijing, China

Yi-Fang Wu, Yu-Kuo Wang, Sheng-Cih Huang, Manoswini Nayak and Tung-Kung Wu
Department of Biological Science and Technology, National Chiao Tung University, Hsin-Chu, Taiwan, Republic of China

Yan-Ren Lin
Department of Biological Science and Technology, National Chiao Tung University, Hsin-Chu, Taiwan, Republic of China
Department of Emergency Medicine, Changhua Christian Hospital, Changhua, Taiwan, Republic of China
School of Medicine, Chung Shan Medical University, Taichung, Taiwan, Republic of China

Yao-Li Chen
Transplant Medicine and Surgery Research Centre, Changhua Christian Hospital, Changhua, Taiwan, Republic of China
School of Medicine, Chung Shan Medical University, Taichung, Taiwan, Republic of China

Keh-Bin Wang
Department of Nuclear Medicine, Kuang Tien General Hospital, Taichung, Taiwan, Republic of China

Tzu-An Liu
Institute of Cellular and System Medicine, National Health Research Institutes, Zhunan, Miaoli County, Taiwan, Republic of China

Bak-Sau Yip
Department of Neurology, National Taiwan University Hospital Hsin Chu Branch, Hsin-Chu, Taiwan, Republic of China

Ralf Weiskirchen
Institute of Clinical Chemistry and Pathobiochemistry, RWTH University Hospital Aachen, Aachen, Germany

Pornwilard M-M
Institute of Clinical Chemistry and Pathobiochemistry, RWTH University Hospital Aachen, Aachen, Germany
Central Division of Analytical Chemistry, Forschungszentrum Jülich, Jülich, Germany
Department of Chemistry and Center for Innovation in Chemistry, Mahidol University, Bangkok, Thailand

J. Sabine Becker
Central Division of Analytical Chemistry, Forschungszentrum Jülich, Jülich, Germany

Nikolaus Gassler
Institute of Pathology, RWTH University Hospital Aachen, Aachen, Germany

Anja K. Bosserhoff
Institute of Pathology, University Hospital of Regensburg, Regensburg, Germany

Gamze Karaca, Marzena Swiderska-Syn, Guanhua Xie, Leandi Krüger, Mariana Verdelho Machado, Katherine Garman, Steve S. Choi, Gregory A. Michelotti and Anna Mae Diehl
Division of Gastroenterology, Department of Medicine, Duke University Medical Center, Durham, North Carolina, United States of America

Wing-Kin Syn
Regeneration and Repair Group, The Institute of Hepatology, Foundation for Liver Research, London, United Kingdom
Department of Hepatology, Barts Health NHS Trust, London, United Kingdom

Linda C. Burkly
Departments of Exploratory Science, Discovery Biology, and Validation Biology, Biogen Idec Inc., Cambridge, Massachusetts, United States of America

Begoña Ochoa
Department of Physiology, Faculty of Medicine, University of the Basque Country, Bilbao, Spain

Sergiu Nedevschi
Department of Computer Science, Technical University of Cluj-Napoca, Cluj-Napoca, Romania

Anca Ciurte
Department of Computer Science, Technical University of Cluj-Napoca, Cluj-Napoca, Romania,
Signal Processing Laboratory (LTS5), E´ cole Polytechnique Fédérale de Lausanne, Lausanne, Switzerland

Jean-Philippe Thiran
Signal Processing Laboratory (LTS5), E´ cole Polytechnique Fédérale de Lausanne, Lausanne, Switzerland
Department of Radiology, University Hospital Center and University of Lausanne, Lausanne, Switzerland

Meritxell Bach Cuadra
Signal Processing Laboratory (LTS5), E´ cole Polytechnique Fédérale de Lausanne, Lausanne, Switzerland
Department of Radiology, University Hospital Center and University of Lausanne, Lausanne, Switzerland
Center for Biomedical Imaging, Signal Processing Core, Lausanne, Switzerland

Xavier Bresson and Olivier Cuisenaire
Department of Radiology, University Hospital Center and University of Lausanne, Lausanne, Switzerland
Center for Biomedical Imaging, Signal Processing Core, Lausanne, Switzerland

Nawal Houhou
Swiss Institute of Bioinformatics (SIB), University Hospital Center and University of Lausanne, Lausanne, Switzerland

Mee Jin Park, So Yeon Kim, Seong Ho Park, Seung Soo Lee, Yedaun Lee and Moon-Gyu Lee
Department of Radiology and Research Institute of Radiology, University of Ulsan College of Medicine, Asan Medical Center, Seoul, Korea

Sang Min Yoon and Jong Hoon Kim
Department of Radiation Oncology, University of Ulsan College of Medicine, Asan Medical Center, Seoul, Korea

Julia Herzen
Institute of Materials Science, Helmholtz-Zentrum Geesthacht, Geesthacht, Germany
Physics Department & Institute of Medical Engineering, Technische Universität München, Garching, Germany

Marian S. Willner and Franz Pfeiffer
Physics Department & Institute of Medical Engineering, Technische Universität München, Garching, Germany

Alexander A. Fingerle, Peter B. Noël and Ernst J. Rummeny
Department of Radiology, Technische Universität München, Munich, Germany

Thomas Köhler
Philips Technologie GmbH, Innovative Technologies, Research Laboratories, Hamburg, Germany

Enken Drecoll
Institute of Pathology, Technische Universität München, Munich, Germany

Wei Xia, Ying Jiang, Yuanyuan Li, Yanjian Wan, Juan Liu, Yue Ma, Zhenxing Mao, Huailong Chang, Gengqi Li, Bing Xu, Xi Chen and Shunqing Xu
Key Laboratory of Environment and Health, Ministry of Education and Ministry of Environmental Protection, and State Key Laboratory of Environmental Health (Incubating), School of Public Health, Tongji Medical College, Huazhong University of Science and Technology, Wuhan, China

Edward Coulstock, Milan Ovečka, Rob Prince, Laura Goodall, Clare Mudd, Armin Sepp, Marie Davies, Gráinne Dunlevy and Adam Walker
Innovation Biopharm Discovery Unit, Biopharm R&D, GlaxoSmithKline, Cambridge, United Kingdom

Jane Sosabowski, Julie Foster and Jerome Burnet
Centre for Molecular Oncology, Barts Cancer Institute, Queen Mary University of London, London, United Kingdom

Rui Li, Meng-Xia Yuan, Chun-Lin Tang and Xiao-Hang Zhang
Department of Ultrasound, Southwest Hospital Affiliated to Third Military Medical University, Chongqing, China

Kuan-sheng Ma and Xiao-Wu Li
Department of Hepato-biliary-Pancreatic Surgery, Southwest Hospital Affiliated to Third Military Medical University, Chongqing, China

De-Yu Guo and Xiao-Chu Yan
Department of Pathology, Southwest Hospital Affiliated to Third Military Medical University, Chongqing, China

András Fülöp, Attila Szijártó,László Harsányi, András Budai, Damján Pekli and Diána Korsós
1st Department of Surgery, Semmelweis University, Budapest, Hungary

Ildikó Horváth and Krisztián Szigeti
Department of Biophysics and Radiation Biology, Semmelweis University, Budapest, Hungary,

Noémi Kovács and Domokos Máthé
CROmed Translational Research Centers, Budapest, Hungary

Kinga Karlinger
Department of Radiology and Oncotherapy, Semmelweis University, Budapest, Hungary

Anneloes E. Bohte, Erik M. Akkerman, Aart J. Nederveen and Jaap Stoker
Department of Radiology, Academic Medical Center, University of Amsterdam, Amsterdam, The Netherlands

Laura van Dussen and Carla E. M. Hollak
Department of Endocrinology and Metabolism, Academic Medical Center, University of Amsterdam, Amsterdam, The Netherlands

Ralph Sinkus
CRB3, UMR 773, Inserm, Universite´ Paris Diderot, Sorbonne Paris Cité, Clichy, France

Peter L. M. Jansen
Department of Gastroenterology and Hepatology, Academic Medical Center, University of Amsterdam, Amsterdam, The Netherlands

Ina Maria Schießl and Hayo Castrop
Institute of Physiology, University of Regensburg, Regensburg, Germany

Sophia Bardehle
Institute of Physiology, Department of Physiological Genomics, Ludwig-Maximilians- University, Munich, Germany
Institute for Stem Cell Research, Helmholtz Zentrum, Munich, Germany

Akiko Hatori, Joji Yui, Lin Xie, Tomoteru Yamasaki, Katsushi Kumata, Masayuki Fujinaga, Hidekatsu Wakizaka, Masanao Ogawa, Nobuki Nengaki, Kazunori Kawamura and Ming-Rong Zhang
Molecular Imaging Center, National Institute of Radiological Sciences, Chiba, Japan

Mattijs Elschot, Bart J. Vermolen, Marnix G. E. H. Lam, Bart de Keizer, Maurice A. A. J. van den Bosch and Hugo W. A. M. de Jong
Department of Radiology and Nuclear Medicine, University Medical Center Utrecht, Utrecht, The Netherlands

Natalia A. Petushkova, Mikhail A. Pyatnitskiy, Olesya V. Larina, Oxana P. Trifonova, Julya S. Kisrieva, Natalia F. Samenkova, Galina P. Kuznetsova and Irina I. Karuzina
V. N. Orekhovich Institute of Biomedical Chemistry, Russian Academy of Medical Sciences, Moscow, Russia

Andrey V. Lisitsa
V. N. Orekhovich Institute of Biomedical Chemistry, Russian Academy of Medical Sciences, Moscow, Russia Postgen Tech LLC, Moscow, Russia

Vladislav A. Rudenko
Postgen Tech LLC, Moscow, Russia

Bettina Maiwald, Donald Lobsien, Thomas Kahn and Patrick Stumpp
Department of Diagnostic and Interventional Radiology, University of Leipzig, Leipzig, Germany

Gaétan Bour, Marc Aprahamian and Jacques Marescaux
Institut de Recherche contre les Cancers de l9Appareil Digestif (IRCAD), Strasbourg, France

Jean-Marc Egly
Institut de Recherche contre les Cancers de l9Appareil Digestif (IRCAD), Strasbourg, France
IGBMC, Department of Functional Genomics and Cancer, CNRS/INSERM/ Université de Strasbourg, BP 163, Illkirch, C. U. Strasbourg, Strasbourg, France

Fernand Martel
IGBMC, Department of Functional Genomics and Cancer, CNRS/INSERM/ Université de Strasbourg, BP 163, Illkirch, C. U. Strasbourg, Strasbourg, France

Laurent Goffin, Bernard Bayle and Jacques Gangloff
ICube laboratory UMR, CNRS 7357, University of Strasbourg, Strasbourg, France

Nobutake Yamamichi, Chihiro Minatsuki, Yu Takahashi, Chiemi Nakayama, Rie Matsuda, Mitsuhiro Fujishiro, Maki Konno-Shimizu, Shinya Kodashima, Satoshi Ono, Keiko Niimi, Satoshi Mochizuki, Yosuke Tsuji, Yoshiki Sakaguchi, Itsuko Asada-Hirayama, Chihiro Takeuchi, Seiichi Yakabi, Hikaru Kakimoto and Kazuhiko Koike
Department of Gastroenterology, Graduate School of Medicine, The University of Tokyo, Tokyo, Japan

Takeshi Shimamoto
Department of Gastroenterology, Graduate School of Medicine, The University of Tokyo, Tokyo, Japan
Department of Gastroenterology, Kameda Medical Center Makuhari, Chiba, Japan

Chigaya Hirano, Ryoichi Wada and Toru Mitsushima
Department of Gastroenterology, Kameda Medical Center Makuhari, Chiba, Japan

Jun Kato and Masao Ichinose
Second Department of Internal Medicine, Wakayama Medical University, Wakayama, Japan

Karen M. Christiansen, Belinda K. Mössner, Janne F. Hansen, Erik F. Jarnbjer, Court Pedersen and Peer B. Christensen
Department of Infectious Diseases, Odense University Hospital, Odense, Denmark

Yong Kwang Park and Won-Jae Lee
Department of Pharmacology and Center for Cancer Research and Diagnostic Medicine, IBST, School of Medicine, Konkuk University, Seoul, Korea

Eun-Sook Park
Department of Pharmacology and Center for Cancer Research and Diagnostic Medicine, IBST, School of Medicine, Konkuk University, Seoul, Korea
KU Open Innovation Center, Konkuk University, Seoul, Korea

Kyun-Hwan Kim
Department of Pharmacology and Center for Cancer Research and Diagnostic Medicine, IBST, School of Medicine, Konkuk University, Seoul, Korea
KU Open Innovation Center, Konkuk University, Seoul, Korea
Research Institute of Medical Sciences, Konkuk University, Seoul, Korea

Jeong Hwa Lee, Ji Hye Hong, Jae Won Lee, Joon Won Lee and Kwang Pyo Kim
Department of Applied Chemistry, Kyung Hee University, Yongin, Gyeonggi, Korea

Index

www.ingramcontent.com/pod-product-compliance
Lightning Source LLC
LaVergne TN
LVHW060553210926
848485LV00005B/1305